WOMEN'S HEALTH CARE HANDBOOK

2nd Edition

Edited by

Bruce E. Johnson, M.D.
Professor of Internal Medicine and
   Family Medicine
University of Kansas School of Medicine
Kansas City, Kansas

Cynda Ann Johnson, M.D., M.B.A.
Professor and Head
Department of Family Medicine
University of Iowa College of Medicine
Iowa City, Iowa

Jane L. Murray, M.D.
Clinical Professor
Department of Family Medicine
University of Kansas School of Medicine
Kansas City, Kansas

Barbara S. Apgar, M.D., M.S.
Clinical Associate Professor
Department of Family Medicine
University of Michigan Medical School
Ann Arbor, Michigan

HANLEY & BELFUS, INC. / Philadelphia

HANLEY & BELFUS, INC.
An Imprint of Elsevier

The Curtis Center
Independence Square West
Philadelphia, Pennsylvania 19106

Note to the reader: Although the information in this book has been carefully reviewed for correctness of dosage and indications, neither the authors nor the editors nor the publisher can accept any legal responsibility for any errors or omissions that may be made. Neither the publisher nor the editors make any warranty, expressed or implied, with respect to the material contained herein. Before prescribing any drug, the reader must review the manufacturer's current product information (package inserts) for accepted indications, absolute dosage recommendations, and other information pertinent to the safe and effective use of the product described.

Library of Congress Cataloging-in-Publication Data

Women's health care handbook / edited by Bruce E. Johnson . . . [et al.].—2nd ed.
    p. ; cm.
Includes bibliographical references and index.
ISBN 1-56053-356-0 (alk. paper)
    1. Women—Medical care—Handbooks, manuals, etc. 2. Women—Diseases—
Handbooks, manuals, etc. 3. Women—Health and hygiene—Handbooks, manuals, etc.
I. Johnson, Bruce E., 1950–
    [DNLM: 1. Women's Health—Handbooks. WA 39 W872 2000]
RA564.85.W66685 2000
616'.0082—dc21

                                                                99-042849

Women's Health Care Handbook, 2nd edition   ISBN 1-56053-356-0

Printed in the United States of America

Last digit is the print number: 9 8 7 6 5 4 3 2

Contents

VI. GYNECOLOGIC PAIN AND SYMPTOMATOLOGY

VII. BREAST ISSUES AND DISORDERS

VIII. MENOPAUSE ISSUES

IX. URINARY TRACT PROBLEMS

X. SEXUAL ISSUES

XI. PSYCHOLOGICAL DISORDERS AND SUBSTANCE ABUSE

XIV. SPECIAL TESTS AND PROCEDURES

Contributors

Elizabeth Alexander, M.D., M.S.
Professor, Department of Family Practice, Michigan State University College of Human Medicine, East Lansing, Michigan

Barbara S. Apgar, M.D., M.S.
Clinical Associate Professor, Department of Family Medicine, University of Michigan Medical School, Ann Arbor, Michigan

Gary E. Bachman, M.S.S.W., L.S.C.S.W.
Assistant Professor, Licensed Specialist Clinical Social Worker, Department of Family Medicine, University of Kansas School of Medicine, Kansas City, Kansas

Richard Bené, M.D.
Clinical Assistant Professor, Department of Family Medicine, University of Kansas School of Medicine, Kansas City, Kansas

Timothy P. Daaleman, D.O.
Assistant Professor, Department of Family Medicine, University of Kansas School of Medicine, Kansas City, Kansas

Diane W. Ebbert, R.N., M.S.N., C.F.N.P.
Clinical Assistant Professor, Department of Family Medicine, University of Kansas School of Medicine, Kansas City, Kansas

Valerie Gilchrist, M.D.
Professor and Associate Program Director, Department of Family Medicine, Northeastern Ohio Universities College of Medicine, Canton, Ohio

Bruce E. Johnson, M.D.
Professor, Departments of Internal Medicine and Family Medicine, University of Kansas School of Medicine, Kansas City, Kansas

Cynda Ann Johnson, M.D., M.B.A.
Professor and Head, Department of Family Medicine, University of Iowa College of Medicine, Iowa City, Iowa

Katherine G. Keller, D.O.
Assistant Professor, Department of Family Practice, Michigan State University College of Human Medicine, East Lansing, Michigan

Mark Larson, M.D.
The Valley Clinic, Ellensburg, Washington

Bruce S. Liese, Ph.D.
Professor, Departments of Family Medicine and Psychiatry, University of Kansas School of Medicine, Kansas City, Kansas

Jane L. Murray, M.D.
Clinical Professor, Department of Family Medicine, University of Kansas School of Medicine, Kansas City, Kansas

Gary R. Newkirk, M.D.
Clinical Professor, Department of Family Medicine, University of Washington School of Medicine, Seattle; Director, Family Medicine Spokane Residency, Spokane, Washington

Moya Peterson, R.N., M.A., C.F.N.P.
Clinical Assistant Professor, Department of Family Medicine, University of Kansas School of Medicine, Kansas City, Kansas

Judith A. Suess, M.D., M.P.H.
Assistant Professor, Department of Family Practice, Michigan State University College of Human Medicine, East Lansing, Michigan

Belinda A. Vail, M.D.
Clinical Associate Professor, Department of Family Medicine, University of Kansas School of Medicine, Kansas City, Kansas

Ginger Vary, A.C.S.W., B.C.S.
Behavioral Science Coordinator, Department of Family Practice, Michigan State University College of Human Medicine, East Lansing, Michigan

Preface to the First Edition

It is with some audacity that one contemplates writing a textbook. The undertaking promises to balloon out of control and consume both time and talents. Well into the writing and organizing, we asked ourselves again, "Why are we writing this book?"

We all have experience practicing, teaching, lecturing and writing in different aspects of women's health. Teaching medical students and residents is the focus of our days. We all organize and present conferences to trainees and practitioners. And we continually find ourselves searching from one source to the next for information practical enough to entice the experienced practitioner while organized and comprehensive enough to direct students and residents. This book hopes to accomplish these goals.

Others who have written textbooks on women's health were not always primary care physicians and may not always have written from the point of view of primary care. This book hopes to encompass most of the aspects of care which are particular to women. Certainly gynecology is included, but also medical diseases found largely, or having unique significance, in women. Psychosocial issues of import to women, such as relationships, abuse, and passages, are included. Being primary care–oriented, we wished also to focus on prevention, hence the inclusion of those chapters toward the beginning of the book.

We drew upon our experience as practitioners in developing a somewhat unique format to each chapter. We start the chapter with a section entitled "The Issues," which outlines the importance in a clinical setting of the topic to be discussed. Highlighting the essence of the topic should allow the reader to see exactly where the topic fits into the field of women's health. "The Issues" section also presents areas of controversy, either in content or interpretation, which are (hopefully) answered later in the chapter.

The second section of each chapter, "The Theory," is a brief review of the important basic information regarding that topic. This may be a review of physiology, psychology, sociology, or even the legal underpinnings of the topic. This section was not meant to be comprehensive—standard textbooks and the current medical literature fulfill that requirement—but to provide a theoretical basis for the topic.

"An Approach" is the section that reflects the doctor in each author. This is designed to be practical and useful for the practitioner in search of immediate and practical information. This section will necessarily reflect the experience (and, to some degree, bias) of the author. Each author was asked to be as fair as possible in including alternative options if there is uncertainty or lack of consensus.

In keeping with the design of this series of books, the chapters are presented in outline format. As we found out, this requires a considerable degree of organization and decision making. An outline format puts an emphasis on the logical flow of information while prizing clarity and brevity. We hope the information is organized in a way that addresses the needs of a busy practitioner trying to make sense of a clinical problem.

In an effort to produce a book which would be optimally useful for the practitioner, we included a complete section on Tests and Procedures. These chapters are meant to be practical and directed in the performance of procedures or in developing approaches to diagnosis and treatment.

We sincerely thank all the contributing authors. We know that authoring a chapter (or several) is demanding and time-consuming. We appreciate the attention to format, content, and deadlines. We also thank Bill Lamsback of Hanley & Belfus for his insight, generosity, and patience.

Finally, we thank our families, specifically Kevin, Drew, Helen, and Chris, for putting up with us during the "birthing." It is to you we dedicate the book.

Cynda Ann Johnson, M.D.
Bruce E. Johnson, M.D.
Jane L. Murray, M.D.
Barbara S. Apgar, M.D.

Preface to the Second Edition

In the preface to the first edition of this textbook, we wrote that it was "with some audacity" that we contemplated writing a book. What to say about approaching the second edition?

It is with pride that we agreed to edit a second edition. *Women's Health Care Handbook* has been well received and we have enjoyed gracious comments from numerous people. It was flattering—and we have responded with an updated edition.

This edition goes beyond flattery, however. What we learned from the first edition has been, we hope, applied here. Since we wanted the book to be even more timely and accurate, we gave all the authors a shorter time frame for completion of their work. Our sincere appreciation goes to the authors for bringing their work to the editors within the agreed deadline.

The publisher asked that the text be somewhat more fluent. We did not want to lose the structure and organization an outline format compels. The compromise is to maintain the outline format but allow a little more prose to make the writing more readable.

We insisted that each chapter be updated, and that recent advances be reflected in the "Suggested Readings." The "Readings" continue to include important concepts, reviews, and advances, but are not necessarily a list of citations for each factual comment in the chapter.

Chapters were rearranged and sections renamed in an effort to make the flow of the book more logical. A few chapters and appendices from the first edition were dropped or merged into other chapters. We added a few chapters, mostly to reflect the increasing interest in pursuing nonpharmacologic or alternative approaches to women's health concerns.

Our efforts were always to make a useful textbook. Each chapter is grounded in theoretical and experimental evidence yet, we hope, is clinically oriented enough to be a favorite text in the clinic or office.

Our sincere thanks again go to Natasha Andjelkovic and Bill Lamsback of Hanley & Belfus, who directed us with insight, encouragement, and patience.

Finally, we recognize the sacrifice of loved ones in allowing the editors time to complete the task. We dedicate this edition to Kevin and Drew, and to Chris.

Bruce E. Johnson, M.D.
Cynda Ann Johnson, M.D., M.B.A.
Jane L. Murray, M.D.
Barbara S. Apgar, M.D., M.S.

Foreword

The Hanley & Belfus *Handbooks* are designed to be both ready references and detailed resources for clinicians, residents, students, and other health professionals. Their outline style concentrates a large quantity of information into a manageable space and presents this information logically and clearly. The format is "user-friendly," with many key issues highlighted in bold print.

In the second edition of *Women's Health Care Handbook*, Bruce and Cynda Johnson, Jane Murray, and Barbara Apgar provide a seamless *Handbook* for the care of the whole woman with sections on all of the developmental, preventive, medical, sexual, and emotional issues which challenge women and the physicians who care for them. As the first edition established itself as one of the leading references on women's health care, I anticipate that this completely revised and updated second edition will further secure its place in the literature. As practicing physicians and teachers, the authors have provided a new tool which will serve colleagues, co-professionals, and students extremely well.

Morris B. Mellion, M.D.
Handbook Series Editor
Omaha, Nebraska

PART I

HEALTH PROMOTION AND DISEASE PREVENTION

1. Preadolescent and Adolescent Health Promotion and Disease Prevention

Jane L. Murray, M.D.

I. **The Issues**
   A. **Early adolescence** (ages 11–14) is a time of rapid body changes, onset of puberty, weight changes, breast development, and eventual onset of menses
      1. Education about bodily changes, and anticipatory guidance are important aspects of a physician's care
      2. At this developmental stage, adolescents usually operate in a concrete cognitive framework, with features of magical thinking. A sexually active 13-year-old, for example, may not comprehend the need for contraception or protection from sexually transmitted diseases (STDs)
   B. **Middle adolescence** (ages 15–17) is a time of seeking independence
      1. Peer support is usually more valuable than parental input
      2. Physicians can be important role models
      3. Health promotion and disease prevention discussions may be effective
      4. Although some features of adult thinking are present, under stress the adolescent reverts to a more concrete level. Physician education and explanation may need to be concrete and given in a step-by-step fashion.
   C. **Late adolescence** (ages 18–21) developmentally is a time of resolution of body image conflicts and of taking more responsibility
      1. Dysfunctional family and personal dynamics may be exposed at this time of bridging into adulthood
      2. A nonjudgmental approach by the physician may facilitate discussion of sexuality, career, and other life choices for the patient
   D. Psychosocial problems may be presented to the physician as physical symptoms
      1. Abdominal pain or dysmenorrhea may mask depression, school phobia, and family stress or violence
      2. Vaginal discharge may mark sexual abuse, ambivalence about sexual activity or sexual identity, or desire or need for contraception
      3. Depression may present as weight changes, recurrent injury, or parental complaints about school failure, truancy, or antisocial behavior
II. **The Theory**
   A. **Most common health-related problems in adolescents**
      1. **Variations in physical growth and development**
         a. Short or tall stature
         b. Precocious or delayed puberty
         c. Delayed menarche
         d. Menstrual irregularities (dysmenorrhea, oligomenorrhea, amenorrhea, excessive bleeding)
      2. **Infectious diseases**
         a. Mononucleosis
         b. Respiratory infections
         c. Genitourinary infections

1

3. **Orthopedic problems**
    a. Scoliosis
    b. Osgood-Schlatter disease
    c. Slipped capital-femoral epiphysis
4. **Endocrine and genetic problems**
    a. Breast disorders
    b. Turner's syndrome
    c. Acne
5. **Chronic medical problems**
    a. Asthma
    b. Diabetes
    c. Headaches
    d. Epilepsy
    e. Collagen vascular disease
6. **Psychosocial problems**
    a. Depression and suicide risk
    b. Alcohol and drug experimentation/abuse
    c. Anorexia/bulimia
    d. Somatization and school phobia
    e. Failure to achieve
    f. Antisocial behavior or "acting out"
7. **Sexuality issues**
    a. Pregnancy and contraception
    b. STDs
    c. Sexual promiscuity
    d. Sexual identity
B. The Department of Adolescent Services of the American Medical Association has made a series of recommendations, based on annual routine health visits, for delivery of health services, health guidance, screening, and immunizations to adolescents between ages 11 and 21. These are referred to as the Guidelines for Adolescent Preventive Services (GAPS). Such visits should address the biomedical and psychosocial aspects of health and focus on preventive services. In fact, data show that health risks in this age group are more social in origin than medical, and that early intervention with unhealthy behavioral choices can reduce adolescent morbidity and mortality.
C. Medical care for adolescents should be confidential, with physician policies regarding when parents should be and should not be involved in care decisions. Such policies should be made clear to adolescents and their parents.
D. Some anticipatory guidance sessions with parents may be in order at least once during early, middle, and late adolescence to discuss normal adolescent behaviors and signs of dysfunction or distress, parenting behaviors, and role modeling
E. Services provided should be developmentally and age-appropriate and sensitive to individual and sociocultural differences
F. Annual (as recommended by GAPS) health guidance activities should promote in adolescents a better understanding of physical growth, psychosocial and psychosexual development, and the importance of becoming actively involved in decisions about their health care
III. **An Approach**
A. **Hints for good communication with adolescents**
    1. Assume an active role in establishing a comfortable, friendly relationship
    2. Take a proactive approach to asking about sensitive issues (e.g., sexuality, drugs, depression)
    3. Have separate discussion with adolescent and parent routinely
        a. Emphasize confidentiality—AAFP statement on confidentiality: *One must attempt to achieve a balance between the rights of the parents and what is necessary to maintain and promote the health and well-being of the adolescent. It is proper and ethical for the family physician to protect an adolescent's confidentiality. Withholding information from third parties, including parents, may be*

appropriate when it pertains to but is not limited to contraception, pregnancy, sexually transmitted diseases, and physical and/or sexual abuse by a parent. Parental involvement, consent, or notification should not be a barrier to care for the adolescent.

   b. Consider an "informed consent" form for parents of adolescents
   4. Recognize "teachable moments"
   5. Enhance your own communication skills: Reflective listening and nonjudgmental responses
   6. Minimize direct questioning
   7. Avoid scientific terms and jargon; use regular language
   8. Give positive feedback; foster a sense of pride in the adolescent's changing body
   9. Facilitate family discussions of developmental issues (e.g., sexuality, identity, experimentation)
   10. Use other professional staff, community agencies, and referrals as appropriate but stay involved and interested

B. **History**
   1. Annual history of substance use (including tobacco, anabolic steroids, alcohol, over-the-counter and prescription drugs, and other substances)
   2. Annual history of high-risk behaviors, sexual activity, activity and exercise level, diet, eating disorders, and body image
   3. Annual inquiry about risk for HIV infection (intravenous drug use, sex with unknown partners or known intravenous drug users or bisexual males, more than one sex partner in last 6 months, exchange of sex for money or drugs)
   4. Annual inquiry about behaviors or emotions that indicate recurrent or severe depression or risk of suicide
   5. Annual inquiry about emotional, physical, and sexual abuse and family violence
   6. Annual inquiry about learning or school problems

C. **Examination**
   1. Complete physical exam recommended once at age 11–14, once at age 15–17, and once at age 18–21 (early, middle, and late adolescence)
   2. Annual screening for hypertension
   3. Consider annual evaluation for scoliosis
   4. Hints for the first pelvic exam
      a. Indications for pelvic exam: vaginal discharge, pelvic pain, history of sexual intercourse, desire for contraception; at age 21, even if not sexually active
      b. Inquire if patient wishes to have a parent or other person present. If the physician is male, a female chaperone is strongly recommended.
      c. Explain carefully each step that will be taken and ensure patient comfort; indicate that exam will go as slowly as patient wishes
      d. Use smallest vaginal speculum possible if cervix is to be visualized; gently stretch introitus with one finger first, and determine axis of uterus if possible.
      e. Consider using a hand-held mirror so patient can see what is being done and learn about her body
      f. Elevate the head of the exam table so that eye contact can be maintained and patient can ask questions during exam
   5. Tanner staging and sexual maturity ratings (Table 1)
      a. Stage 1: prepubertal; elevation of breast papilla; no pubic hair
      b. Stage 2: breast buds, areola slightly widened; straight hair along labia, lightly on pubis
      c. Stage 3: enlargement of entire breast, no protrusion of papilla; pubic hair increased in quantity, darker, present in typical female triangle
      d. Stage 4: enlargement of breast and projection of areola and papilla as secondary mound; pubic hair more dense and curled, present in adult distribution, but less abundant
      e. Stage 5: adult configuration of breast with protrusion of nipple, areola no longer projects separately from breast; abundant adult type pubic hair, possibly extending to medial aspect of thighs

TABLE 1.   Classification of Genital Maturity Stages in Girls (Tanner Ratings)

Stage	Pubic Hair	Breasts
1	Preadolescent	Preadolescent
2	Sparse, slightly pigmented, straight, at medial border of labia	Breast and papilla elevated as small mound, areolar diameter increased
3	Darker, beginning to curl, increased amount	Breast and areola enlarged, without contour separation
4	Coarse, curly, abundant, but amount less than in adult	Areola and papilla form secondary mound
5	Adult feminine triangle, spread to medial surface of thighs	Mature, nipple projects, areola part of genital breast contour

    D. **Tests and procedures** (see chapter 4 for immunization recommendations)
        1. Selected adolescents under age 19 (parents with serum cholesterol greater than 240 mg/dl) should be screened for risk of developing adult hyperlipidemia and all adolescents age 19 and older should have a total cholesterol checked once
          a. If less than 170 mg/dl, screen again in 5 years
          b. If 170–199, repeat test
          c. If greater than 200, do lipoprotein analysis
        2. Sexually active adolescents should be screened for STDs
          a. All patients: gonorrhea, chlamydia
          b. Serology for syphilis if patient
             i. Lives in an endemic area
            ii. Has a history of other STDs
            iii. Has changed sex partners within 6 months
            iv. Has exchanged sex for drugs or money
          c. HIV testing (with proper pre- and posttest counseling and informed consent) in patients with risk factors
            i. Intravenous drug use
            ii. Other STDs
            iii. Residence in area with high prevalence of STDs and HIV
            iv. More than one sex partner in last 6 months
            v. Exchange of sex for drugs or money
            vi. Partner with any risk factors for HIV infection
        3. Sexually active females and all females over 18 should have an annual Pap test for human papillomavirus (HPV) and cancer
        4. Tuberculosis (TB) skin test if the patient
            i. Lives in (or moved from) an endemic area
            ii. Resides in a homeless shelter
            iii. Has been incarcerated
            iv. Works in a health care setting
            v. Has been exposed to active TB
    E. **Patient education and disease prevention**
        1. Annual inquiry about the use of chemical substances (including tobacco and anabolic steroids)
          a. More in-depth history if screening is positive
          b. Referral for treatment if indicated
          c. Recommend that the adolescent stop the use of substances of abuse
          d. Only 1 in 22 self-reports of substance use on standardized questionnaires is revealed in face-to-face encounters with physicians. Samples of these questions are:
            i. Does the adolescent ever use drugs when alone?
            ii. Does the adolescent ever use alcohol when alone?
            iii. Does the adolescent every get drunk or high at social events or have friends who do?
            iv. Does the adolescent ever consume alcohol on school grounds?

       v. Does the adolescent ever miss school because of drinking or hangovers?

      vi. When truant, does the adolescent ever go drinking or get high on drugs?

    e. Use of humor and images (e.g., methods of organizations such as *Doctors Ought to Care*) to convey health messages can be more effective than lectures on the dangers of smoking and taking drugs

2. Counsel about risk-taking behaviors and ways to minimize risk

    a. Use of seat belts, bicycle, and motorcycle helmets

    b. Designated drivers

    c. Athletic protective devices

    d. Safe use of weapons, if adolescent has access to them

3. Annual counseling on the benefits of regular exercise with appropriate physical conditioning before exercising

4. Annual counseling about responsible sexual behaviors

    a. Abstinence

    b. Use of latex condoms to prevent transmission of STDs and HIV

    c. Appropriate birth control methods with counseling in proper use

5. Annual counseling about benefits of a healthy diet and ways to achieve a healthy diet and safe weight management

F. **Special issues in caring for adolescents**

1. **The parent who won't leave the room**

    a. May indicate family dysfunction: overly enmeshed relationship, parental dependence, family violence, or other secret

    b. Meeting first with the parent alone to elicit their concerns and to explain policy of speaking with the adolescent alone and rationale for doing so may be helpful

    c. If the parent is intransigent, ask the adolescent if you have her permission to speak with her and examine her in the presence of the parent

    d. Building a trusting relationship with the parent and the adolescent over time and several visits may be helpful in defusing mistrust.

2. **Adolescents who don't take your advice**

    a. Giving "advice" in the first place may be problematic. Adolescents are developmentally rebelling against authority and asserting independence from parental figures.

    b. If the physician can be seen as providing nonjudgmental information and is willing to discuss the ramifications of various possible choices, the adolescent may make more appropriate choices and take responsibility for herself, thus taking her own "advice" rather than that of an authority figure

3. **The shy or overly modest adolescent**

    a. May reflect emotional immaturity, past or ongoing abuse, poor self-esteem

    b. Building a trusting relationship over time, with minimal physical or psychic interventions unless absolutely necessary, may build confidence in the adolescent and trust of the physician.

4. **Early sexual development**

    a. Most girls do not develop breasts or pubic hair before age 8

    b. Causes of early puberty

        i. Constitutional

        ii. Secondary to central nervous system disease (tumor, infection, trauma, hemihypertrophy)

        iii. Endocrine (adrenal and ovarian tumors, hypothyroidism, androgen-producing teratomas)

        iv. Iatrogenic (hormone administration).

5. **Peer pressure**

    a. Major task of adolescence is identity formation, and group identity (clubs, gangs, special-interest groups) is the norm

    c. Adolescence is the age of experimentation

    d. Individuals frequently have low self-esteem and therefore are subject to group norms and pressures

    e. Parents and physician should encourage activities in groups that tend to experiment safely (e.g., school clubs, drama classes, music activities, sports teams)

      f. The physician should assist parents and adolescents to engage in constructive dialogue about choices the adolescent will make and choice of peer groups whose pressure is likely to be minimally dangerous

6. **Short or tall stature**
   a. Short stature = below 3rd percentile, deceleration from own growth curve, or less than 3 cm growth/year
   b. Causes of short stature without pubertal delay
      i. Familial or constitutional
      ii. Hypothyroidism
      iii. Congenital syndromes (Down, Hurler's)
      iv. Intrauterine growth retardation
      v. Chondrodystrophies
   c. Causes of short stature with pubertal delay include
      i. Congenital (Turner's syndrome, ovarian dysgenesis, Noonan's syndrome)
      ii. Nutritional deprivation
      iii. Hypothalamic/pituitary disorders
      iv. Familial
   d. Causes of tall stature include constitutional/familial etiologies, excessive growth hormone, Marfan syndrome, homocystinuria, neurofibromatosis, gonadal and adrenal tumors, and adrenal hyperplasia

7. **Legal issues and confidentiality**
   a. Parental consent is required for treatment of minors in most situations; reproductive health is an exception in most states, where minors who are capable of making informed consent decisions about contraception, pregnancy, abortion, and STD treatment may do so.
   b. Although legally the physician is usually protected for treating minors for the above conditions, it is always worthwhile to encourage the adolescent to involve her parents in such treatment decisions
   c. A confidentiality policy should be adopted in the physician's practice. In general, all aspects of the adolescent's care should be kept confidential. If confidentiality needs to be broken, the adolescent should first be informed and given an appropriate explanation.

SUGGESTED READING

1. Elster AB (ed): AMA Guidelines for Adolescent Preventive Services (GAPS): Recommendations and Rationale. Baltimore, Williams & Wilkins, 1994.
2. Elster AB, Leavenberg P: Integrative comprehensive adolescent preventive services into routine medical care. Pediatr Clin North Am 44:1365–1367, 1997.
3. Gagliano NJ, Emans SJ, Woods ER: Cholesterol screening in the adolescent. J Adolesc Health 14:104–108, 1993.
4. Montalto NJ: Implementing the guideline for adolescent preventive services. Am Fam Phys 57:2181–2188, 1997
5. Schubiner H, Robin A: Screening adolescents for depression and parent–teenage conflict in an ambulatory medical setting. Pediatrics 85:813–818, 1990.
6. Stevens NG, Lyle S: Guidelines for adolescent preventive services: A critical review. J Am Board Fam Pract Sept–Oct:421–430, 1994.
7. Winters KC: Development of an adolescent alcohol and other drug abuse screening scale: Personal Experience Screening Questionnaire. Addict Behav 17:479–490, 1992.

2. Health Promotion and Maintenance in Adult Women

Bruce E. Johnson, M.D.

I. **The Issues**

Times change and fads come and go. The "yearly physical" is an example in medicine of a "fad" which originally started in the early 1900s, peaked in mid-century and now, though not gone, is largely modified. In retrospect, one sees how this exam was poorly conceived: by performing an exam and ordering tests (typically including yearly blood work, chest x-ray, EKG, sigmoidoscopy and even exercise stress testing), the doctor was searching for extant disease but promising future health; by focusing on tests, the patient was not admonished about preventive issues (often involving difficult lifestyle changes) and came away with an unintended "clean bill of health." Health promotion and maintenance is now promoted as a partnership—the doctor counseling and, yes, testing; the patient modifying and practicing a healthier lifestyle. In addition, modern management practices are not supportive of a "yearly complete physical." Instead, periodic evaluations are often incorporated into visits initiated for other reasons. Finally, physicians are encouraged to broaden the scope of health promotion to include consideration of the multiple issues raised in this chapter.

II. **The Theory**
   - A. To appreciate the recommendations for health promotion and maintenance, one must understand the **underlying concepts and methodology**
   - B. **Definitions**
      1. **Screening**
         - a. A test or examination used to identify a disease or condition
            - i. Screening generally involves persons asymptomatic for the disease under investigation
            - ii. Identifies persons in whom preclinical disease is present
         - b. An effective screening test must be able to identify the disease at an early stage, and treatment must modify the natural history of the disease
         - c. Screening tests ideally directed toward large populations
            - i. Blood pressure in all adults, Pap smear in adult females
         - d. Screening tests can be directed in special populations
            - i. For example, screening for syphilis in an STD clinic
         - e. Ideal screening test
            - i. High sensitivity and specificity with few false-positives and false-negatives (see below)
      2. **Case finding**
         - a. Performing a test in a symptomatic individual to identify a likely disorder
            - i. Symptoms, a family history, exposure makes a positive test likely
         - b. Case finding is directed testing as part of the diagnostic process
      3. **Surveillance**
         - a. Periodic testing in person at high risk or with preclinical disease
            - i. Often searching for recurrence of treated disease
      4. **Purpose of a test depends on the circumstances**
         - a. Performing a Pap smear in all adult women is screening
         - b. Performing a Pap smear in a woman with postcoital bleeding is case finding
         - c. Performing a Pap smear in a woman with previously treated dysplasia is surveillance
   - C. **Evaluation of a test**
      1. **Sensitivity**
         - a. Definitions
            - i. Persons who have a disease and test positive for that disease are true positive; persons who have a disease but test negative are false-negative; persons

who do not have a disease but test positive are false-positive; persons who do not have the disease and test negative are true negative

b. Sensitivity relates to true positive rate, i.e., the assurance that a positive test result means that the person has the disease

c. In virtually any biologic test, there is a range or continuum over which the test is considered "normal"

    i. For many tests, statistical criteria determine the range of normal (e.g., mean ± 2 standard deviations defines the range of normal for hemoglobin)

    ii. For other tests a high degree of interpretive skill enters into the determination of "normal," e.g., chest x-ray, Pap smear

d. Results of a test can be adjusted by varying criteria for "normal," thus improving its sensitivity

    i. Broadening the criteria in order to detect all possible persons with disease increases sensitivity

    ii. Unfortunately, increased sensitivity of a test almost invariably decreases specificity

e. Tests with high sensitivity are often used as screening tests

2. **Specificity**

a. Proportion of persons without a conditions who test negative

b. Specificity of a test relates to true negative rate, i.e., the assurance that a negative test result means that the person does not have the disease

c. Tests with high specificity are often used as confirmatory tests

3. **Positive predictive value**

a. Proportion of persons with a positive test who actually have the condition

b. Positive (and negative) predictive values reflect the prevalence of disease in the population under consideration

c. Even a good test applied to a population with low prevalence of disease has a low positive predictive value. The test is likely to produce more false-positive results than desired

    i. For example, antibody test for human immunodeficiency virus (HIV) is > 99% specific, yet prevalence of HIV disease in general population is low enough (< 0.1%) that false-positive test result is considerable worry. Conversely, HIV test in intravenous drug users in New York (HIV prevalence 50%) has high positive predictive value.

    ii. Any test, no matter how accurate, is more useful in population with high prevalence

4. **Test efficacy** depends on interplay of all these concepts

a. Ideal screening test should have high sensitivity and specificity with no false-positives, even in population with low prevalence

b. Ideal test should be simple, easy to administer, inexpensive, and easily understood

c. There is no ideal test

D. **Methodology to develop recommendations**

1. Criteria accepted to determine whether evidence is adequate to support inclusion in lists of appropriate screening tests

2. Efficacy of a test determined from published reports of sensitivity and specificity

3. Review of medical literature included decision about reliability of data used to draw conclusions

a. Study design becomes important, e.g., randomized controlled trial, historical controls

    i. Weigh adequacy of research design in attempt to avoid bias in conclusions

4. Strength of recommendation relates to adequacy of research design, strength of conclusions, presence of multiple, confirmatory studies, etc.

a. Laborious work but conclusions evidence-based

E. **Areas of recommendations**

1. Screening procedures should be worked into or considered at any patient encounter, not limited to "annual exams"

   2. Screening procedures
      a. Test or examinations performed at episodic or periodic intervals
      b. General recommendations for all persons in certain age group
      c. Specific recommendations for high-risk groups
   3. Counseling
      a. Advice given to persons at episodic or periodic encounters
      b. General or specific, depending on risk
   4. Immunizations
   5. Recommendations appear to some practitioners to be conservative, if not deficient.
      This perception reflects the evidence-based approach employed by most organiza-
      tions formulating recommendations. Actual practice may vary depending on physi-
      cian preference, patient demographics, local factors, etc.
III. **An Approach**
   A. Recommendations consist of screening (including physical exam and tests), **counsel-
      ing**, **immunizations**, and **chemoprophylaxis** (conditions which may be altered by
      supplements)
      1. Critical management issue is implementation and accurate recording of interventions
   B. **Screening**
      1. **Physical exam**
         a. **Height and weight**
            i. Standardized charts (e.g., Metropolitan Life) or body weight index (see
               chapter 5)
            ii. Note low as well as excessive weight
         b. **Blood pressure**
            i. Should be recorded at least every 3 years
         c. **Clinical breast exam**
            i. Breast self-exam should be taught (despite questions regarding efficacy as
               screening procedure)
            ii. Clinical exam by trained, experienced examiner at least every 1–3 years,
               usually in association with mammography (see below)
         d. **High-risk groups**
            i. Complete skin exam (family history of skin cancer, precursor lesions, e.g.,
               dysplastic nevi, or excessive exposure to sunlight)
            ii. Oral cavity exam in tobacco user or alcohol abuser
            iii. Thyroid nodules in persons who were exposed to upper-body irradiation
            iv. Auscultation for carotid bruits
      2. **Laboratory and diagnostic procedures**
         a. Total blood cholesterol, for ages 45–65
            i. If > 200 mg/dl, lipid profile (see Chapter 100)
         b. **Pap smear** (see Chapters 47, 102, 108)
            i. Recommendations vary as to interval
               (a) Initial Pap smear and pelvic exam at first sexual activity or by age 21
               (b) Premenopausal, sexually active woman—probably yearly
               (c) Postmenopausal woman with single partner—probably every 1–3 years
                  after two negative exams at physician discretion
            ii. High-risk circumstances warrant at least yearly exam
               (a) Lifetime history of more than two sexual partners, prior sexually trans-
                  mitted disease, prior abnormal Pap smear, etc.
         c. **Mammogram** (see Chapters 101 and 122)
            i. Highly contentious issue with recommendations by multiple organizations—
               often contradictory
            ii. In women with positive family history for premenopausal cancer, start by
               age 40 and continue yearly until age 60–65
            iii. In women with negative family history and "average" risk, every 1–2 years
               at ages 40–50, yearly at ages 50–65
               (a) Most recommendations suggest continued screening after age 65, usu-
                  ally every 2 years

        iv. Other factors, e.g., fibrocystic breasts, prior breast biopsy, prior breast cancer require individualization

    d. Test for fecal occult blood and sigmoidoscopy

        i. Fecal occult blood test performed yearly

        ii. Flexible sigmoidoscopy recommended at age 50 and, if negative, repeated every 5–10 years

        iii. Family history, especially polyposis, prior genital tract cancer, inflammatory bowel disease compels earlier, more frequent screening

    e. **High-risk groups**

        i. Fasting glucose, for individuals with family history of diabetes with obesity or prior gestational diabetes

        ii. VDRL, chlamydial testing, gonorrhea culture, HIV testing for those engaging in high-risk sexual practices and/or intravenous drug use

        iii. Purified protein derivative test for tuberculosis, for individuals with close household or occupational exposure and health care workers with exposure

        iv. Hearing, for persons exposed to excessive noise

        v. Bone mineral content (see chapter 87)

           (a) Peri- or postmenopausal women with risk factors or if result impacts estrogen replacement decision

           (b) Currently not recommended for all women

C. Counseling

  1. **Substance use**

    a. Tobacco cessation strongly advised to all smokers

    b. Alcohol

        i. For most women, intake should be limited to approximately 15 ml/day, i.e., 12 oz beer, 5 oz wine, 1 oz whiskey

        ii. Special caution regarding drinking and driving

    c. Recreational drugs and associated high-risk behavior

  2. **Diet** (see chapter 5)

    a. Limit intake of fat (especially saturated fat), cholesterol, sodium

    b. Appropriate intake of complex carbohydrates, fiber, fruits, vegetables, calcium

    c. Controversy remains concerning supplements of certain vitamins and minerals, such as vitamins C (immunostimulant), D (osteoporosis prevention), and E (cardiovascular disease prevention), zinc (immunostimulant), selenium (cardiovascular disease prevention), and others

  3. **Exercise** (see chapter 6)

  4. **Sexual practices**

    a. STD prevention/condom use, contraception use, avoid high-risk behavior, unintended pregnancy

  5. **Injury prevention**

    a. Seat belts, smoke detectors, motorcycle/bicycle helmet use, avoid smoking in bed

  6. **Dental health**

    a. Routine brushing, flossing

    b. Referral to dentist if dentition is poor

D. Immunizations (see chapter 4)

  1. Tetanus-diphtheria booster

  2. Rubella (childbearing age)

  3. Pneumococcal if chronic illness

E. Chemoprophylaxis

  1. Folic acid, at least 1 mg/day, if capable of or anticipate pregnancy

  2. Hormone replacement therapy, especially if high risk for osteoporosis or heart disease (see chapter 69)

Acknowledgment

Material in this chapter has been adapted from the U.S. Preventive Services Task Force: Guide to Clinical Preventive Services, 2nd ed. Alexandria, VA, International Medical Publishing, 1996.

SUGGESTED READING

1. American Cancer Society: Summary of Current Guidelines for the Cancer-related Check-up: Recommendations. New York, American Cancer Society, 1996.
2. Carney PA, Dietrich AJ: The periodic health examination provided to asymptomatic older women: An assessment using standardized patients. Ann Intern Med 119:129–135, 1993.
3. Charap MH: The periodic health examination: Genesis of a myth. Ann Intern Med 95:733–735, 1981
4. Han PKJ: Historical changes in the objectives of the periodic health examination. Ann Intern Med 127:910–917, 1997.
5. Hayward RS, Steinberg EP: Preventive care guidelines: 1991. Ann Intern Med 114:758–783, 1991.
6. McPhee SJ, Bird JA: Promoting cancer prevention activities by primary care physicians. JAMA 266:538–544, 1991.
7. Morrison E: Controversies in women's health maintenance. Am Fam Phys 55:1283–1290, 1997.
8. Oboler SK, LaForce FM: The periodic physical examination in asymptomatic adults. Ann Intern Med 110:214–226, 1989.
9. U.S. Preventive Services Task Force: Guide to Clinical Preventive Services, 2nd ed. Alexandria, VA, International Medical Publishing, 1996.
10. Williams RB, Boles M: A patient-initiated system for preventive health care: A randomized trial in community-based primary care practices. Arch Fam Med 7:338–345, 1998

ADDITIONAL SOURCES:

American Cancer Society (http://www.cancer.org)
Centers for Disease Control and Prevention Guidelines (http://www.cdc.gov/prevguid.htm)
Department of Health and Human Services, Office of Disease Prevention and Health Promotion (http://odphp.osophs.dhhs.gov/pubs/guidecps)

3. Health Promotion and Disease Prevention: Special Issues for Older Women

Jane L. Murray, M.D.

I. **The Issues**
   A. Americans are living longer and with improved health status
      1. Fastest growing age group is persons over 100
      2. Women live on average 5 years longer than men
         a. Average life expectancy for women is 77 years
         b. Average life expectancy for men is 72 years
      3. 45% of people aged 65 and over have some limitations of activities of daily living (ADLs)
      4. 60% of people over age 85 have limitations of ADLs
   B. **Guidelines for health promotion and disease prevention** now recommended for all age groups, including older adults
      1. U.S.Preventive Services Task Force
      2. American Geriatrics Society
      3. American Academy of Family Physicians
      4. American Cancer Society
      5. American College of Obstetricians and Gynecologists
   C. **Leading causes of death in persons over age 65**
      1. Heart disease
      2. Cerebrovascular (CV) disease
      3. Obstructive lung disease
      4. Pneumonia and influenza
      5. Lung cancer
      6. Colorectal cancer

TABLE 1.   Conditions Commonly Underdiagnosed in the Elderly

Depression/abnormal bereavement	Dental problems (gingivitis, decay or loss of teeth)
Cognitive changes	Peripheral arterial disease
Physical abuse or neglect	Urinary tract problems (incontinence,
Anemia	infection)
Failing vision	Fecal impaction
Hearing problems	Foot problems
Malignant skin lesions	Locomotor difficulty and falling

II. **The Theory**
   A. **Numerous conditions are commonly underdiagnosed in elderly,** usually because patient does not spontaneously complain about them (Table 1)
   B. **Special groups of elderly at increased risk for health problems**
      1. People over 80–85 years ("frail elderly")
      2. Housebound or isolated
      3. Recently bereaved
      4. Recently hospitalized
      5. Recently relocated
      6. Living in a deprived environment
   C. **Functional status assessment and optimization**—most important aspects of caring for older adults
   D. **Elements of good geriatric care**
      1. Implementation of specific knowledge and skills
      2. True patient advocacy
      3. Accepting legitimacy of death
      4. Emphasis on restoring function
      5. Building and maintaining patient supports
      6. Avoidance of iatrogenesis
      7. Allowing time for healing and repair
      8. Protecting patient from inappropriate recommendations
   E. **Areas important to assess**
      1. Medical status and problems
      2. Functional status
      3. Cognitive status
      4. Affective state
      5. Social and environmental status
      6. Personal values and quality of life
      7. Risk factors
   F. **Reasons to use assessment instruments**
      1. To ensure comprehensiveness
      2. To increase observer accuracy
      3. To save time
      4. To establish baseline measures
      5. To monitor response to therapy
III. **An Approach**
   A. **Medical assessment**
      1. **History**—annually
         a. Medical history and current health status
         b. Presence or absence of abnormal uterine bleeding
         c. Family history: especially cardiovascular disease, diabetes mellitus, cancer of breast, ovary or colon.
         d. Medication use (prescription and nonprescription)
         e. Symptoms of transient ischemic attacks (TIAs), hearing loss, memory loss
         f. Dietary intake, especially adequate protein, calcium, calories and nutrients
         g. Physical activity
         h. Sexual history including safer sexual practices
         i. Tobacco, alcohol and drug use

  j. Functional status at home

  k. Screening for domestic violence, elder abuse or neglect, depression

 2. **Physical exam**—annually

  a. Height and weight

  b. Blood pressure—at least every 2 years

  c. Visual acuity

  d. Hearing and hearing aids

  e. Cardiac auscultation

  f. Clinical breast exam

  g. Abdominal exam

  h. Digital rectal exam

  i. Pelvic exam

  j. Auscultation for carotid bruits—at high risk for CV disease (hypertension, smoking, coronary artery disease, atrial fibrillation, diabetes) or those with neurologic symptoms (TIAs) or history of CV disease

  k. Complete skin exam—persons with family or personal history of skin cancer, increased exposure to sunlight, clinical evidence of precursor lesions

  l. Complete oral cavity exam—in people with exposure to alcohol or tobacco or with suspicious symptoms or lesions detected through self-examination

  m. Palpation for thyroid nodules—in people with history of upper-body irradiation

B. **Functional assessment**

 1. Katz Activities of Daily Living (ADL) instrument (Appendix A)

  a. Screens for physical ability to perform daily personal functions: bathing, dressing, toileting, transfer, continence, feeding

  b. Helps to determine needs for home help, physical and occupational therapy, assistive devices

 2. Lawson and Brody Instrumental Activities of Daily Living (IADL) instrument (Appendix B)

  a. Screens for ability to use common tools in everyday environment: telephone, walking, shopping, preparing meals, housework, handy work, laundry, take own medication, manage money

  b. Helps to determine need for assistance to comply with medical interventions

C. **Cognitive assessment**

 1. Pfeiffer Short Portable Mental Status Exam

  a. 10 questions, 10 points

  b. Mainly memory assessment

  c. Easy to administer

  d. Screens normal from cognitive impairment

  e. Not for global cognitive impairment

 2. Folstein Mini-Mental State (Appendix C)

  a. 11 questions, 30 points

  b. More global than Pfeiffer

  c. Good only for screening for cognitive impairment

 3. DAT Inventory (Appendix D)

  a. Under investigation as clinical tool to differentiate Alzheimer's disease from other types of dementia

 4. Set Test

  a. 4 sets: fruits, animals, colors, towns

  b. Patient asked to list as many items in each set as possible

  c. 10 points per set; possible total of 40 points

  d. Score should be greater than 15 in nondemented adults.

D. **Affective state assessment**

 1. Beck Inventory—long used for measuring depression in adults

 2. Hamilton Inventory—another depression scale

 3. Zung Depression Scale—self-rating depression scale

 4. Yesavage Depression Scale—(Appendix E)

  a. First depression scale developed for and validated in older adults

E. **Environmental context assessment**
  1. Social contacts and activities
  2. Life satisfaction: sexual, physical, emotional
  3. Home environment—safety and basic necessities
     a. Visiting nurses often provide excellent information about physical home environment
     b. Home visits by physician sometimes useful to understand full context of patient's life and circumstances
     c. Formal environmental assessment tools are available (Appendix F) which evaluate stairs, ramps, handrails, heating and air conditioning, plumbing/bathroom accessibility, lighting, telephone, floor covering, thresholds, obstacles, assistive devices, hazards, water temperature, medicine cabinet contents, cupboard and refrigerator contents, cooking facilities
F. **Health promotion and disease prevention activities** (per U.S. Preventive Services Task Force, 1996)
  1. **Screening**
     a. Blood cholesterol (fasting or nonfasting)—at least every 5 years
     b. Mammogram—every year for ages 50–65; after 65, frequency controversial
     c. Fasting plasma glucose (annual if markedly obese, family history of diabetes mellitus (DM) or personal history of gestational DM; otherwise no routine screening)
     d. PPD test for tuberculosis (TB)—annual if high-risk (e.g., household members of persons with TB, recent immigrant from country with high TB rate, nursing home residents, residents of correctional facilities, HIV-positive persons); otherwise none
     e. Papanicolaou smear—annually for patients with a cervix, unless documented lifelong screening with consistently negative results, to age 70
     f. Annual fecal occult blood testing and/or flexible sigmoidoscopy. Full colonoscopy for people having first-degree relatives with colorectal cancer; personal history of endometrial, ovarian, or breast cancer; or previous diagnosis of inflammatory bowel disease, adenomatous polyps, or colorectal cancer
  2. **Counseling**
     a. Diet and exercise
        i. Low saturated fat, cholesterol and sodium; high complex carbohydrates, sodium, calcium
        ii. Selection of exercise program: at least 30 minutes 3 times a week of aerobic exercise for cardiovascular benefit, and weight bearing exercise, including weight training, for osteoporosis prevention
     b. Substance use: tobacco cessation; alcohol and other drugs (limiting intake, not driving); treatment for abuse
     c. Safer sexual practices, sexuality, loss of partner/masturbation, lubrication
     d. Injury prevention: prevention of falls, use of seat belts, smoke detector, not smoking near bedding and upholstery, hot water heater temperature (under 120°F), safety helmets for biking/motorcycling, childhood safety issues if children in home
     e. Dental health: regular tooth brushing, flossing; annual dental visits, properly fitting dentures
     f. Other primary preventive measures: discuss hormone replacement therapy; advance directives and living will; skin protection from ultraviolet light
  3. **Immunization and chemoprophylaxis** (see chapter 4)
     a. Tetanus-diphtheria booster every 10 years
     b. Influenza vaccine—annually
     c. Pneumococcal vaccine (once)
     d. Hepatitis B vaccine for household and sexual contacts of HBV carriers, multiple sexual partners
G. **Preventing iatrogenesis**
  1. Careful assessment; use tools as indicated
  2. Use nonpharmacologic therapies whenever possible

3. Minimize number of medications
   a. Exponential rise in adverse drug interactions with more than 3 drugs
   b. Stop unnecessary drugs
4. Simplify the drug regimen
5. Use the lowest effective dose and gradually increase as needed
6. Obtain a complete drug history, including over-the-counter drugs and alcohol
7. Provide careful and complete patient education
8. Maintain good office records
9. Maintain a healthy awareness of sensitivity of the elderly to iatrogenic problems.

SUGGESTED READING

1. U.S. Preventive Services Task Force: Guide to Clinical Preventive Services, 2nd ed. Baltimore, Williams & Wilkins, 1996.
2. American Cancer Society: Guidelines for the Cancer-related Check-up. Atlanta, American Cancer Society, 1996.
3. Fleischman C, Honebrink A, Sherif K, et al: Guidelines for preventive health screening in women. Women's Health Prim Care 1:413–423, 1998.
4. National Cancer Institute: Statement from the National Cancer Institute on the National Cancer Advisory Board recommendations on mammography. NCI Press Office, March 27, 1997.
5. National Heart, Lung and Blood Institute: Recommendations regarding public screening for measuring blood cholesterol. NIH Publication No. 95-3045, September 1995.
6. Winawer SJ, Fletcher RH, Miller L, et al: Colorectal cancer screening: Clinical guidelines and rationale. Gastroenterology 112:594–642, 1997.

APPENDIX A

Activities of Daily Living (ADL) Scale

Name _____ Day of evaluation _____

For each area of functioning listed below, check description that applies. (The word "assistance" means supervision, direction, or personal assistance.)

Bathing—either sponge bath, tub bath, or shower

☐	☐	☐
Receives no assistance (gets in and out of tub by self, if tub is usual means of bathing)	Receives assistance in bathing only one part of the body (such as back or a leg)	Receives assistance in bathing more than one part of the body (or not bathed)

Dressing—gets clothes from closets and drawers, including underclothes, outer garments, and using fasteners (including braces, if worn)

☐	☐	☐
Gets clothes and gets completely dressed without assistance	Gets clothes and gets dressed without assistance, except for assistance in tying shoes	Receives assistance in getting clothes or in getting dressed, or stays partly or completely undressed

Toileting—going to the "toilet room" for bowel and urine elimination; cleaning self after elimination and arranging clothes

☐	☐	☐
Goes to "toilet room," cleans self, and arranges clothes without assistance (may use object for support such as cane, walker, or wheelchair and may manage night bedpan or commode, emptying same in morning)	Receives assistance in going to "toilet room" or in cleansing self or in arranging clothes after elimination or in use of night bedpan or commode	Doesn't go to room termed "toilet" for the elimination process

Transfer

☐	☐	☐
Moves in and out of bed as well as in and out of chair without assistance (may be using object for support, such as cane or walker)	Moves in and out of bed or chair with assistance	Doesn't get out of bed

(Continued on following page.)

APPENDIX A *(Cont.)*

Activities of Daily Living (ADL) Scale

Continence

☐ Controls urination and bowel movement completely by self

☐ Has occasional "accidents"

☐ Supervision helps keep urine or bowel control; catheter is used or person is incontinent

Feeding

☐ Feeds self without assistance

☐ Feeds self except for getting assistance in cutting meat or buttering bread

☐ Receives assistance in feeding or is fed partly or completely using tubes or intravenous fluids

Source: Courtesy of Sidney Katz, MD. Reprinted with permission.

For additional information on administration and scoring refer to the following references:
1. Katz S: Assessing self-maintenance: Activities of daily living, mobility, and instrumental activities of daily living. J Am Geriatr Soc 31:721–727, 1983.
2. Katz S. Akpom CA: A measure of primary sociobiologic functions. Int J Health Services 6:493–508, 1976.
3. Katz S, Downs TD, Cash HR, et al: Progress in development of the index of ADL. J Gerontol 10:20–30, 1970.

APPENDIX B

Instrumental Activities of Daily Living (IADL) Scale

Self-Rated Version Extracted from the Multilevel Assessment Instrument (MAI)

1. Can you use the telephone:
   without help, 3
   with some help, or 2
   are you completely unable to use the telephone? 1

2. Can you get to places out of walking distance:
   without help, 3
   with some help, or 2
   are you completely unable to travel unless special arrangements are made? 1

3. Can you go shopping for groceries:
   without help, 3
   with some help, or 2
   are you completely unable to do any shopping? 1

4. Can you prepare your own meals:
   without help, 3
   with some help, or 2
   are you completely unable to prepare any meals? 1

5. Can you do your own housework:
   without help, 3
   with some help, or 2
   are you completely unable to do any housework? 1

6. Can you do your own handyman work:
   without help, 3
   with some help, or 2
   are you completely unable to do any handyman work? 1

7. Can you do your own laundry:
   without help, 3
   with some help, or 2
   are you completely unable to do any laundry at all? 1

8a. Do you take medicines or use any medications?
   (If yes, answer Question 8b) Yes 1
   (If no, answer Question 8c) No 2

(Continued on following page.)

APPENDIX B *(Cont.)*

Instrumental Activities of Daily Living (IADL) Scale

8b. Do you take your own medicine?
without help (in the right doses at the right time),   3
with some help (take medicine if someone prepares it for you and/or reminds you to take it),   2
or (are you/would you be) completely unable to take your own medicine?   1

8c. If you had to take medicine, can you do it?
without help (in the right doses at the right time),   3
with some help (take medicine if someone prepares it for you and/or reminds you to take it),   2
or (are you/would you be) completely unable to take your own medicine?   1

9. Can you manage your own money:
without help,   3
with some help, or   2
are you completely unable to handle money?   1

Source: Lawton MP, Brody EM: Assessment of older people: Self-maintaining and instrumental activities of daily living. Gerontologist 9:179–185, 1969; reprinted with permission.

For additional information on administration and scoring refer to the following references:
1. Lawton MP: Scales to measure competence in everyday activities. Psychopharm Bull 24:609–614, 1988.
2. Lawton MP, Moss M, Fulcomer M, et al: A research and service-oriented multilevel assessment instrument. J Gerontol 37:91–99, 1982.

APPENDIX C

Mini-Mental State Examination (MMSE)

Add points for each correct response

Orientation		Score	Points
1. What is the:	Year?	_____	1
	Season?	_____	1
	Date?	_____	1
	Day?	_____	1
	Month?	_____	1
2. Where are we?	State?	_____	1
	County?	_____	1
	Town or city?	_____	1
	Hospital?	_____	1
	Floor?	_____	1

Registration
3. Name three objects, taking one second to say each. Then ask the patient   _____   3
to repeat all three after you have said them.

Give one point for each correct answer. Repeat the answers until patient learns all three.

Attention and calculation
4. Serial sevens. Give one point for each correct answer. Stop after five   _____   5
answers. Alternate: Spell WORLD backwards.

Recall
5. Ask for names of three objects learned in question 3. Give one point for   _____   3
each correct answer.

Language
6. Point to a pencil and a watch. Have the patient name them as you point.   _____   2
7. Have the patient repeat "No ifs, ands, or buts."   _____   1
8. Have the patient follow a three-stage command: "Take a paper in your   _____   3
right hand. Fold the paper in half. Put the paper on the floor."
9. Have the patient read and obey the following: "CLOSE YOUR EYES."   _____   1
(Write it in large letters.)

(Continued on following page.)

APPENDIX C *(Cont.)*

Mini-Mental State Examination (MMSE)

Language *(Cont.)*   Score   Points

10. Have the patient write a sentence of his or her choice. (The sentence should   _____   1
    contain a subject and an object and should make sense. Ignore spelling
    errors when scoring.)
11. Have the patient copy the design. (Give one point if all sides and angles   _____   1
    are preserved and if the intersecting sides form a quadrangle.)

_____ = Total 30

In validation studies using a cut-off score of 23 or below, the MMSE has a sensitivity of 87%, a specificity of 82%, a false positive ratio of 39.4%, and a false negative ratio of 4.7%. These ratios refer to the MMSE's capacity to accurately distinguish patients with clinically diagnosed dementia or delirium from patients without these syndromes.

Source: Courtesy of Marshall Folstein, MD. Reprinted with permission.

For additional information on administration and scoring refer to the following references:

1. Anthony JC, LeResche L, Niaz U, et al: Limits of "Mini-Mental State" as a screening test for dementia and delirium among hospital patients. Psych Med 12:397–408, 1982.
2. Folstein MF, Anthony JC, et al: Meaning of cognitive impairment in the elderly. J Am Geriatr Soc 33:228–235, 1985.
3. Folstein MF, Folstein S, McHugh PR: Mini-Mental State: A practical method for grading the cognitive state of patients for the clinician. J Psych Res 12:189–198, 1975.
4. Spenser MP, Folstein MF: The Mini-Mental State Examination. In Keller PA, Ritt LG: Innovations in Clinical Practice: A Source Book 4:305–310, 1985.

APPENDIX D

Alzheimer's Disease
Dementia of the Alzheimer Type (DAT): Assessment Inventory

Clinical Features	Criteria for Scores 0 to 2*		
	0	1	2
Mental Functions			
Memory	Normal or forgetfulness that improves with cues	Recalls 1 or 2 of 3 words spontaneously; incompletely aided by prompting	Disoriented; unable to learn 3 words in 3 min; recall not aided by prompting
Visuospatial	Normal or clumsy drawings; minimal distortions	Flattening, omissions, distortions	Disorganized, unrecognizable copies of models
Cognition	Normal or impairment of complex abstractions and calculations	Fails to abstract simple proverbs and has difficulty with mathematic problems	Fails to interpret even simple proverbs or idioms; acalculia
Personality	Disinhibition or depression	Appropriately concerned	Unaware or indifferent irritability not uncommon
Language	Normal	Anomia; mild comprehension deficits sometimes present	Fluent aphasia with anomia, decreased comprehension, paraphasia
Motor Functions			
Speech	Mute, severely dysarthric	Slurred, amelodic, hypophonic	Normal

(Continued on following page.)

APPENDIX D *(Cont.)*

Alzheimer's Disease
Dementia of the Alzheimer Type (DAT): Assessment Inventory

	Criteria for Scores 0 to 2*		
Clinical Features	0	1	2
Motor Functions *(cont.)*			
Psychomotor speed	Slow, long latency to response	Hesitant responses	Normal, prompt responses
Posture	Abnormal, flexed, extended, or distorted	Stooped or mildly distorted	Normal, erect
Gait	Hemiparetic, ataxic, apractic, or hyperkinetic	Shuffling, dyskinetic	Normal
Movements	Tremor, akinesia, rigidity, or chorea	Imprecise, poorly coordinated	Normal

* A score of > 14 indicates DAT.
Adapted from Cummings JL, Benson DF: Dementia of the Alzheimer type: An inventory of diagnostic clinical features. J Am Geriatr Soc 34:12–19, 1986.

APPENDIX E

Geriatric Depression Scale (Short Form)

Choose the best answer for how you felt over the past week.

1. Are you basically satisfied with your life? yes/no
2. Have you dropped many of your activities and interests? yes/no
3. Do you feel that your life is empty? yes/no
4. Do you often get bored? yes/no
5. Are you in good spirits most of the time? yes/no
6. Are you afraid that something bad is going to happen to you? yes/no
7. Do you feel happy most of the time? yes/no
8. Do you often feel helpless? yes/no
9. Do you prefer to stay at home, rather than going out and doing new things? yes/no
10. Do you feel you have more problems with memory than most? yes/no
11. Do you think it is wonderful to be alive now? yes/no
12. Do you feel pretty worthless the way you are now? yes/no
13. Do you feel full of energy? yes/no
14. Do you feel that your situation is hopeless? yes/no
15. Do you think that most people are better off than you are? yes/no

This is the scoring for the scale. One point for each of these answers. Cut-off: normal (0–5), above 5 suggests depression.

1. no	6. yes	11. no
2. yes	7. no	12. yes
3. yes	8. yes	13. no
4. yes	9. yes	14. yes
5. no	10. yes	15. yes

Source: Courtesy of Jerome A. Yesavage, MD. Reprinted with permission.

For additional information on administration and scoring refer to the following references:
1. Sheikh JI, Yesavage JA: Geriatric Depression Scale: Recent evidence and development of a shorter version. Clin Gerontol 5:165–172, 1986.
2. Yesavage JA, Brink TL, Rose TL, et al: Development and validation of a geriatric depression rating scale: A preliminary report. J Psych Res 17:27, 1983.

APPENDIX F

Architectural Assessment Check List

1. Entries/Exits
   a. Location(s): Front _____ back _____ side _____
   b. Stairs: yes _____ no _____ front _____ back _____
   c. Ramp: yes _____ no _____ slope _____ width _____
   d. Rail: yes _____ no _____ which side? L _____ R _____ both _____ height _____
   e. Door width: front _____ back _____
   f. Threshold height: _____

2. General
   a. Number of stories: _____
      If 2 stories, are essential rooms on first? yes _____ no _____
      If 2 stories, number of stairs _____
   b. Heating type: _____
   c. Air conditioning type: _____
   d. Indoor plumbing? yes _____ no _____

3. Kitchen
   a. Lighting: number, type ____
      adequate light? yes _____ no _____ glare? yes _____ no _____
   b. Color scheme: _____
   c. Stove type: _____ location of controls _____
   d. Refrigerator? yes_____ no _____ contents: _____
   e. Cupboards: height _____ accessible? yes _____ no _____
   f. Counter height: _____ sink height _____ type of faucet handles _____
   g. Telephone? _____
   h. Table/chairs: _____
   i. Nearest bathroom: _____ ft.
   j. Entry/exit door width: _____
   k. Threshold height: _____
   l. Type of floor covering: _____

4. Bedroom?
   a. Lighting: number, type _____
      adequate light? yes _____ no _____ glare? yes _____ no _____
   b. Color scheme: _____
   c. Door width: _____
   d. Threshold height: _____
   e. Type of floor covering: _____
   f. Bed height: _____
   g. Furnishings: _____
   h. Closets: shelf height _____ hanging height _____
   i. Width of passages: _____
   j. Window height: _____
   k. Telephone? yes _____ no _____
   l. Distance to bathroom: _____ ft.
   m. Assist devices used: _____
   n. Hazards: _____

5. Hallway
   a. Width: _____
   b. Threshold(s) height(s) _____
   c. Door width(s) _____

6. Bathroom
   a. Door width _____ threshold height _____ aisle width _____
   b. Tub yes ____ no ____ shower yes ____ no ____ glass door yes ____ no ____
      faucet handles _____
   c. Sink: faucet handle type _____
   d. Toilet height: _____

(Continued on following page.)

APPENDIX F

Architectural Assessment Check List

6. Bathroom *(cont.)*
   e. Lighting adequate?   yes _____   no _____   glare?   yes _____   no _____
   f. Water heater temperature: _____
   g. Medicine cabinet contents: _____
   h. Special adaptive devices: _____
   i. Hazards: _____

7. Living room
   a. Sofa height _____   depth _____
   b. Chair (1) height _____   depth _____   width _____   arm height _____   leg type _____
      chair (2) height _____   depth _____   width _____   arm height _____   leg type _____
      chair (3) height _____   depth _____   width _____   arm height _____   leg type _____
   c. Table(s), height: _____
   d. Television: yes _____   no _____   radio: yes _____   no _____
   e. Color scheme: _____   lighting adequate _____   yes _____   no _____
   f. Width of passages: _____
   g. Distance to bathroom: _____ ft.
   h. Nearest telephone: _____

8. Laundry
   a. Washing machine?   yes _____   no _____
   b. Dryer?   yes _____   no _____
   c. Accessibility: poor _____   fair _____   good _____
   d. Storage shelf height _____

9. Special assistance devices _____
   _____
   _____

Source: Courtesy of Michael S. Vernon, MD, and Harold Kallman, MD.

4. Immunizations for Adolescents and Adults

Cynda Ann Johnson, M.D., M.B.A.

I. The Issues

For years, adolescent and adult immunization was a dull topic—nothing much was new, and the only concern in offices and emergency departments was to ask patients presenting with a wound, "Is your tetanus shot up-to-date?" Within the last decade, however, issues of adult immunization have taken on a new importance: new vaccines have been developed, revision of the childhood immunization schedule has affected the recommendation for boosters in adolescence and adulthood, and some elective vaccines have increased in popularity among health care providers and the public. Physicians who practice primary care need to keep abreast of such trends and to be prepared to offer appropriate vaccines to their patients as well as to answer any questions patients may have about safety, efficacy, side effects, and cost.

II. The Theory

A. Active immunization

1. Defined as administration of all or part of a microorganism or modified product of that microorganism (e.g., toxoid)
2. Goal: to evoke an immunologic response mimicking that of natural infection without the risk
3. Depending on immunizing agent, protection may be complete for life or partial and in need of boosters

B. **Definition of vaccine effectiveness**
1. Evidence of protection against natural disease
2. Induction of antibodies is an indirect measure, but serum antibody concentrations are not always predictive of protection
3. Boosters often required for vaccines that incorporate nonliving substances
4. Vaccines incorporating inactivated (killed) infectious agents may not elicit the range of immunologic responses provided by live, attenuated agents
    a. Example: inactivated polio vaccine (IPV), which may evoke sufficient serum antibody response but not local antibody (immunoglobulin A), as does the live, attenuated oral polio vaccine (OPV)
    b. Result is possible (though rare) local infection or colonization if IPV is used, although systemic infection is prevented or ameliorated
    c. Advantages to killed vaccine, however, are safety in immunosuppressed host and no viral excretion by vaccinee

III. **An Approach**
   A. **General guidelines**
   1. **Current immunization history** is essential part of routine (or yearly) exam
       a. Women often present for yearly Papanicolaou smear
       b. Review immunization history
           i. Encourage routine boosters
           ii. Offer appropriate elective immunizations
           iii. Describe new vaccines if potential candidate
   2. **Obtain informed consent** for immunizations
   3. **Follow recommended guidelines** for site and route of administration (Table 1)
   4. **Vaccine storage**
       a. Guidelines for storage should be followed carefully
       b. A recent study indicates that majority of vaccines in the community have been exposed to conditions that could reduce or destroy their potency
   5. **Simultaneous administration** of multiple routine vaccinations is not contraindicated and helps compliance
       a. Exception: separate cholera and yellow fever vaccines by 3 weeks for optimal antibody response
       b. Vaccines commonly associated with local or systemic reactions (e.g., cholera, parenteral typhoid, plague) can accentuate reaction; should administer on separate occasions, if possible
   6. Lapse in immunization schedule—do not start over
   7. Patient with unknown immunization status is assumed to be susceptible
   8. Active immunization of person who recently received immune globulin depends on type of immune globulin received
       a. **Mumps, measles, and rubella immune globulin**
           i. Do not give vaccine within 3 months
       b. **Hepatitis immune globulin** (HBIG), **tetanus immune globulin** (TIG), **rabies immune globulin** (RIG)
           i. Corresponding inactivated vaccine or toxoid may be administered at any time
           ii. Useful in postexposure prophylaxis
           iii. Immune response not impaired
           iv. Provide immediate protection and active/passive immunity
           v. Administer at different site from immune globulin
       c. **Varicella vaccine** should not be administered for at least 5 months after receipt of immune globulin preparation
       d. Immune globulin for travel may be administered concurrently with OPV and yellow fever vaccines (both live virus vaccines) if departure is imminent
   9. **Tuberculin testing**
       a. Not a prerequisite before administration of live virus vaccines
   10. **Accurate record keeping** for immunizations
       a. Month, day, and year of administration
       b. Vaccine administered

TABLE 1.   Vaccines Licensed in the U.S. and Their Routes of Administration

Vaccine	Type	Route
Adenovirus[¶]	Live virus	Oral
Anthrax	Inactivated bacteria	SC
BCG	Live bacteria	ID (preferred) or SC
Cholera	Inactivated bacteria	SC, IM, or ID
DTP	Toxoids and inactivated bacteria	IM
DTaP	Toxoids and inactivated bacteria component	IM
Hepatitis A	Inactivated virus	IM
Hepatitis B	Inactivated viral antigen	IM
Hib conjugates	Polysaccharide-protein conjugate	IM
Influenza	Inactivated virus (whole-virus)	IM
Japanese encephalitis	Inactivated virus	SC
Measles	Live virus	SC
Meningococcal	Polysaccharide	SC
MMR	Live viruses	SC
Pertussis	Inactivated bacteria	IM
Plague	Inactivated bacteria	IM
Pneumococcal	Polysaccharide	IM or SC
Poliovirus		
OPV	Live virus	Oral
IPV	Inactivated virus	SC
Rabies	Inactivated virus	IM or ID[§]
Rubella	Live virus	SC
Tetanus	Toxoid	IM
Tetanus-diphtheria (Td)	Toxoids	IM
Typhoid		
Parenteral	Inactivated bacteria	SC
Parenteral	Capsular polysaccharide	SC
Oral	Live bacteria	Oral
Varicella	Live virus	SC
Yellow fever	Live virus	SC

From American Academy of Pediatrics: Active and passive immunizations. In Peter G (ed): 1997 Red Book: Report of the Committee on Infectious Diseases, 24th ed. Elk Grove Village, IL, American Academy of Pediatrics, 1997, p 5.

BCG, Bacille Calmette-Guérin vaccine; DTP, diphtheria and tetanus toxoids and pertussis vaccine, adsorbed; DTaP, diphtheria and tetanus toxoids and acellular pertussis vaccine, adsorbed; Hib, *Haemophilus influenzae* type b vaccine; MMR, live measles-mumps-rubella vaccine; OPV, oral poliovirus vaccine; IPV, inactivated poliovirus vaccine; Td, tetanus and diphtheria toxoid; DT, diphtheria and tetanus toxoids. SC, subcutaneous; ID, intradermal; IM, intramuscular.

¶ Available only to U.S. Armed Forces

§ Human diploid cell rabies vaccine for intradermal use is different in constitution and potency from the intramuscular vaccine; it should be used for preexposure immunization only.

   c. Manufacturer, lot number, and expiration date
   d. Site and route of administration
   e. Health care provider administering the vaccine
  11. Sources of vaccination information
   a. *The Red Book* by the American Academy of Pediatrics
   b. *Morbidity and Mortality Weekly Report* (MMWR) by the Centers for Disease Control and Prevention (CDC)
   c. *Health Information for International Travel* by the CDC (www.cdc.gov/travel/travel.html)
 B. Tetanus toxoid/adult diphtheria toxoid (Td)
  1. Pertussis vaccine is not given after age 7
  2. Adult diphtheria toxoid contains less toxoid than child's variety and results in fewer adverse reactions

TABLE 2.   Simplified Primary Immunization Schedule for Adolescents and Adults
Not Immunized in Childhood

Recommended Time	Immunization
First visit	IPV,[¶] Td, MMR
1–2 months after first visit	IPV, Td, MMR
6–12 months after second visit	IPV, Td

IPV, inactivated polio vaccine; Td, tetanus and adult diphtheria toxoids; MMR, live measles, mumps, and rubella viruses vaccine

[¶] Adults partially immunized against polio may have the series completed with either IPV or OPV (oral polio vaccine)

    3. Immunization schedule
      a. See Table 2 for schedule of immunizations for people not immunized in infancy
      b. Td booster required every 10 years
        i. See Table 3 for Td prophylaxis
        ii. Do not give tetanus toxoid only as often happens in emergency departments as part of wound management
        iii. Administer after 5 years in conjunction with dirty wound
    4. Td booster not contraindicated in pregnancy
      a. Schedule for unimmunized pregnant women
        i. Two doses of Td at least 4 weeks apart
        ii. Second dose at least 2 weeks before delivery
        iii. Prevents neonatal tetanus
C. **Polio vaccine**
    1. Risk of poliomyelitis is small in U.S.; potential problem if wild virus is introduced into susceptible populations in communities with low immunization levels
    2. Two types of trivalent vaccine available
      a. **Live oral poliovirus vaccine** may rarely be associated with paralysis in healthy recipients and contacts
        i. Greatest risk with first dose
        ii. Immunocompromised persons at highest risk
      b. **Inactivated poliovirus vaccine**
      IPV with enhanced potency, available in U.S., induces seroconversion rates equal to that of OPV
        i. No serious side effects from IPV; preparation contains trace amounts of streptomycin and neomycin; hypersensitivity reactions to these antibiotics are possible
        ii. IPV preferred in unimmunized adults because the risk of vaccine-associated paralysis after OPV is slightly higher in adults than in children
    3. **Immunization recommendations** for adolescents and adults (see Table 2 for primary series)

TABLE 3.   Guide to Tetanus Prophylaxis in Routine Wound Management

History of Absorbed Tetanus Toxoid (doses)	Clean, Minor Wounds		All Other Wounds*	
	Td[†]	TIG[†]	Td	TIG
Unknown or < 3	Yes	No	Yes	Yes
≥ 3[‡]	No[§]	No	No[¶]	No

From American Academy of Pediatrics: Tetanus. In Peter G (ed): 1997 Red Book: Report of the Committee on Infectious Diseases, 24th ed. Elk Grove Village, IL, American Academy of Pediatrics, 1997, p 520.

* Such as, but not limited to, wounds contaminated with dirt, feces, soil, and saliva; puncture wounds, avulsions; and wounds resulting from missiles, crushing, burns, and frostbite
[†] Td, adult-use tetanus and diphtheria toxoids; TIG, tetanus immune globulin (human)
[‡] If only 3 doses of fluid toxoid have been received, a fourth dose of toxoid should be given
[§] Yes, if more than 10 years since last dose
[¶] Yes, if more than 5 years since last dose

    a. Routine primary poliovirus vaccination of previously unvaccinated adults (18 years of age or older) residing in the U.S. is not indicated

    b. Immunization is recommended for adults at greater risk of exposure to wild polioviruses than the general population

       i. Travelers to areas or countries where poliomyelitis is or may be epidemic or endemic

       ii. Members of communities or specific populations experiencing disease caused by wild polioviruses

       iii. Laboratory workers handling specimens that may contain polioviruses

       iv. Health care workers in close contact with patients who may be excreting polioviruses

    c. Schedule for primary series

       i. Two doses of IPV at intervals of 1–2 months

       ii. Third dose 6–12 months after second dose

    d. Immunization during pregnancy should be avoided (although no convincing evidence indicates that either OPV or IPV has adverse effect); if immediate protection against poliomyelitis is needed, either OPV or IPV is recommended

D. **Mumps, measles, rubella (MMR) vaccine**

1. Two doses given at least one month apart are required for people born after 1956

    a. Older people generally immune by having contracted the disease

    b. Immunization before college entry is important

    c. Measles outbreaks, which included vaccinated people, led to recommendation of second vaccination

    d. Mumps also occurs in highly vaccinated populations

    e. Rubella is always a concern because of potential for congenital rubella syndrome

    f. No contraindication to vaccination of people who are already immune

       i. Routine serologic testing not indicated

       ii. Consider serologic testing as part of prepregnancy evaluation—less important in women having received two vaccinations

2. **Adverse reactions**

    a. **Mumps vaccine**—previously reported adverse reactions may not have been causally related

    b. **Measles vaccine** (also attributed to MMR)

       i. 5–15% develop fever of 39.4°C or higher

         (a) Begins 7–12 days after vaccination

         (b) Lasts 1–2 days, occasionally up to 5 days

       ii. Rash in 5%

       iii. Rare reports of thrombocytopenia within 2 months after vaccination

    c. **Rubella vaccine**

       i. Rash, fever, and lymphadenopathy, generally only in children

       ii. Joint involvement

         (a) Small peripheral joints involved in 1–3% of adolescent females over 12 years of age

         (b) Arthritis (up to 10%) and arthralgia (up to 25%) more common in unvaccinated postpubertal females; if occurs, begins 7–21 days after vaccination though generally transient (1 day to 3 weeks)

         (c) Persistent or recurrent arthritic complaints occasionally reported in vaccinated adult women, but true relationship to vaccination is unclear

       iii. Transient peripheral neuritis occurs rarely

3. **Special groups**

    a. **Women with altered immunity**—in general MMR should not be given, except that those infected with HIV need measles immunization

    b. **Pregnant women should not be given MMR** based on theoretical risk of fetal infection with live virus

       i. Accidental rubella immunization during pregnancy or within 3 months before pregnancy must be reported

E. **Influenza vaccine**
1. Protects against both influenza A and influenza B
   a. Antiviral medications, such as amantadine hydrochloride, prevent or reduce symptoms of influenza A only
2. Administer yearly for protection against influenza
   a. High levels of influenza activity generally do not occur before the month of December in the U.S.
      i. Vaccine may be offered as early as September
      ii. Organized vaccination campaigns optimally undertaken in November
   b. Any person > 6 months of age who wishes to reduce chance of becoming infected with influenza may be vaccinated
      i. Restrict to high-risk groups when vaccine in short supply
      ii. May vaccinate during pregnancy
3. Influenza epidemics cause excessive mortality attributable to influenza pneumonia and cardiopulmonary disease
4. **Groups at high risk for influenza-related complications**
   a. Persons 65 years of age or older
   b. Residents of nursing homes or chronic care facilities
   c. People with chronic disorders of the pulmonary or cardiovascular system (including those with asthma)
   d. People who have required regular medical follow-up or hospitalization during the preceding year
   e. Children and teenagers who receive long-term aspirin therapy who may be at risk for developing Reye's syndrome during an influenza infection
5. Groups who are potentially capable of transmitting influenza to high-risk persons also should be vaccinated
   a. Physicians, nurses, and other personnel in hospital and outpatient care settings who have contact with high-risk patients
   b. Employees of nursing homes and chronic care facilities who have contact with patients or residents
   c. Providers of home care to high-risk persons
   d. Household members of high-risk persons
6. **Contraindications**
   a. Persons with acute febrile illness should not be vaccinated until symptoms have abated
   b. Influenza vaccine should not be given to anyone with known hypersensitivity to eggs
7. **Adverse reactions**
   a. Influenza vaccination does not cause the flu
   b. Most frequent side effect is soreness at the injection site
   c. Fever, malaise, and myalgia are possible
      i. Especially in persons who have had no exposure to the influenza virus antigens
      ii. Symptoms occur 6–12 hours after vaccination and last 1–2 days

F. **Pneumococcal vaccine**
1. Polysaccharide vaccine contains 23 types of *Streptococcus pneumoniae*
2. Not effective against otitis media
3. One-time vaccination, but highest-risk groups may be reimmunized after 5 years, including:
   a. Persons 65 years of age and older
   b. Immunocompetent adults with chronic disease
   c. Immunocompetent adults with alcoholism, CSF leak, asplenia
   d. Immunocompromised adults
   e. Adults with HIV infection
   f. People living in special environments or social settings with an identified increased risk of pneumococcal disease or its complications, including Native American and Alaskan populations

4. **Urgent vaccination**
   a. Unvaccinated hospitalized patients from high-risk groups should be immunized before hospital discharge
   b. At least 2 weeks before elective splenectomy or initiation of chemotherapy
5. **Safety in pregnancy has not been evaluated**—vaccinate high-risk women before or after pregnancy
6. **Adverse reactions**
   a. Half of vaccinees experience mild side effects such as erythema and pain at the injection site
   b. Fever, myalgias, and severe local reactions occur in < 1%

G. **Hepatitis B virus vaccine**
   1. Two recombinant hepatitis B vaccines currently available in U.S.; equally immunogenic when administered in recommended doses
   2. Vaccinate in deltoid muscle—injection in the hip results in lower response rate
   3. **Dosage schedule**
      a. Three injections at 0, 1, and 6 months (or sometimes at 0, 2, and 4 months)
   4. Adequate antibody response is > 10 mIU/ml
      a. Adequate response in 90–95% of patients
      b. Although 10–60% of patients lose detectable antibody within 10 years, protection against viremic infection and clinical disease appears to persist
         i. Need for revaccination except in hemodialysis patients is unknown
      c. Postvaccination antibody testing not routinely required except in: hemodialysis patients (measure antibody titer yearly and revaccinate when level falls below 10 mIU/ml); staff of hemodialysis units; patients with HIV; people who received their vaccination in the buttocks; health care workers at high risk for needlestick exposure
   5. Table 4 lists those who should be considered for hepatitis B immunization
   6. Follow hospital protocols for postexposure prophylaxis
   7. Pregnancy is not a contraindication to hepatitis B vaccination; prenatal testing for hepatitis B antigen is recommended for all pregnant women

TABLE 4. People Who Should Receive Hepatitis B Immunization

- All infants—infants of HBsAg-positive mothers require postexposure immunoprophylaxis with HBIG and vaccine
- Infants and children at risk of acquisition of HBV by person-to-person (horizontal) transmission should be immunized by 6–9 months of age
- Adolescents*—special efforts should be made to vaccinate adolescents at high risk for HBV infection
- Users of intravenous drugs
- Sexually active heterosexual persons with more than 1 sex partner in the previous 6 months or with a sexually transmitted disease
- Sexually active homosexual or bisexual males
- Health care workers at risk of exposure to blood or body fluids
- Residents and staff of institutions for developmentally disabled persons
- Staff of nonresidential child care and school programs for developmentally disabled persons if attended by a known HBV carrier
- Hemodialysis patients
- Patients with bleeding disorders who receive certain blood products
- Household contacts and sexual partners of HBV carriers
- Members of households with HBsAg-positive adoptees from countries where HBV infection is endemic
- International travelers who will live for more than 6 months in an area of high HBV endemicity and who otherwise will be at risk
- Inmates of long-term correctional facilities

HBsAg = hepatitis B surface antigen; HBIG = hepatitis B immune globulin; HBV = hepatitis B virus.
* Implementation may be initiated before children reach adolescence.

TABLE 5.   Recommended Doses and Schedules for Hepatitis A Virus (HAV) Inactivated Vaccines

Age (yrs)	Vaccine	Antigen Dose	Volume (ml/dose)	No. of Doses	Schedule
2–18	Havrix (SKB)	360 ELU	0.5	3	Initial, 1, and 6–12 mo later
	Havrix (SKB)	720 ELU	0.5	2	Initial and 6–12 mo later
	Vaqta (Merck)	25 U	0.5	2	Initial and 6–18 mo later
19 and older	Havrix (SKB)	1440 ELU	1.0	2	Initial and 6–12 mo later
	Vaqta (Merck)	50 U	1.0	2	Initial and 6–12 mo later

From American Academy of Pediatrics: Hepatitis A. In Peter G (ed): 1997 Red Book: Report of the Committee on Infectious Diseases, 24th ed. Elk Grove Village, IL, American Academy of Pediatrics, 1997, p 242.
U, units; ELU, enzyme-linked immunoassay units; SKB, SmithKline Beecham.

8. **Adverse reactions**—most common side effect is soreness at injection site
9. Future of hepatitis vaccination
   a. Vaccination of high-risk individuals has not greatly affected the incidence of hepatitis B infection
   b. Universal vaccination of neonates and adolescents is currently recommended
   c. Ultimately universal hepatitis B vaccination will probably be recommended

H. **Hepatitis A virus vaccine**
   1. Description of vaccine
      a. Two inactivated HAV vaccines are available in U.S.
      b. 80–98% of vaccinees seroconvert by day 15—virtually 100% 1 month after second dose
   2. Dosing schedule—see Table 5
      a. Primary series should be administered at least 2 weeks before expected exposure to hepatitis A virus
      b. Duration of protection not known; at least 20 years expected
      c. Postimmunization serologic testing not needed due to high rate of seroconversion
      d. May be administered with hepatitis A immune globulin if both immediate and long-term protection needed
   3. Recommendations for use
      a. Anyone > 2 years of age desiring protection against hepatitis A infection, in whom the vaccine is not otherwise contraindicated, may be immunized
      b. Persons traveling or working in countries with high or intermediate endemicity
      c. Persons living in communities with high endemic rates of HAV infection and periodic hepatitis A outbreaks (e.g., Native American, Alaskan Native)
      d. Men who have sex with men
      e. Persons with chronic liver disease
      f. Users of injection and illicit drugs
      g. Laboratory workers who handle HAV
      h. Handlers of primate animals that may be harboring HAV
   4. Pregnancy—no studies available but risk considered low
   5. It is not known whether the vaccine is excreted in human milk
   6. Adverse reactions
      a. Injection site soreness in 56%
      b. Headache in 14%

I. **Varicella zoster vaccine** (VZV)
   1. Live, attenuated for use in individuals 12 months of age and older who have not had varicella
   2. Persons age 13 and older require two doses of vaccine, 4–8 weeks apart

    3. Conversion rates
       a. 82% after one dose; 94% after both doses
       b. Antibodies still present in 95% of converters for 8–20 years after vaccination
       c. Routine postexposure testing to document seroconversion is not indicated, but desirable in certain circumstances, e.g., newly immunized health worker who will be exposed to immunocompromised individuals
    4. Performance of serologic testing for immunity to chickenpox is optional before administration of the vaccine if no history of the disease
       a. Cost of serologic testing must be considered
       b. No adverse effects if the vaccine is inadvertently administered to an individual already immune to the virus
    5. Potential for development of herpes zoster no greater (and probably less) than after natural varicella infection
    6. Contraindications to routine administration of VZV
       a. Immunocompromised persons; vaccines may be given, however, to other susceptible individuals in the household
       b. Persons with hypersensitivity to any component of the vaccine, including gelatin
       c. Persons with a history of an anaphylactic reaction to neomycin (trace amounts are found in the vaccine)
       d. Because of incomplete data as to whether there will be interference with the development of immunity
          i. Individuals with moderate or severe illness of any kind
          ii. Within 5 months of receipt of immune globulin
       e. Pregnancy (though varicella immune globulin may be used within 96 hours of exposure)
    7. Cautions
       a. Pregnancy should be avoided for one month after administration of the vaccine
       b. May be given to the susceptible nursing mother if risk for exposure to natural VZV is high
       c. Not FDA-approved for postexposure vaccination but may be effective if given within 3 days of exposure
    8. Adverse reactions
       a. Tenderness and erythema at the injection site in about 25–35% of vaccinees
       b. Sparse, maculopapular or varicelliform rash
          i. Occurs in 5% of vaccinees
          ii. Onset within one month of vaccination
    9. Storage of VZV
       a. Must be stored in a freezer of +5°F or colder
       b. Must be used within 30 minutes once reconstituted

J. Vaccinations and travel to developing countries
    1. Mumps, measles, and rubella
       a. Remain uncontrolled in most countries
       b. Vaccination status must be up-to-date
    2. Wild poliovirus and diphtheria
       a. Exposure likely in developing countries
       b. Check Td status
       c. Single dose of OPV or IPV should be given, assuming initial series was complete
    3. Varicella vaccination status should be up to date if patient has not had chickenpox
    4. Influenza for people at risk for complications (should receive a second vaccination in the spring if traveling to the southern hemisphere during April through September)
    5. Selective vaccination against yellow fever, typhoid, plague, meningococcal disease, rabies, hepatitis A and B, or administration of immune globulin to prevent hepatitis A and B
       a. Recommended on the basis of disease-specific risks in the countries to be visited
       b. Type and duration of travel
       c. Biyearly updates in Summary of Health Information for International Travel from CDC

SUGGESTED READING

1. ACP Task Force on Adult Immunization and Infectious Diseases Society of America: Guide for Adult Immunization, 3rd ed. Philadelphia, American College of Physicians, 1994.
2. American Academy of Pediatrics: Active and passive immunizations. In Peter G (ed): 1997 Red Book: Report of the Committee on Infectious Diseases, 24th ed. Elk Grove Village, IL, American Academy of Pediatrics, 1997.
3. Bia FJ: Medical considerations for the pregnant traveler. Infect Dis Clin North Am 6:371–387, 1992
4. Center for Disease Control and Prevention. Immunization of Health-Care Workers: Recommendations of the Advisory Committee on Immunization Practices (ACIP) and the Hospital Infection Control Practices Advisory Committee (HICPAC). MMWR 46(No. 66-18), 1997.
5. Dejonghe J, Parkinson B: Benefits and costs of vaccination. Vaccine 10:936–939, 1992.
6. Long J, Kyllonen K: Adult vaccinations: A short review. Cleveland Clin J Med 64:311–317, 1997.
7. Margolis HS: Prevention of acute and chronic liver disease through immunization: Hepatitis B and beyond. J Infect Dis 168:9–14, 1993.
8. Thanassi WT: Immunizations for international travelers. West J Med 168:197–202, 1998
9. U.S. Preventive Services Task Force. Guide To Clinical Preventive Services, 2nd ed. Alexandria, VA, International Medical Publishing, 1996.
10. Woodyard E, Woodyard L, Alto WA: Vaccine storage in the physician's office: A community study. J Am Board Fam Pract 8:91–94, 1995.

5. Nutrition in Adult Women

Bruce E. Johnson, M.D.

I. The Issues

Probably few aspects of contemporary medical care involve more misconceptions than nutrition. Adequate nutrition is essential to proper functioning of virtually all organ systems as well as to maintenance of psychological well-being. The problem is one of balance. The early advances in defining nutritional deficiencies (calories, protein, vitamins, and minerals) were significant and relatively easy to address. Nutritional excesses that result in disease states also may be identified, especially when they occur over a short time (e.g., neuropathy associated with megadoses of pyridoxine). A greater challenge facing nutritionists is to define the more subtle risks that may be present in modest deficiencies or excesses. Confirming an association between dietary supplement and disease prevention is laudable but strikingly difficult in experimental design. Because this chapter cannot cover all advances in nutritional aspects of women's health, it focuses on a few conditions of deficiency and a few controversies about prevention of diseases of particular import to women. Obesity, one of the greatest diseases of excess, and certain eating disorders (anorexia nervosa and bulimia) are covered in other chapters.

II. The Theory

A. Calorie determination

1. Caloric intake remains remarkably stable on day-to-day basis
   a. Sensors and metabolic or even genetic controls on calorie intake are unclear but manifested through sensations of hunger and satiety
   b. Incomplete recognition of satiety leads to overingestion of calories and obesity
   c. Other psychological issues are involved in anorexia nervosa or bulimia (binge/purge) syndromes
   d. Fluctuations in daily weight reflect water shifts more than calorie intake
2. **Sources of energy (calorie) expenditures**
   a. **Basal metabolic rate**
      i. Energy expended to maintain body functions at rest and varies with sex, age, weight, height, and body habitus
   b. **Activity**
      i. Variable energy expenditure results from physical activity demands

    c. **Diet-induced thermogenesis**
      i. Calories produced as heat in absorption, digestion, and metabolism of food
    d. Additional expenditures
      i. Disease or other unusual states may increase energy requirements, e.g., inflammatory illness, trauma, surgery, pregnancy and lactation
  3. Rough calculation of calorie requirements
    a. **Basal metabolic rate** (BMR) in kcal (method of Harris and Benedict)
      BMR = 655 + (9.5 × W) + (1.8 × H) − (4.7 × A), where W = usual weight in kg, H = height in cm, and A = age
    b. **Diet-induced thermogenesis**
      i. Caloric utilized in digestion and metabolism calculated at 6–10% of BMR (i.e., added to BMR)
    c. **Activity expenditures**
      i. In general, sedentary activities expend an additional 400–800 kcal; office work, 600–1000 kcal; moderate work/exercise 1200–1600 kcal. All estimates assume relatively constant activity level throughout entire day.
    d. Using these guidelines, the caloric requirement for a 40-year-old woman, 5'4", 132 lbs in office job is 1800–2000 kcal/day
B. **Dietary recommendations** (see Fig. 1)
  1. In 1992, the U.S. government modified its recommendations for appropriate diet
    a. Previously focused on the four major food groups
  2. **Food guide pyramid** emphasizes decreased fat intake, some decrease in protein, and proportionally increased intake of complex carbohydrates
    a. Sets goal of 30% calories from fat, including 10% from saturated fat with about 300 mg cholesterol daily
      i. Limit simple sugars, salt and alcoholic beverages
    b. Suggests number of servings of several types of foods to balance vitamin and mineral intake, and to provide fiber
      i. Daily servings of several food groups: e.g., 6–11 servings/day of bread, pasta, rice; 2–4 servings of fruit; 3–5 servings of vegetables; 2–3 servings of meat, poultry, fish, beans, nuts; 2–3 servings of milk, cheese; and sparing use of fats, oils, sweets

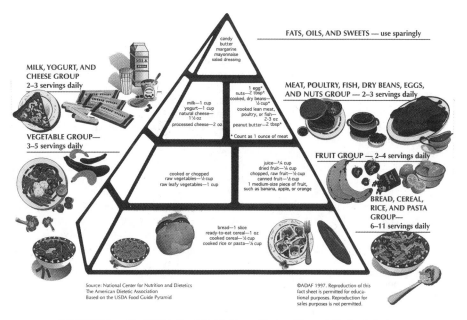

FIGURE 1. The USDA Food Guide Pyramid: A guide to daily food choices.

TABLE 1. Recommended Dietary Allowances for Healthy Women

Vitamin A μg retinol equivalents	800	Calcium, mg	800–1200
Vitamin D, μg	5–10	Phosphorus, mg	800–1200
Vitamin E, mg alpha-tocopherol equivalents	8	Magnesium, mg	280–300
		Iron, mg	10–15
Vitamin K, μg	45–65	Zinc, mg	12
Vitamin C, mg	50–60	Iodine, μg	150
Thiamine, mg	1–1.1	Selenium, μg	45–55
Riboflavin, mg	1.2–1.3	Copper, mg	1.5–3
Niacin, mg	13–15	Manganese, mg	2–5
Vitamin B$_6$, mg	1.4–1.6	Fluoride, mg	1.5–4
Biotin, μg	50–100	Chromium, μg	50–200
Pantothenic acid, mg	4–7	Molybdenum, μg	75–250

    c. Designed to be more relevant to dietary choices in language understandable by public

C. **Vitamins and minerals**
1. Recommended daily allowances (RDA) set for wide range of vitamins and minerals (Table 1)
2. Differing technologies involved in establishing RDAs
   a. Typically recommend 3–10 times more vitamin and mineral intake than needed to prevent obvious deficiency state
   b. Recommendations stop short of amount known to cause abnormalities due to excess
3. Recommendations make allowances for differences in age, sex, and, if appropriate, pregnancy and lactation
   a. Requirements with aging not certain
      i. Aging probably results in incomplete absorption of several nutrients
      ii. May recommend larger RDAs for many vitamins and minerals in elderly
4. RDAs assume healthy individual
   a. Illnesses may profoundly affect demands for vitamins and minerals
5. In the U.S., classic diseases of deficiency are rare
   a. Occasional diagnoses of **thiamine deficiency** (cardiovascular beri-beri and Wernicke's syndrome in alcoholics) and **vitamin C deficiency** (scurvy in pediatric urban poor)
   b. Some deficiencies are less dramatic but cumulative
      i. For example, **deficiency of iron** with iron-deficient anemia; and **deficiency of calcium** with osteoporosis
   c. Other deficiencies associated with diseases of abuse (e.g., folate deficiency in alcoholism), and medical treatment (e.g., pyridoxine deficiency in isoniazid use)
6. **Diseases of vitamin and mineral excess** are typically iatrogenic or due to health fads or misguided dietary adventures
   a. Peripheral neuropathy with excessive pyridoxine;
   b. Fluorosis (mottled teeth, possibly brittle bones) may occur naturally with high fluoride content of drinking water (even if not supplemented) or with excess vitamin supplement
7. Putative benefits proposed for intake of some vitamins and minerals in excess of established RDAs (e.g., some suggest that vitamin E may decrease incidence of heart disease and that vitamins C and E and selenium function as antioxidants)

III. **An Approach** (selected nutrients only)
  A. **Calcium**
1. Important cation for many biochemical and physiologic reactions, and bone metabolism
2. 99% of body calcium in bone
   a. 10–15% of bone is being remodeled at any one time
   b. Deficient ingestion of calcium over time results in less calcium deposition and reduced bone density

    c. Calcium balance significantly affected by loss of estrogen levels at menopause (see Chapter 87)
3. **Total bone mass** determined in women by age 30
    a. Contributing factors include family history, body size, race (blacks tend to have more bone mass than other racial groups), and lifetime calcium intake
    b. Gradual decline in bone density up to time of menopause
        i. Thereafter, bone density declines rapidly (2–5% loss per year in first several years)
4. **Calcium intake often deficient, at least in U.S. women**
    a. Milk, yogurt, cheese richest sources
        i. Other foods relatively rich in calcium include some fish (canned salmon, herring eaten with bones), rhubarb, spinach, nuts
    b. Ingestion of milk products declines in teenage years and rarely recovers
    c. Not uncommon to see otherwise nutritionally sound women ingesting less than 500 mg calcium daily
5. **Calcium intake most critical at three times:**
    a. **Childhood and young adulthood**—to build maximal bone density
    b. **Perimenopause**—to ameliorate losses otherwise experienced through estrogen deficiency
    c. **Advanced age**—loss of estrogen stimulus, poor calcium absorption
6. **Dietary recommendations** for daily calcium intake (in mg elemental calcium/day)
    a. Adolescents and young adults: 1200–1500 mg/day
    b. Adult women (25–50): 1000 mg/day
        i. 1200–1500 mg/day during pregnancy and lactation
    c. Perimenopausal women: 1000–1200 mg/day
    d. Postmenopausal women
        i. 1000 mg/day on estrogen replacement
        ii. 1000–1500 mg/day without estrogen replacement
7. If woman cannot ingest enough calcium through diet, supplements should be recommended
    a. Calcium carbonate is least expensive but varies in dissolvability and absorption
    b. Choice of supplement frequently based on lack of side effects with most women complaining of gastric distress or constipation
    c. Instruct patient to calculate milligrams elemental calcium, not the calcium salt

B. **Vitamin D**
  1. As vitamin engaged in calcium absorption, often considered in relationship to osteoporosis
  2. Occasional deficiency in clinical settings
    a. Poor nutrition in general; homebound (e.g., with chronic illness), elderly, and institutionalized people
    b. Bowel disease especially malabsorption syndromes, small bowel inflammatory disease
    c. Difficult to tell "clinically;" must measure if suspicious
  3. Supplemental dose varies from 400 IU/day to 10,000 IU/week
    a. Monitoring of serum calcium appropriate at early stages of supplementation
    b. Little added value in more expensive calcitriol (1,25-dihydroxyvitamin D3) over cholecalciferol (vitamin D3) except in patients with renal disease

C. **Vitamin E**
  1. A fat-soluble vitamin absorbed in the small intestines and stored in body tissues
  2. Widespread in foods
  3. Difficult, if not impossible, to produce vitamin E deficiency in adults eating general diet
    a. Unusual cases of childhood cholestatic liver disease may have manifestations of vitamin E deficiency
        i. Neurologic symptoms with gait abnormalities, decreased proprioception, and changes in posterior column of spinal cord

4. Believed to be **antioxidant rather than cofactor**
   a. Intracellular prevention of toxic oxidation products
   b. Interacts with low-density lipoprotein (LDL) cholesterol
      i. Oxidized LDL believed to be major contributor to atherosclerosis; vitamin E increases resistance of LDL to oxidation
5. Proposed as **cancer-preventive agent**
   a. Based on function as antioxidant rather than epidemiological observations
   b. Belongs to group of antioxidants, including vitamin A, beta-carotene, vitamin C, and selenium thought to have cancer preventive properties
   c. Little evidence to date that ingestion of levels above RDA prevents cancer
6. Studied in **prevention of atherosclerosis**, specifically coronary artery disease
   a. Recent report from Nurses' Health Study of over 80,000 women comparing highest intake (through supplements) with lowest dietary intake showed substantial decreased risk of coronary artery disease
      i. Relative risk among high vitamin E users was 0.59–0.66
      ii. Additional confirmation may come from ongoing Women's Health Study
   b. Other studies that examined vitamin E in prevention or treatment of peripheral vascular disease (including men and women) are inconclusive
7. **Current RDA for women**—8 IU/day
   a. Common dietary intake 2–8 IU/day
   b. Supplements range from 20–30 IU in multivitamins to 400 IU in megadose gelcaps
   c. No described complications of megadose vitamin E usage
D. **Selenium**
   1. Ubiquitous in soil and ingested via fruits and vegetables
      a. Absorption mechanisms unknown
      b. Recognized deficiency state in province of China where soil is low in selenium
         i. Cardiomyopathy with arrhythmias as well as, occasionally, peripheral myopathy in children and women of childbearing age
   2. Component in glutathione peroxidase, clearing free radicals and functioning as antioxidant
   3. In animal studies, selenium appears to protect against cancer-causing chemicals and viruses
      a. Similar function not proven in humans
   4. Selenium mentioned, along with other antioxidants, as **cancer-protective**
      a. Epidemiological studies suggest protective effect by ingestion of vegetables high in these nutrients, including cancer of lung, colon, bladder and cervix
      b. Not conclusive and could be due to other factors
   5. No clearly identified selenium toxicity syndrome described
   6. RDA for selenium set at 45–55 µg/day
E. **Iron**
   1. Essential component of heme and certain enzymes such as cytochrome oxidase
   2. Deficiency state is related to fall in iron stores and heme production and eventually leads to anemia
   3. **Physiologic demands and losses**
      a. Iron requirements increase substantially during growth spurts of infancy and adolescence
         i. Amounts to about 1–2 mg/day in adult men and women
      b. Typical menstrual period results in loss of 30–40 mg iron
      c. Pregnancy transfers approximately 500 mg iron to fetus
      d. Iron lost through sloughing of senescent gastrointestinal (GI) cells and desquamation of skin cells
   4. **Pathologic losses**
      a. GI loss from peptic disease, gastritis, angiodysplasia, polyps, and carcinoma
      b. Genitourinary tract, pulmonary hemosiderosis, intravascular hemolysis
      c. In tropical areas, parasites (especially hookworm) frequently cause substantial blood and iron loss

5. **Problems with absorption**
   a. Poor access to iron-rich foods, primarily meats
      i. Worldwide this is most common dietary reason for iron deficiency
   b. Gastric disorders, including achlorhydria (with aging) and gastrectomy
   c. Intestinal malabsorption of many causes
   d. Ingestion of material that chelates iron
      i. Tannates (such as in tea), phylates, and phosphates bind iron and decrease absorption
      ii. Rarely, geophagia (clay eating) binds iron
6. When all sources of iron loss and poor absorption are included, **up to 40% of all women of childbearing age worldwide may be iron deficient and 20% frankly anemic**
7. Sources of dietary iron include meats (especially red meat), whole grains, nuts, dark-green leafy vegetables
   a. Usually only 10% dietary iron absorbed though in iron deficiency, efficiency can climb to 20–30%
      i. Iron as heme (i.e., meats) more efficiently absorbed than inorganic forms
   b. Citrates and ascorbates (e.g., vitamin C) bind iron so that absorption improves
8. **Manifestations of iron deficiency**
   a. Inconsistent symptoms related to decreased iron stores without anemia
   b. Once anemic, **typical symptoms** include fatigue, lassitude, exertional dyspnea
   c. Some athletes report decreased endurance and fitness with iron deficiency even without frank anemia
   d. **Physical findings**, if present, include glossitis, angular stomatitis, koilonychia (spoon-shaped nails), gastric achlorhydria, and menorrhagia
      i. Of interest, achlorhydria and menorrhagia may be both cause and consequence of iron deficiency
   e. **Special symptom of pica**
      i. Compulsive eating of unusual material or foodstuffs
         (a) Ice (pagophagia), clay (geophagia), starch (ambylophagia)
         (b) Celery, potatoes, carrots, or similar foods
      ii. Cause of pica unknown, but considered a consequence, not cause, of iron deficiency
      iii. More common in women; may be detected in as many as 50% of women with iron deficiency anemia
      iv. Patients often embarrassed; sometimes concerned
      v. Once iron therapy started, patients occasionally develop abhorrence to previously desired material
9. **Treatment with iron preparations**
   a. Ferrous sulfate, 325 mg (60 mg elemental iron), 1–3 times daily
      i. Side effects include GI upset, distention, occasional gastric erosions
      ii. Because constipation so common, lubricating agent (e.g., docusate) is routinely added
      iii. Warn patient about appearance of black stool—not hemoccult positive
   b. If iron sulfate not tolerated, ferrous gluconate or ferrous lactate may be used
   c. If oral route unsuccessful, iron dextran may be given either intramuscularly (using Z-tract to prevent skin discoloration) or intravenously
      i. Test dose mandatory (50 mg subcutaneously or 1 ml intravenously) to check for allergy
      ii. Total dose calculations included in drug package insert
F. **Folic acid**
   1. Adequate intake strongly protects against neural tube defects
   2. Folic acid widespread in vegetables, fruits but dietary intake of these often deficient and supplementation advised
   3. For women capable of pregnancy, recommend 0.4 mg/day supplement (for unplanned pregnancy); for women planning pregnancy, recommend 0.4–0.8 mg/day supplement at least 1month before conception; for women with previous neural tube defect pregnancy, recommend 4 mg/day supplement 1–3 months before conception

SUGGESTED READING

1. American Academy of Pediatrics: Folic acid for the prevention of neural tube defects. Pediatrics 92:493–494, 1993.
2. Centers for Disease Control and Prevention: Recommendations to prevent and control iron deficiency in the United States. MMWR 47(RR-3):1–27, 1998.
3. Chlebowski RT, Grosvenor M: The scope of nutrition intervention trials with cancer-related endpoints. Cancer 74(Suppl 9):2734–2738, 1994.
4. Corman LC (ed): Clinical Nutrition. Med Clin North Am 77:711–938, 1993.
5. Monteleone GP, Browning DG: Nutrition in women: Assessment and counseling. Primary Care 24:37–51, 1997.
6. Morley JE (moderator): Nutrition in the elderly. Ann Intern Med 109:890–904, 1988.
7. National Institutes of Health Consensus Development Panel on Optimal Calcium Intake: Optimal calcium intake. JAMA 272:1942–1948, 1994.
8. Oakley GP: Eat right and take a multivitamin. N Engl J Med 338:1060–1061, 1998.
9. Stampfer MJ, Hennekens CH, Manson JE, et al: Vitamin E consumption and the risk of coronary disease in women. N Engl J Med 328:1444–1449, 1993.
10. U.S. Department of Agriculture: Food Guide Pyramid. Washington, DC, U.S. Government Printing Office, 1992.

6. Exercise

Bruce E. Johnson, M.D.

I. **The Issues**

A book written on women's health 100 or more years ago would not have needed a chapter on exercise. Exercise was omnipresent and unavoidable. The daily chores of agrarian societies required almost endless work in the house, the fields, with children. Exercise was part of a woman's (and man's) expectations—and lacked today's quasi-glamorous image. Today, purposeful exercise is given recognition and value as a personal and societal symbol. Given the otherwise sedentary nature of present-day life, the medical benefits of exercise are well worth recounting, taking note of the cautions to be acknowledged in the evaluation of any woman's exercise plans.

II. **The Theory**
  A. **Types of exercise**
    1. Aerobic
       a. Exercise in which lactate does not build up in blood
       b. Sustained for longer periods of time
    2. Anaerobic
       a. Exertion at intensity that requires use of anaerobic pathways for energy generation
          i. Byproduct is generation of lactate in sufficient quantities that enter bloodstream
       b. Associated with extraordinary demands; most competitive sports operate on anaerobic level to some degree
       c. Cannot be sustained for long period
    3. Isotonic
       a. Movements that involve shortening and lengthening of muscles, e.g., running, swimming
    4. Isometric
       a. Strength development of muscles with little movement, e.g., weightlifting
       b. Most sports have components of both isometric and isotonic movement
    5. Exercise frequently muscle group specific
       a. Running is mostly lower extremity; swimming, upper extremity
       b. Relatively few sports involve equal use of all muscle groups though specific exercise programs are designed to be equal throughout the body (some so-called aerobic exercises, circuit-type weightlifting)

6. Exercise does not have to involve competitive sports
   a. Gardening, stair climbing at work/home, housework
B. **Anatomy**
   1. Wider hip
      a. Slight anterior placement of femoral neck compared to males
      b. Gives varus at hip with resultant valgus at knees
         i. Increases angle which femur meets tibial plateau
      c. Leads to swinging motion of leg more than straightforward thrusting at knee
         i. Raises possibility of strain on ligaments, tendons, certain muscle groups
   2. Center of gravity slightly lower
   3. In general, strength in women is more in lower than upper extremities
      a. Muscle fiber size slightly greater in lower than upper extremities
   4. Women have somewhat larger number of fast-twitch than slower-twitch muscle fibers (with unknown significance)
   5. Laxity in tendons and ligaments
      a. Women more than men; younger women more than older women
      b. Probably relates to certain injury patterns
      c. Accentuated in pregnancy with production of "relaxin" hormone
   6. Percent body fat relatively high
      a. Decreases in highly trained athletes
      b. Unclear if relevance to performance characteristics
C. **Physiology and menstrual changes**
   1. Menstrual cycle abnormalities
      a. Prevalence of menstrual irregularity widespread
         i. 20% of physically active women and up to 50% of competitive athletes experience irregular menses
         ii. Amenorrhea as much as 10 times more common in competitive athletes than general female population
   2. Cause of menstrual changes not entirely known
      a. Changes in diet, body fat, energy utilization, and hormonal milieu
         i. Exercise-induced changes in estradiol, progesterone, testosterone, prolactin, catecholamines, cortisol, beta-endorphin and beta-lipotropin
   3. Relationship to body fat
      a. Previously thought that menstruation was related to percent body fat
         i. At one time, thought that 17% body fat needed for menarche, 20% or more to maintain regular menstrual cycles
      b. Recent studies discount a specific percent body fat as sole factor regulating menses
      c. Athletes tend to have lower body fat, yet some athletic women with as little as 4% body fat continue to have regular menstruation
   4. **Types of menstrual abnormalities**
      a. **Luteal phase deficiency**
         i. Shortening of luteal phase (progesterone effect) without significant change in total cycle length resulting in occasional skipped periods
         ii. Related to decreased progesterone production?
         iii. Reported in runners, swimmers among others
         iv. Associated with decreased bone density and infertility
      b. **Anovulation**
         i. Almost normal estrogen production but low progesterone and, in contrast to luteal phase deficiency, irregular periods
         ii. More often delays between periods (> 35 days) rather than more frequent (< 21 days)
         iii. When menses occur, may be quite heavy (reflecting "unopposed" estrogen)
      c. **Exercise-associated amenorrhea**
         i. Hypoestrogen state with loss of periods
         ii. Described most frequently in runners, ballet dancers, gymnasts
         iii. Appears to be hypothalamic disorder with alterations in release of gonadotropin-releasing hormone

5. Greatest risk from menstrual abnormality is loss of bone density
   a. Although exercise generally encourages bone formation, lack of estrogen (and probably progesterone) counterbalances beneficial effect
      i. Bone loss occurs despite exercise
   b. Athletes with normal menstrual cycles consistently have bone density greater than athletes in same sport with abnormal menstrual pattern
      i. One study documented 17% decrease in bone density in runners with irregular periods
6. Unfortunately, many women athletes view menstrual irregularity as sign of fitness attainment; even strive for loss of menses

D. **Benefits of exercise**
   1. **Functional ability**
      a. Fit women seem able to accomplish daily tasks without fatigue and are more productive, while daily tasks often leave sedentary persons tired
   2. **Mortality**
      a. Long-term studies in men suggest lower overall mortality in those who exercise; assumption is that same applies to women
         i. Related to alteration in disease risk factors, especially cardiovascular disease, diabetes, hypertension, obesity
   3. **Weight loss**
      a. Multiple studies confirm additive benefit of exercise compared with diet alone
         i. Weight loss tends to be faster and sustained (as long as exercise maintained)
      b. Exercise effects contributing to weight loss
         i. Increased caloric use during exercise
         ii. Mild anorexiant due to endorphin production
         iii. Increased muscle bulk provides overall boost to body caloric need, since muscle cells have higher basal metabolic requirements than fat cells—truly results in "higher metabolism"
         iv. Healthy lifestyle, emphasizing balanced diet, avoidance of snacks, decreased alcohol
   4. **Cardiovascular effects**
      a. Most studies to date demonstrate significantly lower risk for myocardial infarction
         i. More conclusive studies in men
         ii. Studies that include women show benefit although not to same degree as in men
      b. Meta-analysis of > 30 studies concludes that inactivity is as great a risk factor as smoking and hyperlipidemia
      c. Cardiovascular benefit results from almost any intensity of exercise, but most substantial with frequent (> 4 sessions/week), vigorous exercise (running, racket sports, swimming)
   5. **Hypertension**
      a. Multiple studies, including several in women, confirm that regular exercise reduces high blood pressure
         i. May allow borderline hypertensive woman to control blood pressure without medication
      b. Combined effect of weight loss and exercise enhances likelihood of blood pressure reduction
      c. Generally requires at least 3 exercise sessions/week of > 30 minutes and attainment of a degree of fitness
      d. Ability to sustain high level of exercise greatest impediment to long-term control of hypertension
   6. **Hyperlipidemia**
      a. Improvement in lipids seen even after modest exercise
      b. May be related in part to weight loss
      c. Changes in lipid profile include reduction in total cholesterol, LDL, triglycerides (perhaps related to increased insulin sensitivity) with beneficial increase in HDL
         i. Exercise one of few effective nonpharmacologic interventions that raise HDL

7. **Osteoporosis**
    a. Prevention one of the primary benefits of regular exercise
        i. Bone density may increase with regular exercise as only intervention
        ii. Women in societies which require physical labor have low incidence of osteoporosis; this effect persists even with other risk factors such as low calcium intake, ethnic predisposition, no estrogen replacement
    b. Effect of gravity may be necessary to promote maximal bone formation
        i. Swimmers have slightly less bone density than athletes in running or racket sports
8. **Pulmonary disease**
    a. Regular exercise increases functional capacity even in advanced obstructive lung disease
        i. Walking or other aerobic exercise an important aspect of pulmonary rehabilitation
    b. People with asthma can be helped by regular exercise (except, of course, exercise-induced asthma)
        i. Swimming better than other forms of exercise; this may be related to humidity of inspired air
9. **Diabetes mellitus**
    a. Exercise improves management of both diabetes type I and type II for several reasons
        i. Weight reduction
        ii. Reduced insulin secretion by pancreas (alpha-adrenergic inhibition of beta cells)
        iii. Increased insulin sensitivity by enhanced binding to receptors on muscle cells (increased number of receptor sites maintained > 24 hours after exercise)
    b. Counterregulatory hormones, especially cortisol and glucagon, prevents exercise-induced hypoglycemia
    c. Overall benefit may be greater in type II than type I diabetes
        i. Exercise prescription still valuable in both
10. **Breast cancer**
    a. Regular exercise may reduce risk of breast cancer
        i. Related to known relationship between anovulation (as induced by exercise) and reduced breast cancer (?)
    b. Effect also may be consequence of lifestyle changes with weight control, decreased fat intake, no smoking, less alcohol
11. **Other cancers** (rectal/colon, bladder) also modestly reduced
12. **Psychological effects**
    a. Exercise decreases anxiety
    b. Depression less severe and shorter duration in women who exercise
    c. Commonly accepted that exercise induces endorphins, giving mild opioid effect ("runner's high")
    d. Sense of well-being, feeling of greater energy during day, pride in activity
13. **Pregnancy**
    a. In general, women exercising before pregnancy may continue to exercise during pregnancy
        i. Regular running, even marathons accomplished in late stages of pregnancy
    b. No increase in spontaneous abortion, shorter labor, less likelihood of cesarean section, less meconium staining
    c. Drawbacks to exercise in pregnancy
        i. Slightly lower birthweight (due to less fetal fat)
        ii. No difference in pregnancy-induced hypertension or preeclampsia
        iii. No change in risks to multiple fetus pregnancy
        iv. Should not be recommended to women with moderate-to-severe heart disease
    d. Women who had previously been sedentary should not begin vigorous exercise program
        i. Risk of orthopedic injuries probably outweighs benefits

E. **Cautions with exercise**
1. **Cardiovascular disease**
   a. Congenital abnormalities
      i. Autopsy studies of athletes dying suddenly while exercising suggest that congenital abnormality of heart is most likely cause
      ii. Hypertrophic cardiomyopathy
         (a) Symptoms, if present, of exercise-related fatigue, syncope, chest pain relieved by squatting
         (b) Frequently have systolic flow murmur
         (c) Frequently have left ventricular hypertrophy on EKG, even in teen years
      iii. Other congenital abnormalities include absent coronary arteries, coronary artery tunnel (artery in myocardium, often passing under other artery), aberrant coronary ostia
         (a) Very difficult to diagnose before onset of symptoms
   b. Marfan syndrome
      i. While not solely a cardiovascular disease, death while exercising often from cardiac/aortic source
         (a) Dissection of aorta common, often proximal (as opposed to the more common distal dissection of atherosclerosis)
         (b) Dissection at aortic root may rapidly occlude coronary ostia, leading to angina, sudden death
      ii. Suspicion due to appearance
         (a) Tall, thin women with arm span greater than height
         (b) Joint laxity
         (c) Frequent lens dislocation
      iii. Autosomal dominant inheritance
2. **Sudden death**
   a. Cardiac death from unsuspected coronary artery disease
      i. Virtually no information specifically relating to risk of sudden death in women
      ii. In men, may be modest increase in sudden death by men who exercise compared to matched sedentary controls
      iii. Subacute or ignored symptoms
   b. Recent, heightened concern of sudden death in women using, or having used, performance enhancing drugs (e.g., androgenic steroids)
      i. Induced changes in lipids
      ii. Development of left ventricular hypertrophy
   c. Occasional instances of sudden death attributed to myocarditis, presumably viral
      i. Recommendation against vigorous exercise while suffering viral illness such as influenza
   d. Even with these cautions, overall cardiovascular mortality in women who exercise much lower than in sedentary people
3. **Orthopedic injuries**
   a. In some instances, risk of orthopedic damage outweighs anticipated benefits
      i. Extreme obesity, previously sedentary elderly, preexisting arthritis
4. **Stress fractures**
   a. More common in women than men
   b. Strongly associated with menstrual irregularity and decreased bone density
   c. In addition to osteopenia, stress fractures are indication of overuse injury or poor training/coaching
5. **Degenerative joint disease** (DJD)
   a. Concern that constant trauma to joints, especially knees, hips, will result in arthritis
      i. Running/jogging considered highest risk
      ii. Swimming often touted as relatively nontraumatic
   b. Fortunately, several long-term studies, looking both at symptoms and radiographs, find no increase in development of DJD, even with jogging
      i. Could be selection bias; that is, women who have or are likely to develop DJD are unable to jog

6. **Concussion**
    a. More common in contact sports which, heretofore, have been male-dominated
    b. Safety issue related to wearing of helmets
        i. Football, baseball, cycling, ice hockey, equestrienne, goalie, boxing
    c. Prior history of concussion important
        i. High risk of serious consequences with subsequent concussions
        ii. Quintessential example is dementia pugilistica in boxers without helmet (similar, milder syndrome reported in quarterbacks, soccer players)
7. **Heat-related disease**
    a. Heat stroke is a serious systemic disease with relatively high mortality
    b. Prevention involves common sense, delay or cancellation of athletic events planned during conditions of excessive heat
    c. Particular risk with certain medications (antihypertensives, antidepressants, anticholinergics), recent viral or diarrheal illness
    d. Previous attack of heat stroke makes woman much more likely for subsequent episodes in compatible environmental circumstances
8. **Trauma, accidents, attacks**
    a. Sad fact of life that women must protect themselves from attacks while exercising
        i. Typically secluded area of public trail/park
9. **Skin**
    a. With outdoor exercise, increased risk of actinic damage
        i. Skin cancer, melanoma increased in women with exposure to sun
        ii. Actinic damage results in "old skin"
            (a) Wrinkles, leathery skin, actinic keratoses
F. **Female athlete triad:** eating disorders, amenorrhea, osteoporosis
    1. Triad of three conditions in female athletes (Table 1)
    2. Most frequent in competitive runners, gymnasts, skaters, ballet dancers
        a. Common feature is perceived emphasis on lean, thin look
            i. In some sports (e.g., gymnastics) scoring is in part subjective; impression is that "thin is better"
        b. One study of college athletes found 32% used at least one weight-control practice, such as self-induced vomiting, laxative purging, use of diet or diuretic pills
            i. Practice detected in 72% of gymnasts, almost 50% of runners, and even 20% of softball players
        c. Also noted in recreational "jogging addicts"

TABLE 1. Identification of the Female Triad Syndrome

Historical features	Physical findings
Preoccupation with weight	Body weight below normal
Patient's perception that she is not thin enough to achieve desired athletic level	Especially if > 15% below normal
	Sallow, yellowish appearance to skin
Frequent dieting	Loss or thinning of hair
Preoccupation with food, diet fads	Lanugo hair
Use of drugs to control weight	Swollen salivary glands
Laxatives, diet pills, diuretics	Bradycardia, cardiac arrhythmias
Declining athletic performance	Hypotension, orthostatic
Excessive exercise not part of training	Sores or calluses on knuckles (rubbing on teeth while gagging during self-induced vomiting)
Frequent injuries	
Amenorrhea, menstrual irregularities	**Initial laboratory tests**
Complaints related to electrolyte abnormalities	Anemia
Muscle cramps	Leukopenia
Palpitations	Electrolyte abnormalities (especially potassium)
Dizziness, weakness	Low uric acid
Tingling, numbness in extremities	
	Other studies
	Hormone levels, especially low estrogen, low gonadotropins
	Radiographs or bone scans of stress fractures

3. Relatively common disorder with three components
   a. **Eating disorders**
      i. Anorexia nervosa
         (a) Altered body perception in which patient perceives body to have too much fat
         (b) Self-induced starvation
         (c) Frequent vomiting, diuretic use
         (d) Multiple endocrine and metabolic abnormalities, e.g., virtually undetectable estrogen levels, flattened FSH curve
      ii. Bulimia
         (a) Desire to be thin though weight often at normal level
         (b) Episodes of binge-eating followed by guilt and purging through self-induced vomiting or laxative abuse
         (c) Compared to anorexia nervosa, not as likely to self-starve
         (d) Menstrual irregularities occur but less than in patients with anorexia nervosa
   b. **Amenorrhea**
      i. Usually hypoestrogenism
      ii. In disordered thinking, menses a sign that training not intensive enough
   c. **Osteoporosis**
      i. Occurs at young age (often early 20s)
      ii. Probably related to combination of dietary deficiency of calcium and hypoestrogenism
      iii. Most frequent manifestation is stress fractures
         (a) Typically lower extremity but reported in ribs, clavicle, sternum, vertebrae
4. Female athlete triad is the coincidence of three conditions, two of which (amenorrhea, osteoporosis) may be consequences, in part, of the first (eating disorder) but exacerbated by the underlying presence of excessive exercise

III. **An Approach**
   A. **Preexercise evaluation** (Table 2)
      1. Generally, risks of exercise in most young women do not warrant extensive evaluation
         a. Counseling and advice worthwhile
         b. Evaluation useful in older women (> 45–50 years)
      2. **Nutrition**
         a. Because many women exercise to assist in weight control, proper nutrition is balance between adequate intake yet not so many calories that weight loss does not ensue
         b. Proper balance includes carbohydrates, protein, fat
            i. For most female athletes, no need for protein supplements
            ii. Reduction of fat in diet helps significantly in weight loss
         c. **Vitamins**
            i. While balanced diet should supply enough vitamins, little harm in multiple vitamin supplement
         d. **Calcium**
            i. Important because exercise is meant, in part, to promote maintenance of bone
            ii. Peak bone density occurs in 20s and early 30s, a time of considerable interest in exercise
            iii. With adequate estrogen, nonlactating woman of this age should ingest approximately 1000 mg/day
            iv. Typical "American" diet (with includes few dairy products) provides only 500 mg/day—supplement almost universally recommended
         e. **Iron**
            i. Iron loss from menstruation, excessive sweating, GI bleeding, even traumatic hemolysis
            ii. Women who refrain from meat may not get enough iron from remainder of diet
            iii. Iron deficiency presents as fatigue or inability to achieve previous levels of performance

TABLE 2. Components of a Preexercise Evaluation*

Historical information
Current medical history
Concurrent illnesses
Especially cardiovascular,
pulmonary/asthma, diabetes,
osteoporosis
Disabilities and injuries
Known absence of one of paired
organ (e.g., eye, ear [hearing],
kidney, ovary)
Symptoms
Especially chest pains, breath-
lessness, dizziness
Medications
Allergies
Medicines
Pollens, weeds, environmental
(hay fever)
Bee or wasp stings
Menstrual history
Current pregnancy
Dysmenorrhea
Amenorrhea or missed periods
Past medical history
Serious illnesses
Injuries, fractures, joint trauma
Concussion
Heat stroke
Family history
Sudden death at early age in close
family member

Nutrition
Overweight, underweight
Perception of weight appropriate to
appearance
Adequate calories, vitamins, minerals,
especially iron, calcium
Dieting, fads
Skipped meals, vomiting
Careful search for suggestions of
anorexia or bulimia

Physical examination
General
Appearance of Marfan syndrome, anorexia, other
undiagnosed illness (e.g., Cushing's disease)
Cardiovascular
Blood pressure (including equal in both arms and legs
Cardiomegaly
Gallops, especially +S4
Murmurs, especially aortic (e.g., hypertrophic
cardiomyopathy) or mitral valve prolapse
Pulmonary
Wheezing
Cough
Phlegm production
Skin
Present changes or risk for actinic injury
Neurologic
Deficits
Gait, balance abnormalities
Musculoskeletal
Laxity ("double-jointed," genu recurvatum)
Leg length
Scoliosis
Degenerative changes

Laboratory tests and radiography
(Young, healthy women probably do not need more studies
than recommended for routine health maintenance)
In certain circumstances or with risk factors, consider:
Complete blood count
Iron and iron-binding capacity
Electrolytes
Glucose[†]
Lipid profile[†]
Endocrine tests (e.g., thyroxine, follicle-stimulating
hormone, estradiol)
Urinalysis
Electrocardiogram[†]
Echocardiogram
Exercise stress test
Chest radiograph
Bone mineral analysis
Pulmonary function tests

* These suggestions should be considered as basic and probably incomplete for any one person. Modifications must be included for special circumstances, such as young or elderly women, women with concurrent illnesses, handicaps, or other conditions.
[†] Reasonable tests to consider for previously sedentary, peri- or postmenopausal women.

     f. The physician may need assistance from nutritionist for complicated problems,
       e.g., exercise and diabetes, exercise and weight loss, exercise and pregnancy
     g. Questioning about nutrition should include questions about eating disorders, if
       body habitus or certain injuries heighten suspicion
  3. **General physical exam**
    a. Should be thorough, including gynecologic exam
    b. Cardiovascular (see below)
    c. Pulmonary
      i. Evidence of chronic lung disease or inducible asthma that limits exercise
     ii. Good time to highlight smoking cessation
    d. Neurologic
      i. Particular concern about seizure disorders with certain sports (e.g., scuba diving)

  e. Musculoskeletal
   i. Evidence for preexisting joint injury or laxity
4. **Cardiovascular risk evaluation**
  a. Assess risk for heart disease
   i. For women under age 30–35, concern directed to hereditary conditions at high risk for sudden death (hypertrophic cardiomyopathy, coronary artery abnormalities, CAD, Marfan syndrome, mitral valve prolapse)
   ii. For women over age 35–40, concern directed to coronary artery disease and/or other conditions at high risk for sudden death (CAD, anomalous coronary arteries, hypertrophic cardiomyopathy, myocarditis)
  b. History and physical exam
   i. Athletic heart tends to be larger (volume rather than muscle), with frequent flow murmurs and not infrequent S3 sound
  c. If suspicions, either from history, family history or exam, proceed with diagnostic studies
   i. Lipid studies (include both LDL and HDL)
   ii. Electrocardiogram
    (a) Many normal athletes have resting bradycardia, often < 50
    (b) Mild changes in ST-T segments or T waves seen commonly but LVH does not occur normally in athletes
   iii. Echocardiogram
    (a) Athletic heart has increased stroke volume and mildly increase ventricular wall without hypertrophy
    (b) Valves typically not affected
   iv. Exercise stress test
    (a) Difficult decision in women because false-positive tests in premenopausal women high
    (b) Equivocal test frequently leads to thallium or stress-echo, which drives up costs for false-positive test
5. **Counseling**
  a. **Safety issues**
   i. Helmet for multiple sports (goalkeepers, boxing, etc.)
   ii. Protective clothing, e.g., padding for ice hockey
   iii. Avoiding locations at which assault possible while jogging or walking
  b. **Equipment**
   i. Proper shoes for walking/jogging
    (a) Can be difficult to fit since women's feet tend to be narrower and shoes designed for men too wide
    (b) Seek specialty store
   ii. Clothes appropriate for sport, weather
    (a) Dress warm enough during cold weather, cool enough in warm weather
   iii. Bra
    (a) Essential for all female athletes, even with small breasts
    (b) Should support without binding, chafing
    (c) Many inexpensive bras do not provide adequate support
    (d) Underwiring, poor fit may cause chafing and irritation; seams may rub or irritate nipples
    (e) Specially made bra ("sports bra") provides excellent support, broad distribution of weight, leaves shoulders free for movement
  c. Effects of exercise on concurrent disease or medication
B. **Exercise prescription**—critical factors for successful exercise are choosing the right exercise and choosing the right time for exercising
 1. **Choosing the right exercise**
  a. Appropriate limits
   i. Not too strenuous, nor too simple
   ii. Walking may be appropriate for older, previously sedentary woman; younger, trimmer woman often desire more vigorous activity

    b. Orthopedic considerations
        i. Anticipate possible orthopedic consequences and guide woman away from high-risk activities
        ii. For example, water aerobics may be perfect for older, heavier, arthritic woman
    c. An exercise that is fun
        i. Exercise is often perceived as boring; one needs something that is fun, or at least distracting
        ii. Try several activities before committing to purchase of equipment or joining athletic club
        iii. Consider whether exercise has "built-in" distractions such as change of scenery (jogging) or access to television/radio (treadmill)
    d. An exercise that can be done with someone else
        i. Incentive to show up when the woman is "counted on" by another person
          (a) Walking in neighborhood, aerobic classes, dance, team or racket sports

2. **Choosing the right time**
    a. One reason women fail to continue to exercise is that it interferes with other commitments
        i. Need to establish privileged exercise time
        ii. Unlikely woman will exercise regularly if chosen time clashes with fixed commitments such as meal preparation or taxi-service
    b. Should be a time that will almost consistently be free
        i. Early in morning before family arises, lunch hour if usually without luncheon commitments, immediately after work if it does not delay family or social commitments
    c. If exercising with a partner, schedule with partner as well
    d. Unless person adept at several exercises, may be difficult to continue outdoor exercise all year round
        i. May need to change time of exercise during different season
          (a) Jogging in morning during summer when cool, in afternoon during winter when warmer
    e. Avoid late evenings
        i. Interferes with evening activities (which often take precedence)
        ii. Exercise just before bed occasionally causes difficulty in falling asleep
        iii. If exercise involves outside settings, increases likelihood of assault

3. **Beginning the exercise**
    a. Recommend for first several weeks that exercise be done daily at the chosen time
        i. Imprinting of time for exercise; other activities should not interfere
    b. For most women, start slow and advance gradually
        i. Do not try to achieve fitness in 1 or 2 weeks
        ii. Set initial goals for 6–8 weeks
        iii. Be realistic—aim to feel better, lose a little weight, and achieve an increase in sustained heart rate
    c. Goal heart rate can be individualized
        i. Simple formula for fitness heart rate is 80% times (220 – age)
        ii. Ideally achieve and sustain fitness heart rate for 20–30 minutes
        iii. Even this is too strenuous for many previously sedentary women
    d. Alternatively, choose distance traveled or time elapsed, e.g., after 6 weeks, swim 40 laps or after 8 weeks, jazzercise for 25 minutes
    e. Aim for 3–5 sessions/week, each achieving an accelerated heart rate for 25–40 minutes

C. **Female athlete triad**
    1. Health care provider needs suspicion to identify
        a. Not so difficult when patient is obviously semistarved
        b. More difficult when person denies symptoms
    2. Table 1 lists certain diagnostic clues
    3. Recommended to cut back on intensity of exercise and allow weight to increase (it often corrects amenorrhea and halts further loss of bone density)

    4. Treatment directed at all components of syndrome

      a. Eating disorder most intractable

        i. Often requires psychological or psychiatric referral

          (a) Effectiveness of drug therapy variable

      b. Amenorrhea requires complete evaluation

        i. Rule out pregnancy

        ii. Evaluation of hormonal status complicated but essential

        iii. Generally responds to oral contraceptives or estrogen replacement

          (a) If luteal phase disorder identified and pregnancy desired, may respond to clomiphene or progesterone

      c. Osteoporosis

        i. Document stress fractures, decreased bone mineral analysis

        ii. Most important step is to replace estrogen

        iii. Supplement calcium

        iv. Unfortunately, lost bone density may not be completely recovered

D. Special musculoskeletal syndromes

    1. Trochanteric bursitis

      a. Due to modest varus at hip

      b. Pain with abduction of leg

      c. Often mistaken for arthritis of hip

        i. Check for unequal leg length

      d. Treated with NSAIDs, ice massage, ultrasound

        i. Occasionally requires corticosteroid injection

    2. Patellofemoral dysfunction

      a. Due to modest valgus at knee with slight genu recurvatum resulting in abnormal tracking of patella

      b. Knee pain, especially with climbing or descending stairs

        i. Occasional presence of effusion, but this sign should also suggest meniscal or ligamentous injury to knee

      c. Use NSAIDs, specific knee rehabilitation

        i. Involves strengthening of vastus medicalis, quadriceps

    3. Anterior cruciate ligament injuries

      a. Occur at 2–6 times greater frequency in women than men (especially in running sports, such as soccer and field hockey, and skiing)

      b. Probably due to biomechanical and anatomic differences at knee, but cause not determined

      c. Surgery required with greater frequency than in men

SUGGESTED READING

1. Bernstein L, Henderson BE: Physical exercise and reduced risk of breast cancer in young women. J Natl Cancer Inst 86:1403–1408, 1994.
2. Buress J, Christiani D: Counseling to Promote Physical Activity. In U.S. Preventive Services Task Force: Guide to Clinical Preventive Services, 2nd ed. Alexandria, VA, International Medical Publishing, 1996, pp 611–624.
3. Cumming DC: Exercise-associated amenorrhea, low bone density, and estrogen replacement therapy. Arch Intern Med 156:2193–2195, 1996.
4. Curfman GD: The health benefits of exercise: A critical reappraisal. N Engl J Med 328:574–576, 1993.
5. Greene JW: Exercise-induced menstrual irregularities. Comp Ther 19:116–120, 1993.
6. Kohrt WM, Spina RJ: Prescribing exercise intensity for older women. J Am Geriatr Soc 46:129–133, 1998.
7. Peterson DM: Exercise and physical activity in the adult population: A general internist's perspective. J Gen Intern Med 8:149–160, 1993.
8. Putukian M: The female triad: Eating disorders, amenorrhea and osteoporosis. Med Clin North Am 78:345–356, 1994.
9. Svendsen OL, Hassager C: Effect of an energy-restrictive diet, with or without exercise, on lean tissue mass, resting metabolic rate, cardiovascular risk factors, and bone in overweight postmenopausal women. Am J Med 95:131–140, 1993.
10. Tanner SM: Preparticipation examination targeted for the female athlete. Clin Sports Med 13:337–353, 1994.

11. Tofler IR, Stryer BK: Physical and emotional problems of elite female gymnasts. N Engl J Med 335:281–283, 1996.
12. Wiggins DL, Wiggins ME: The female athlete. Clin Sports Med 14:687–707, 1997.

7. Alternative Therapies in Women's Health Care

Jane L. Murray, M.D.

I. The Issues

The fact that patients seek and use alternative therapies with increasing frequency is commonly recognized in medicine today. Physicians and other health care providers are expanding their own education to learn about these modalities so that they can be intelligently discussed with patients and used safely when indicated. More research is being conducted on the efficacy and safety (or lack thereof) of a variety of complementary and alternative therapies. This chapter has been added to help clinicians understand some of the modalities commonly in use, and to have as a ready reference for discussion with patients.

II. Types of Alternative Therapies

A. Herbs commonly in use

1. A variety of herbal/botanical substances are being used by women for a variety of gynecological and other health-related symptoms. Table 1 lists the common name, botanical name(s), common uses of the plant, usual doses (if known), active pharmacologic ingredients and toxicities.

2. A major problem in the U.S. at this time is that herbal products are unregulated, and potencies and contaminants are often uncertain. Many reputable companies offer products which are standardized and contain what the label indicates. Contacting the American Botanical Council or the Herb Research Foundation may be helpful for clinicians who desire further information.

3. Herbs can be administered as bulk herbs, teas, tincture, fluid extracts, tablets, or capsules. **Teas** are actually infusions with the hot water serving as a solvent for removing some of the medicinal properties from the herb. Teas are generally weaker than tinctures, fluid extracts, and solid extracts. **Tinctures** are usually made using an alcohol and water mixture as the solvent. The herb is soaked for several hours or days, the solution then is pressed out, resulting in the tincture. **Fluid extracts** are more concentrated than tinctures, often using solvents such as vinegar, glycerin, propylene glycol, etc. A **solid extract** is produced by methods described above, as well as techniques such as thin layer evaporation. The dry solid extract can be ground into granules or fine powder. It can also be diluted with alcohol and water to form a fluid extract or tincture.

B. Nutritional approaches—Dietary Changes and Nutritional Supplements

In some ways it seems odd that nutritional approaches have been considered "alternative" by mainstream medical practitioners. However, most physicians receive little training in nutrition, and often feel unprepared to discuss dietary manipulation with patients in detail. For many medical conditions, there is ample evidence that supplemental vitamins and nutrients can be quite beneficial in the prevention and even treatment of disease. This knowledge becomes more commonplace every day.

1. **Antioxidants** are being recommended for conditions ranging from cardiovascular disease to cancer prevention. Commonly recommended antioxidants include vitamins E and C, coenzyme Q10 (also known as ubiquinone), mixed carotenoids (alpha and beta carotenes), and pycnogenols.

2. **Megavitamins** (i.e., higher amounts than the current RDA)—frequently recommended to prevent viral illnesses (vitamin C), skin and hair problems (vitamin A),

TABLE 1. Herbs Commonly Used in Alternative Therapies

Common Name	Latin Name	Dose	Uses	Active Ingredients	Toxicity
Angelica	*Angelica radix* *A. atropurpurea*	Tincture (11:5) 1.5 g/day Fluid extract (1:1) 1.5–3 g/day Solid powder 4.5 g/day	Menstrual regulation, gas, diuretic, dyspepsia	Furocoumarins, psoralens	Anticoagulation, photosensitivity
Astragalus	*Astragalus membranaceus*	Various	Immune stimulant, enhances macrophage activity topically: heals burns	Polysaccharides	Loose stools
Blueberry	*Vaccinium myrtillus*	25% anthocyanidin 80–160 mg tid	Atherosclerosis, cataracts, diabetes, neuropathy, peptic ulcer, vascular fragility, macular degeneration	Anthocyanocides	None
Black cohosh	*Cimifuga racemosa*	40–200 mg/day, not to exceed 6 months	Hot flashes, PMS, dysmenorrhea	Salicylic, tannic, and ioferulic acid	Uterine contractions, nausea, bradycardia
Bromelain (pineapple extract)	*Anans camosus*	1,800–2,000 mcu 250-750 mg/day on an empty stomach	Digestive aid, arthritis, inflammation, athero-sclerosis, wound healing, infection, cancer	Proteases	Possible allergy in sensitive individuals, possible nausea, vomiting, diarrhea, menorrhagia
Chamomile	*Matricaria recutita*	1.5–2 g/day as tea 3% infusion for topical use	Anti-inflammatory sedative, anxiolytic	Phenols, terpenes	None
Chaparral	*Larrea tridentata*	**Do not use**	Anticancer	Pyrrolizidine alkaloids	**Hepatitis—not recommended**
Chasteberry	*Vitex agnus-castus*	Tincture: 20 mg/day	PMS, mastalgia, menopausal symptoms, poor lactation	Antiprolactins	Rash, GI distress
Comfrey	*Symphytum* sp.	Poultice of ground herb, topical use only	Wound healing	Allantoin, pyrrolizidine alkaloids	**Liver toxicity if taken internally; topical use only**
Cranberry	*Vaccinium oxycoccus* *V. macrocarpon*	16 oz juice/day	UTI, kidney stones	Hippuric acid, others (?)	None known
Dong quai	*Angelica polymorpha* *A. sinensis*	Dried root: 1–2 g tid Tincture (1:5) 3–5 ml tid Fluid extract (1:1) 0.5–2 ml Solid extract (4:1) 125–500 mg tid	Menstrual regulations, PMS, dysmenorrhea	Coumarin derivatives phytoestrogens, psoralens	Photosensitivity

	Scientific name	Maximum daily dose	Uses	Active constituents	Cautions/side effects
Echinacea	*Echinacea purpurea* *E. augustifolia*	Maximum daily dose (given tid): dried root: 5 g; freeze-dried plant: 1–2 g; tincture (1:5) 6–12 ml; fluid extract (1:1) 3–6 ml; solid extract (3.5% echinacoside) 300–750 mg	Immune stimulation	Polysaccharides, flavenoids, alkamides, essential oils	Should not be taken longer than 8 weeks, no documented toxicity, interactions, or side effects
Evening primrose	*Oenothera biennis*	240 mg GLA: 3 g/day	PMS, menopause, weight loss, anti-inflammatory	Gamma-linolenic acid (GLA), cis-linoleic acid, tannins	None
Feverfew (European)	*Tanacetum parthenium*	125 mg/day of standardized extract (0.4% parthenolide)	Migraine headache prophylaxis	Parthenolide	Not to be taken during pregnancy, (anticoagulation ?), no documented problems
Garlic	*Allium sativum*	4–12 mg allicin or 0.4–12 g dried powder or 2–5 g fresh bulb daily	Atherosclerosis, hypertension, infection, cancer, allergy, immunosuppression, hyperlipidemia	Allicin	Inhibits platelet function, possible postoperative bleeding, some GI distress, contact dermatitis
Germander	*Teucrium chamaedrys*	**Do not use**	Weight loss	Diterpenoids	**Liver toxicity—unsafe**
Ginger	*Zingiber officinale*	1–2 g/day	Atherosclerosis, headache, nausea, inflammatory pain, inner ear dysfunction	Sesquiterpenes, mono-terpenes, gingerols, shogaols	None
Ginko	*Gingko biloba*	120–160 mg/d standardized extract (24% flavone glycoides and 6% terpene lactones)	Increased blood flow, dementia	Flavenoids, ginkolides, bilobalides	Transient headache, caution with concurrent NSAIDs and ASA, no documented severe side effects
Ginseng (Chinese or Korean)	*Panax ginseng*	10 mg ginsenoside 4–6 g/day	Antistress, fatigue, anxiety, cancer, menopausal symptoms	Saponins (ginsenoside)	Hypertension, anxiety, irritability, insomnia, breast pain, menstrual irregularities
Siberian Ginseng	*Eleutherococcus senticosus*	1% eleutheroside E: 100–200 mg tid	Fatigue, immunosuppression	Eleutherosides	High doses: insomnia, anxiety, melancholy irritability
Hawthorn	*Crataegus oxyacantha* *C. monogyna*	10% procyanidins: 120–240 mg tid; 18% procyanidolic oligomers: 240–480 mg/day	Atherosclerosis, arrythmias, CHF, hypertension, vascular disease	Flavenoids: procyanidins (has Ca^{2+} channel-blocking activity)	Agitation, depression

(Table continued on following page.)

TABLE 1. Herbs Commonly Used in Alternative Therapies (*Cont.*)

Common Name	Latin Name	Dose	Uses	Active Ingredients	Toxicity
Lemon balm	*Melissa officinalis*	Dried herb 2–3 teaspoons bid Tincture 2–6 ml tid	Tension, anxiety, stress, depression	Essential oils, sesquiterpenes	None known
Licorice	*Glycyrrhiza glabra*	Powdered root: 1–2 g tid Fluid extract: (1:1) 2–4 ml tid Solid extract (4:1) 250–500 mg tid Deglycyrrhinizinated locorice (DGL) 80–760 mg 20 min before meals	Anti-inflammatory, mineralo-corticoid, peptic ulcer, menopausal symptoms	Glycyrrhizin, flavenoids, saponins	Hypertension, pseudoaldo-steronism, edema
Ma huang	*Ephedra sinica*	Dried herb: 0.5–1 g tid 10% alkaloid content extract: 125–300 mg tid	Stimulant, asthma, weight loss	Ephedrine	Mania, psychosis, hypertension, tachycardia, anxiety, insomnia **Do not use with anti-depressants or antihypertensives**
St. Johns' wort	*Hypericum perforatum*	300 mg tid of standardized extract (0.13–0.30% hypericin)	Antidepressant	Hypercin	Photosensitivity in high doses, exercise caution with other antidepressants, no major side effects
Stinging nettle	*Urtica dioica*	8–12 g/day	Diuretic	Acetylcholine, formic and gallic acid, vitamins A and C, 5-hydroxytryptamine	Skin irritation
Uva ursi	*Arctostaphylos uva ursi*	2 g powdered herb boiled in water, filtered 1 cup tid	Diuretic, UTI, bladder irritability, antifungal, antibacterial	Phenol, flavenoids, arbutin (releases hydroquinone)	Tinnitus, vomiting, seizures in high doses
Valerian	*Valeriana officinalis*	Dried root: 1–2 g hs Tincture (1:5): 4–6 ml hs Fluid extract (1:1) 1–2 ml ha Solid extract (1–1.5% valtrate) 150–300 mg hs	Sedative, hypnotic	Valerenic acid (has GABA-like activity)	Dystonic reactions, liver toxicity (rare)

lower homocysteine, and protect from cardiovascular disease (vitamins B6, B12, and folic acid).

3. **Elimination diets**—to avoid allergic responses in patients with a variety of symptom complexes, such as asthma, rhinitis, dermatitis, irritable bowel syndrome, etc. Most commonly recommended food groups to eliminate include dairy products, wheat products, citrus fruits, corn, nitrates, pork, simple sugars.

C. **Mind-body therapies**

The science of psychoneuroimmunology has brought insights into the effect of the mind on the body and vice versa. Immune and endocrine function are tightly tied to the nervous system and largely controlled by its neurohormonal communication.

1. **"Relaxation response"**—popularized in recent years by Herbert Benson, MD, of Harvard University and others for prevention of stress-related illnesses, and treatment of cancer and other serious disease. Various methods are employed (special breathing techniques, guided imagery, progressive muscle relaxation) which assist in tapping into the autonomic nervous system to lower blood pressure and heart rate and mobilize immune factors to fight disease.

2. **Meditation**—a variety of methods including mindfulness meditation, transcendental meditation, yoga, and other techniques which connect the mind and body through the autonomic nervous system. Used to manage chronic pain, hypertension, anxiety, headache, stress disorders, etc.

3. **Biofeedback**—utilizes similar techniques of relaxation training connected to an objective feedback loop for the subject to verify the physiologic activity being altered (e.g., finger temperature probe, brain wave monitoring, muscle tension, etc.) Biofeedback has been found useful for treating substance abuse, hypertension, headache, temporomandibular joint (TMJ) syndrome, anxiety.

4. **Hypnosis**—generally employed by psychologists, helps patient achieve a deep state of relaxation where usual mental inhibitions and "screens" may be lowered, thus allowing the therapist to suggest that the patient begin to remember or experience long suppressed memories and feelings. Hypnosis has been found useful for treating addictive behaviors, including overeating, smoking and substance abuse.

D. **Energy therapies**—operate on a paradigm quite different from our usual western model of anatomy and physiology. However, the energy fields surrounding the body and each cell are measured and utilized regularly in conventional medicine: electromagnetic forces are measured via EEGs, EKGs, EMGs, and nerve conduction studies. Changes in tissue via differential magnetic resonances are studied utilizing MRIs. These energy fields around both the patient and therapist are essential in the effectiveness of the various energy therapies.

1. **Acupuncture**

a. The Chinese concept of qi ("chi") is actually the concept of energy flow throughout the human body. Through each organ and system is a complement of yin and yang energy, which, when unbalanced, can produce disease and symptoms. Balancing the energy flow by accessing the qi via acupuncture points is the primary mechanism by which acupuncture operates. Practitioners of Oriental Medicine typically utilize Chinese herbal treatments along with acupuncture, or even in preference to needling, depending upon the condition being treated and the individual patient's situation.

b. The National Institutes of Health convened a consensus conference on acupuncture in November 1997 and concluded that acupuncture is proven effective for a variety of medical conditions (acute and chronic pain of various types, nausea of pregnancy and chemotherapy, among others). Numerous research studies are being conducted to further evaluate its efficacy in many health conditions.

2. **Therapeutic touch**

a. A practice popularized by Dolores Kreiger has become a widespread therapy taught in most U.S. nursing schools and throughout the world today. This system utilizes the energy field between the practitioner and patient to provide a "smoothing" of ruffled energy, which can result in an enhanced sense of well being, decreased pain, and faster healing after surgery.

      b. Therapeutic touch is used for a variety of pain problems including headache, back pain, arthritis pain.

3. **Craniosacral therapy**
   a. This therapeutic method was developed by an osteopathic physician, John Upledger, DO, who observed during spinal surgery that the cerebrospinal fluid (CSF) had a definite pulsation. He postulated that if the flow of CSF was disturbed or perturbed, that the energy flow throughout the nervous system could be disrupted and symptoms and disease could result. He developed a method for sensing the CSF pulse at the occipital and sacral areas, and for teaching practitioners to perform subtle movements at these areas which would assist the flow to normalize.
   b. Little research has been published in mainstream medical journals to document the effectiveness of this technique. Testimonials abound, and the method appears to have a high safety profile.

4. **Homeopathy**
   a. Homeopathy was developed by Samuel Hahnemann in Germany in the 1880s. It was at one time a poplar form of treatment in the U.S., but now is much more widespread in western Europe than in the U.S.
   b. Even homeopathic practitioners admit that they do not understand the mechanism at work in homeopathic treatments. However, it is thought to occur through the energetic activation of molecules of a given substance, that when diluted and shaken at a certain frequency, leads to increased potency. Therefore the most dilute solutions have the strongest therapeutic effect. In addition, the substance being used for a given condition is one which would actually cause the problem being treated if it were given undiluted.
   c. While research on the effectiveness of homeopathy is lacking, it is generally felt to be safe and nontoxic. A recent meta-analysis indicated that there is an effect separate from the placebo effect occurring, but that more study is needed.

E. **Structural/manipulative therapies**
   1. **Osteopathic manipulative medicine** (OMM)—is really quite a mainstream method of managing a variety of musculoskeletal problems, with a wide body of research literature to support its use for musculoskeletal disturbances.
   2. **Chiropractic**—a method developed by David Palmer in the late 1800s which characterizes most ailments as being related to derangements in spinal alignment. For some musculoskeletal pain complaints, there is a body of research evidence to support the safety and efficacy of chiropractic care. For other organ-based symptoms and illnesses, there is little evidence to suggest efficacy of chiropractic adjustments.
   3. **Massage therapies**—especially the more rigorous methods such as Rolfing and Hellerwork could be considered "manipulative" therapies. The soft tissues of muscle, fascia, tendons, and ligaments are moved, massaged, stretched in order to work out painful musculoskeletal conditions.

III. **Conditions**
Many of the subjects covered elsewhere in this book have been rearranged alphabetically by condition. Listed after each condition or symptom are some commonly recommended nutritional, botanical, mind-body, energy medicine or structural/manipulative approaches for which there appears to be evidence of effectiveness and safety. An exhaustive bibliography is not possible, but overview texts and articles providing evidence about these modalities are listed in "Suggested Reading".

A. **Acute viral illness**
   1. Herbs: astragalus, berberine, bromelain, echinacea, garlic, angelica
   2. Nutritional: megavitamins, especially vitamin C
   3. Mind-body: to the extend the immune system can be influenced by these methods, they may be useful (?)

B. **Allergies/asthma**
   1. Herbs: astragalus, stinging nettle (allergic rhinitis), ginko biloba, ma huang (asthma—*CAUTION: not to be taken by persons with hypertension, heart disease, urinary retention, thyroid disease, diabetes, taking antidepressants or antihypertensives),* eucalyptus (inhaled, for rhinitis, not internally)

    2. Nutritional: elimination of allergens, anti-inflammatory foods (omega-3 and -6 fatty acids)

    3. Mind-body: hypnosis, biofeedback, yoga

    4. Energy methods: acupuncture, homeopathy

C. **Anxiety**

    1. Herbs: ashwaganda ("Indian ginseng"), kava kava, valerian, chamomile

    2. Nutritional: eliminate caffeine, sugar

    3. Mind-body: meditation, biofeedback, hypnosis

    4. Energy methods: acupuncture, craniosacral technique

D. **Arthritis**

    1. Herbs: boswellia, bromelain, devil's claw, feverfew, ginger, licorice root, cayenne (topically)

    2. Nutritional: evening primrose oil, elimination diets

    3. Mind-body: yoga, meditation

    4. Energy methods: acupuncture, craniosacral, homeopathy

    5. Structural/manipulative: chiropractic, OMM

E. **Cancer**

    1. Herbs: astragalus, berberine (may help support WBC during chemotherapy or radiation), chapparal (*dangerous hepatotoxicity*), echinacea (may enhance T cell function), garlic (may increase natural killer cell activity), green tea (potent antioxidant/anticancer properties), shiitake mushroom (immune enhancing/anticancer properties)

    2. Nutritional: antioxidants

    3. Mind-body: imagery, meditation

    4. Energy methods: acupuncture (pain, nausea), homeopathy (?)

F. **Cardiovascular disease/atherosclerosis**

    1. Herbs: bromelain, ginger (antiplatelet aggregation), garlic (cholesterol lowering)

    2. Nutritional: antioxidants; vitamins B_6, B_{12}, folic acid (lower homocysteine), CoQ10 (CHF), pycnogenols (lower cholesterol, antiplatelet)

    3. Mind-body: meditation, biofeedback (hypertension, angina)

    4. Energy methods: acupuncture (?)

G. **Depression**

    1. Herbs: St. John's wort, ginko biloba

    2. Nutritional: L-tryptophan, elimination diets

    3. Mind-body: all

H. **Fatigue**

    1. Herbs: panax ginseng, Siberian ginseng, licorice

    2. Nutritional: elimination diet, megavitamin

    3. Mind-body: meditation

I. **Fibromyalgia**

    1. Herbs: valerian

    2. Nutritional: magnesium, malic acid, elimination diet

    3. Mind-body: meditation

    4. Energy methods: acupuncture, craniosacral

    5. Structural/manipulative: chiropractic, massage

J. **Headache**

    1. Herbs: feverfew (migraine), ginger

    2. Nutritional: elimination diet

    3. Mind-body: meditation, biofeedback

    4. Energy methods: acupuncture, craniosacral, therapeutic touch, homeopathy Structural/manipulative: OMM, chiropractic (?), massage

K. **Hyperlipidemia**

    1. Herbs: garlic, ginseng (?)

    2. Nutritional: essential fatty acids, high fiber, pycnogenols

L. **Hypertension**

    1. Herbs: garlic, hawthorn, valerian, feverfew

    2. Nutritional: calcium, magnesium

    3. Mind-body: meditation, biofeedback
    4. Energy methods: acupuncture
M. **Irritable bowel syndrome**
    1. Herbs: peppermint oil
    2. Nutritional: elimination diet
    3. Mind-body: any
    4. Energy methods: any
N. **Insomnia**
    1. Herbs: passion flower, valerian, lemon balm
    2. Nutritional: avoid caffeine, magnesium
    3. Mind-body: relaxation training, meditation
    4. Energy methods: any
O. **Liver disease**
    1. Herbs: milk thistle, licorice root
P. **Mastalgia/fibrocystic breasts**
    1. Herbs: evening primrose
    2. Other: topical natural progesterone
Q. **Menopausal symptoms**
    1. Herbs: black cohosh, evening primrose oil,
    2. Nutritional: phytoestrogens, especially soy and flax seeds, vitamin E
    3. Mind-body: meditation, yoga, t'ai chi
    4. Energy methods: any
    5. "Natural" hormones: natural estrogens, progesterone, testosterone, dehydroepi-androsterone (see chapter 70)
R. **Nausea**
    1. Herbs: ginger
    2. Energy therapies: acupuncture
S. **Premenstrual syndrome**
    1. Herbs: black cohosh, chaste tree,
    2. Nutritional: magnesium, vitamins B_6 and E, omega-6 fatty acids
    3. Mind-body: any
T. **Substance abuse**
    1. Nutritional: elimination diets, whole foods, vitamin/mineral supplements
    2. Mind-body: hypnosis, biofeedback, meditation, hypnosis

SUGGESTED READING

1. Blumenthal M, Goldberg A, Gruenwald J, et al (eds): German Commission E Monographs. Austin, TX, American Botanical Council, 1997.
2. Ernst E: Harmless herbs? A review of the recent literature. Am J Med 104:1170–1178, 1998.
3. Israel D, Youngkin EQ: Herbal therapies for perimenopausal and menopausal complaints. Pharmacotherapy 17:970–984, 1997.
4. Fugh-Berman A: Clinical trials of herbs. Prim Care 24:889–903, 1997.
5. Lewith G, Kenyon J, Lewis P: Complementary Medicine: An Integrated Approach. New York, Oxford University Press, 1996.
6. NIH Consensus Development Panel on Acupuncture: Acupuncture. JAMA 280:1518–1524, 1998.
7. Werbach MR, Murray MT: Botanical Influences on Illness: A Sourcebook of Clinical Research. Tarzana, CA, Third Line Press, 1994.
8. Watkins A: Mind-Body Medicine: A Clinician's Guide to Psychoneuroimmunology. New York, Churchill Livingstone, 1997.
9. Zink T, Chaffin J: Herbal "health" products: What family physicians need to know. Am Fam Phys 58:1133–1140, 1998.

OTHER SOURCES

American Botanical Council web site: http://www.herbalgram.org
Cochrane Library: http://www.archie.cochrane.co.uk
Herb Research Foundation: (303) 449-2265
Homeopathic Pharmacopoeia Convention of the United States: (202) 362-8943
Office of Alternative Medicine Clearinghouse: (888) 644-6226; http://www.altmed.od.nih.gov

PART II
LIFESTYLES

8. Sexual Orientation

Elizabeth Alexander, M.D., M.S.

I. The Issues

At some point, most health professionals provide health care for lesbians. It is difficult to establish the proportion of the population that is lesbian; estimates vary, in part, because of differing sampling methods and concern about the social consequences of revealing a lesbian orientation. Part of the variability also results from differing definitions of lesbian orientation. Some definitions include only sexual behavior persistently oriented toward the same gender over time. More loosely applied definitions allow lesbians to define themselves, and they may do so in terms of political or affectional preference rather than primary sexual behavior with women. The issues that arise in the health care setting are variable, including self-definition, self-acceptance, isolation from extended family and the larger society, and conflicts between being closeted versus being open, with all of the risks inherent in either choice. Health professionals must be sensitive to the unique life and health issues of lesbians if they are to deliver the best possible care and to avoid the unknowing perpetuation of oppression.

II. The Theory

- A. **Definition:** Lesbians are women who define themselves as having a predominant sexual and affectional attraction for members of their own gender that remains over a significant period of time, whether or not they are sexually involved with women at a behavioral level. By this definition, a lesbian may be celibate, may at times have sex with men for any number of reasons, may be in a monogamous relationship with a woman, or may have multiple relationships.
  1. Sexual orientation involves three variables (sexual behavior, sexual fantasy, and nurturance) on a continuum between homosexual and heterosexual (Fig. 1)
- B. **Prevalence:** 4–7% of all adult women have identified a same gender partner at some point in their lives, according to some studies
- C. **Etiology**
  1. Currently sexual orientation is thought to be determined by complex interaction of genetic, early (intrauterine) hormonal, and early behavioral influences
  2. Theories about domineering mothers or absent fathers as causative have been thoroughly disproved

Exclusively Homosexual 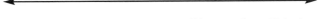 Exclusively Heterosexual

- A) Sexual behavior: how one expresses oneself in terms of sexual behaviors with others.
- B) Sexual fantasy: the object of sexual fantasy, either when a person is alone, or engaging in sexual behavior.
- C) Nurturance needs: with whom and how one meets one's needs for emotional closeness (which may include physical, but not sexual nurturance)

Example: A woman might be at various points on the continuum, changing over time, for each of the variables (i.e., exclusively homosexual in terms of meeting needs for nurturance, in the middle of continuum in terms of sexual fantasy, and at various points, over a lifetime, in terms of sexual behavior).

FIGURE 1. Variables in the definition of sexual orientation.

    3. No proof of significant increase in same-sex orientation among children of lesbian mothers, although clusters of gay and lesbian relatives are found in many extended families

D. **Cultural variation**
    1. Similar prevalence of same-sex behavior across cultures
    2. Same-sex orientation variably accepted as normal or abnormal in different cultural and ethnic groups, with part of this variation attributable to differences in definition

E. **Lifelong issues**
    1. Decision to be closeted or open with family and friends about sexual orientation must be made repeatedly throughout life
    2. Ongoing societal oppression that occurs in social, economic, and workplace settings
    3. Decisions about bearing, adopting and raising children, including those from previous partnerships
    4. Absence of rituals for societally nonsanctioned family units, which help mark change and bind family identity over time

F. **Common causes of conflict** in lesbian couples
    1. Difference within couple in ability to be open about sexual orientation, causing stress and fear in relationship
    2. Differing levels of internalized homophobia
    3. Issues with extended families
    4. Issues involving raising children of one or both partners
    5. Differing access to resources, especially economic
    6. Sexual concerns with limited resources for help/information
    7. Being a couple in society that often does not recognize this relationship as viable or socially sanctioned, including the inability to be publicly affectionate, exclusion from social functions of larger society

G. **Prevalent myths vs. facts**
    1. Myth: lesbians are promiscuous
    Fact: in one recent study, 64% had 1 partner in past year, 12% had no partners in past year, 12% had 2 partners in past year, and 12% had more than 2 partners in past year
    2. Myth: women become lesbians because they are unable to find male partner
    Fact: most lesbians have been in relationship(s) with men prior to self-identification as lesbian
    3. Myth: lesbians typically take "butch-femme" roles
    Fact: this is more common in lesbians over age 60; among younger women acceptance of traditional male–female boundaries not prevalent
    4. Myth: lesbians hate men
    Fact: true only insofar as environment provides justification

III. **Approach in Health Care Setting**
A. **Expressed reasons for delays in seeking health care**
    1. Perception that health care system is hostile and unsafe (expressed by lesbians in numerous studies)
      a. Two recent studies indicate that > 50% of nursing students and instructors expressed negative attitudes toward lesbians
      b. Four large studies document negative physician attitudes toward gay patients
    2. Expectation of invisibility and awareness that for patient to have her needs met she may need to counter provider's assumption of heterosexuality by self-disclosing as a lesbian—an irrevocable decision
    3. Financial limitations
    4. Concerns about information in medical records and potential for misuse

B. **Expressed expectations of lesbians of health care settings** include affordable care, holistic, and preventive care, respect, clear communication and women-managed clinics and providers

C. **Disclosure of sexual orientation in health care setting**
    1. Health professional should not assume heterosexual orientation
    2. Comfortable way of asking most patients about orientation is simply to say, "Tell me about your significant intimate relationships"

      3. Woman thought to be lesbian should not be pressured into self-disclosing
      4. Quality care and supportive environment can be provided by addressing patient's life situation without labeling her
      5. Acknowledgment of health risks associated with decision to be open or closeted
      6. Important to know whether patient is open and to whom she discloses lesbian identity, including friends, coworkers, and extended family

D. **Discussion of charting:** provider and patient should discuss and negotiate what will be recorded in chart prior to recording, with the awareness that such information can be misused to oppress gays and lesbians

E. **Discussion of family issues**
      1. Acceptance or rejection by parents, siblings, and other significant family members
      2. Who should be notified in case of health care crisis
        a. Who patient considers her most important family
        b. Who should not be given information (since estrangement from family of origin is common)
      3. Information may be shared about durable power of attorney or "living wills"
      4. Acceptance by, or disclosure to, children (if relevant)
      5. How holiday times are spent (e.g., separate from partner and with extended family)

F. **Issues of oppression** as they relate to health should be explored
      1. Workplace concerns and possible consequences of disclosure or nondisclosure, such as isolation, verbal or physical violence, and invisibility
      2. Past history of abuse
        a. In one study 43% of lesbians report history of sexual assault
        b. 57% report some form of victimization attributable to sexual orientation
      3. Ongoing abuse
        a. Lesbians who depend on family of origin or on others may be vulnerable to abuse
        b. Some lesbians also experience violence from female partners and may feel shame in disclosure
      4. Unequal access to resources
        a. Lesbians often lack access to health care and insurance, because women in general earn less money than men
        b. Lesbians rarely covered by family health benefits available to married heterosexual women, unless working for a company with domestic partner benefits

G. **Particular health risks**
      1. Health risks more common among lesbians than heterosexual women include:
        a. Alcoholism: self report of 23% compared with 8% in heterosexual women
        b. Marijuana use: 67% compared with 7% in heterosexual women
        c. Cocaine use: 23% compared with 2% in heterosexual women
        d. Smoking: 27% compared with 13% in heterosexual women
        e. Depression
        f. Successful suicide attempts: especially high among gay and lesbian youth
        g. Sexual assault, including history of incest
        h. Other victimization
        i. Illness related to artificial insemination, including possibility of infection with human immunodeficiency virus (HIV) from untested sperm donor
        j. Low access to health care resulting in delayed diagnoses: 13% uninsured compared with 9% of adult heterosexual women
        k. Accidental injuries
        l. Increased risk factors for breast cancer: childlessness, obesity, and smoking
        m. Higher rates of obesity
      2. HIV infection among lesbians not thoroughly understood
        a. Woman-to-woman transmission rates are considered very low
        b. Lesbian may acquire HIV through sharing needles or sexually from man
        c. Combination of lesbian identity and HIV result in double oppression

H. **Legal issues**
      1. Need for advance directives and designated patient advocate more important for lesbians because of few legal protections for woman and her partner

2. Wills are essential if patient wants to designate as her heir a partner or other person who is not a relative
3. Access to health insurance
4. Protection of privacy of information recorded in chart; potential for misuse of information
   I. **Referral resources** need to be developed to specialists who have evidenced supportive attitude toward lesbians

SUGGESTED READING

1. Alexander, C: Gay and Lesbian Mental Health: A Sourcebook for Practitioners, Binghamton, Harring Park Press, 1996.
2. Bell AP, Weinberg MS: Homosexualities: A Study of Diversity Among Men and Women. New York, Simon & Schuster, 1978.
3. Clausen J, Duberman M: Beyond Gay or Straight: Understanding Sexual Orientation. Philadelphia, Chelsea House Publishers, 1997.
4. Ford CS, Beach FA: Patterns of Sexual Behavior. New York, Harper, 1951.
5. Harrison AE: Comprehensive care of lesbian and gay patients and families. Prim Care 23:31–46, 1996.
6. McKirnan DJ, Peterson PL: Alcohol and drug use among homosexual men and women: Epidemiology and population characteristics. Addict Behav 14:545–553, 1989.
7. Michigan Organization of Human Rights: Michigan Lesbian Health Survey: Results Relevant to AIDS, August 1991.
8. Rankow EJ: Lesbian health issues for the primary care provider. J Fam Pract 40:486–493, 1995.
9. Roth S: Psychotherapy with lesbian couples: Individual issues, female socialization, and the social context. In McGoldrick M, Anderson CM, Walsh F (eds): Women in Families. New York, W.W. Norton, 1989.
10. Stevens PE: Lesbian health care research: A review of the literature from 1970 to 1990. Health Care Women Int 13:91–120, 1992.

9. Women in the Workplace

Katherine G. Keller, D.O.

I. **The Issues**

The huge influx of women into the workforce during the last half century has had a profound effect on women's health. At least 57% of all American women work outside the home, half of them mothers; 70% of working mothers with preschool children had full-time employment in March 1992, and the number of single working mothers is increasing.[9] Changing family dynamics and increasingly significant life stresses pull women in many directions. Societal expectations that women will meet the needs of parents, children, and partners in addition to job expectations leave little time for self and have a major effect on health. The health issues that arise from the multiple and increasing roles of women stem from both social and medical factors; the former often are responsible for the latter.

II. **The Theory—Social Issues**
  A. **Combining work and home**
    1. **Increased stress levels**
       a. Societal demands that women "do it all" have increased greatly over past 20–30 years
       b. Most women must work to keep family financially viable, whether they are single or have a working partner, especially if children are in the family
       c. Often married women no longer have choice of remaining full-time homemakers, which may increase stress in marriage
       d. Working women feel pulled between demands of family and work and may feel that they do neither job well

    e. It is important to encourage women to take time for themselves, even 5 minutes in a busy schedule, to do something they enjoy

    f. Exercise is great stress reliever; even walking on the lunch hour helps

2. **Childcare issues**

    a. Childcare is necessary but often suboptimal, with little one-on-one supervision

    b. Full-time childcare tends to be expensive, with more intimate settings (in-home or small family groups) the most expensive

    c. Trust is major issue; it is difficult for many families to find trustworthy and reliable caregiver

    d. Guilt is another concern; it is painful to acknowledge that someone other than parent has more time with child

    e. Reliability is important; repeated changes of caregiver are disruptive for children

    f. Back-up plans are essential in anticipation of illness and other emergencies; daycare outside the home often has no provision for ill children

    g. **Advantages of daycare**

        i. Woman who wants to pursue a career and chooses to work

        ii. Improved socialization for children

        iii. Accelerated learning as children are exposed to preschool setting with older children

    h. Some workplaces have on-site daycare, which allows parents to easily visit children during breaks and is especially convenient for breastfeeding mothers

B. **Reproductive impact**

1. **Hazards to fertile women in workplace**

    a. Historical rationale for excluding women from certain jobs; real hazards to conception and normal fetal development at some work sites

    b. Premarital and preconception counseling should include careful analysis of current and past workplace exposures

    c. Potential toxins are numerous[3]

        i. Anesthetic agents

        ii. Arsenic

        iii. Lead

        iv. Mercury

        v. Polybrominated biphenyls (PBBs)

        vi. Polychlorinated biphenyls (PCBs)

        vii. Insecticides

        viii. Paint and ink

        ix. Petroleum products

        x. Solvents

        xi. Agents used in plastics, rubber, paper, and pharmaceutical industries

        xii. Infectious diseases

    d. More is known about spermatotoxicity than ovarian toxicity (because of accessibility for study), but it seems clear that toxins play role in hormonal disruption of normal menstrual cycle and events necessary for conception

    e. Fertilization and implantation may be impaired, leading to early pregnancy losses

    f. Critical period of embryonic vulnerability—days 18–55 after conception, when women may not realize that they are pregnant

    g. However, fetus is vulnerable to toxins until birth, especially nervous system

    h. **Strategies for risk reduction**

        i. Careful family planning

        ii. Preconception risk assessment with attention to behavior modification in other areas that increase risk, such as alcohol and tobacco use, and stabilization of medical problems (especially hypertension and diabetes)

        iii. Job monitoring or modification[3]

            (a) Male partner should minimize potential harmful exposures about 3 months before attempting conception

            (b) Female partner should minimize risk beginning with cycle during which conception is attempted; known teratogens should be completely avoided in first trimester of pregnancy

            (c) All attempts should be made to minimize maternal exposure throughout pregnancy and breastfeeding

    i. Health care providers should familiarize themselves with state and local law covering occupational exposures

    j. **Resources for women concerned about occupational exposure**
       i. Local occupational health clinics
      ii. REPROTOX (a computer database on reproductive and developmental hazards), Columbia Hospital for Women Medical Center, 2425 L Street, NW, Washington, DC 20037, 202-293-5137
     iii. National Institute of Environmental Health Sciences, PO Box 12233, Research Triangle Park, NC 27709, 919-541-3345
     iv. National Institute for Occupational Safety and Health (NIOSH) resource line: 1-800-356-4674
      v. Occupational Safety and Health Administration (OSHA) has offices in many larger cities (check government listing in phone book under Department of Labor); toll-free hotline: 1-800-321-OSHA

2. **Maternity leave**
    a. United States lags behind all other industrialized countries in length of parental leave granted to workers; in Britain 18 weeks are allowed; in Sweden, 12 months
    b. Standard maternity leave in U.S. is 6 weeks for vaginal delivery and 8 weeks after cesarean section
    c. Most authorities believe that this is the minimum for physical recuperation after delivery; it does not address after factors that affect work performance, such as sleep deprivation
    d. New parents are encouraged to take as much leave as possible to encourage bonding and stability in newly expanded family
    e. While pregnancy is not pathologic condition, employed women have some protection under Pregnancy Discrimination Act; pregnancy must be treated as any other temporary disability at workplace
    f. No law mandates paid maternity leave; before passage of Family Medical Leave Act in 1993, workers not covered by a disability leave policy had no protection
    g. Family Medical Leave Act mandates up to 12 weeks of unpaid, job-protected leave for birth or adoption of a child; acquiring foster child; serious illness of child, spouse or parent; and serious illness of the employee; covers only public agencies and private sector employers of 50 or more employees within 75 miles[4]

3. **Breastfeeding** (see Chapter 63, Breastfeeding)

C. **Economics and division of labor by gender**
  1. Compensation inequity
    a. 1991 figures show women employed full-time in the U.S. earn 70% of median male income[9]
    b. Women in the same jobs tend to earn less than men; women are also more prevalent in lower-paying jobs
    c. Trend justified by outdated beliefs that women are not primary breadwinners, that women give less to jobs because of devotion to family, and that women are less experienced than male counterparts
    d. Inequity is narrowing with time but probably will persist because of higher numbers of women in service jobs as well as part-time, seasonal, and temporary work

2. **Sexual harassment** (see Chapter 77)

3. **Glass ceiling**
    a. As more women entered supervisory roles in executive management and academia, phenomenon called "glass ceiling" was recognized
    b. Women found that for not clearly visible reason, career advancement was halted short of upper levels
    c. Recent documentation of inequity in advancement and promotion as well as several lawsuits regarding gender bias have focused some attention on problem but have failed to break through completely; barriers are still widespread

4. **Work hours and flexibility of scheduling**
    a. Because of family responsibility, many women seek employment with flexible hours or choose first shift so they can be home when children return from school
    b. Part-time work is feasible for many women
    c. Newer option is job sharing

        i. Two persons work part-time

       ii. Employer still has a full-time job role filled

  5. **Benefits**

    a. Women hold more service-oriented jobs than men and are more likely to work part-time, seasonally, or on temporary basis

    b. Common to such job situations is lack of comprehensive employer-paid benefits

    c. Overall, more women than men in U.S. are covered by medical insurance (73.2% vs. 70.2%), but this reflects higher percentage of women receiving Medicare and Medicaid[9]

    d. Working women not covered through spouse or employer may seek insurance privately, but this is significantly more expensive than comparable group plans

    e. Many women find themselves choosing a job on the basis of medical coverage and retirement benefits alone or stay on job that is unrewarding to maintain benefits

III. **An Approach—Social Issues**

  A. **Social problems that plague women workers are complex and may seem overwhelming**

  B. **No easy solutions**, but options help women to cope as well as to develop skills for advancement in job market

    1. Know the law

      a. If woman is victim of gender-based harassment or "glass ceiling," there may be legal recourse

      b. Health care providers may recommend that patient contact Equal Employment Opportunity Commission if rights are infringed

    2. Be familiar with local community resources for working women

    3. Identify feminist therapists in community

    4. Recommend assertiveness training and stress management courses

    5. Most importantly, validate patient's concerns and let her know that she is valued member of society in all roles she fills

IV. **The Theory and Approach—Medical Problems**

  A. **Illness or injury directly due to work activity**

    1. **Physical problems**

      a. Work-related injuries traditionally were seen in women whose work is physical but now are more common in office settings, especially with prolonged computer usage

      b. Careful history and thorough documentation are important for worker's compensation

      c. Treatment guided by proper diagnosis

      d. Types of injuries

        i. **Acute trauma**

          (a) Sprains, strains, lacerations and fractures treated with standard protocols

          (b) Low back injuries[1]

            (i) In absence of signs of dangerous underlying conditions (such as possible fracture, tumor or infection, cauda equina syndrome) special studies unnecessary; 90% of patients recover spontaneously within 4 weeks

            (ii) Careful history and physical exam are important, with special attention to neurologic screening

            (iii) Initial care

              • Patient education

              • Reassure patient that there is no sign of dangerous condition

              • Recovery anticipated with few weeks (may be longer with sciatica)

              • Patient comfort, including medication (acetaminophen or nonsteroidal antiinflammatory drugs)

              • Literature demonstrates no evidence of benefit of muscle relaxants, but may be helpful

              • Manipulation via physical therapy or manual medicine is both safe and effective in first month of acute symptoms without radiculopathy

              • Ice massage or alternating heat and ice affords some symptom relief

(iv) Alteration of activity
- Avoid activities that increase stress on back
- More than 4 days of bed rest is harmfully debilitating
- Gentle conditioning exercise may be started within first 2 weeks and increased incrementally
- Patient should be encouraged to return to normal activity as soon as possible

(v) Work restrictions
- Historical information as well as patient's perception of safe limits are best guide
- Recognize that even moderate unassisted lifting may aggravate back symptoms
- Restrictions intended to allow spontaneous recovery or to build activity tolerance with exercise

(vi) Reassessment is indicated if back symptoms do not improve within 4 weeks

(vii) Evidence of dangerous underlying condition should suggest further diagnostic studies and possible referral

ii. **Repetitive stress injuries or cumulative trauma disorders**
   (a) Carpal tunnel syndrome is most common
      (i) Antiinflammatory agents useful
      (ii) Wrist splints worn at work and bedtime
      (iii) Alteration in work habit to avoid inciting activities
      (iv) Computer users often find wrist rest helpful
      (v) Adjusting work surface and chair height
      (vi) Frequent breaks to stretch (at least once an hour)
      (vii) Physical therapy in more severe cases
      (viii) Occasionally surgery is indicated with persistent symptoms or signs of muscle atrophy
   (b) Other repetitive stress injuries are treated much the same way; the key is prevention through changes in work habit

iii. **Exposure to toxins or chemicals**
   (a) Mostly seen in industrial work or laboratories
   (b) May present as puzzling constellation of symptoms that patient does not associate with work
   (c) Careful history essential, especially temporal association with occupational changes
   (d) Treatment of occupational toxin exposures is highly specific; best sources of information are local occupational health clinic and OSHA

e. **Disability**
   i. Complicated and often emotionally loaded topic
   ii. Some patients find it impossible to return to work after injury because of persistent physical symptoms
   iii. Job change may be only solution when injury precludes return to same job or worker's position is so untenable that secondary gain emerges after injury
   iv. Primary care physicians in particular face burden of forms for certification of disability
      (a) Best strategy is to complete forms to best of ability
      (b) Ask patients directly if they can perform listed tasks
      (c) Almost all states have independent disability examiners; primary care physician rarely makes final determination
   v. Conflicts may arise between employer and patient
      (a) Physicians may serve as advocates
      (b) Clear description of signs and symptoms as well as diagnosis is helpful in resolving disputes about work capability

2. **Emotional problems**
   a. **Depression** (see Chapter 78, Depression)
   b. **Panic disorder** (see Chapter 79, Anxiety)

B. **Health issues indirectly related to work**
   1. **Obesity and deconditioning**
      a. Many work environments promote sedentary habits for women
      b. Often working woman has little time for organized exercise or even daily stretching
      c. Combined with poor eating habits (either fast food on the run or snacks available in the office), lack of activity puts women at risk for both obesity and deconditioning
      d. Workers should be encouraged to increase physical activity in any way possible
         i. Exercise before or after work
         ii. Join coworkers in walking at lunch time
         iii. Get up and stretch at least once an hour while working at desk or computer
         iv. Physician can help by making it clear that exercise is commitment to long-term health that every woman needs to make, just as she receives annual health maintenance exams
      e. Encourage better eating habits, especially low fat foods
         i. Planning meals in advance, appropriate shopping, and packing lunch night before
         ii. Limit eating out, especially fast food
         iii. Request nutritional information at fast food restaurants and choose items low in fat as well as calories
         iv. Try to avoid word "diet" and discuss "meal planning"
   2. Tobacco exposure
      a. Smokers
         i. Smoking is significant cause of morbidity and mortality
         ii. Smoking cessation needs to be urged by primary care physician at every opportunity
         iii. Many workplaces are now smoke-free or limit locations at which employees may smoke, which may help smoking cessation
      b. Nonsmokers
         i. Nonsmokers have increased risk of smoking-related illness due to passive smoke exposure
         ii. Workplaces that have smoke-free policies often do so to protect nonsmokers
         iii. Workers exposed to tobacco smoke in workplace should discuss issue with employers

SUGGESTED READING

1. Acute Low Back Problems Guideline Panel: Acute low back problems in adults: Assessment and treatment. Am Fam Physician 51:469–484, 1995.
2. Ayers L, Cusack M, Crosby F: Combining work and home. Occup Med 8:821–832, 1993.
3. Filkins K, Kerr M: Occupational reproductive health risks. Occup Med 8:733–754, 1993.
4. Freedman J: Maternity leave: Rights, rules and regulations. J Am Med Wom Assoc 47:85–95, 1992.
5. Headapohl D: Sex, gender, biology and work. Occup Med 8:685–707, 1993.
6. Snapp MB: Occupational stress, social support, and depression among black and white professional-managerial women. Wom Health 18:41–79, 1992.
7. Rosenfeld JA: Maternal work outside the home and its effects on women and their families. J Am Med Wom Assoc 47:47–53, 1992.
8. Unger K: Working women: Economic and social considerations. Occup Med 8:859–868, 1993.
9. United States Department of Labor: 1993 Handbook on Women Workers: Trends and Issues. Washington, DC, U.S. Department of Labor, 1993.
10. Wollersheim J: Depression, women and the workplace. Occup Med 8:787–796, 1993.

10. Marriage

Timothy P. Daaleman, D.O.

I. The Issues

Most women experience their primary dyadic relationship within the context of marriage. The married state usually connotes a relationship that is committed, monogamous, and either legitimized by religious or secular authorities, or recognized by the couple's peer or reference group. As a provider of care that is comprehensive, longitudinal and inclusive, the generalist physician has an advantageous perspective from which he or she can observe and potentially influence the marital relationship.

II. The Theory

A. Marriage and health

1. Married persons have fewer physician visits and report being sick less often than unmarried persons. In addition, unmarried persons are more likely to use more tobacco and alcohol products, and have greater risk factors for accidents (i.e., not use seat belts) and illness than their married counterparts.
2. Through the provision of routine habits, social support and intimacy, and adequate nutrition, marriage has a protective effect on spouses from stress. Many spouses monitor and attempt to control their spouse's health behaviors. Women are more likely to attempt to control health behaviors than men.
3. Marriage has beneficial effects on health for women who are not employed, either through the provision of financial resources or social support

B. Public and private domain

1. Marriage is a private enterprise with a social structure and value system that is unique and specific to the relationship
2. Both civil and religious authorities recognize the importance of the marital relationship as a locus of socialization into larger reference groups (i.e., family, community), and have an interest in validating the union or dissolution of the relationship

C. A long and coupled life

1. There are several characteristics that spouses in long-term marriage (>20 years) possess: loyalty to spouse, lifetime commitment to marriage, strong moral values, commitment to sexual fidelity, desire to be a good parent, faith in God and spiritual commitment, desire to please and support spouse, good companion to spouse, willingness to forgive and be forgiven
2. **In older couples**, there is a stronger relationship between marital satisfaction and health for women than for men
   a. Wives report more mental and physical health problems in dissatisfied marriages than their husbands
   b. When compared to middle-aged couples, older couples exhibit: a reduced potential for conflict and greater potential for pleasure in several areas, equivalent levels of overall mental and physical health, and lesser gender differences in sources of pleasure

III. An Approach

The primary care physician should: recognize and identify sources of dysfunction within a marital relationship; be appreciative of the association between marriage and health and well-being; and intervene appropriately to promote a mutually satisfying relationship.

A. Assessment

Providers can screen for potential sources of conflict, identify undifferentiated problems, and clarify existing difficulties within a marital relationship by examining three areas: communication, roles and responsibilities, and sexuality/intimacy.

1. **Communication**

   Couples with a greater degree of marital dissatisfaction are more likely to display the following communication behaviors:

    a. Partner manipulation

    b. Avoidance of conflict and conflict resolution: couples who terminate their marriages tend to display communication behaviors characteristic of avoidance, indirectness, and decreased involvement with the relationship

    c. Coercion

        i. Couples who communicate to each other that they have equal control in the relationship experience fewer problems in interpersonal perceptions

        ii. Couples that communicate in self-disqualifying and egocentric ways perceive their marriages as less satisfying and each other's feelings and behaviors less accurately, than those without such interactive patterns

    d. Destructive interactive patterns:

        i. The withdrawal behavior, which is generally exhibited by men, in the demand/withdrawal pattern, enables them to maintain power in the relationship

        ii. Within the context of domestic violence, the batterer acquires power of a moral nature while the victim plays the role of the accused

        iii. After violence occurs, reconciliation with the batterer relieves the victim of his/her role as the suspect

2. **Roles and responsibilities**

    a. **Work outside the home**

        i. Women's participation in the labor force has increased dramatically in the last 50 years; in 1990 up to 56% of married women returned to work within the first year of their infants' lives.

        ii. There are several variables that affect women's participation in the labor force: the more children a women has, the less likely she is to work outside the home; the higher the woman's educational level, the more likely she is to work; African-American women are more likely to work than white women.

        iii. Working is associated with; lower fertility, longer first birth intervals, and earlier use of birth control.

        iv. Women employed in higher-status jobs generally marry at an older age

        v. There is little difference in marital satisfaction between full-time housewives and working women, although in marriages where the husband disapproves of the woman's employment, there is more reported marital discord

        vi. Employed women are more likely to think about separation or divorce than housewives, but the divorce rate between the two groups is not significantly different

    b. **Domestic responsibilities**

        i. Women who view themselves as coproviders with their husbands spend 2.5 times as many minutes per week performing household tasks as their husbands

        ii. Wives who are not employed outside the home work on domestic chores eight times as much as their husbands; women who see their careers as secondary to their husbands' work five times as much.

        iii. Economic decision-making power increases for women who work

        iv. Decisions about meals, household maintenance, and children are more likely to be shared if both parents are employed

        v. The working mother is still responsible for over 70% of child care responsibilities; employed women assume primary responsibility for the physical and emotional well-being of their children.

        vi. Nearly three-fourths of family caregivers for the elderly and disabled are women

        vii. Older couples tend to have well defined and rigid patterns of interaction, based on gender roles, poor health in either spouse can lead to a reorganization of responsibilities and a redefinition of a dominant and caretaker role for the well spouse

3. **Sexuality and intimacy**

    a. Lack of sexual activity can be a warning sign of an unsatisfactory or unstable marriage; sexually inactive marriages are associated with: unhappiness with the marital relationship, increased likelihood of separation, lack of shared activity, few arguments over sex, lack of physical violence, increased age, fewer children, the presence of preschoolers, poor health/physiologic changes.

    b. The physician can explore issues surrounding sexuality and intimacy through open-ended and non-threatening questions pertaining to sexual practices, orientation, and satisfaction; the initial information may be best obtained through an individual approach.

    c. A thorough history, comprehensive review of systems—with attention to medications—and a directed physical exam will help the clinician classify the presenting problem into one of three areas; organic/physical, medication-related, and psychologically based dysfunction.

    d. After the initial individual assessment is performed, the clinician should meet with the couple to clarify, validate, or supplement information, assess the dyadic relationship and interpersonal dynamics, and outline a preliminary plan

B. **Intervention**

The decision to intervene within a marriage should be made after a careful and comprehensive assessment. Although preliminary information obtained can be fragmented, unilateral, and inexact, the clinician is obligated to pursue issues regarding the marital relationship if there are presenting problems regarding: violence or the threat of violence (physical, emotional, sexual), activities of daily living, sexual dysfunction, psychiatric or emotional disturbances. The provider should always be cognizant of his/her own bias and belief systems, and assume a neutral and open-minded position prior to any intervention.

  1. **Premarital education and screening**

    a. The generalist is often the provider of required serologic and other premarital screening tests for an engaged couple, in addition to contraceptive counseling; this role allows the physician an entree to address larger issues regarding marriage and any potential sources of conflict.

    b. Many religious denominations have preparation classes as a prerequisite for marriages that will be sanctioned within the respective faith traditions

  2. **Domestic violence**

    a. Couples who present with physical finding inconsistent with their clinical histories should be suspect for domestic abuse or violence; in this setting, the physician's primary responsibility is for the safety and well-being of the victim.

    b. Civil authorities and community and family resources should be notified and coordinated

    c. The physician should be aware that the victim may refuse any and all interventions, including protective custody

  3. **Sexual dysfunction**

    a. Many couples with an identified organic/physical dysfunction benefit from minor interventions (i.e., medication changes, prostheses, lubrication); in areas of uncertain diagnosis or treatment, consultation with specialty colleagues (i.e., gynecology, urology) is recommended.

    b. Couples with a psychologically based sexual dysfunction are candidates for psychotherapy; with appropriate education and experience, the primary physician may elect to begin a therapeutic relationship with the parties involved, however, many generalists choose to refer to therapists with expertise in this area.

  4. **Marriage counseling**

    a. As a neutral observer, the primary care physician can reflect back to the married couple; identified areas of conflict or hidden agendas of each partner, functional and dysfunctional patterns of communication, the impact of the marital relationship on health and well-being.

    b. There are several systems of therapy available (i.e., cognitive, behavioral, marital, family); the clinician should be familiar with the strengths and limitations of each system or consult a mental health specialist in order to choose the most appropriate therapy for the presenting problem.

    c. Some generalist physicians have advanced training in marital therapy and provide this service as a routine part of their care.

SUGGESTED READING

1. Ayers L, Cusack M, Crosby F: Combining work and home. Occup Med 8:821–831, 1993.
2. Baxter LA, Dindia K: Marital partners' perceptions of marital maintenance strategies. J Soc Pers Relat 7:187–208, 1990.
3. Cupach WR, Comstock J: Satisfaction with sexual communication in marriage: Links to Sexual Satisfaction. J Soc Pers Relat 7:179–186, 1990.
4. Donnelly DA: Sexually inactive marriages. J Sex Res 30:171–179, 1993.
5. Fenell DL: Characteristics of long-term first marriages. J Ment Health Counsel 15:446–460, 1993.
6. Fowers BJ: His and her marriage: A multivariate study of gender and marital satisfaction. Sex Roles 24:209–221, 1991.
7. Gove WR, Style CB, Hughes M: The effect of marriage on the well-being of adults: A theoretical analysis. J Fam Issues 1:1–35, 1990.
8. Levenson RW, Carstensen LL, Gottman JM: Long-term marriage: Age, gender, and satisfaction. Psychol Aging 8:301–313, 1993.
9. Noller P: Gender and emotional communication in marriage: Different cultures or differential social power? Special Issue: Emotional Communication, Culture, and Power. J Language Soc Psych 1:132–152, 1993.
10. Noller P, Feeney JA, Bonnell D, Callan VJ: A longitudinal study of conflict in early marriage. J Soc Pers Relat 1:233–252, 1994.
11. Rosenfeld J: Maternal work outside the home and its effect on women and their families. J Am Med Wom Assoc 47: 47–53, 1992.
12. Serra P: Physical violence in the couple relationship: A contribution toward the analysis of the context. Fam Process 32:21–33, 1993.
13. Sperry L, Carlson J: The impact of biological factors on marital functioning. Am J Fam Therapy 20:145–156, 1992.
14. Umberson D: Gender, marital status, and the social control of health behavior. Soc Sci Med 34:907–917, 1992.
15. Waldron I, Hughes ME, Brooks TL: Marriage protection and marriage selection: Prospective evidence for reciprocal effects of marital status and health. Soc Sci Med 43:113–123, 1996.
16. Wickstrom L, Holte A: Relationship control and interpersonal perception in marriage. Scand J Psychol 34:149–160, 1993.

11. Parenting

Belinda A. Vail, M.D.

I. The Issues

Following the "women's liberation movement" a greater number of women continue to move into positions of greater authority, higher-paid positions, and into the professional field. Yet, they still continue to bear the burden of housework and child rearing. However, of all the jobs they have, the one at which most women want most to succeed is parenting. Despite the plethora of information in every imaginable medium, women often feel anxious and inadequate at a job that their gender has performed for thousands of years. The basic job of parenting is teaching children to leave, and to become self-sufficient and responsible adults, capable of caring for themselves and others. Hundreds of books on the subject present as many different theories. Each parent and child is different, and parenting must be tailored to the individual relationship. Physicians often recognize poor parenting behaviors in their patients, but may have trouble helping those patients to become better parents. As school violence escalates and teenage pregnancy and drug abuse continue to rise, there is an ever increasing need to learn to assist mothers in parenting, their most important occupation.

II. The Theory

    A. **The first responsibility of parenting is to provide children's basic needs**

        1. Children need love, affection, and touching

        2. They need to feel that they are cared about and that they belong

        3. They need security

        4. They need to develop their own sense of identity and a healthy self-esteem

    5. They need a sense of power or the feeling that they have some control over people and events around them

    6. Children also need to have fun: "The business of childhood is play"

B. **Responsible parenting builds healthy families, which have several characteristics in common:**

    1. Parents care for and set limits for their children and act as teachers, modeling appropriate behavior

    2. Children are always loved, even if their behavior is unacceptable. Each person's personal boundaries are respected.

    3. All feelings (but not all behaviors) are accepted

    4. Children are expected to contribute to the family at a level appropriate to their age

    5. Children are respected and praised appropriately

    6. Even busy families find some time for family activities and to have fun together

III. **An Approach**

A. **Providing basic needs and teaching children how to separate and move into the world** on their own are the responsibilities of parenting. The following are a compilation of parenting techniques to achieve these goals.

    1. The parents as a couple (or the single parent) should be more important than the parent–child relationship

        a. Children need to see that parents value their own lives and relationships

        b. Parents who have high self-esteem help their children to develop self-esteem

        c. Family as a whole must be a greater priority than each individual child; this starts with the parents as a couple.

        d. Parents who are happy with their lives and jobs are good role models for their children

        e. Children need to learn to occupy themselves while adults are interacting with each other; children do not need constant attention.

    2. **Children need clear expectations and limitations**

        a. Children should be expected to obey their parents and teachers. Families do not work as true democracies, because the children are not equal to the parents in experience or power.

        b. Children should have tasks to perform that contribute to the functioning of the family. Chores teach children responsibility, build self-esteem, teach citizenship, and they help the child to feel as a part of the family.

        c. Expect children to finish what they started; it teaches persistence and self-motivation.

        d. Expect caring and responsible behavior in dealing with others

        e. Limits and expectations should be important

        f. Setting too many limits detracts from the more important ones and makes enforcement very difficult

        g. Limits need to be within the child's ability to comprehend and to comply

    3. Modeling

        a. Children learn more from what their parents do than from what they say

        b. Parents whose behavior contradicts what they say model deception and dishonesty for their children

B. **Parents need to communicate with their children**

    1. Listening is the first tool of communication

        a. Teaches the child good listening skills;

        b. Shows the child that the parents care and that they respect the child's thoughts and feeling

        c. Allows the child to have power and importance

    2. **Empathy**—when parents understand the feelings of the child, the child's behavior becomes more understandable, and the child becomes more likely to attempt a behavioral change

    3. **Repeating or rephrasing** what the child has said lets the child know that the parent is listening and creates fewer misunderstandings

    4. **Allowing the child to ask questions** after the parents state their position leaves room for negotiation and further communication

5. Be patient
6. **Negotiation** is a skill that can be developed by allowing children to participate in setting limits, with each side giving in a little when an impasse is met. This skill must be developed over the life of the child in an age-appropriate manner.
7. Lectures, threats, and warnings are poor examples of communication and rarely bring about the wanted results

C. **Discipline**
1. Discipline is a form of teaching that involves the 4 Cs:
   a. **Consensus**—agree on the expectations prior to an explanation to children
   b. **Clarity**—be clear and concise in an explanation of the rules; sometimes "because I said so" will have to suffice.
   c. **Consequences**—natural consequences are the best, but any predetermined and agreed upon consequences with severity appropriate to the transgression will be adequate
   d. **Consistency**—if children break the rules or do not behave as expected, they need to suffer the consequences. Do not rescue them, or they will push the limits again and again.
2. **Punishment**
   a. Punishments are power-based and do not allow children to exert power or to make their own choices (control is external—by the parent)
   b. Punishment teaches children to obey but does not teach responsibility
   c. Physical punishment (e.g., spanking) implies that hitting is acceptable and should be used sparingly or not at all
   d. Punishments are most appropriate for situations in which the child is in danger (e.g., running into the street or sticking keys in electrical outlets)
3. Consequences
   a. Are related to the rule or limitation and teach internal control
   b. Are related to the future and so give long-term results
   c. Usually build self-esteem and respect

D. **Infants and toddlers**
1. "Catch them being good"
   a. Pick up infants and play with them or talk to them before they cry
   b. Praise children often when they are exhibiting appropriate behavior rather than waiting for inappropriate behavior that requires negative feedback. Praise should be frequent but concise. If children are ignored during appropriate play, they quickly learn that inappropriate behavior draws the parent's attention.
   c. Frequent quiet touching of children who are behaving appropriately encourages continued good behavior
2. Expect children to be able to occupy themselves for periods of time appropriate to age
   a. It is not the job of the parent to entertain the child
   b. Television should be limited
   c. Toys should be limited and should encourage imagination. The more complex the toy, the less imagination is required and the sooner the child will become bored. Too many toys seem to overwhelm children, limit their attention span, and create a bigger mess for the parent.
   d. Younger children (< 15–18 months) require the parent to be in sight most of the time
3. **Discipline**
   a. Infants and toddlers are very dependent on attention from their caregiver. Removing the child from attention is a highly effective form of discipline. "Time out": the child must sit quietly in a chair outside the area of activity for about 1 minute for each year of age. Sending a child to his or her room functions much like "time-out."

E. **School-aged children**
1. School-aged children develop a sense of industry and internal motivation
   a. Children learn to participate in more structured and orderly routines (school and organized activities, such as scouting and sports)

      b. They need to learn skills necessary to interacting with many others outside the home
      c. School-aged children are anxious to help and can be given appropriate tasks or chores

  2. **Discipline**
      a. "Time-out" will still work, although sending the child to his or her room is more often used for older ages
      b. Natural consequences should be used at this age because the child is developing reasoning skills

F. **Adolescents**
  1. Adolescents are simultaneously narcissistic, idealistic, and endowed with sudden great knowledge. Adolescence is a time to accomplish many tasks.
      a. Establishing an identity and self-esteem
      b. Developing self-sufficiency and independence
      c. Establishing peer relationships
      d. Establishing relationships with the opposite sex and becoming comfortable with their sexuality
      e. Deciding on career goals and how to train for them

  2. Parenting the teenager
      a. Continue to listen and enhance self-esteem
      b. Negotiation is important for enhancing life skills and for just surviving the wrath of the teen
      c. "Tolerate much, but sanction little"
      d. Encourage self-reliance
      e. Develop family rituals and routines
      f. Provide social support
      g. Respect privacy
      h. Learn to let go. That's what parenting is all about—preparing children to leave the home.
      i. Do not give in to peer pressure
      j. Continue to parent—to provide support, guidance, and discipline
      k. Do not make big issues of small ones. Shaved heads, torn clothing, and earrings may be embarrassing to the parents, but do not represent a long-term problem.

G. **Parenting and divorce**
  1. About 30% of children experience divorce in their family before the age of 18. Single-parent households are now almost as common as two-parent families. Single parenting after divorce brings unique challenges.

  2. **Common pitfalls to avoid:**
      a. Do not make drastic changes in the child's lifestyle, if at all possible. For example, it is best if the child can stay in the same house and school with the same friends.
      b. Do not fight in front of children
      c. Do not denigrate spouse to the children
      d. Do not use the children to "spy," to take sides in an argument, or to convey adult messages (i.e., child support is late)
      e. Do not use the child as a friend or confidante to relate fears or request support. The child will have enough fears of his or her own.
      f. Do not undermine the other parent's discipline; this quickly leads to a manipulative child.

  3. **Positive parenting in divorce**
      a. Reassure the children that the divorce is not their fault and that even though the parents are no longer married, the children still have two parents
      b. Try to maintain consistent discipline, and do not undermine the other parent
      c. Maintain frequent and consistent visitation with the noncustodial parent
      d. Be civil
      e. Seek professional help if things seem to be out of control

4. **Step-parenting**
   a. Allow the children to express their feelings, even if you do not agree with the way they feel
   b. Respect their feelings and love for the original parent
   c. As in the original family, make the marriage the most important relationship
   d. Decide on discipline and follow through. Support the spouse in discipline issues
   e. Maintain a healthy attitude—you know it is difficult for everyone, but with time things will work out
   f. Step-parents have increased satisfaction with their role if they (1) have previous experience as a parent; (2) have good relationships with other family members; (3) share similar values with the other parent; and (4) are included in the discipline process.

IV. **Role of the Physician**
   A. **Recognizing parental problems**
      1. Physicians should recognize signs of poor parenting
         a. Behavior problems in children are often evident during the exam, especially when it occurs at each visit
         b. Parents' use of verbal and corporal punishment is the strongest predictor of behavior problems
         c. Parents who develop a perspective on their own early negative relationships do not reenact poor parenting practices on their own children
         d. In adolescent mothers, self-esteem is a good predictor of parenting skills knowledge
      2. Physicians should actively search for parenting problems
         a. Simple questions to the parents starting with first well child exams about their own impressions, fears, and concerns about their parenting abilities. An early pattern of inquiry will make parents more comfortable with discussing problems with parenting as they occur.
         b. Parental assessments of children's behaviors can be used as an early screening tool
   B. **Teaching parenting skills**
      1. Teaching skills as part of routine office visits or well child exams
         a. Parents respond best to information that focuses on their area of concern. (If the mother is concerned about the child sleeping in his own bed, an opportunity presents to reinforce consistency by repeatedly returning the child to his own bed)
         b. Media such as posters or videos can help to widen the range of interests of the mothers
         c. Verbal suggestions are best for brief, concrete information
         d. Written material is better for more complex information
      2. Expanding beyond the clinic visit
         a. Nurses, patient educators, physician assistants, nurse practitioners can all be used to provide or augment patients' education
         b. Referral for parenting classes
         c. Counseling referral for both the mother and child, especially when early behavior problems no longer seem to be a transient "phase".

SUGGESTED READING

1. Bettelheim B: A Good Enough Parent. New York, Vintage Books, 1987.
2. Bodenburg DA: Overachieving Parents, Underachieving Children. Los Angeles, Lowell House, 1992.
3. Bradley FO, Stone LA: Parenting Without Hassles. Salt Lake City, Olympus, 1983.
4. Brenner V, Fox RA: Parental discipline and behavior problems in young children. J Genetic Psychology 159:251–256, 1998.
5. Christophersen ER: Beyond Discipline. Kansas City, MO, Westport, 1990.
6. Christophersen ER: Little People. Shawnee Mission, KS, Overland Press, 1977.
7. Cline F, Fay J: Parenting with love and logic. Colorado Springs, CO, Pinon Press, 1990.
8. Curwin RL, Mendler AN: Am I in Trouble? Santa Cruz, CA, Network Publications, 1990.
9. Dreikurs R, Cassel P: Discipline without Tears. New York, Hawthorne Books, 1972.

10. Everett LW: Factors that contribute to satisfaction or dissatisfaction in stepfather–stepchild relationships. Perspect Psychiatric Care 34:25–35, 1998.
11. Glascoe FP, Oberklaid F, Dworkin PH, Trimm F: Brief approaches to educating patients and parents in primary care. Pediatrics 101:E10, 1998.
12. Helmstetter S: Predictive Parenting. New York, William Morrow, 1989.
13. Hurlbut NL, Culp AM, Jambunathan S, Butler P: Adolescent mothers' self-esteem and role identity and their relationship to parenting skills knowledge. Adolescence 32:639–654, 1997.
14. Joslin KR: Positive Parenting. New York, Fawcett Columbine, 1994.
15. Kulner L: Parent and Child. New York, William Morrow, 1991.
16. Nelson J, Lott L, Glenn HS: Positive Discipline A–Z. Rocklin, CA, Prima Publishing, 1993.
17. Phelps JL, Belsky J, Crnic K: Earned security, daily stress, and parenting: A comparison of five alternative models. Dev Psychopathol 10:21–38, 1998.
18. Polland BK: Parenting Challenge. Berkeley, CA, Tricycle Press, 1994.
19. Pruett MK, Hoganbruen K: Joint custody and shared parenting: Research and interventions. Child Adolesc Psychiatr Clin North Am 7:273–294, 1998.
20. Rimm S: How to Parent so that Children Will Learn. Watertown, WI, Apple Publishing, 1990.
21. Rosemond J: Six-Point Plan for Raising Happy, Healthy Children. Kansas City, MO, Andrews & McMeel, 1989.
22. Strasburger VC: Getting Your Kids to Say "No" in the '90s When You Said "Yes" in the '60s. New York, Simon & Schuster, 1993.
23. Taffel R: Parenting by Heart. Reading, MA, Addison-Wesley, 1992.
24. Wahler RG, Meginnis KL: Strengthening child compliance through positive parenting practices: What works? J Clin Child Psychol 26:433–440, 1997.
25. Woititz JG: Healthy Parenting. New York, Simon & Schuster, 1992.

12. Divorce

Belinda A. Vail, M.D.

I. The Issues

Every year thousands of women in the U.S. endure the physical, psychological, and financial stress of divorce. Over the past three decades the divorce rate has more than doubled and now shows signs of leveling off only because the number of marriages has continued to decline. Currently about half of marriages end in divorce, usually placing the women at a social disadvantage and often straining social resources. Despite the rise of women in the work force, they continue to earn less than their male counterparts, and they still continue to bear the major burden of child care after the divorce. Primary care practitioners should be aware of the number and complexity of stressors that divorcing women face and help them to adjust to their new living situation as expediently as possible.

II. The Theory

A. Epidemiology

1. Currently almost 50% of marriages end in divorce
2. Highest divorce rates are for women who marry before 20 years of age and who were pregnant or had a child at the time of the marriage
3. Lowest divorce rates are for women who marry after 30 years of age and have at least 16 years of education
4. Likelihood of divorce decreases with increasing number of children, increasing age of couple, and increasing length of marriage
5. Remarriages
   a. 4 of 10 marriages involve a remarriage of at least one partner
   b. 5% of all women are divorced at least twice
   c. 29% of women who remarry divorce again
   d. Second marriages end in fewer years
   e. Median duration of divorce before remarriage is 2.5 years

B. **Trends**
  1. Age at first marriage is rising
     a. In 1975, 87% of women in their late 20s had been married
     b. In 1990, only 69% of women in their late 20s had been married
  2. Divorce rate is leveling off and is expected to stabilize with about 40% of marriages ending in divorce
  3. Percentage of women marrying a second time is decreasing
  4. The gap between whites and minorities continues to widen
     a. Only 61% of black women in their late 30s have been married
     b. 70% of first births to black women were out of wedlock
  5. Length of marriages is decreasing
C. **Increasing development of single-parent families**
  1. Economic burden is still primarily borne by the woman, but both partners may suffer financially
  2. Impact on child development is still felt in single-parent homes, although these children have fewer problems than those from violent two-parent homes
  3. Increased impact on minorities
     a. 54.8% of black children in single-parent homes
     b. 30% of Hispanic children in single-parent homes
     c. 19.2% of white children in single-parent homes
D. **Factors related to increased divorce rate**
  1. National economic affluence: as more women have the ability to support themselves, they no longer stay in an unhappy relationship because it is a necessity
  2. Civil rights and affirmative action have given women more opportunities to support themselves
  3. Less social stigma against divorce: as the number of divorced families grow it becomes the norm
  4. College students who come from divorced families have more difficulty with intimate relationships, indicating that the difficulty with forming long term relationships may be self-perpetuating
  5. "Me" decade of the 70s: some emphasis has shifted from the family to the rights and wants of the individual
  6. No-fault divorce laws have made it easier and cheaper to obtain a divorce
  7. Studies showing less serious impact on children help women feel less guilt
E. **Sociologic factors related to increased likelihood of divorce**
  1. Marriage before age 20
  2. High school dropout or failure to attain degree at any level
  3. Premarital pregnancy
  4. Instability of husband's work or income
  5. Marked year-to-year increase in husband's income
  6. Wives with higher incomes
F. **Stages of divorce**
  1. Threat of separation—deliberation and despair
  2. Decision to divorce
     a. 85% of divorces not by mutual agreement
     b. More women than men (57.5%) initiate divorce
     c. Decision usually made:
        i. As result of "last straw" (infidelity, drinking, major life event)
        ii. After psychotherapy
        iii. With realization that security and gratification are markedly outweighed by accumulation of grievances and psychological toll
  3. Divorce—legal maneuvering
  4. Separation shock
  5. Rollercoaster of emotions—marked highs and lows; lows often brought on by encounters with ex-spouse
  6. Work on identity
  7. Recentered self—growing self-esteem

G. **Social fallout for women**
   1. Financial
      a. Average post-divorce income for women is $15,000–$18,000
      b. 90% have no long-term financial goals
      c. Difficulty in obtaining loans and credit
   2. Career
      a. Many women have no job training or skills
      b. Many have been unemployed for significant periods of time
      c. Working women often in low-paying jobs
   3. Return to school
      a. May be necessary to obtain job skills
      b. Helps sense of accomplishment and self-esteem
      c. Increases already high financial burden
   4. Social stigmata
      a. Women often embarrassed to become "a statistic"
      b. Women often excluded from engagements with their former "couple" friends
   5. Sexuality
      a. Difficulty communicating about sex
      b. Fear of new sexual relationships/health concerns
   6. Children
      a. Decreased affluence and ability to support children financially make payment of child support a priority—most states are making it much harder for men to ignore child support payments
      b. Every effort should be made to avoid other significant changes in children's lives
      c. Consistent discipline is very important
      d. Single parenting—close relationship between mother and children (without role reversals) is necessary to decrease long-term effects of divorce
      e. Children should not be used as messengers or spies or be privy to arguments or fights
   7. Psychiatric stability
      a. The incidence of psychiatric diagnoses increases by 2.5-fold in women who are divorcing
      b. Women seem to develop problem during the divorce which persist after the divorce is over. Men's psychiatric problems seem to resolve with the completion of the divorce

H. **Legal issues**
   1. Property division
   2. Spousal support
   3. Child support
   4. Custody and visitation
   5. Living arrangements and possession of house

I. **Remarriage**
   1. Resolution of first marriage issues is imperative
   2. Remarriages have high divorce rate and shorter span than first marriages

III. **An Approach**

A. **Recognition of divorce and its place in life cycle**
   1. Women must first deal with immediate emotions of guilt, anger, and self-pity
   2. Grieving: Divorce should be recognized as an ending, much like death. Women need permission to mourn, acknowledgment of their feelings, and permission to let go.

B. **Dealing with social issues**
   1. Social worker can help with finances and educate them about government agencies and programs. They can also assist with women who are in abusive relationships.
   2. Abuse: A significant number of women are leaving abusive relationships; verbal and physical abuse both become more common during divorce. A significant number of women will be in serious danger. Physicians should always inquire about abuse
   3. Sexuality
      a. Do not assume that divorced women of any age simply quit having sex
      b. Discuss issues of sex and communication

      c. Premenopausal women—discuss birth control; many women may have come from marriages in which husband had vasectomy

      d. Postmenopausal women—discuss issues of new sexual relationships and lubrication

      e. All women—discuss sexually transmitted diseases, including acquired immunodeficiency syndrome

C. **Dealing with psychological and family issues**

  1. Crisis intervention may be necessary if the woman is in some way unable to care for herself and her children or is in physical danger

      a. Establish relationship and explore dimensions of problem

      b. Encourage exploration of feelings and emotions

      c. Assess suicidal risk

      d. Explore and assess past coping attempts and current alternatives and solutions

      e. Develop plan of action including follow-up

  2. Cognitive therapy

      a. Helps to put patient back in control

      b. Must be able to empathize with patient and ask open-ended questions

      c. In some cases helps couples to view divorce as a positive step

D. **Divorce mediation**

  1. Decreases financial cost (much cheaper than legal fees)

  2. Decreased emotional cost

  3. Protection of children's rights

  4. Sense of empowerment

E. **Avoiding post-divorce traps**

  1. Psychological traps

      a. Self-blaming—feeling responsible for entire situation

      b. Catastrophizing—exaggerating potential difficulties

      c. Mind-reading—assumptions about feelings, attitudes, and motivation of others

      d. Filtering—focusing on worst aspects of situation

      e. Global labeling—generalizing negative qualities into negative label of ex-spouse

      f. Overgeneralizing—all-or-none thinking

      g. Blaming others

      h. Shoulds—feeling obligated to certain actions

  2. Behavioral traps

      a. Withdrawal

      b. Dependency

      c. Clinging to ex-spouse

      d. Living for others (i.e., children)

      e. Escape from self

      f. Don Juanism—thinking they have to have perfect appearance

      g. Searching for "the other half"

SUGGESTED READING

1. Barber BL, Eccles JS: Long-term influence of divorce and single parenting on adolescent, family, and work-related values, behaviors, and aspirations. Psychol Bull 111:108–126, 1992.
2. Conger RD, Rueter Ma, Elder GH Jr: Couple resilience to economic pressure. J Pers Soc Psychol 76:54–71, 1999.
3. Ensign J, Scherman A, Clark JJ: The relationship of family structure and conflict to levels of intimacy and parental attachment in college students. Adolescence 33:575–582, 1998.
4. Hayes CL, Anderson D, Balu M: Our Turn: The Good News about Women and Divorce. New York, Simon & Schuster, 1993.
5. Kelly JB: Marital conflict, divorce, and children's adjustment. Child Adolesc Psychiatr Clin North Am 7:259–271, 1998.
6. Liese B: Integrating Crisis Intervention, Cognitive Therapy, and Triage. In Roberts AR (ed): Crisis Intervention and Time-limited Cognitive Treatment. Thousand Oaks, CA, Sage Publications, 1995, pp 28–56.
7. McKay M, Rogers PD, Blades J, Gosse R: The Divorce Book. Oakland, CA, New Harbinger, 1984.
8. National Vital Statistics Report: Births, marriages, divorces, and deaths: Provisional data for May 1998. Natl Vital Stat Rep 47:1–2, 1998.

9. Norton AJ, Miller LF: Marriage, Divorce, and Remarriage in the 1990s: Current Population Reports, Special Studies. U.S. Department of Commerce, Economics, and Statistics Administration, Bureau of the Census, 1992, pp 23–180.
10. Patford J: The doctor's role in separation: Reflections on some preliminary data. Aust Fam Physician 27:573–576, 1998.
11. Radford B, Travers-Gustafson D, Miller C, et al: Divorcing and building a new life. Arch Psychiatr Nurs 11:282–289, 1997.
12. Ruggles S: The rise of divorce and separation in the United States, 1880–1990. Demography 34:455–466, 1997.
13. Summers P, Forehand R Armistead L, Tannenbaum L: Parental divorce during early adolescence in Caucasian families: The role of family process variables in predicting the long-term consequences for early adult psychosocial adjustment. J Consult Clin Psychol 66:327–336, 1998.
14. Svedin CG, Wadsby M: The presence of psychiatric consultations in relation to divorce. Acta Psychiatr Scand 98:414–422, 1998.
15. Vansteenwegen A: Divorce after couple therapy: An overlooked perspective of outcome research. J Sex Marital Ther 24:123–130, 1998.
16. Wallerstein JS: The long-term effects of divorce on children: A review. J Am Acad Child Adolesc Psychiatry 30:349–360, 1991.

13. Abandonment

Judith A. Suess, M.D., M.P.H.,
and Ginger Vary, A.C.S.W., B.C.S.

I. The Issues

Abandonment is not a phenomenon that happens only to babies or old people; most women experience it repeatedly over the course of their life. Sequelae have an impact on health, quality of life, and the ability to form and maintain meaningful relationships.

II. The Theory

A. **Definition:** abandonment is loss of supportive presence of family member or significant other
   1. May be due to volitional or involuntary act
   2. May result from death, illness, emotional betrayal, or cessation of fulfilling a particular role
   3. Loss of cultural or societal milieu are also forms of abandonment

B. **Risk factors for health sequelae**
   1. Every woman at risk
   2. The more tenuous the woman's support system, the lower her self-esteem
   3. The more marked the dependency needs, the higher the risk that abandonment(s) will adversely affect her physical and/or emotional health

C. **Categories of abandonment**
   1. Abandonment at birth or in childhood
      a. Death of parent(s), sibling(s), grandparent(s), pet(s)
      b. Divorce or threat of divorce of parents
      c. Given up for adoption, additional loss of biologic family members, especially in case of twins
      d. Abandonment of parental role
         i. Physical, emotional, and/or sexual abuse
         ii. Substance abuse by parent (may result in role reversal or child may be forced into specific roles such as hero or scapegoat)
         iii. Illness of parent (e.g., diabetes, chronic pain, multiple sclerosis) may result in role reversal or parental inaccessibility
         iv. Parental inaccessibility or emotionally unavailable parent for any reason. This may be due to large family size, fatigue, teen mother, or other competing demands such as a debilitating treatment regimen for breast cancer.

v. Not providing a safe environment, permitting abuse or neglect to occur, e.g., secondary smoke from mother's boyfriend adversely affecting child's asthma or one parent ignoring the other's abusive behavior

2. **Abandonment during adulthood**
   a. Death of parents
   b. Death or illness of spouse—especially difficult if due to suicide, accident, mental illness (e.g., Alzheimer's disease, depression)
   c. Absence of anticipated support from children or other family members (e.g., during illness, old age)
   d. Physical illness or alteration of body image of woman resulting in abandonment by significant other or family member
   e. Mental illness of woman resulting in abandonment (e.g., severe depression resulting in inability to communicate)
   f. Religious, political, and ethical disagreements resulting in abandonment by family, society and/or religious institution
      i. Abortion
      ii. Pregnancy
      iii. Sexual orientation
      iv. Conversion to other religion
   g. Sexual misconduct by someone in professional role is betrayal of trust in context of power differential
      i. Clergy
      ii. Therapist
      iii. Teacher
      iv. Physician
   h. Divorce
   i. Failure of biological parent to acknowledge role in life of their child after adoptee has found her and/or him

3. **Abandonment either during childhood or adulthood**
   a. Fear of abandonment can be as detrimental as actual abandonment in its effects; greater effect on women and children than on men because of power differential
   b. Disruption of social fabric
      i. Epidemics, e.g., acquired immunodeficiency syndrome
      ii. War
      iii. Diaspora (Jews, Kurds, African Americans)
      iv. Inappropriate acculturation efforts (Native American children were forced to go to boarding schools to learn white culture)
      v. Famine
      vi. Poverty
      vii. Lack of societal validation of culture, traditions, or rites of passage, e.g., Native American rituals outlawed, gay/lesbian developmental milestones, partner status not recognized

D. **Health sequelae of abandonment**
   1. Abandonment in all of its forms may cause rupture of interpersonal trust and loss of sense of personal control and personal worth
   2. Mental illnesses and emotional states
      a. Depression
      b. Anxiety
      c. Eating disorders—especially binge eating; act of eating, not consumption of food, is pathology
      d. Posttraumatic stress disorder
      e. Guilt
      f. Shame, feeling of worthlessness
      g. Insomnia
      h. Irritation and anger
      i. Loneliness
   3. Low self-esteem; may result in low achievement or overachievement

    4. Sexual dysfunction, including sexual acting out
    5. Substance abuse or addiction
    6. Somatizing, e.g., low back pain, headaches
       a. May be homeostatic mechanism, compensatory, way to get care
    7. Fear of intimacy
    8. Domestic violence
    9. Self-destructive behaviors, e.g., perpetual victim status, masochism, sabotaging success
   10. Loss of self, personhood
   11. Loss or bereavement may result in atypical grief, extended grief, or "frozen grief"
      a. Frozen grief occurs when acute process is interrupted before completion
      b. Unresolved grief results in inability to reestablish relationships or to regain former sense of well-being
        i. Woman doesn't feel sad but is emotionally dead
        ii. Nothing makes her happy
   12. Codependency, i.e., woman is focused on something or someone outside herself with unrealistic expectations of change
      a. May result in inability to end relationship when needs are not being met or relationship is abusive
   13. Lack of autonomy in thinking or behavior
   14. Homelessness

III. **An Approach**
  A. **Common presenting complaints**
    1. Inability to accomplish change or task
    2. Somatization, e.g., fatigue, chest pain, low back pain, or cluster of somatic complaints
    3. Depression and/or suicidal ideation
    4. Insoluble problems with current relationship
  B. **History taking and interviewing**
    1. Bring up possible contributions of abandonment issues in any conditions enumerated in health sequelae of abandonment (II.D.)
    2. Elicit how woman dealt with abandonment
      a. Closure with person who abandoned her
      b. Finding alternatives for personal support in her life
      c. Inability to develop and/or fear of subsequent relationships
      d. Grieving the loss
        i. American culture does not encourage grieving; it encourages "moving on"
        ii. Physician must be sensitive to stages of bereavement
        iii. Suggestions and interventions need to be appropriate to stage of bereavement
    3. Discuss body-mind unity concepts, i.e., presenting symptoms may have originated more from stress of abandonment than from physical cause
    4. Discuss how to go about finding alternative sources of support
    5. Be careful not to frighten patients with overly strong reactions to history
      a. Physician's response should also not minimize importance of what patient says
      b. Physician's response needs to be based on and appropriate to patient's needs or patient may feel more abandoned and alone
  C. **Tasks of provider**
    1. Solidify therapeutic relationship
      a. Assure woman explicitly you will not abandon her, regardless of whether she fulfills your expectations
      b. Clarify your availability and limits
      c. Give adequate notice if you are moving or leaving practice
    2. Validate connection between past or present abandonment and ongoing physical or emotional problems; acknowledge anniversary date of loss
    3. Expiate guilt (conscious or unconscious) that it is her fault that the abandonment occurred
    4. Affirm that anger and other strong emotional reactions are appropriate even if the abandonment was involuntary

    5. Acknowledge the commonality of abandonment issues and resulting sequelae

    6. Refer to appropriate mental health professionals when the primary provider lacks the competence or time to adequately address the issues

  D. **Treatment options:** see Chapter 77, Gender-based Sexual Harrassment, for advantages of individual vs. group therapy

    1. Individual therapy

    2. Support groups

    3. Group therapy

    4. Bibliotherapy, i.e., providing appropriate reading materials

    5. Modalities that have been efficacious in individual and group settings

      a. Stress reduction

      b. Biofeedback

      c. Nutrition

      d. Massage

      e. Meditation

      f. Prayer

SUGGESTED READING

1. Armsden GC, Lewis FM: Behavioral adjustment and self-esteem of school-age children of women with breast cancer. Oncol Nurs For 21:39–45, 1994.
2. Asper K: The Abandoned Child Within. New York, Fromm International, 1993.
3. Bernporad JR, Beresin E, et al: A psychoanalytic study of eating disorders. I: A developmental profile of 67 index cases. J Am Acad Psychoanal 20:509–531, 1992.
4. Clayton PJ: Bereavement and depression. J Clin Psychiatry 51:39–40, 1990.
5. Crow-Dog M: Lakota Woman. New York, Harper Collins, 1990.
6. Draucker CB: Childhood sexual abuse: Sources of trauma. Issues Mental Health Nurs 14:249–262, 1993.
7. Farberow NL, Gallagher-Thompson D, Gilewski M, Thompson L: The role of social supports in the bereavement process of surviving spouses of suicide and natural deaths. Suicide Life-threat Behav 22:107–124, 1992.
8. Fortune MM: Is nothing sacred? San Francisco, Harper, 1989.
9. Goodman L, Saxe L, Harvey M: Homelessness as psychological trauma. Am Psychol 46:1219–1225, 1991.
10. Hammerschlag A: The Dancing Healers. San Francisco, Harper & Row, 1989.
11. Herman JL: Trauma and Recovery. New York, Harper Collins, 1992.
12. Kaplan H, Sadock B (eds): Comprehensive Textbook of Psychiatry, vol. II, 5th ed. Baltimore, Williams & Wilkins, 1989.
13. Kaschak E: Engendered Lives. New York, Harper Collins, 1992.
14. Kuh D, Maclean M: Women's childhood experience of parental separation and their subsequent health and socioeconomic status in adulthood. J Biosoc Sci 22:121–135, 1990.
15. Lerner HG: The Dance of Intimacy. New York, Harper & Row, 1989.
16. Meshot CM: Adolescent mourning and parental death. Omega J Death Dying 26:287–299, 1992–1993.
17. Orback S: Fat Is a Feminist Issue. Berkeley, Paddington Press, 1978.
18. Parker G, Manicavasagar V: Childhood bereavement circumstances associated with adult depression. Br J Med Psychol 59:387–391, 1986.
19. Patton CJ: Fear of abandonment and binge eating. J Nerv Mental Dis 180:484–490, 1992.
20. Rieder I, Ruppert P (eds): AIDS: The Women. San Francisco, Clies Press, 1988.
21. Sable P: Attachment, anxiety and loss of a husband. Am J Orthopsychiatry 59:550–556, 1989.
22. Sieqel K, Gorey E: Childhood bereavement due to parental death from AIDS. J Develop Behav Pediatr 15:566–570, 1994.

14. Living Alone

Mark Larson, M.D.

I. The Issues

The number of American adults living alone has risen steadily since the early 1950's. The proportion of single-person households in all age groups is rising, with the fastest rise among persons over 85. Almost 50% of this group live alone. Women are more likely in all stages of life to live alone. The impact of living arrangements on health and mortality probably changes over the life cycle.

II. The Theory

A. Children and adolescents
1. Usually live with others
2. Consider runaways and homeless
3. Problems encountered by children living alone
   a. Poor school performance; malnutrition; sexual abuse; prostitution; sexually transmitted disease; substance abuse; teenage pregnancy; and poverty

B. Young adults
1. Living alone can be positive step
   a. Independence; freedom; autonomy; and self-reliance
2. Negative issues similar to those of children can occur with young adults

C. Middle age
1. Never married
   a. Generally mentally and physically less healthy
   b. Higher rates of mortality than married people
2. Divorce
   a. Men—increased cancer and cardiovascular mortality linked to poor social support
   b. Women—no evidence of increased health risks related to divorce alone

D. Old age
1. Factors that increase probability of living alone
   a. Decreased number of kin
   b. Disability decreases probability
   c. Higher income
2. Elderly prefer living independently (i.e., alone)
3. As people age, differential between men and women changes dramatically
   a. Ages 65–69 years: 81 men/100 women
   b. Ages 85+: 39 men/100 women
4. Most men live with someone
   a. Less need for social support
   b. Less willing to accept help
   c. Experience difficulty coping with change late in life
   d. Most men their age still married
5. Most women live alone
   a. 10% women married: two-thirds live alone
   b. Most elderly women are poor: 23% live at poverty level compared with 16% of men
   c. Women experience more disabling effects of chronic illness
   d. Elderly women are better able than elderly men to form new intimate relationships
   e. Women more easily accept assistance
   f. Women often widowed earlier and have more time to adjust to living alone
   g. Women experience increased difficulty with household maintenance

III. An Approach

A. Consider variability among patients problems in regard to living situation
1. **Widowhood**
   a. Women are widowed longer and better adapted to independent living

  b. Women expect to be widowed
  c. Encourage involvement in domestic and community activities
2. **Poverty**
  a. Offer suggestions for money management
  b. Refer for community services
3. **Social isolation**
  a. Social networks
    i. Can be positive or negative
    ii. Consider both structure and composition of social networks
  b. Recommend that elderly living alone remain active
4. **Depression and suicide**
  a. Counseling to reduce risk
  b. Decrease social isolation
  c. Treat depression
5. Inquire about **living arrangements**
6. **Activities of daily living**
  a. Assess ADL (personal care) or IADL scale
  b. Obtain household assistance
  c. Encourage use of social services
7. Consider **adverse health outcomes of living alone**
  a. Encourage cessation of smoking
  b. Treat alcohol abuse
    i. Address alcohol as health issue
    ii. Alcohol use higher among those living alone
  c. Obesity/physical activity
    i. Discuss low-fat diet and weight-bearing exercise program. Develop exercise prescription
  d. Nutrition
    i. Encourage meal preparation services (e.g., meals on wheels)
    ii. Prescribe vitamin supplementation
    iii. Refer to dietitian

SUGGESTED READING

1. Barer BM: Men and women aging differently. Int J Aging Hum Dev 38:29–40, 1994.
2. Bondevik M, Skogstad A: Loneliness among the oldest old: A comparison between residents living in nursing homes and residents living in the community. Int J Aging Hum Dev 43:181–197, 1996.
3. Davis MA, Moritz DJ, Neuhaus JM, et al: Living arrangements, changes in living arrangements, and survival among community dwelling older adults. Am J Public Health 87:371–377, 1997.
4. Gliksman MD, Lazarus R, Wilson A, Leeder SR: Social support, marital status and living arrangement correlates of cardiovascular disease risk factors in the elderly. Soc Sci Med 40:811–814, 1995.
5. Mack R, Salmoni A, Viverais-Dressler G, et al: Perceived risks to independent living: The views of older, community-dwelling adults. Gerontologist 37:729–736, 1997.
6. MacNeill SE, Lichtenberg PA: Home alone: The role of cognition in return to independent living. Arch Phys Med Rehabil 78:755–758, 1997.
7. Nagatomo I, Takigawa M: Mental status of the elderly receiving home health services and the associated stress of home helpers. Int J Geriatr Psychiatry 13:57–63, 1998.
8. Oxman TE, Berkman LF: Assessment of social relationships in elderly patients. Int J Psychiatry Med 20:65–84, 1990.
9. Pagel MD, Erdly WW, Becker J: Social networks: We get by with (and in spite of) a little help from our friends. J Pers Soc Psychol 53:793–804, 1987.
10. Sarwari AR, Fredman L, Langenberg P, Magaziner J: Prospective study on the relation between living arrangement and change in functional health status of elderly women. Am J Epidemiol 147:370–378, 1998.
11. Wilmoth JM: Living arrangement transitions among America's older adults. Gerontologist 38:434–444, 1981.

15. Developing New Relationships

Mark Larson, M.D.

I. The Issues

New relationships span the female life cycle. The process begins with parents and expands to friends, dating, marriage, work and old age. Some relationships are voluntary, such as friendships and love relationships, whereas others are not, such as parents and family, certain work relationships, neighbors, and in-laws. A new relationship may be a source of stress in a woman's life.

II. The Theory

A. On the classic **Social Readjustment Rating Scale**, developed by Holmes and Rahe in 1967, almost every stressor is associated with changes in relationships and, ultimately, the formation of new relationships. For example, the following is a list of the first 10 of 43 items on the Holmes and Rahe Scale:

1. Death of a spouse
2. Divorce
3. Marital separation
4. Jail term
5. Death of a close family member
6. Personal injury or illness
7. Marriage
8. Fired from work
9. Marital reconciliation
10. Retirement

B. Such changes and resulting new relationships may have important implications for health status and health care

1. Changes in marital status have the potential to lead to loneliness and depression
2. Death of a spouse occurs with a higher frequency among women. Pursuit of new relationships exposes women to potential medical problems, such as sexually transmitted diseases.
3. **Involuntary new relationships,** such as those encountered in jail or at work, may result in substantial emotional stress and psychiatric symptoms
4. The marital engagement of a young woman provides the family physician the opportunity to discuss family planning

C. The most significant new relationships occur within the structure of the family system (e.g., marriage, birth of child). Each of the **family life cycle stages** is characterized by important new relationships.

1. Between families: the unattached young woman
   a. Wide range of changes in dating and friendship relationships
2. Joining of families through marriage
   a. Results in multiple new relationships that bring increased stress as new demands are placed on the couple
3. Family with young children
   a. **With the birth of the first child, a couple form the most important new relationship of their lives.** Furthermore, as young children enter school, the couple discover numerous other new relationships in their lives.
      i. Teachers
      ii. Students
      iii. Other parents
4. Family with adolescents
   a. Dating
   b. School
   c. Outside activities
5. Launching children and moving on
   a. More time to develop and nurture new relationships outside the family
6. Family in later life
   a. Become grandparents, meet new older couples and other people through traveling and other activities

III. **An Approach**
  A. **Each new relationship carries with it potential medical implications**
  B. Practitioners should inquire about the patient's new relationships and ask how they are affecting the patient's health:
    1. Diet
    2. Exercise
    3. Mental status
    4. Personal hygiene
    5. Sexuality
  C. **Health maintenance interventions** can be directly linked to family life cycle stages
    1. **Contraception** and sexually transmitted diseases
       a. Women in new dating relationships should be counseled about safe-sex behaviors and contraceptive choices
    2. **Prenatal care**
       a. Pregnant women and their partners should consider the effect of this new relationship on their relationship as a couple
    3. **Parent education**
       a. Anticipatory guidance: child-rearing issues
          i. Child car seats
          ii. Discipline
          iii. Basic child health
          iv. Immunizations
    4. **Counseling**
       a. Couples counseling in all life cycle stages
       b. Sexual counseling
          i. The annual female exam is a good time to address sexual functioning
       c. Family counseling
          i. Address during appointments for well-child checks and school physicals
          ii. Women often bring children to the physician for such visits.

SUGGESTED READING

1. Aune KS, Aune RK, Buller DB: The experience, expression, and perceived appropriateness of emotions across levels of relationship development. J Soc Psychol 134:141–150, 1993.
2. Duncan LE, Agronick GS: The intersection of life stage and social events: Personality and life outcomes. J Pers Soc Psychol 69:558–568, 1995.
3. Hauser ST, Borman EH, Powers SI, et al: Paths of adolescent ego development: Links with family life and individual adjustment. Psychiatr Clin North Am 13:489–510, 1990.
4. Holmes TH, Rahe RH: The social readjustment rating scale. J Psychosom Res 11:213–218, 1967.
5. Gould RL: Transformations: Growth and Change in Adult Life. New York, Simon & Schuster, 1978.
6. Liese BS, Price JG: The family life cycle. In Rakel RE (ed): Textbook of Family Practice, 4th ed. Philadelphia, W.B. Saunders, 1990.
7. Miller MA, Rahe RH: Life changes scaling for the 1990s. J Psychosom Res, 43:279–292, 1997.
8. Sheehy G: Passages: Predictable Crises of Adult Life. New York, Dutton, 1976.

16. "Sandwich Generation"

Jane L. Murray, M.D., and
Gary E. Bachman, M.S.S.W., L.S.C.S.W.

I. **The Issues**
   A. Middle-aged adults, mainly women, who must care for both their own families and their aging parents, are a growing cohort of Americans
      1. 71% of family members providing care to aging relatives are women
      2. 75% of such caregivers are over 50 years of age
      3. 79% of caregivers are married
      4. 48% are caring for a homebound spouse; 34% for an aging parent; 15% for another relative
      5. Nearly one-half (48%) spend over 50 hrs/week in caretaking
      6. Many caregivers are single heads-of-households
      7. Many caretakers work full time outside the home
      8. $11.4 billion annual productivity loss to employers of family caregivers
   B. This so-called sandwich generation (sandwiched between responsibilities for their own children and their parents and/or grandparents) is at risk for significant health problems, mainly related to stress and fatigue
      1. 58% of caregivers report a variety of personal health problems:
         a. Hypertension—20%
         b. Arthritis—14%
         c. Anxiety—11%
         d. Back pain—7%
         e. Indigestion—7%
         f. Depression—7%

II. **The Theory**
   A. Since the mid-1960s, public policy in America has favored institutionalization of the frail elderly over maintaining them in the home and may have penalized "sandwich generation" caregivers
      1. Such providers of in-home services for no remuneration were at risk of impoverishment as they aged
      2. Typically, such caregivers could not afford institutionalization for their aging parent, yet were not eligible for public assistance
   B. More recent changes in public policy have recognized that increasing resources are channeled into more expensive long-term care services, mainly in institutional settings
      1. More and more states are requiring elderly patients to be screened before admission into a long-term care setting, and efforts are made to determine whether community-based resources are available
      2. Family providers of in-home care are frequently unaware of resources that may provide financial and service support for the demanding tasks that they have assumed
      3. Families often feel pressured to make uneducated choices
      4. Young children in sandwiched families may be frightened or confused by the stresses facing their parents and by medical activities in the home
      5. Conversely, children in such families may develop a close relationship with their grandparent or great grandparent at a time when an elderly relative may provide role modeling and nurturing
      6. The opportunity to participate in end-of-life activities and dying may either frighten or enhance family cohesion, depending on family circumstances and relationships
   C. Some families may not wish to institutionalize their frail elderly for various reasons:
      1. Guilt
      2. Previous promises "never" to institutionalize
      3. Fear of the unknown in institutional settings

4. Personal sense of satisfaction and reward; family honor
5. Cultural norms
6. Dependence on elder's resources; greed
7. Pressure from other family members
8. Gradual increase in required degree of caregiving and support
9. Strength of family relationships—caregiving may not be a "burden"

III. **An Approach**
   A. Women who become caretakers should be encouraged to:
      1. Find back-up caregivers for respite, vacations—get other family members involved
      2. Be careful not to neglect their own diet, exercise, medical problems, health care visits, family needs
      3. Participate in support groups for caregivers
      4. Be aware of and seek support and counseling for signs of stress, depression, and burnout
      5. Identify appropriate community resources
      6. Ask questions and get as much information as possible about such issues as the elder's condition, recommendations, and prognosis
   B. Physicians caring for women in the "sandwich generation" should be alert to insidious symptoms of depression, anxiety and fatigue and be aware of the influence of long-standing family conflicts, fear of inheriting some aging condition (e.g., Alzheimer's disease), and guilt
      1. May be helpful in identifying support services in the local community
      2. May give "permission" to such patients to request, seek, and accept help when needed and not to feel guilt about needing to tend to their own health and personal needs
      3. May encourage awareness of signs of family stress, such as marital discord, loss of intimacy, disruptive or other worrisome childhood behavior
      4. May encourage healthy lifestyle: diet, exercise, avoidance of drugs and tobacco, appropriate use of alcohol
      5. Must be aware of potential for elder abuse, neglect, or financial exploitation by family members
      6. Should be aware of typical family responses to the elder's physical or mental deterioration: denial, overinvolvement, anger, guilt, acceptance
   C. Public policy should be influenced to assist in-home caregivers as appropriate to sustain quality of life for the aging relative and caregiver alike
      1. New federal Family Medical Leave Act allows some employer support for employees needing time off to care for sick family members
      2. Increasing numbers of employers are recognizing the need for workplace assistance to employees providing care to family members (e.g., cafeteria benefit plans with options for respite care, day care, flexible working hours, emergency elder care)
   D. Resources
      1. Children of Aging Parents (CAPS): 1-800-227-7294
      2. Well Spouse Foundation: 1-800-838-0879
      3. National Family Caregivers Association: 1-800-896-3650
      4. Family Caregiver Alliance: (415) 434-3388
      5. American Association of Retired Persons: (202) 434-2277
      6. Eldercare Locator—Federal Administration on Aging: 1-800-677-1116

SUGGESTED READING

1. Bergen R: Expanding options in the long-term care of our elderly. Caring Mag March:66–68, 1992.
2. Eubanks P: Hospitals face the challenge of "sandwich generation" employees. Hospitals 65:60–62, 1991.
3. Kiecolt-Glaser JK, Glaser F, Shuttleworth EC, et al: Chronic stress and immunity in family caregivers of Alzheimer's disease victims. Psychosom Med 49:523–535, 1987.
4. King AC, Brassington G: Enhancing physical and psychological functioning in older family caregivers: The role of regular physical activity. Ann Behav Med 19:91–100, 1997.
5. Schulz R, Newsom J, Mittelmark M, et al: Health effects of caregiving: The caregiver health effects study. Ann Behav Med 19:110–116, 1997.

17. Growing Older

Jane L. Murray, M.D., and
Gary E. Bachman, M.S.S.W., L.S.C.S.W.

I. **The Issues**
Evidence suggests that women do not adequately plan for retirement, and may discover financial inadequacies as retirement approaches. Loneliness and isolation are common companions of aging women, who typically outlive their spouses. Coping with solitude can be a major task of aging, especially in women. Serial losses of physical vigor, spouse and other loved ones, health status, and economic status are common with aging in America. Such loss provides a backdrop for the development of significant depression in the elderly.

II. **The Theory**
    A. **Health problems commonly missed in elderly**—depression, incontinence, nutritional deficits, hearing problems, vision problems, falls, undesirable drug effects of prescription medication, misuse or nonuse of prescription medication, cognitive decline and impaired memory, mistreatment, abuse, exploitation, substance abuse
    B. **Most older adults are reasonably healthy and independent**
        1. Only 5–7% of people over age 65 are in nursing home at any given time; vast majority are women, who tend to outlive men significantly
        2. Only 5% of elderly are homebound
        3. Fastest growing age group in America are people over 85 years (with women having longer life expectancy than men)
    C. **Successful aging**
        1. Ability to share distress with others
        2. Avoiding or minimizing depression
        3. Maintaining high levels of physical and mental activity
        4. Avoiding social isolation

III. **An Approach**
    A. **Be prepared for greater commitment of staff and time**, as older patients may take longer to undress and may not wish to do so until they know physician is about ready to see them. Also, elder patients may take longer to "tell their story" and benefit from patient, attentive listener. A full physical assessment is important, even if history takes longer than expected. Appropriate checklists to ensure complete evaluation may be helpful, and save time, and a series of appointments may be preferable to one extremely long session.
    B. **Perform age- and condition-appropriate health promotion, risk reduction, and disease screening** for aging patients (see Chapter 3 for health maintenance details in older women). Assess cognitive function, affective status, functional status, and perform appropriate history and physical exam with elderly, focusing especially on frequently missed areas.
    C. **Avoid introducing iatrogenic problems** by minimizing the use of drugs, simplifying drug regimens and using appropriate doses in elderly; providing careful patient education; keeping good records; using standardized assessment tools as needed.
    D. **Promote healthy aging behaviors** through preretirement counseling, encouraging the development of a large social network and hobbies, multiple interests, and physical activity
    E. **Talk with patients and families**, explaining diagnosis, procedures, prognosis; ask patient to repeat information to confirm understanding. Ask about the patient's personal interests and activities. Often simple inquiries lead toward conceptualization of the patient as an individual and enhances the physician's understanding of her functional and social capacity.
    F. **Be aware of patients' financial and insurance resources**, as many seniors live on fixed or predictable income that affects compliance and well-being. Medicare and most

supplemental insurance provides no coverage for prescriptions; assistive devices may not be covered or require prior approval from carrier. Acceptance of Medicare assignment is often the single most influential factor in patient's choice of a physician as accepting assignment reduces the financial burden on the patient and reduces confusion associated with filing claims, promotes understanding of billing and ultimately payment for services.

G. **Be aware of environmental barriers in office.** Walk around building and office, viewing it from perspective of frail elderly patient: Do doors open easily? Is room well lit? Does traffic "flow"? Does carpet interfere with walkers? Are rooms wheelchair-accessible? Are forms written in style, color, and size that are readable? Are chairs firm with straight backs and easy to get in and out of?

H. **Facilitate, encourage, and ensure continuity of care.** Many elderly patients place high value on their personal relationship with their physician. Also remember that physical illness is often preceded by emotional turmoil and that presenting complaints may mask psychosocial problems. Previous knowledge of the patient and family, i.e., continuity of care, in such instances may facilitate appropriate intervention.

I. **Try not to stereotype elder patients and remain attentive to:** substance abuse; depression and undiagnosed or untreated chronic mental illness; change in mental status and forgetfulness; hearing loss; weight loss and dental problems; environmental barriers in home; immobility; impairment of vision; sexual problems. Remember that while hypochondriacal complaints may mask underlying physical or emotional concerns, elderly patients may underreport disease and other specific problems unless specifically asked (see Table 1, Chapter 3).

J. **Touch patient to establish trusting relationship**

K. **Assess activities of daily living** (ADLs) (see Chapter 3)
   1. How did you get here today?
      (Access to transportation, social support, ambulation)
   2. Did you have difficulties scheduling this appointment?
      (Use of telephone, skill at complicated tasks, ability to remember and follow through on plans)
   3. Do you do your own shopping?
   4. Do you prepare your own meals? What do you eat?
   5. Any problems taking care of your home?
   6. Do you have access to and do your own laundry?
   7. Do you take any medications? Can you explain what they are for and how you are supposed to take them?
   8. Do you have problems making ends meet? Do you handle your own money and expenses?

L. **Evaluate mental status** to establish a baseline of functioning; be aware of literacy/educational level

M. **Encourage patient self-determination**
   1. Is there an advance health care directive (e.g., living will)?
   2. Is there an existing durable power of attorney for health care decisions? A desire for same?
   3. Are patient's desires and wishes known and documented in event of occurrence that may require one of these documents?

N. **Ask about factors or circumstances in home that raise concerns about patient's safety**
   1. Ask about issues of abuse, mistreatment, financial exploitation
      a. Does the patient feel threatened or unsafe?
      b. Have they been touched in way that makes them uncomfortable?
   2. Ask about friends or family to whom patient can turn for help
      a. Would patient feel comfortable asking for help if needed?
   3. Physicians should be familiar with community resources, such as local Area Agency on Aging, State Division of Aging, Adult Protective Services, and advise patient to call physicians if help needed
   4. Office staff should be aware of basic community resources and encourage them to share concerns that may arise from their interactions with patient

SUGGESTED READING

1. Harris MB: Growing old gracefully: Age concealment and gender. J Gerontol 49:149–158, 1994.
2. Murray JL: Health maintenance. Prim Care 16:289, 1989.
3. Perkins K: Psychosocial implications of women and retirement. Soc Work 37:526–532, 1992.
4. Rockwood K, Silvius JL, Fox RA: Comprehensive geriatric assessment. Postgrad Med 103:247–264, 1998.
5. Sorenson KD: To grow old: From a socio-medical epidemiological intervention study among old citizens of Copenhagen. Dan Med Bull 39:211–213, 1992.
6. Tombaugh TN, McIntyre NJ: The mini-mental state examination—a comprehensive review. J Am Geriatr Soc 40:922–935, 1992.

18. Special Populations

Timothy P. Daaleman, D.O.

I. **The Issues**

Women with either physical or mental disabilities present a special challenge to the generalist physician. These patients have historically been managed in an institutional setting with a multi-specialty approach to their care. Recently there has been a shift in the locus of their care to the community setting, with an emphasis on integration into the community. The primary care physician will take on a greater role as the provider of the majority of medical services to these patients.

II. **The Theory**

  A. **Mental and developmental disability**

   1. There are many etiologies of mental or developmental disability in women; Down syndrome, cerebral palsy, autism, congenital anomalies, schizophrenia, mental retardation, mood disorders, substance abuse.
   2. The mentally or developmentally disabled have **higher incidences of diseases that go either undetected or untreated**
   3. There is a **greater prevalence of chronic disease and a higher proportion of multiple medical problems** among these women. The major prevalence of conditions by system includes neurologic, ophthalmologic, dermatologic, psychiatric-emotional, and musculoskeletal. Seizure disorders are the most frequently cited problem.
   4. These populations are heavily dependent on publicly financed health programs since the disabled are considered to be high users of services by most insurers
   5. A majority of these women require home health services or are involved with community-based resources

  B. **Physical disability**

   1. There are several causes to physical disability in women: paralysis (including hemiplegia, paraplegia, and spinal injuries), multiple sclerosis, spina bifida, polio and post-polio sequelae, juvenile and adult arthritis (osteoarthritis and rheumatoid arthritis), Guillain-Barré syndrome, unspecified neuromuscular disorders
   2. Most physically disabled women are able to live independently with little or no assistance in their activities of daily living
   3. These women are generally involved in fulfilling relationships and remain active in their roles as mothers, wives, and significant others

III. **An Approach**

The health care needs of the physically or mentally disabled woman can be managed by the generalist physician. The successful management of these patients incorporates four perspectives in a comprehensive approach; reproductive health issues, well maintenance and preventive care, coordination of care, the role of the caretaker.

  A. **Reproductive health issues**

   1. **Contraception**

a. **Mentally disabled**

Contraception and the prevention of sexually transmitted disease (STD) remain a significant challenge in the mentally handicapped female. Women with chronic mental illness are particularly vulnerable to STDs and AIDS.

  i. Oral contraceptives are effective, although many patients cannot swallow pills and caretakers must be relied on to monitor compliance

  ii. Barrier methods (condoms, diaphragms, sponges) provide some measure of protection against STDs; however they require significant amount of manual dexterity, comprehension, motivation, and partner compliance.

  iii. Intrauterine devices require little post-placement intervention, yet can result in increased menstrual flow, dysmenorrhea, and greater risks of infection

  iv. Injectable progesterone agents may be best suited for the mentally disabled female; depo-medroxyprogesterone (150 mg every 3 months) or Norplant are safe, efficacious, and practical modalities; several side effects, particularly depressive mood swings, and weight gain, should be considered prior to implementation.

  v. Surgical intervention (tubal ligation or hysterectomy) remains as a consideration for the severely mentally impaired; ethical issues which include patient autonomy and informed consent should be addressed and clarified by committee review.

b. **Physically disabled**

Women with physical deformities, paralysis, or impaired motor dysfunction are not routinely offered contraceptive counseling. Those disabled after menarche are less likely to be satisfied with the contraceptive method or counseling they receive than those disabled prior to menarche.

  i. Contraceptive counseling needs to be specific to the physical disability and reasonable for the level of sexual activity; periodic reassessment is recommended.

  ii. Oral contraceptives are favored due to their safety, efficacy, and ease of use

  iii. Partner-dependent methods (condoms, vasectomy) and sterilization (tubal ligation, hysterectomy) are reasonable choices among women in sustained relationships

  iv. Methods that require physical dexterity (diaphragm, use of inserter, vaginal foam/gel) may be difficult for these women to use

2. **Sexuality**

a. **Mentally disabled**

Educational programs for both the disabled and their caretakers should be directed toward improving social behavior, enhancing self-respect, and facilitating communication skills. These multidisciplinary (social workers, health educators, physicians) programs should be capable of providing group and individual counseling.

  i. Parents or caretakers of the mentally handicapped tend to be very protective and restrictive of any expression of sexuality by their children; counseling within a caretaker group should focus on gaining an understanding of their charges as sexual beings, on improving communication skills regarding developmental sexuality, and on establishing reasonable goals.

  ii. Counseling within the patient group should promote an understanding of one's own sexual identity and development, and on learning appropriate social behavior (i.e., the concept of public versus private body parts); role playing, visual aids, and group discussions can facilitate the presentation of sexuality as part of normal growth and development.

  iii. Sexual abuse is a significant problem, especially for the mildly disabled, due to their passive, obedient, and oftentimes affectionate behavior; counseling sessions within both the caretaker and patient group should focus on identification and avoidance of situations that may lead to sexual abuse.

  iv. Education and counseling for the severely mentally disabled is best done on an individual basis with a focus on teaching personal hygiene, controlling unacceptable public behavior, and avoiding self-abuse

v. Menstrual hygiene can cause problems for patients and their caretakers; behavioral modification programs and injectable progesterone agents (Depo-Provera) have been successful in the management of menstruation; low-dose oral contraceptives and hysterectomy are also alternatives.

b. **Physically disabled**

Many disabled women receive little or no information regarding their sexuality. This may be due to a discomfort level with discussions involving sexuality by both providers and patients. Health care providers need to be both comfortable and knowledgeable regarding both the medical and psychosexual aspects of disability.

i. A clear explanation of the anatomic and physiologic aspects of reproductive medicine can assist patients in understanding their own physical capabilities and limitations

ii. Counseling with these patients should: promote communication skills in both the patient and significant other, develop an appreciation of the plurality of noncoital, physical, and nonphysical means of expression; cultivate a forum where issues of sexuality (i.e., masturbation, homosexuality) can be discussed; and discuss the prevention and treatment of sexually transmitted diseases.

iii. Issues regarding fertility, pregnancy, and parenting need to be raised and clarified in disabled women of reproductive age

B. **Well maintenance and preventive care**

Both physically and mentally disabled women require care that is comprehensive, periodic, and longitudinal. Screening for unrecognized disorders is essential since these women are at a higher risk for chronic health problems.

1. **Detailed and comprehensive history** and physical is recommended on all new patients

2. List of all concurrent providers and old medical records should be obtained and reviewed

3. Problem list should be generated with medication information listed

4. **Complete physical examination**, including a breast and pelvic examination, should be performed

5. In patients where pelvic examinations are difficult, pelvic sonography or a virginal speculum may be options

6. Sedation has been used to assist in pelvic exams in women with severe mental disabilities; however, ethical issues and the clinical importance of the exam need to be assessed prior to the use of anesthesia.

7. **Papanicolaou smears** should be obtained in those patients with abnormal bleeding, those over 30, and women who are sexually active; the frequency of Papanicolaou smears should be directed by established guidelines (ACOG, ACS).

8. **Breast self-examinations**, annual breast examinations, and mammography remain important screening tools; in those patients who cannot perform monthly breast examinations, a chaperoned caretaker may be an alternative in the high-risk female.

9. The **immunization status** of each patient should be reviewed and updated

10. Patients who are involved in community living settings should be periodically screened (PPD, chest x-ray) for tuberculosis

11. Women with **mental or developmental disabilities** should be screened for diabetes mellitus, hypertension, hypo- and hyperthyroidism, anemia, deafness, hepatitis, mood disorders, and arthritis

12. Women with **physical disabilities** occasionally have indwelling catheters or require self-catheterization and are at risk for urinary tract infections and disseminated sepsis; these patients may have alternating periods of bacteriuria and sterile urine; although the cost-effectiveness of screening asymptomatic women remains unclear, all symptomatic episodes of infection should be treated.

13. In addition, the physically disabled should be routinely assessed for decubitus ulcers, depression, and problems with motor or sensory function (i.e., spasticity)

C. **Coordination of care**

The primary care physician must assume multiple roles and responsibilities in the care of the mentally and physically disabled. These women generally have had multiple levels of care and numerous providers, and are at risk for care that is fractured, duplicative, and discontinuous.

1. The generalist is responsible for the overall care of the patient; a complete list of all providers and their respective domains of care needs to be outlined and clarified with the patient and the providers.
2. The primary care physician should be the physician of first contact for acute and new, undifferentiated problems
3. Polypharmacy is a frequent problem with these women; a routine medication review that is discussed with the patient and documented in the medical record is essential.
4. Scheduled, periodic office visits can assist in health surveillance and disease prevention
5. As both advocate and educator, the physician can assist the patient in health care decisions (advanced directives, organ donation, etc.)

D. **Role of the caretaker**

The disabled are frequently dependent upon caretakers to assist them in activities of daily living. The caretaker can be a family member, a significant other, or a custodian who is charged with the responsibility of the disabled individual. Physicians must be cognizant of the central role that caretakers play.

1. In patients with communication limitations, caretakers are the primary historians
2. Caretakers have considerable stressors which have the potential of leading to abuse; the physician must be vigilant in assessing the effect of these stressors on the caretaker/patient relationship.
3. Caretaker anger toward the patient is occasionally directed at the physician or other provider; the physician's facility in handling these situations can clarify sources of anger and frustration, and diffuse potential litigation.
4. Caretakers are oftentimes responsible for initiating and monitoring therapy (i.e., medicine administration, diet); they should be included in the decisions concerning their charges.

SUGGESTED READINGS

1. Beange H, Bauman A: Caring for the developmentally disabled in the community. Aust Fam Phys 19:1555, 1558–1563, 1990.
2. Beckmann CR, Gittler M, Barzansky BM, Beckmann CA: Gynecologic health care of women with disabilities. Obstet Gyn 74:75–79, 1989.
3. Coverdale JH, Bayer TL, McCullough LB, Chervenak FA: Sexually transmitted disease prevention services for female chronically mentally ill patients. Comm Ment Health J 31:303–315, 1995.
4. Egan TM, Siegert RJ, Fairley NA: Use of hormonal contraceptives in an institutional setting: Reasons for use, consent, and safety in women with psychiatric and intellectual disabilities. N Z Med J 106:338–341, 1993.
5. Elkins TE, Gafford LS, Wilks CS, et al: A model clinic approach to the reproductive health concerns of the mentally handicapped. Obstet Gyn 68:185–188, 1986.
6. Hankoff LD, Damey PD: Contraceptive choices for behaviorally disordered women. Am J Obstet Gyn 168:1986–1989, 1993.
7. Huovinen KJL: Gynecological problems of mentally retarded women. Acta Obstet Gyn Scand 72:475–480, 1993.
8. Jones KP, Wild RA: Contraception for patients with psychiatric or medical problems. Am J Obstet Gyn 170:1575–1580, 1994.
9. Minihan PM., Dean DH: Meeting the needs for health services of persons with mental retardation living in the community. Am J Public Health 80:1043–1048, 1990.

19. Domestic Violence

Gary E. Bachman, M.S.S.W., L.S.C.S.W.

I. **The Issues**
   A. **Domestic violence has been described as the single most significant source of illness and injury to women in the U.S.**
      1. 2–4 million women are physically battered by husbands, former husbands, boyfriends, or lovers each year
      2. Adolescents are physically assaulted by a parent at rates approaching one in ten
      3. Approximately 1 million women seek emergency medical care for injuries that are directly the result of violence each year
      4. One in five women who present to emergency rooms has injuries inflicted by her partner
      5. Battered women further comprise a significant percentage of rape victims (30–50%), suicide attempts by women (26%), psychiatric patients, mothers of abused children (45%), alcoholics, and women who miscarry (20%)
      6. Rates of domestic violence toward women across the life span have been estimated from 25 to 50%
         a. The elderly face far greater risk of physical harm, intimidation and exploitation from family members than from strangers (80% vs. 20%)
         b. Women between 18 and 20 accounted for 42% of the "identified" victims of violence" in one emergency department study
      7. Leaving, or attempting to leave the relationship is the single greatest predictor of homicide
      8. In 85–95% of domestic homicides, police have been called to the home at least once in the preceding year. In more than half of these cases, they had been called five times or more.
   B. **The majority of battered women have sought medical attention for injuries resulting from violence at least once**
      1. Medical education has generally avoided the topic of domestic violence
      2. Treatment has tended to focus on injuries and complaints as isolated incidents rather than as symptoms of an ongoing risk
      3. Absence of recognition contributes to the erroneous belief that violence is relatively rare and that it is most often random and anonymous
      4. Most victims (68–75%) indicate they would have acknowledged the violence if their physicians had asked
      5. Spontaneous disclosure of violence, particularly to a health care provider, is relatively uncommon, primarily because of:
         a. Fear
         b. Guilt
         c. Embarrassment
      6. Explanations for injuries may be inconsistent with physical findings. This may be the ideal opportunity for the provider to express concern about domestic violence.
II. **The Theory**
   A. **Definitions**
      1. **Physical abuse** is slapping, hitting, punching, kicking, biting, pushing, shoving, choking, or the use of any instrument or weapon to inflict injury
      2. **Sexual abuse** is any forced or coerced sexual activity or performance
      3. **Psychological or emotional abuse** is often described by victims as feeling worse than physical abuse and has been compared to brainwashing in its effect. Examples include:
         a. Deprivation of sleep, food, clothing, or shelter
         b. Continuous criticism and undermining of self worth

      c. Unpredictability of response (for example, the woman may be awakened in middle of night, unsure whether to expect intimacy or unprovoked violence)

      d. Threats of violence toward victim, loved ones, property, or pets

      e. Destruction or damage to property or pets

      f. Forced isolation from family, friends, neighbors, and health care providers

      g. Withholding of affection

      h. Manipulation with changing demands, lies, and contradictions

      i. Interference with employment

   4. Laws in most states define "domestic" violence as that occurring between individuals who do currently or have ever resided together

B. Cycle of violence

   1. Women and children historically have been relegated to the status of private property; thus the physical consequences of family violence are viewed as "private matters." Spontaneous disclosure of violence is rare. Victims have often met with blame, disbelief and scorn.

      a. Laws that support the reporting, investigation, and prosecution of domestic violence now exist in most states

      b. The Catholic Bishops Council now advocates a policy that encourages recognition of **safety** concerns as primary in family counseling

      c. Shelters, counseling centers, and toll-free hotlines are now available as resources for women and potential helpers throughout the nation

   2. Violent relationships commonly demonstrate a **cyclical or spiraling pattern** that is typified by:

      a. A period of calm giving way to **increasing tension** that builds to an episode of violence that is inevitably followed by a period of restored calm

      b. **Repetition** of the cycles ranges from hours to months

      c. **Escalation** of the incidence and severity of violence is common as the pattern spirals

C. Physical indicators of violence

   1. The most frequent physical injuries are to the **head** and **neck**:

a. Bruises	g. Fractured jaw
b. Abrasions	h. Broken nose
c. Strangle marks	i. Pulled hair
d. Black eye	j. Permanent hearing loss
e. Fractured orbital ridge	k. Facial lacerations
f. Eye damage	

   2. Injuries consistent with **blunt trauma to the trunk** are almost as common:

a. Bruising of the breasts, abdomen, perineum	c. Bruised ribs
	d. Broken ribs
b. Broken collarbones	e. Internal hemorrhage

   3. **Multiple injuries, bilateral distribution, or injuries at different stages of healing**

   4. Abrasions consistent with "rug rash" may be evident

   5. **Injuries consistent with forced restraint.** Severe injuries to the extremities occur least often and are usually reflective of the victims' efforts to shield themselves or flee:

      a. Muscle strains

      b. "Crescent moon" shape of finger nail marks

      c. Spiral fractures

      d. Bruises reflecting image of a hand or other instrument

      e. Rope burns

   6. **Pregnancy** appears to be a period of great risk for the escalation of violence

      a. Evidence of old injuries not disclosed in history

      b. History of unexplained or repeated miscarriages

      c. Frequent "accidental" injuries

      d. Requests for termination of pregnancy

   7. **Intentional disfigurement**

      a. Cigarette burns

      b. Human bites

      c. Repeated lacerations

    d. Unusual injuries

    e. Burns or scalding from splashed liquids

  8. **Sexual assault or rape**

D. **Physical symptoms**—women who have been battered describe significantly more somatic concerns than women who have not. Domestic violence belongs on the differential diagnosis list when considering such presentations.

  1. **Headaches, back and rib pain** (chronic or acute)

    a. Presentation of pain that is vague or inconsistent

    b. Pain related to previous or undisclosed injuries

  2. **Gastrointestinal disturbances**—abdominal pain and discomfort have been strongly associated with history of sexual assault or abuse

  3. **Chronic pain** of any type has been strongly associated with history of prolonged sexual and/or physical abuse

  4. Physiologic concerns related to **anxiety and depression** may include:

    a. Weight loss

    b. Sleep disturbances

    c. Hyperventilation

    d. Numbness and "tingling" of extremities

    e. Palpitations

    f. Dizziness

    g. Malaise, generalized weakness

    h. Choking sensations

    i. Allergic skin reactions

    j. Difficulty with speech

    k. Tearfulness

  5. **Hearing loss** related to trauma

  6. **Cognitive impairment, confusion, or mental status changes**

E. **Behavioral and familial indicators**

  1. Psychiatric considerations

    a. **Posttraumatic stress disorder and acute stress disorders** as defined in the DSM-IV. Criteria i –iv must be present:

      i. Exposure to traumatic event or events in which the following factors were present

        (a) Death, or threatened death, or serious injury to self or others and

        (b) Experience of intense fear, helplessness, or horror in response to event

      ii. Persistent reexperience of a traumatic event (1 of the following)

        (a) Recurrent and intrusive recollections

        (b) Recurrent distressing dreams

        (c) Dissociative flashbacks

        (d) Intense emotional distress to events symbolic of or similar to past traumatic events

        (e) Physiologic reactivity to these symbolic or similar events

      iii. Persistent avoidance of associated stimuli and numbing of responses (3 of the following)

        (a) Avoidance of thoughts, feeling, or discussion of the trauma

        (b) Avoidance of people, places, and events that may provoke memories

        (c) Inability to recall important aspects of the trauma

        (d) Markedly diminished interest in significant activities

        (e) Detachment or estrangement

        (f) Restricted range of affect

        (g) Sense of foreshortened future

      iv. Persistent symptoms of increased stimulation (2 of the following)

        (a) Sleep disturbances

        (b) Irritability or explosive anger

        (c) Difficulty in concentrating

        (d) Hypervigilance

        (e) Exaggerated startle response

    b. Battered women have often been misdiagnosed psychiatrically. Common misdiagnoses include:

      i. Schizophrenia

      ii. Borderline personality

      iii. Antisocial personality

      iv. Dependent personality disorders

    c. **Suicidal thoughts**, gestures, or attempts
        i. The attempt may not reflect a desire to die but rather a desperate attempt to escape
        ii. Inquiry about suicidal risk should be made of all victims of violence
    d. **Alcohol and drug abuse**
        i. Shelters for battered women routinely do not accept women who are intoxicated or actively drinking or using drugs
        ii. Patients should be questioned about patterns of recreational drug and alcohol use
        iii. Referral or admission to substance abuse treatment or detoxification center if indicated
        iv. Requests for pain medications may suggest addiction or self-medication for undisclosed trauma

2. **Behavioral considerations**
    a. Victims may seem uncooperative or "noncompliant." Such behavior may be a very basic function of survival within their social circumstances.
        i. Inconsistent or unreliable historians
        ii. Shame or embarrassment about their circumstances
        iii. Evasive and untrusting about any inquiries
        iv. Impaired ability to trust may be the learned response to chronic victimization
    b. **Apprehension and fear**
        i. For their own lives
        ii. For lives of their children
        iii. Of rejection by friends, family, or helpers
        iv. Of emotionally hurting children
        v. Of legal process and possibly losing custody of their children
        vi. Of retaliation against friends, family, helpers, pets, and property
        vii. Of capacity for independence
        viii. About the spouse's safety
        ix. Of harassment and violence wherever they go
    c. Expressions of **guilt** for "causing" the violence or **responsibility** for failure of marriage
    d. **Denial** is common. Victims may try to minimize or normalize the violent event.
    e. **Thought disorganization or forgetfulness.** Early onset of organic brain syndromes.
    f. **Passivity, dependency, rigid adherence to traditional sex roles, and a broad sense of insecurity** results in:
        i. Social isolation
        ii. Lack of employment skills
        iii. Lack of access to financial resources
        iv. Lack of transportation
        v. Reluctance to speak in presence of partner
        vi. Ambivalence about taking concrete action
    g. **Low self-esteem** may be a response to:
        i. Constant ridicule and criticism that she is stupid, worthless, incompetent, a poor partner or a poor parent
        ii. Hopelessness at failure of previous attempt to seek help or escape
        iii. History of victimization that dates from childhood abuse and neglect or from previous relationships
    h. **Hope** that a partner will somehow change their behavior
    i. **Reluctance** to take interpersonal risks. Restricted disclosure may be the response to having been doubted, criticized, or even endangered by poorly guided good intentions of others.
    j. **Repressed anger:** Hostility may be misdirected toward potential helpers or "intruders," whose interventions may be perceived as a threat
    k. **Homicidal thoughts and gestures**

3. **Family risk factors** are common in homes where violence has been identified. The presence of multiple factors suggests a need to assess the potential for harm:

a. History of violence within family
b. History of violence in previous relationships
c. Rigid, stereotyped sex roles/expectations
d. Low self-esteem
e. Idealization of marriage
f. Exaggerated sense of personal responsibility for success of relationship
g. Child abuse
h. Witness of violence between parents
i. Abusive or neglectful of children
j. Rigid family boundaries
k. Inadequate parenting skills (role conflicts, inadequate education, unrealistic expectations of child)
l. "Special needs" children in home (hyperactive, handicapped, mentally retarded)
m. Blended families (children from previous relations)
n. Poor or dysfunctional communication skills (incongruent/irrelevant messages, blaming, placating, yelling, and screaming)
o. Social and emotional isolation from neighbors and extended family (language and / or cultural barriers)
p. Unreasonable or extreme jealousy (particularly when there is an identified target of the jealousy, regardless of validity)
q. Geographic isolation (rural location, lack of phone or transportation)
r. Involvement in illegal activities
s. Financial stress
t. Extremely dependent (financially or emotionally) on each other
u. Alcohol or drug abuse
v. Pregnancy (particularly when unwanted or unplanned)
w. Repeated runaway episodes by children in family
x. Presence of physically dependent/cognitively impaired adult or elder
y. Separation or divorce

F. **Impact on provider behavior.** The physician's reactions to a patient may be useful diagnostic tools. When the physician consistently pursues or distances self from a patient, it is a signal that "a problem exists." Compassion and empathy are valuable tools. They are often more efficient if the physician can maintain objectivity. Be conscious of:

1. **Anger**
   a. At the assailant who inflicted harm
   b. At the victim for having allowed or provoked violence
   c. At "the system" that has not effectively intervened
   d. At a culture that tolerates such behavior
   e. At self for feeling angry
2. **Helplessness and frustration** based on past experience with victims
   a. Rebuffed offers of help
   b. Refusal of patients to admit cause of injury in spite of obvious signs
   c. Failure of patients to follow through on promises to get help
   d. Recurrence of injuries
   e. Increasing severity of injuries
   f. Victim's acceptance of responsibility for violence
   g. Doubt of victim's sincerity
   h. Failure of legal or social services to provide desired assistance
3. **Labeling of patients** as
   a. "Difficult" to diagnose with vague or changing complaints
   b. "Hysterical"—exaggerated behavioral response
   c. "Troublemakers"—always complaining, never satisfied,
   d. "Noncompliant"—not doing what the provider wants
4. **Fear** of
   a. Making things worse
   b. Becoming a victim

5. **Concerns**
   a. Having to "take sides" (particularly when both partners are one's patients)
   b. The risk of chasing away patient or family
   c. Angering the patient
   d. Commitment of time (fiscal responsibility) and legal implications
      i. In exam room
      ii. In court as a witness in civil or criminal case
      iii. In court as a defendant in civil case
6. **Personal thoughts or experiences** with violence as victim, witness, or even as batterer may emerge
   a. Personal vulnerability
   b. Anger
   c. Guilt
   d. Remorse
   e. Responsibility for rescue
7. Guilt for not having recognized the signs earlier
8. **Uncertainty** about what to do next

III. An Approach
A. Recognition
1. Diagnosis is generally determined 85% by history, 10% by physical exam, and 5% by laboratory tests
2. Patient's chart should be reviewed before entering the room. Look for patterns of behavior or injury that may be overlooked as isolated events. Pertinent history may have been previously obtained.
3. All patients, both male and female, should be asked about threats to their safety
   a. Inquiry is the single most valuable tool in discovering the presence of domestic violence
   b. The acronym **SAFE** is both easy to remember and gets to the basic issues that are common to most violent relationships. It is also useful for addressing other risk reduction issues, such as work and home safety.
      i. **S**: Do you feel safe in your home, relationships, work, and/or school? (Homicide is the number one cause of workplace fatalities.) Any particular stressors in your life?
      ii. **A**: Have you ever felt abused in a relationship? Are you ever afraid that you might be abused in a relationship? Are you ever concerned that someone (parent, child, sibling, friend) is being abused? How do you handle anger?
      iii. **F**: Do you have friends or family to turn to for support? Do you or your partner come from families where there is a history of violence?
      iv. **E**: What would you and your family do in an emergency? Have you thought about what you might need in order to escape from the house or what to do in a fire, tornado, or other emergency? Do your children know where to go and who to call for help? And would they do it?
   c. In incidents where violence is described, particularly when it is recent or ongoing, a risk assessment must be made and shared with the patient. Ask very specific questions to clarify any concerns.
4. **Genograms**
   a. Useful tool for normalizing the review of family history and health issues
   b. May reveal patterns of family interaction associated with increased risk
5. **Healthy suspicions:** assume all injures are non-accidental until demonstrated otherwise
6. Nursing and other support staff should:
   a. Learn warning signs of domestic violence (including child and elder abuse, neglect and mistreatment)
   b. Be aware of community resources
   c. Be familiar with laws regarding confidentiality, mandated reporting, and domestic violence
   d. Practice interpersonal and business communication skills to reduce staff's exposure to violence

7. Physicians should be receptive to input from staff about observations of patients and families
8. Establish relationships with community resources or shelters who may be willing to respond immediately to calls for assistance.

B. **Intervention**
1. Provide assurances of **privacy, safety, and comfort** in which patients may feel secure in sharing their circumstances
    a. Interview and examine in private room. Avoid treatment rooms separated only by curtains.
    b. Respect personal space and modesty. Limit the number of staff involved.
    c. limit any unnecessary touching as it may be unwelcome
    d. Inform patients of treatment options and plans. Invite questions.
    e. Model positive styles of communication. Sit down. Talk slowly, clearly, and calmly. Be patient.
2. If the patient is accompanied by her partner:
    a. Observe interactions between partners
    b. Assess temperament of each
    c. Maintain nonjudgmental attitude toward both partners
    d. The abusive partner who accompanies his spouse to the clinic is likely to have moved into the calm stage of the cycle. He may be feeling extremely guilty and remorseful. Acknowledge these appropriate feelings and behaviors.
    e. Facilitate cooperation with specific concrete requests:
        i. "I'm going to perform my physical evaluation now. I need you to step out of the room. I'll let you know when we are done."
    f. Most batterers have a very clear awareness of who they can get away with hitting and who they cannot
    g. **If violence is threatened or emerges, or if the physician or staff feel threatened, contact law enforcement immediately**
        i. Do not threaten this action. Take action or do not bring it up. The immediate safety of staff and patients supersedes matters of confidentiality.
        ii. Facilitate safety of patients and staff by evacuation if necessary
3. **Assure confidentiality.** The concept of confidentiality may need to be explained.
4. Use specific and common descriptive language
    a. A hematoma is a bruise
    b. A laceration is a cut
    c. Ask specific questions to clarify responses: "Did someone hit you here?"
5. Share your suspicions or concerns with the patient
6. Be aware of the factors that may influence the victim's decision to remain in a dangerous situation
    a. Acknowledge issues raised by the patient, i.e., fear, guilt, confusion
    b. Separation and divorce are the events most strongly associated with homicide
7. Ask the patient what she would like to do about the violence
8. Offer reassurance of willingness to work with the patient:
    a. Become familiar with the issues of violence, abuse, and victimization
    b. Acknowledge that decisions about what to do remain patients
    c. Affirm that you will not abandon or refuse care based on a decision either to leave or remain in the relationship
9. **Education**
    a. Educate patients about cyclical behavior in relationships and particularly about the spiraling cycle of violence
        i. Educate patients to anticipate and identify warning signs that precede episodes of violence
    b. Questions that may encourage insight include:
        i. "How has this situation changed over the years?"
        ii. "What does the future hold for you?"
        iii. "How is the violence affecting your children?"
    c. How to safely access community resources

      i. Invite resource staff to meet with patients
      ii. Patient should memorize important phone numbers or hide them
      iii. Patient education materials on domestic violence are best left in a location where it is unlikely to be found by an abusive partner

  d. Encourage patient to make plans for an emergency. Ask:
      i. Under what circumstances would she decide to leave?
      ii. How would she do it?
      iii. Where would she go?
      iv. What would she need to take with her? (cash, identification, clothing, etc.)

10. **Facilitate continuity**
  a. Encourage patient to return to see you, or link her with a provider who is sensitive to the issue of violence
  b. Obtain signed "release of information" for records from other physicians or facilities

C. **Risk assessment and plan for follow-up.** Most urban communities and an increasing number of rural areas have established **battered women's hotlines and shelters**. Become familiar with local community resources. A counselor or advocate may be available to meet with patients immediately.

1. Ask, "Are you safe tonight?"
2. Assess risk for homicide and suicide and share your assessment with the patient. Factors associated with increased risk:
  a. Separation and divorce
  b. Revelation that previous "accidental injuries" resulted from intentional acts
  c. Absence of or loss of boundaries between private and public display of violence
  d. Expressed threats to kill, particularly when there is access to weapons or a specific plan
  e. Use of a weapon to threaten
  f. Batterer previously hit only when drinking, now batters when he is sober
  g. Batterer fears showing weakness
  h. Excessive jealousy, particularly with identified third party
  i. Batterer's increased use of alcohol/drugs
  j. Batterer's unpredictable mood swings and behavior
  k. Recent or sudden unemployment, serious illness, or death in the family
  l. law enforcement or social agencies are involved in or investigating allegations of violence or neglect
3. A written history and physical exam should reflect accurately any information revealed about presence or absence of violence in patient's past and present. Record in the medical record:
  a. Date, time, and place of the exam
  b. What you were told about the incident and how the injuries were sustained
  c. Description of all injuries. Use a body map. Differentiate evidence of old or healing injuries from acute injuries.
  d. If sexual assault has been alleged, gather evidence in accordance with state laws. This may best be referred to an emergency department where staff may be more familiar with the process and have access to sealed "sexual assault evidence collection kits."
  e. Document that safety was assessed (for children in the home as well as for the patient) and what referrals and recommendations for follow-up were offered
4. **Collaboration.** Identify and use local resources:
  a. Battered women's shelter
  b. Law enforcement (many jurisdictions now enforce "domestic violence" laws that include mandated arrest of the assailant.)
  c. Hospital social work staff
  d. Child protection and welfare agencies
  e. Adult protective services (in cases of elder abuse)
  f. Community mental health centers
  g. Clergy
  h. County attorney (for protective orders)

5. Be aware of the **state laws** about the reporting of certain injuries or mechanisms of injury
6. Maintain a **problem list** in patient charts
   a. Identify domestic violence as a medical problem
   b. Note any concerns about violence that may have surfaced on reflection after the patient has already left
   c. Note safety issues that may warrant follow up
   d. Problem lists are particularly valuable where others may provide subsequent care
7. **Continuity** is important for successful and effective intervention
   a. Have a long-term view of success. There is no quick fix.
   b. Follow up on concerns identified in the problem list
   c. Be supportive and encouraging. Remain available
   d. **Relapse and setbacks are common**
   e. The choice to take or leave any particular recommendation at any particular time, ultimately remains the patients
   f. Ask every patient at every visit if they have concerns for their SAFEty.

SUGGESTED READINGS

1. American Medical Association. Diagnostic and Treatment Guidelines on Domestic Violence. Pamphlet #AA:22-406 20M. Chicago, American Medical Association, 1992.
2. Bolin L, Elliott B: Physician detection of family violence: Do buttons worn by doctors generate conversations about domestic violence? Minn Med 79:42–45, 1996.
3. Burge S: Violence against women as a health care issue. Fam Med 21:368–373, 1989.
4. Brennan SJ, Bradshaw RD, Hamlin ER, et al: Spouse abuse: A physicians guide to the identification, diagnosis, and management in the uniformed services. Military Med 164:30–36, 1999.
5. Caralis PV, Musialowski R: Women's experiences with domestic violence and their attitudes and expectations regarding medical care of abuse victims. South Med J 90:1075–1080, 1997.
6. Covington DL, Dalton VK, Diehl SJ, et al: Improving detection of violence among pregnant adolescents. J Adolesc Health 21:28–34, 1997.
7. Delahunta EA: Hidden trauma: The mostly missed diagnosis of domestic violence. Am J Emerg Med 13:74–76,1995.
8. Elliott BA, Johnson MM: Domestic violence in a primary care setting: Patterns and prevalence. Arch Fam Med 4:113–119, 1995.
9. Glander SS, Moore ML: The prevalence of domestic violence among women seeking abortion. Obstet Gynecol 91:1002–1006, 1998.
10. McAfee RE: Guidelines for the care of abused women: The least we can do. Home Healthcare Nursing 12:47–53, 1994.
11. McGrath ME, Hogan JW: A prevalence survey of abuse and screening for abuse in urgent care patients. Obstet Gynecol 91:511–514, 1998.
12. Mehta P, Dandrea LA: The battered woman. Am Fam Physician 37:193–199, 1988.
13. Muelleman RL, Lenaghan PA: Battered women: Injury locations and types. Ann Emerg Med 28:486–492, 1996.
14. Oriel KA, Fleminf MF: Screening men for partner violence in a primary care setting: A new strategy for detecting domestic violence. J Fam Pract 46:493–498, 1998.
15. Reid SA, Glasser M: Primary care physicians' recognition of and attitudes toward domestic violence. Acad Med 72:51–53, 1997.
16. Roberts GL, Lawrence JM: Domestic violence in the emergency department: Two case-control studies of victims. Gen Hosp Psychiatry 19:5–11, 1997.

20. Social, Cultural, and Behavioral Influences

Timothy P. Daaleman, D.O.

I. The Issues

Cultural, socioeconomic, and behavioral influences have a significant impact on health and disease. Primary care providers must recognize and be appreciative of these influences in their own patients and in the communities they serve. This sensitization requires an orientation toward medical care that transcends the traditional biomedical model, and often tests the limits of acceptance and tolerance in the generalist.

II. The Theory

A. The influence of culture

1. Culture, a concomitant of the human condition, is the product of assimilated values, behaviors, and experiences shared by a specific group. Various groups act as sources of reference for normative behavior, value systems, and interpretation of meaning for life events.
2. It is a common misassumption that culture is static and monolithic, and that behavioral norms are uniform. Education, income, religion, and locus are a few of the key social factors that create heterogeneity within specific groups. The process of acculturation by the individual is fluid and is influenced by the interplay of dominant and subcultural norms.

B. The biopsychosocial model

1. The biopsychosocial model was developed as an alternative approach to the biomedical model for the study of disease. As a traditional scientific model, the biomedical model involved a shared set of assumptions and rules about disease based on the scientific method. Disease was viewed as a deviation of the norm of quantifiable, biologic variables that were independent of social, behavioral, or psychological influences.
2. The biopsychosocial model integrates biomedical and psychosocial perspectives in a general systems approach. This orientation conceptualizes the person as being comprised of multiple, interconnected dimensions (i.e., molecules, cells, organisms, persons, families, society, biosphere). Since systems theory holds that all dimensions or levels of organization are linked to each other, change in one dimension affects change in the others.
3. Disease can be due to a multiplicity of causes and can affect various dimensions within the person
4. The physician must accept the responsibility to evaluate the patient's presenting problem by using his or her professional knowledge base and skill level to examine the social, psychological, and biologic determinants of the problem

C. Culture and the experience of illness

1. Illness has been defined as the patient's perception, experience, expression, and pattern of coping with symptoms, while disease is the way health care providers view symptomatology in a biomedical context
2. An active process of selection and interpretation frames the experience of illness in a cultural milieu
3. Both patients and providers are grounded in culture belief systems regarding illness and health and are active coparticipants in the process

III. An Approach

The generalist physician recognizes the cultural, socioeconomic and behavioral aspects and determinants of health and disease. The ability to accept and conceptualize the perspective of patients, and the social and cultural groups in which they dwell, is facilitated by effective communication skills, and a self awareness of one's own attitudes and value systems regarding well-being, and illness. Cultural, socioeconomic, and behavioral influences in this setting can be clarified by examining four domains: access to care, resource use and provision, perceptions of health and disease, and cultural epidemiology.

A. **Access to care**
   Financial and non financial boundaries affect the ability of patients to enter into and continue in the health care delivery system
   1. **Financial boundaries**
      a. Since the enactment of the Medicaid program, the poor use physicians' services at rates that are comparable to non indigent patients; the uninsured poor, however, have use rates that continue to lag behind all other populations.
      b. Patients that are covered by Medicaid do not have the same level of access to physicians in private practice, due to a diminishing participation among providers; the poor continue to rely on institutional care (clinics, emergency departments).
      c. The reliance on non–office-based care increases the risk of fragmented care, and results in less preventive and primary care, and higher costs to the system
      d. The generalist should be cognizant of a patient's financial constraints and influences regarding his/her care; the use of laboratory and radiographic studies, pharmaceuticals, and diagnostic and therapeutic interventions may need to be reassessed.
   2. **Non-financial boundaries**
      a. The health care system is oriented around a western biomedical model, and entry into the system is facilitated by a familiarity with that model; cultural and language differences are two factors which can impede access and negotiation of the system.
      b. Physicians should take an ethnographic approach when encountering patients with cultural or language differences; in many instances disclosure of personal information (including current symptoms or health history) by the patient is not always appropriate when a new provider is met.
      c. The use of interpreters and a sufficient allotment of time during patient encounters can facilitate language and cultural differences between providers and patients
      d. Transportation, child care, and employment responsibilities are a few additional factors that can affect access to care
B. **Resource use and provision**
   The decision to use medical resources is dependent upon the availability and accessibility of those and other non-medical resources
   1. **Providers of care**
      a. Medical pluralism and non-allopathic medicine is practiced and accepted among many populations
      b. Self-care practices are a predominant option for many women, even in areas where western allopathic services are available
      c. Different resources are used either alternatively for different ailments and/or multiple resources can be used at the same time for one problem
      d. Women may rely on different providers (e.g., midwives, herbalists, chiropractors) for different areas of their health care; the primary care physician should assess and document all providers of care for his or her patient; in addition, domains of health care influence and responsibility should be clarified.
   2. **Support structures**
      a. Decision making, regarding appropriate treatment can be dependent on multiple, sometimes conflicting reference groups (e.g., family, community, religious or faith affiliations.)
      b. Various networks can: make available financial resources, provide emotional and psychological support, promote or inhibit lifestyle choices that affect health and well-being, and delay or encourage access to health care
      c. The family and other larger cultural groups can influence the quality of the therapeutic process by the way these groups respond to illness in their members
      d. Established clinical models (genogram, family APGAR) can be used to assess the structure and function of patients in relation to their support structures
C. **Perceptions of health and disease**
   Patients do not define illness and well-being through their symptoms alone, but by an active process of selection and interpretation of their symptoms

1. **Illness and health behavior**
   a. Patient can enter into a sick role if: a physician confirms that the patient is ill; the family, or larger cultural reference group defines the patient as being ill.
   b. As a result of adopting the sick role, the individual is exempt from routine obligations (e.g., work, social responsibilities) and must accept certain responsibilities (e.g., expectation to cooperate with others to get well)
   c. The physician may be asked to arbitrate and legitimize a patient's adoption of the sick role and concomitantly support the illness behavior
   d. The assignment of a specific diagnosis by the physician can carry non medical repercussions for both patient and the larger community; providers should be cognizant of the social, ethnic, and religious meanings with disease processes that involve reproductive health, infectious disease, and mental health.
   e. There are multiple factors that cause people to exhibit illness behavior: the individual's ability to recognize the symptoms; the number, persistence, and perceived seriousness of the symptoms; the extent of social and physical disability resulting from the symptoms; the availability of medical and non medical resources.
   f. Several triggers may affect the decision of patient to seek care: symptoms that interfere with a valued social activity (e.g., work); an interpersonal crisis that draws attention to the symptoms; others sanction or encourage the patient to seek care; symptoms are perceived as threatening in nature.
   g. The concept of wellness defines not only the absence of disease, but an active process in which patients seek to improve their health; wellness promotion emphasizes that there are multiple aspects of a person's lifestyle that affect well-being, and tends to focus on healthy ways of living.
   h. The generalist must learn to understand and incorporate the health belief systems of these patients into his/her approach to care
   i. Physicians may encounter health beliefs or practices that are harmful or detrimental to well-being; the establishment and maintenance of an effective, longitudinal patient–physician relationship is critical to facilitating this dilemma.
      i. The provider should seek to clarify practices/beliefs that are harmful versus practices/beliefs that are culturally or socially unacceptable
      ii. Practices/beliefs that are detrimental should be identified to the patient and reflected in the larger social context (i.e., family, community); a family or community member may be helpful in this process.
      iii. If an impasse is reached, the provider should negotiate and clearly document his/her responsibilities and domains of care with the patient
2. **Sources of information**
   a. There are multiple factors that influence patients' interpretation of symptoms and their responses to them; the conceptualization of illness and illness behavior is made within a learned cultural context.
   b. Most illness behaviors are the result of cultural and social conditioning that begins in childhood
   c. The generalist should seek to identify the significant cultural/ethnic, socioeconomic, and religious/faith influences regarding medical and health care in their patients
   d. A respected family or community member (folk healer, clergy), or reference text or doctrine (Torah, Koran), can give insight to these factors
   e. The poor are exposed to less information about disease than those with higher socioeconomic status
   f. Providers can gain a greater understanding into patient perspectives by framing these influences around issues of preventive health care, acute and emergent problems, chronic medical problems, reproductive health issues, and mental health
D. **Cultural epidemiology**
   Providers should be familiar with the prevalence and disease pattern of the their patients in the context of the communities they dwell. By examining cultural, ethnic, religious, and socioeconomic sets of beliefs and behaviors, the generalist can anticipate potential patterns of disease and screen accordingly.

1. **Socioeconomic factors**
   a. Patients in the lower socioeconomic strata access health care through public or institutional gateways, and are usually more seriously ill than entrees who used private means
   b. Lack of health information, limited resources, and patient fears regarding public health care providers all contribute to a delay in treatment
   c. The poor have higher rates of chronic illness (diabetes mellitus, hypertension) that are more severe, uncontrolled, and result in greater incidences of complications
   d. Primary care providers should optimize encounters with these patients by practicing preventive health care (e.g., blood pressure checks) and routine gynecologic care (e.g., Papanicolaou smears, mammography)
   e. The homeless are a population that has increased risk factors for tobaccoism, drug and alcohol abuse, violence, and environmental hazards; many disorders that can be prevented in a domiciled population are exacerbated due to conditions of homelessness.
   f. Homeless women are often single mothers or heads of households
2. **Religious factors**
   a. Religious prescriptions or proscriptions affect the health practices of many patients; abstention from meat, alcohol, stimulants, tobacco, and the practice of meditation have direct outcomes on well-being.
   b. Some religious traditions have specific guidelines and prohibitions in areas of contraception and reproductive health
   c. There is a growing interest in the relationship between clergy, religious institutions, and medical practice in promoting the therapeutic process
3. **Cultural and ethnic factors**
   a. Many practices that are linked to health care outcomes are encouraged or prohibited within a given cultural or ethnic context
   b. Lifestyle or culturally influenced behavior is a major determinant of community health
   c. The physical environment (e.g., urban vs. rural), social climate (e.g., violence), and patterns of human relationship (e.g., family, community) need to be assessed to examine the effects of culture on parameters of health and disease.

SUGGESTED READING

1. Barker JC: Cultural diversity—changing the context of medical practice. West J Med 157:248–254, 1992.
2. Burkett GL: Culture, illness, and the biopsychosocial factors in disease etiology. Fam Med 23:287–91, 1991.
3. Cassel J: An epidemiological perspective of psychosocial factors in disease etiology. Am J Public Health 64:1040–1043, 1974.
4. DiMatteo MR: Social Psychology and Medicine. Cambridge, MA, Oelgeschlager, Gunn & Hain, 1982.
5. Engle GL: The need for a new medical model: A challenge for biomedicine. Science 196:129–136, 1977.
6. Heggenhougen HK, Shore L: Cultural components of behavioral epidemiology: Implications for primary health care. Soc Sci Med 22:1235–1245, 1986.
7. Henderson GE, King NMP, Strauss RP, et al (eds): The Social Medicine Reader. Durham, NC, Duke University, 1997.
8. Hodnicki DR, Horner SD, Boyle S: Women's perspective of homelessness. Public Health Nurs 9:257–262, 1992.
9. Leven JS, Schiller PL: Is there a religious factor in health? J Religion Health 26:9–36, 1987.
10. Rowland D, Salganicoff A: Commentary. Lessons from Medicaid: Improving access to office-based physician care for the low-income population. Am J Public Health 84:550–552, 1994.
11. Vredevoe DL, Brecht M, Shuler P, Woo M: Risk factors for disease in a homeless population. Public Health Nurs 9:263–269, 1992.
12. Wedding D: Behavior and Medicine, 2nd ed. St. Louis, MO, Mosby, 1995.

21. Gender Issues in Caring for Female Patients

Jane L. Murray, M.D.

I. **The Issues**
   A. **Male and female communication styles are often different** and pose challenges to different-gender physician–patient encounters
   B. Literature about **male/female physician differences in practice patterns and attitudes** reveals several differences
      1. Women more often work part time, in groups, in salaried positions, and in urban areas than men and overall work fewer hours per week
      2. Women physicians tend to see fewer patients, spend more time per patient, and care for a greater percentage of female patients than do men physicians
      3. Women physicians make less money but tend to be more satisfied with their incomes than men physicians
      4. Women make more gynecologic and reproductive health diagnoses and more diagnoses related to endocrine problems and psychosocial issues
      5. Women perform fewer complex procedures and feel less prepared in surgical areas
      6. Studies of medical students' attitudes toward caring for underserved populations reveal significant erosion in students' positive attitudes between the first and fourth years of medical school for men, but not for women
   C. **Gender disparities in clinical decision making** and medical research have recently been reported
      1. Evidence that women's complaints of dizziness, headache, back pain, chest pain, and fatigue are not evaluated and treated as aggressively as men's similar complaints
      2. Differences in treatment of serious illness, such as coronary artery disease, end-stage renal disease, and lung cancer reveal that male patients overall receive significant interventions (e.g., kidney transplants, open heart surgery) more frequently than women
      3. Hospitalized men receive more laboratory and radiologic procedures than do women, even after adjusting for potential confounders
      4. Research into women's health issues and inclusion of women in large studies have recently been emphasized at national level
   D. **Sexual harassment** of patients by physicians, particularly male physician/female patient incidents, has been topic of ethical discussion for generations; more recent evidence indicates sexual harassment of female physicians by male patients
      1. More than 75% of female physician respondents to recent survey indicated some experience with sexual harassment by male patients at some time during training or practice
II. **The Theory**
   A. **Men and women in U.S. grow up in quite different cultures**
      1. Men tend to have played in large groups as children, with winners and losers, elaborate rules, and clear hierarchy of power relationships
      2. Women tend to grow up playing in small groups or pairs, in games that did not involve winning and losing, and with communication and talk used to create intimacy and sense of belonging
   B. Because there are so many more women in medicine today (40% of all U.S. medical students are female), **patients now have choices about gender of physician**
      1. Female patients frequently report that they want physician who will listen to their story, understand them, and treat them in context of human, personal relationship
      2. They want care that is more patient-centered than doctor-centered
      3. Women are more likely to visit physician for problems related to reproductive health, family, and emotional concerns and vague symptoms. Such complaints and situations usually require trust between physician and patient, they are more time-consuming, they require empathetic listener, and they benefit from attributes more generally cultivated in social upbringing of girls

C. **Literature reveals that physicians interrupt patients after average of 18 seconds into clinical encounter**
   1. In male physician–female patient interactions, such interruptions are frequently used to get information more quickly so that physician can make therapeutic decision
   2. In female physician–female patient encounters, such interruptions often serve to show that one speaker understands the other, not to direct conversation
D. Studies of female physician practices reveal that women tend to spend more time with patients; this time is spent talking
   1. Female patients more readily reveal personal information to female physician than to male physician
   2. Female physicians spend more of their practice day engaged in counseling, guidance and discussion of psychosocial issues than do male physicians
   3. Female physicians are more accepting of multidisciplinary, social, and humanistic aspects of patient care
E. Some evidence suggests that **women physicians may perform preventive procedures more consistently for women patients than male physicians**, although such research is controversial

III. **An Approach**
   A. **Skills that facilitate communication** can be learned
      1. Understanding some of potential differences in male–female communications styles is helpful
      2. Reading books, such as Deborah Tannen's *You Just Don't Understand: Women and Men in Conversation* may be first step
   B. **Office procedures**
      1. Greet patient while she is dressed
      2. Ask patient if she wishes female chaperone for pelvic, breast, and rectal exams
   C. **Become reflective listener** by letting the patient tell her story uninterrupted, trying to understand her in her own context, realizing that telling story is partially therapeutic— the physician does not have to have all answers. Involve patient in decision making, be sensitive to psychosocial issues and stressors, and become familiar with community resources that can assist in long-term management of common psychosocial problems
   D. **Ensure that standard health maintenance and preventive procedures are followed**
   E. **Ask routinely about problems that occur more frequently in women** and may significantly affect patient's health: childhood abuse, sexual assault, stress, depression, domestic violence

SUGGESTED READING

1. Allen D, Gilchrist V, Levinson W, et al: Caring for women: Is it different? Patient Care Nov:183–199, 1993.
2. Benderly BL: In Her Own Right: The Institute of Medicine' Guide to Women's Health Issues. National Academy Press, Washington, DC, 1997.
3. Bennett JC: Inclusion of women in clinical trials—policies for population subgroups. N Engl J Med 328:288–291, 1993.
4. Council on Ethical and Judicial Affairs, American Medical Association: Sexual misconduct in the practice of medicine. JAMA 266:2741–2745, 1991.
5. Council on Ethical and Judicial Affairs, American Medical Association: Gender disparities in clinical decision making. JAMA 266:559–562, 1991.
6. Crandall SJS, Volk RJ, Loemker V: Medical students' attitudes toward providing care for the underserved. JAMA 269:2519–2523, 1993.
7. Jha AK, Kuperman GJ, Rittenberg E, et al: Gender and utilization of ancillary services. J Gen Intern Med 13:476–481, 1998.
8. Lurie N, Slater J, McGovern P, et al: Preventive care for women and the sex of the physician. N Engl J Med 328:478–482, 1993.
9. Majeroni BA, Karuza J, Wade C, et al: Gender of physicians and patients and preventive care for community-based older adults. J Am Board Fam Pract 6:359–365, 1993.
10. Mandelbaum-Schmid J: Are women physicians changing the practice of medicine? MD March:69–76, 1993.
11. Phillips SP, Schneider MS: Sexual harassment of female doctors by patients. N Engl J Med 329:1936–1939, 1993.
12. Tannen D: You Just Don't Understand: Women and Men in Conversation. New York, William Morrow, 1990.

PART III

MENSTRUAL DISORDERS

22. Abnormal Vaginal Bleeding

Cynda Ann Johnson, M.D., M.B.A.

I. **The Issues**

The menstrual cycle is a pervasive element much of a woman's adult life. For most women, it is an expected, if also bothersome, monthly event. If it goes awry, it is a source of consternation. Menstrual irregularities are the chief complaint in many women's visits to a generalist's office. Thus, it is essential that the generalist be aware of both the range of normal bleeding patterns and clues to abnormal patterns, knowing when to reassure the patient and when further investigation and/or intervention is indicated.

II. **The Theory**

  A. **Menstrual cycle** (Fig. 1)

    1. Follicular phase—an orderly sequence of events results in the maturation of usually a single follicle

      a. Under the influence of follicle-stimulating hormone (FSH), one follicle dominates by day 7

      b. Estradiol takes over as the predominant hormone

      c. Process complete in 10–14 days

    2. **Ovulation**

      a. Onset of luteinizing hormone (LH) surge 34–35 hours before rupture of follicle from ovary

      b. With LH surge, levels of progesterone continue to rise; estradiol levels plummet at LH peak

      c. Ovulation occurs 10–12 hours after LH peak and 24–36 hours after peak estradiol levels

      d. Increase in progesterone and midcycle progesterone-influenced rise in FSH result in freeing of egg from attachments

    3. **Luteal phase**

      a. Normal luteal function requires optimal preovulatory follicular development and stable levels of LH after surge

      b. Progesterone suppresses growth of new follicle

      c. Degeneration of corpus luteum mediated by prostaglandins and luteolytic action of its own estrogen production

      d. Menses occur approximately 14 days after LH midcycle surge; luteal phases of 12–17 days may be normal

  B. **Descriptors of menstrual cycle**

    1. **Normal menstrual cycle**

      a. Length: 2–6 days

      b. Blood loss: maximum of 80 ml; average is 35 ml

      c. Interval: maximum of 35 days

    2. **Abnormal bleeding cycles** (Table 1)

      a. Length: > 7 days

      b. Blood loss: > 80 ml

      c. Interval: < 21 days or > 35 days

  C. **Causes of abnormal vaginal bleeding** (Tables 2 and 3)

    1. Goal is to rule out causes other than dysfunctional uterine bleeding (DUB)

    2. In DUB bleeding source is uterine and mechanism is hormonal

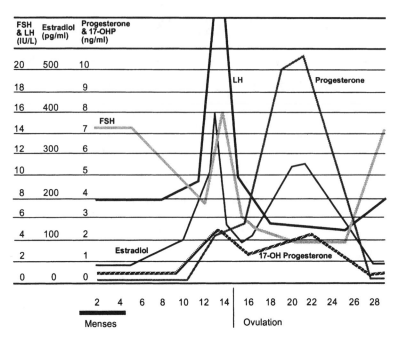

FIGURE 1.   Hormonal shifts during the menstrual cycle. (Adapted from Speroff L, Glass RH, Kase NG: Clinical Gynecologic Endocrinology and Infertility, 5th ed. Baltimore, Williams & Wilkins, 1994.)

    a. Causes 80% of cases of menorrhagia
    b. Results from any of five hormonal states
        i. **Progesterone and estrogen withdrawal**
           (a) Mechanism for bleeding in normal menstrual cycle
           (b) May result from estrogen and progesterone withdrawal in some hormone replacement regimens
           (c) Expected occurrence of each cycle of combined oral contraceptive pills (OCPs)
           (d) May also cause ovulatory DUB
        ii. **Estrogen withdrawal**
           (a) May cause midcycle spotting as estrogen levels drop just before ovulation
           (b) Results from destruction of ovaries (e.g., surgical bilateral oophorectomy or radiation)
           (c) May occur whenever estrogen therapy is stopped
        iii. **Progesterone withdrawal**
           (a) May occur whenever progestin therapy is stopped, usually 2–4 days later

TABLE 1.   Patterns of Abnormal Uterine Bleeding

Menorrhagia: prolonged or excessive uterine bleeding at regular intervals; the term **hypermenorrhea** is synonymous.

Menometrorrhagia: prolonged uterine bleeding at irregular intervals.

Metrorrhagia: uterine bleeding at irregular but frequent intervals; amount is variable.

Intermenstrual bleeding: bleeding of variable amounts between regular menstrual periods.

Polymenorrhea: uterine bleeding at regular intervals of less than 21 days.

Oligomenorrhea: uterine bleeding in which the interval between bleeding episodes may vary from 35 days to 6 months.

Amenorrhea: no uterine bleeding for at least 6 months.

TABLE 2.   Causes of Abnormal Vaginal Bleeding

Pregnancy states	**Systemic diseases**
Intrauterine	Coagulopathies
Spontaneous abortion	Blood dyscrasias
Threatened	Endocrinopathy
Inevitable	Renal/liver failure
Complete	**Neoplasia**
Incomplete	Vulvar
Ectopic	Vaginal
Molar-trophoblastic disease	Cervical
Inflammatory/infectious conditions	Uterine corpus
Vulvitis	Fallopian tube
Vaginitis	Ovarian
Cervicitis	**Drug effects**
Endometritis	Prescribed
Salpingitis	Self-medicated
Pelvic inflammatory disease	**Other**
Trauma	Endocervical polyps
Foreign body	Endometrial polyps
Direct trauma	Endometriosis
	Dysfunctional uterine bleeding

     iv. **Estrogen breakthrough**

        (a) High or moderately high estrogen states, such as high-dose OCPs or anovulatory patients with persistent estrogen secretion, often result in heavy bleeding because of excessive build-up of endometrium

     v. **Progesterone breakthrough**

        (a) May result from continuous administration of progestins alone such as: progestin-only contraceptive pill (minipill); subcutaneous progestin implants (Norplant); long-acting, injectable progestin (Depo-Provera)

        (b) Bleeding is intermittent and of variable duration, similar to low-estrogen breakthrough bleeding

        (c) Also results from inappropriate balance of estrogen and progestin, such as high-progestin OCPs or multiphasic OCP (in which the progestin cycle may not support the endometrial lining)

III. **An Approach**

  A. **Menstrual history**

    1. **Essential information**

      a. **Menarche**

        i. Age—8–16 years; average 12 years

        ii. Large caloric storage of fat before cycling begins; minimum weight for height required to stimulate onset of menstrual cycles

TABLE 3.   Bleeding Patterns with Tumors of the Reproductive Tract

Condition	Menorrhagia	Metrorrhagia	Postmenopausal Bleeding
Vulvar cancer	–	+ +	+ +
Vaginal cancer	–	+ +	+ +
Cervical cancer	–	+ +	+ +
Cervical polyp	–	+ +	+
Uterine myoma	+ +	+	–
Endometrial carcinoma	–	–	+ +
Fallopian tube cancer	–	–	+
Ovarian cancer	–	±	±

From Herbst AL, Mishell DR, Stenchever MA, Droegemueller W: Comprehensive Gynecology, 2nd ed. St. Louis, Mosby, 1992, with permission.

         iii. Light affects reproductive process via pineal gland and hypothalamus to control outpouring of gonadotropin-releasing factor

    b. **Characteristics of menstrual cycle**
        i. First day of last menstrual period
        ii. Duration of bleeding
        iii. Amount of bleeding
        iv. Interval
        v. Regularity of bleeding

    c. **Menopausal status**
    d. **Bleeding of other-than-vaginal origin**

  2. Other historical questions to uncover pathologic causes of abnormal vaginal bleeding
    a. Weight problems, stress, and recent use of hormonal agents support DUB as cause
    b. Hormonal regimens must be described in detail, including periods of noncompliance

B. Physical examination
  1. **Pelvic examination**
    a. Adolescents
        i. Not indicated for postpubertal patients who are sexually inactive, oligomenorrheic, and within 18 months of menarche
        ii. Indicated with pattern of increased bleeding, with even one episode of very heavy bleeding, or if hormonal therapy is considered
    b. All other women with abnormal vaginal bleeding
        i. Pelvic exam, Papanicolaou smear, and endometrial biopsy (may judiciously restrict endometrial biopsy in younger age group and treat empirically)

C. Laboratory evaluations
  1. Hemoglobin or hematocrit
  2. Coagulation studies in adolescent with continuous DUB or episode of heavy bleeding
    a. Coagulation defects in up to 20% of adolescents who require hospitalization for bleeding
  3. If patient with chronic anovulation becomes persistently oligomenorrheic or amenorrheic, draw prolactin level, thyroid function studies, and androgen studies
  4. Other studies depending on patient history might include pregnancy test, tests for infective agents including gonorrhea, chlamydia, herpes, trichomonas, yeast, or liver and renal function tests

D. Classification of patients with DUB
  1. **Chronicity**
    a. Acute—1–3 episodes
        i. One-time therapy
        ii. Follow-up treatment of no more than 3 months
        iii. May resolve spontaneously
    b. Chronic
        i. Long-term or repeated treatment
        ii. Requires endometrial sampling
  2. **Quantity of bleeding**
    a. Very heavy—requires prompt treatment, usually with hospitalization
    b. Moderately heavy
    c. Light to moderate
        i. No therapy may be required in women with light irregular bleeding, e.g., women on low-dose oral contraceptives
  3. **Phase of reproductive life**
    a. Postpubertal
        i. Occasionally have short ovulatory cycles, but usually anovulatory cycles with irregular menses
        ii. Full maturation of the hypothalamic–pituitary– ovarian axis usually within 18 months of menarche (but may be up to 5 years)
    b. Reproductive (all other postpubertal women who do not have menstrual irregularities of perimenopausal years)

TABLE 4. Classification of Ovulatory Dysfunctional Uterine Bleeding

Corpus luteum insufficiency	Prolonged corpus luteum activity	Mixed etiologies
Luteal phase defect	Persistent corpus luteum	Short proliferative and/or
Premenstrual spotting	Irregular shedding	secretory phases
Menorrhagia	Menorrhagia	Midcycle spotting
	Oligomenorrhea	Polymenorrhea

      i. DUB often from hormonal contraception
     ii. DUB from anovulation
        (a) Polycystic ovary syndrome, stress, weight change, excess exercise
    iii. Subgroups of reproductive group
        (a) Women desiring pregnancy
        (b) Women preferring hormonal contraception
        (c) Women not preferring hormonal contraception in whom pregnancy would be accepted; however, hormonal regimens are not necessarily contraindicated
  c. Perimenopausal
      i. Anovulatory or short ovulatory cycles
4. Functional state
  a. Ovulatory DUB (Table 4)
      i. 15–30% of patients with DUB
     ii. Difficult group to treat; bleeding hard to control
    iii. Often results from aberrations of corpus luteum function
    iv. Includes patients with midcycle spotting
  b. Anovulatory DUB
      i. Patients not on hormonal therapy
        (a) Estrogen production without counterbalancing effect of progesterone
        (b) Endometrial sloughing not regular or complete without ovulation
     ii. Patients on hormonal therapy
        (a) Patients on combined oral contraceptives are expected to be anovulatory; an ovulatory endometrium may indicate noncompliance or missed pills
        (b) Patients on progestin-only pills or who have subdermal implants ovulate occasionally
    iii. Endometrial biopsy to determine definitively if patient is ovulatory
        (a) Dilatation and curettage not indicated
        (b) Time sample late enough in cycle for ovulation to have taken place
        (c) Day 21 is reasonable compromise for short or long cycles
        (d) Basal body temperatures and serum progesterone levels help to guide timing for sample if ovulation is suspected
5. Endometrial thickness
  a. Abundant or scant
  b. Determine with endometrial biopsy
  c. Thickness of endometrium as demonstrated on ultrasound of uterus may be helpful
E. **Treatment options for DUB**
  1. Patient should keep menstrual calendar to monitor success of therapy
  2. **Hormonal regimens** (Table 5)
    a. Not all-inclusive
    b. May use comparable dosages of other estrogens and progestins than those listed in table
    c. Choose appropriate hormonal regimen on basis of patient profile (Table 6)
    d. **Patient with acute, very heavy, uncontrolled bleeding**
      i. Often requires hospitalization
     ii. In nearly all cases, there is time to perform an endometrial biopsy
    iii. Intravenous estrogen, 25 mg every 4 hours, until bleeding abates; maximum of 3 doses

TABLE 5.   Hormonal Medication Options for Treatment of DUB

1. Intravenous estrogen—25 mg every 4 hours. Maximum of 3 doses. Follow with conjugated estrogens, 1.25–2.5 mg/day orally, plus medroxyprogesterone acetate, 10 mg/day orally for 7–10 additional days; then stop.
2. Conjugated estrogens, 0.625–1.25 mg orally on calendar days 1–25 each month with medroxyprogesterone acetate, 10 mg orally on days 16–25
3. Combined oral contraceptives, 1 pill orally up to 4 times/day for 3–5 days to stop bleeding; then 1 pill/day until pill pack is finished.
4. Conjugated estrogens, 1.25 mg/day orally for 7–10 days; then stop.
5. Medroxyprogesterone acetate, 10 mg/day orally for 10 days or progesterone in oil, 100–200 mg intramuscularly
6. Clomiphene citrate
7. Medroxyprogesterone acetate, 10 mg/day orally for 10 days; repeat monthly.
8. Combined oral contraceptives, 1 pill daily
9. Progesterone-containing intrauterine device or progesterone-only birth control pill
10. Depo-Provera, 150–300 mg intramuscularly every 3 months

    iv. Oral conjugated estrogens (e.g., Premarin) in divided doses up to 10 mg/day; not well-tolerated by patients
    v. If bleeding somewhat less heavy, use lower doses of oral estrogen and allow bleeding to abate over 24–48 hours
    vi. Follow any of above regimens with oral medroxyprogesterone acetate, 10 mg/day, along with oral conjugated estrogen, 1.25–2.5 mg/day for 7–10 days; then stop both hormones and withdrawal bleeding will take place within a few days

TABLE 6.   Medication Options Based on Patient Profiles

Profile Categories	Medication Option*									
	1	2	3	4	5	6	7	8	9	10
Chronicity										
Acute	+	+	+	+	+	o	o	o	o	o
Chronic	o	+	o	o	o	+	+	+	+	+
Quantity of bleeding										
Very heavy	+	o	o	o	o	o	o	o	o	o
Moderately heavy	o	+	+	o	+	+	+	+	+	+
Light to moderate	o	+	o	+	+	+	+	+	+	o
Phase of reproductive life										
Postpuberty	+	o	+	+	+	o	+	+	o	o
Reproductive—pregnency desired	+	o	+	o	+	+	o	o	o	o
Reproductive—hormonal contraception preferred	+	o	+	+	+	o	o	+	+	+
Reproductive—hormonal contraception not preferred	+	o	+	+	+	o	+	+	o	+
Perimenopausal	+	+	o	+	+	o	+	o	+	+
Functional state										
Ovulatory	+	+	+	+	+	o	o	+	+	+
Anovulatory	+	+	+	+	+	+	+	+	+	+
Endometrial thickness										
Abundant	+	+	o	o	+	+	+	+	+	+
Scant	+	+	+	+	o	+	o	+	o	o

+ = appropriate option, o = inappropriate option.
* Option numbers correspond to options listed in Table 3.
To use Table 6: Start with chronicity. Identify treatment options appropriate for the patient's profile. Working downward through the other categories, eliminate the options that are not appropriate for her profile in one or more categories. The final options are only those that are appropriate for the patient in every category of her profile. For example: 21-year-old, nonsmoking woman, G_2P_2, with heavy, irregular periods who desires no more children. Endometrial biopsy reveals abundant tissue and indicates anovulation. Appropriate options are 8, 9, and 10. The best option depends on other characteristics of the patient, including acceptability and whether any of the appropriate regimens has been tried successfully in the past.

  e. **Patient with acute, moderately heavy bleeding**
    i. Administration of any of the combined oral contraceptive pills
      (a) May be given up to 4 times/day, but fewer doses are better tolerated
      (b) Continue for several days until bleeding clearly subsided; then finish the
        pill pack at 1 pill/day; this delays withdrawal bleeding in patient who has
        just experienced heavy bleeding
    ii. Administration of a progestational agent alone
      (a) Preferred for patient with excessive endometrial tissue
      (b) Medroxyprogesterone acetate, 10 mg/day for 10 days, or 100–200 mg
        (depends on patient's weight) intramuscularly of progesterone in oil
      (c) One-time regimen is desirable for the patient who is anxious to become
        pregnant soon
  f. **Patient with midcycle spotting**
    i. Conjugated estrogens, 1.25 mg daily for 5–10 days
      (a) Also useful for patient with denuded endometrium
      (b) Patient on long-term oral contraception who begins to have intermenstrual
        spotting
      (c) Patient with progesterone breakthrough bleeding
      (d) Use for 1–3 cycles
  g. **Patient with chronic DUB who desires pregnancy**
    i. Clomiphene citrate
  h. **Other patients with anovulation**
    i. If no contraception preferred: medroxyprogesterone acetate, 10 mg/day for
      10 days each month
      (a) Bleeding decreases over about 3 months
      (b) Patient has fewer estrogenic symptoms (common with anovulation)
      (c) Progestins provide some protection against uterine cancer in patients ex-
        periencing unopposed estrogen effect
      (d) Some patients prefer options listed below despite the fact that contracep-
        tion is also afforded
    ii. If contraception preferred:
      (a) First choice usually low-dose combined oral contraceptive
        (i) Results in decreased menstrual flow by as much as 60% to as little
          as 20 ml/cycle
        (ii) May use for 3 months in patient not desiring hormonal contraception
          to slough and stabilize the endometrium progressively
      (b) Progestin-only contraception—usually results in less quantity of blood
        loss, but bleeding pattern is irregular
  i. **Patient with DUB on combined oral contraceptive pills**
    i. Change to a different pill (see Chapter 37)
    ii. Use a different form of birth control
  j. **Patient with ovulatory DUB**
    i. Depot medroxyprogesterone acetate
    ii. Combined oral contraceptive pill
    iii. Often requires adjunct therapy such as nonsteroidal antiinflammatory agent
  k. **Perimenopausal patient with DUB**
    i. Conjugated estrogens 0.625 mg daily on days 1–25 each month, adding
      medroxyprogesterone acetate, 10 mg, on days 16–25; withdrawal bleeding is
      expected
    ii. Combined oral contraceptive pills containing only 20 µg ethynil estradiol are
      an excellent choice for the nonsmoking perimenopausal woman with DUB
3. **Nonhormonal medical therapy**
  a. Nonsteroidal antiinflammatory drugs (NSAIDs)
  b. Androgenic steroids, such as danazol, have extensive side effects, including
    weight gain and acne, and are expensive
  c. Antifibrinolytic agents, including aminocaproic acid and tranexamic acid, should
    be reserved for patients with hemorrhagic conditions

    d. Gonadotropin-releasing hormone (GnRH) agonist
       i. Induces hypoestrogenism and amenorrhea
      ii. Includes leuprolide acetate, nafarelin, goserelin
     iii. Especially useful in treating patients with menorrhagia due to leiomyomas
     iv. May be used in perimenopausal women with uncontrolled DUB until menopause in lieu of surgical intervention
    e. Consider consultation before using any of these agents other than NSAIDs

4. **Surgical options**
    a. Dilatation and curettage
       i. Rarely needed
      ii. Removes hyperplastic tissue in anovulatory patient, but rarely curative over the long term
     iii. Consider in life-threatening hemorrhage, hypovolemic patient, or if response to intravenous estrogen is inadequate
    b. Hysterectomy
       i. Consider in patients with chronic DUB who have completed their families
         (a) If repeated hormonal therapy required
         (b) If patient repeatedly anemic
    c. Endometrial ablation
       i. Destroys the endometrium
      ii. Laser photovaporization or electrosurgical technique
     iii. Successful in 85% of patients
         (a) Success rate may be improved by presurgical treatment with GnRH agonist
     iv. Alternative for women who are not optimal surgical candidates
      v. Outpatient procedure
     vi. May be cost-effective
    vii. Preserves uterine organ
   viii. Remaining tissue may result in vaginal bleeding; cancer of the endometrium has been reported

5. **Patients given appropriate therapy who continue to bleed need further investigative studies**
    a. Hysteroscopy
    b. Pelvic sonography
    c. Hysterosalpingography
    d. Possible causes include submucous myomas and endometrial polyps

SUGGESTED READING

1. Apgar BS: Dysmenorrhea and dysfunctional uterine bleeding. Prim Care 24:161–178, 1997.
2. Cowan BD, Morrison JC: Management of abnormal genital bleeding in girls and women. N Engl J Med 324:1710–1714, 1991.
3. Johnson CA: Making sense of dysfunctional uterine bleeding. Am Fam Physician 44:149–157, 1991.
4. Mints M, Rådestad A: Follow-up of hysteroscopic surgery for menorrhagia. Acta Obstet Gynecol Scand 77:435–438, 1998.
5. Valle RF: Endometrial ablation for dysfunctional uterine bleeding: Role of GnRH agonists. Int J Gynaecol Obstet 41:3–15, 1993.
6. Vercellini P, DeGiorgi O: Menstrual characteristics in women with and without endometriosis. Obstet Gynecol 90:264–268, 1997.

23. Amenorrhea

Cynda Ann Johnson, M.D., M.B.A.

I. **The Issues**

When a woman complains of skipped menstrual periods, several issues must be considered: when to make the diagnosis of amenorrhea, the cause of the condition, patient's age and desire for fertility, and protection from unopposed estrogen or, on the other hand, from estrogen deficiency. Because amenorrhea is a condition with a clear-cut symptom but often varied and complicated causes that require time and dedication to investigate, the patient must be an active partner in the process.

II. **The Theory**

 A. Definition of amenorrhea

  1. No menstrual period by age 14 years in absence of growth or development of secondary sexual characteristics

  2. No menstrual period by age 16 years, regardless of development of secondary sexual characteristics

  3. No menstrual period for 6 months in a woman who usually has normal periods or for a length of time equivalent to 3 cycle intervals in a woman whose cycle is less regular

 B. **Categories of amenorrhea**

  1. Primary vs. secondary

   a. Primary includes definitions 1 and 2

   b. Secondary includes definition 3

  2. Newer system abandons such terms

   a. Compartment I: disorders of the outflow tract or uterine target organ

   b. Compartment II: disorders of the ovary

   c. Compartment III: disorders of the anterior pituitary

   d. Compartment IV: disorders of the hypothalamus

III. **An Approach**

 A. **Complete history**

  1. Growth and development; previous menstrual history; pregnancy; methods of contraception; medications, including hormonal; lifestyle such as emotional stress, nutritional status, exercise; galactorrhea; thyroid history

 B. **Complete physical exam**

  1. Height and weight; hair distribution; development of secondary sexual characteristics and Tanner staging; evidence of central nervous system disease; galactorrhea (must not be tentative in trying to elicit on exam); pelvic exam

 C. **Initial laboratory examination** for cost-effective evaluation

  1. Pregnancy test; serum prolactin level; thyroid-stimulating hormone level; other tests only as indicated after careful history and physical exam

 D. **Progesterone challenge test**

  1. Administer progesterone in oil, 200 mg intramuscularly or medroxyprogesterone acetate, 10 mg/day orally for 5 days

  2. Wait for evidence of withdrawal bleeding which usually occurs 2–7 days after administration of the medication

  3. **Positive test** (any withdrawal bleeding) indicates:

   a. Functional outflow tract

   b. Uterus has been primed with endogenous estrogen

   c. Minimally reactive endometrium, at the least

   d. Patients who have only minimal spotting in response to the progesterone challenge test

    i. Test is still positive

    ii. Immediate further testing not indicated

    iii. Watch carefully; liberal use of repeat progesterone challenges

    iv. If no withdrawal bleeding at any time, proceed with further work-up

    e. Diagnosis of anovulation (Compartment IV) if thyroid and prolactin levels are normal

    f. If galactorrhea is also present, obtain an x-ray with a coned-down view of the sella turcica

4. **Treatment of anovulation**

    a. Previously patients were not treated unless: they desired pregnancy; were treated only every few months; or if they experienced symptoms of estrogen excess

    b. Current recommendations are based on evidence that untreated patients are at risk for endometrial cancer and possibly breast cancer

    c. Perform endometrial biopsy before treatment

    d. Specific treatment regimen is based on patient's age, contraceptive needs, and lifestyle

        i. For anovulation only: medroxyprogesterone acetate, 10 mg orally for the first 10 days of each month

        ii. For women also desiring contraception: combined oral contraceptive pills or any progesterone-only contraception

        iii. For women desiring pregnancy: clomiphene citrate or other hormonal regimens to stimulate ovulation

        iv. For perimenopausal women: regimen of estrogen and progesterone replacement therapy

5. **Negative progesterone challenge test** with no vaginal bleeding

    a. Two rare clinical syndromes in which amenorrheic patients with adequate endogenous estrogen have a negative progesterone challenge test

        i. High levels of circulating androgen, although most women with androgen excess syndrome (e.g., polycystic ovary syndrome) will have withdrawal bleeding, a few will not because of the decidualizing effect of androgen on the endometrium

        ii. Specific adrenal enzyme deficiency causing high endogenous progesterone levels

    b. **Proceed to next step in work-up**

E. **Priming the endometrium with estrogen**

1. Differentiates women with target organ outflow tract dysfunction from those with inadequate endometrial proliferation

2. Administer equivalent of 2.5 mg of conjugated estrogen orally for 21 days; common error is to administer inadequate amount of estrogen

3. Add 10 mg of oral progesterone acetate for the last 5 days

4. Repeat the process if no withdrawal bleeding occurs

5. **Negative test (withdrawal bleeding absent)—diagnosis is Compartment I abnormality**

    a. Asherman's syndrome—destruction of the endometrium

    b. Müllerian anomaly (structural)

    c. Testicular feminization syndrome

6. **Positive test**—patient has withdrawal bleeding in response to estrogen and progesterone challenge

    a. **Check gonadotropins**—both follicle-stimulating hormone (FSH) and luteinizing hormone (LH)

    b. **If FSH is elevated and LH normal**—a normal finding periodically during perimenopausal years

    c. **If both FSH and LH are elevated—diagnosis is Compartment II abnormality**

        i. Ovarian failure

           (a) Physiologic menopause

           (b) Premature menopause

           (c) Destruction of the ovary by radiation or chemotherapy

           (d) Resistant ovary syndrome: follicles in ovary do not respond to even high levels of circulating gonadotropins

        ii. Abnormal karyotype

           (a) Turner's syndrome

           (b) Mosaicism

           (c) Gonadal dysgenesis

    d. **If both FSH and LH are normal or low**
       i. Further evaluation by primary care physician in consultation with endocrinologist or other specialist
      ii. Evaluation of sella turcica
         (a) Patients with prolactin level greater than 100 ng/ml—pituitary tumor is more likely and should proceed to computerized tomography (CT) with enhancement or magnetic resonance imaging (MRI)
         (b) Patients with prolactin level < 100 ng/ml—pituitary tumor is unlikely and, while plain films with coned view of sella turcica are probably adequate, most doctors proceed with CT or MRI because of fear of missing disease
     iii. **Empty sella syndrome**
         (a) Congenital abnormality of sella turcica
         (b) X-ray picture similar to tumor
         (c) Similar appearance after surgery or radiotherapy
         (d) Clarify with further scanning

F. **Identification of pituitary adenoma by any technique is Compartment III diagnosis**
  1. Follow-up and treatment depend on tumor size, patient's desire for pregnancy, and significance of galactorrhea
  2. Determine options in consultation with endocrinologist
    a. Yearly surveillance with prolactin level and examination of sella turcica
  3. Treatment with a dopamine agonist such as bromocriptine (2.5 mg 2 times/day orally) for patients who wish to become pregnant or have uncomfortable galactorrhea
  4. Surgery

G. Patients with low or normal gonadotropins, normal prolactin levels, normal-appearing sella turcica, and who experience positive withdrawal bleeding response to estrogen priming have a Compartment IV diagnosis (as do patients with anovulation)
  1. Mechanism is probable suppression of pulsatile function of gonadotropin-releasing hormone (GnRH)
  2. Includes patients who are amenorrheic as a result of anorexia nervosa, stress, high-level exercise, being underweight in general
  3. Annual follow-up exam
    a. Prolactin level, x-ray of sella turcica
    b. Decrease frequency to every 2–3 years when results remain unchanged
  4. Return to menstrual function
    a. Normal return of GnRH function at 15% below ideal body weight
    b. Menstruation returns secondarily
    c. Correlates with percent of body fat necessary to sustain menstruation
      i. 17% body fat adequate to initiate menarche at age 13 years
     ii. 22% body fat necessary after age 16 to sustain normal menstrual function
  5. **Treatment of hypothalamic amenorrhea (Compartment IV disorder)** with estrogen replacement
    a. Any regimen otherwise used as postmenopausal hormone replacement

SUGGESTED READING

1. Baird D: Amenorrhoea. Lancet 350:275–279, 1997.
2. Frisch RE: Body fat, menarche, and reproductive ability. Semin Reprod Endocrinol 3:45–46, 1985.
3. Kiningham RB, Apgar BS: Evaluation of amenorrhea. Am Fam Physician 53:1185–1194, 1996.
4. McIver B, Romanski SA: Evaluation and management of amenorrhea. Mayo Clin Proc 72:1161–1169, 1997.
5. Speroff L, Glass RH, Kase NG (eds): Clinical Gynecologic Endocrinology and Infertility, 5th ed. Baltimore, Williams & Wilkins, 1994.
6. Warren MP: Evaluation of secondary amenorrhea. J Clin Endocrinol Metab 81:437–442, 1996.

24. Premenstrual Syndrome

Cynda Ann Johnson, M.D., M.B.A.

I. **The Issues**

No longer do physicians dispute the existence of a constellation of cyclic symptoms that can be categorized as premenstrual syndrome (PMS). But even now, its true prevalence, cause and optimal treatment remain unclear. Many women come to their physicians seeking help for PMS, and although most women experience some premenstrual discomfort, fewer than 10% meet current diagnostic criteria. Women's groups, as well as the lay press, have led women to be skeptical (appropriately in most cases) of physicians' empathy with, interest in, and knowledge of diagnosis and treatment of PMS. Primary care physicians must keep abreast of current literature on PMS—both lay and scientific—to assist with this enigmatic syndrome.

II. **The Theory**
  A. **Definition of premenstrual syndrome**
      1. Cyclic recurrence
      2. Luteal phase of the menstrual cycle
      3. Combination of physical, psychological, and behavioral symptoms
      4. Symptoms sufficiently severe to result in deterioration of interpersonal relationships and/or interference with normal activities
      5. Symptom-free interval (follicular phase) follows in which patient feels and functions well
  B. **Pathophysiology not understood**
      1. Probable biologic trigger, compounding psychosocial factors
      2. Probable increase in genetically determined sensitivity of one or more neurotransmitter systems (e.g., gamma-aminobutyric acid, serotonin) to effects of cyclical fluctuations in ovarian steroid levels
      3. Women with PMS have a reduction in urinary prostaglandin excretion
      4. Beta-endorphin levels throughout the periovulatory period have been shown to be lower in women experiencing PMS
      5. Women with PMS and high stress levels have high luteal phase cortisol levels

III. **An Approach**
  A. **Diagnosis**
      1. **Historical clues**
          a. History of maternal PMS
          b. Low levels of exercise
          c. Younger age
          d. Higher parity
      2. **Typical pattern**
          a. At midcycle up to 7 days before menses
              i. Breast tenderness, abdominal bloating, fatigue, emotional lability, depression, thirst, appetite changes, edema of extremities
          b. 1–2 days before menses
              i. Anxiety and hyperactivity, resulting in: marital and relational discord; social isolation; work absenteeism
              ii. Dysmenorrhea is separate phenomenon
          c. Onset of menses
              i. Relief of psychological symptoms
              ii. Dysmenorrhea may continue
      3. Women with PMS have stability of symptoms across cycles
          a. Individualized constellation of symptoms highly reproducible in each woman across cycles
          b. Mood symptoms, especially anxiety, irritability and mood lability, account for more functional impairment than somatic symptoms

4. Self-rating scale for PMS
   a. **Chart symptoms** for at least 2–3 cycles (Fig. 1)
   b. Diagnose PMS if number of "yes" responses ≤ 5 in follicular phase and ≥ 15 in premenstrual phase

---

Name _____ Date _____

Instructions: The following questions are concerned with the way you feel or act today. Please answer *all* questions by circling YES or NO as indicated.

1. Do you find yourself avoiding some of your social commitments?	YES	NO
2. Have you gained 5 or more pounds during the past week?	YES	NO
3. Is your coordination so poor that you are unable to use kitchen utensils, garden tools, or unable to drive?	YES	NO
4. Do you feel more angry than usual?	YES	NO
5. Do you avoid family activities and prefer to be left alone?	YES	NO
6. Do you doubt your judgment or feel that you are prone to hasty decisions?	YES	NO
7. Do you feel more irritable than usual?	YES	NO
8. Is your efficiency diminished?	YES	NO
9. Do you feel tense and restless?	YES	NO
10. Do you feel a marked change in your sexual drive or desire during the last week? If YES, is it *increased* or *decreased?*	YES ↑	NO ↓
11. Are your present physical symptoms causing so much pain and discomfort that you are unable to function?	YES	NO
12. Have you recently canceled previously scheduled social activities?	YES	NO
13. Do you feel as if you were unable to relax at all?	YES	NO
14. Do you feel confused?	YES	NO
15. Do you suffer from painful or tender breasts?	YES	NO
16. Do you have an increased desire for specific kinds of food (e.g., cravings for candy, chocolate, etc.)?	YES	NO
17. Do you scream/yell at family members (friends, colleagues) more than usual? Are you "short-fused"?	YES	NO
18. Do you feel sad, gloomy, and hopeless most of the time?	YES	NO
19. Do you feel like crying?	YES	NO
20. Do you have difficulty completing your daily household/job routine?	YES	NO
21. Was there a marked change in your sexual drive with definite change in your sexual behavior during the last week? If YES, is it *increased* or *decreased?*	YES ↑	NO ↓
22. Do you find yourself being more forgetful than usual or unable to concentrate?	YES	NO
23. Do you happen to have more "accidents" with your daily housework/job (cut fingers, break dishes, etc.)?	YES	NO
24. Have you noticed significant swelling of your breasts and/or ankles and/or bloating of your abdomen?	YES	NO
25. Does you mood change suddenly without obvious reason?	YES	NO
26. Are you easily distracted?	YES	NO
27. Do you think that your restless behavior is noticeable by others?	YES	NO
28. Are you clumsier than usual?	YES	NO
29. Are you obviously negative and hostile toward other people?	YES	NO
30. Are you so fatigued that it interferes with your usual level of functioning?	YES	NO
31. Do you tend to eat more than usual or at odd irregular hours (sweet, snacks, etc.)?	YES	NO
32. Do you become more easily fatigued than usual?	YES	NO
33. Is your handwriting different (less neat than usual)?	YES	NO
34. Do you feel jittery or upset?	YES	NO
35. Do you feel sad or blue?	YES	NO
36. Have you stopped calling or visiting some of your best friends?	YES	NO

FIGURE 1. Self-rating scale for premenstrual syndrome (From Steiner M, Haskett RF, Carroll BJ: Acta Psychiatr Scand 62:177–190, 1980, with permission.)

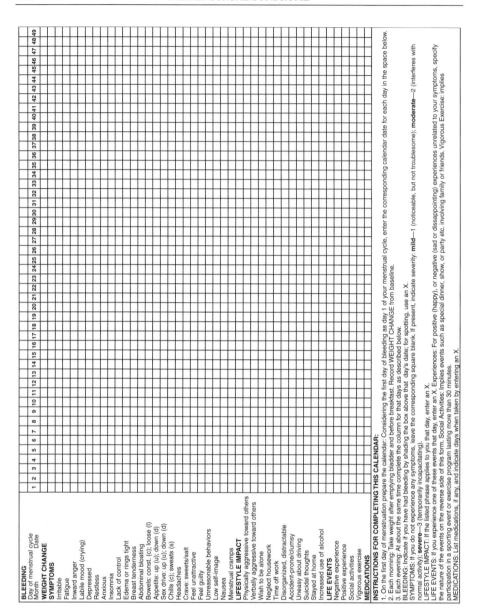

FIGURE 2. PRISM Calendar developed by R. L. Reid and S. Maddocks.

5. See Figure 2 for example of Prospective Record of the Impact and Severity of Menstrual Symptomatology (PRISM calendar)
   a. A score of < 8 on day 9 and > 12 on day 27 will accurately diagnose PMS 90% of the time
6. See Table 1 for diagnostic criteria for premenstrual dysphoric disorder (PMDD)
   a. Strict criteria
   b. Can probably be considered to be a subset of PMS, affecting 2.5–4% of women
   c. More closely related to other mood disorders than to PMS

B. **Treatment**
   1. High placebo response in most studies

TABLE 1. Research Diagnostic Criteria for Premenstrual Dysphoric Disorder

A. In most menstrual cycles during the past year, five (or more) of the following symptoms were present for most of the time during the last week of the luteal phase, began to remit within a few days after the onset of the follicular phase, and were absent in the week postmenses, with at least one of the symptoms being either 1, 2, 3, or 4:
   1. Markedly depressed mood, feelings of hopelessness, or self-deprecating thoughts
   2. Marked anxiety, tension, feelings of being "keyed up," or "on edge"
   3. Marked affective lability (e.g., feeling suddenly sad or tearful or increased sensitivity to rejection)
   4. Persistent and marked anger or irritability or increased interpersonal conflicts
   5. Decreased interest in usual activities (e.g., work, school, friends, hobbies)
   6. Subjective sense of difficulty in concentrating
   7. Lethargy, easy fatigability, or marked lack of energy
   8. Marked change in appetite, overeating, or specific food cravings
   9. Hypersomnia or insomnia
   10. A subjective sense of being overwhelmed or out of control
   11. Other physical symptoms, such as breast tenderness or swelling, headaches, joint or muscle pain, a sensation of "bloating," weight gain

B. The disturbance markedly interferes with work or school or with usual social activities and relationships with others.

C. The disturbance is not merely an exacerbation of the symptoms of another disorder, such as major depressive disorder, panic disorder, dysthymic disorder, or a personality disorder (although it may be superimposed on any of these disorders).

D. Criteria A, B, and C must be confirmed by prospective daily ratings during at least two consecutive symptomatic cycles.

From American Psychiatric Association: Diagnostic and Statistical Manual of Mental Disorders, 4th edition (DSM-IV). Washington, DC, American Psychiatric Association, 1994.

   2. Most interventions do not show clear-cut benefit over placebo
   3. **Patient-generated interventions**
      a. Self-charting is therapeutic
         i. Provides sense of empowerment for the woman who feels out of control and at the mercy of symptoms
         ii. Allows prospective planning to deal with symptoms
            (a) Family, work, and social responsibilities, when feasible, may be limited during time of most severe symptoms
      b. Regular exercise
         i. Boosts mood and energy level
         ii. Helps to eliminate water
         iii. Aerobic exercise may also help women with mild premenstrual symptoms
      c. Eating habits
         i. Complex carbohydrates in frequent, small feedings
         ii. High magnesium-containing foods (nuts, seeds, whole grains, legumes)
         iii. Low-salt diet
         iv. Minimize intake of caffeine and alcohol
      d. Rest
      e. Stress reduction
      f. Avoidance of situational or behavioral triggers
   4. **Physician-initiated interventions**
      a. Reassurance
         i. Patients who fit criteria for PMS
            (a) Many women have PMS—it is a real entity
            (b) No cure at this time
            (c) Treatment based on symptom relief
            (d) Counseling may be adjunct to other treatment
         ii. Patients not fitting criteria for PMS
            (a) Menstrual distress patients—symptoms throughout month with premenstrual exacerbation (also known as premenstrual magnification)

  (b) Episodic distress patients—fluctuating symptoms throughout cycle, unrelated to menses
  (c) Acknowledge that the symptoms are real
  (d) Conservative therapy with attention to lifestyle issues
  (e) Counseling
b. **Medications shown to be effective** in some placebo-controlled, crossover studies
  i. Serotonergic antidepressants—perform the best in the greatest number of trials
    (a) Fluoxetine 5–20 mg (maximum 60 mg) daily
      (i) Start with 20 mg daily
      (ii) Titrate up or down to lowest effective daily dose
      (iii) When an effective daily dose is established, consider a trial of luteal phase–only treatment
    (b) Sertraline 25–50 mg daily (try luteal)
    (c) Paroxetine 5–20 mg daily (try luteal)
    (d) Fluvoxamine 25–50 mg daily (try luteal)
    (e) Clomipramine 25–75 mg daily (luteal only—more side effects than other serotonergic antidepressants)
  ii. Alprazolam
    (a) Anxiolytic and antidepressant
    (b) 0.25 mg orally 2 or 3 times/day during premenstrual period, reducing the dosage at time of menses; some investigators suggest a maximal total dose of 4 mg/day
    (c) Warn about sedative effect; may not be compatible with operating machinery
    (d) Relief of anxiety and depression
  iii. Buspirone (anxiolytic) 5–30 mg daily in divided dose (luteal)
  iv. Antiprostaglandins (nonsteroidal antiinflammatory drugs)
    (a) Administer premenstrually and menstrually
    (b) Relieves dysmenorrhea and premenstrual mood changes
  v. Spironolactone
    (a) 25 mg 4 times/day orally during premenstrual interval
    (b) May alleviate psychological symptoms and symptoms related to fluid retention
  vi. Pyridoxine
    (a) 200–800 mg/day orally
    (b) Avoid high doses (> 1 g/day), which are associated with sensory neuropathy
  vii. Gonadotropin-releasing hormone agonists
    (a) Inhibit cyclical gonadotropin release
    (b) Create pseudomenopausal state
    (c) Abolish all symptoms of PMS
    (d) Cause problems of hypoestrogenemia
  viii. Danazol
    (a) 100–200 mg/day orally during luteal phase
    (b) General improvement in symptoms
c. **Medications of questionable or variable efficacy**
  i. Combined oral contraceptive pills
    (a) Hormonal side effects
    (b) Symptoms during placebo pills
    (c) Triphasic pills simulate menstrual cycle and may produce similar symptoms
    (d) Alternative is continuous use of pill with fixed low dosage, stopping for withdrawal every 3 or 4 months
  ii. Progestational agents
    (a) Depression is significant side effect of progestins
    (b) Progestin-only contraception
    (c) Medroxyprogesterone acetate, 10–30 mg/day orally
  iii. Natural progesterone
    (a) Scientific support lacking
    (b) Still preferred by many patients

(c) 50–100 mg rectal or vaginal suppositories or aqueous rectal suspension twice daily during luteal phase (up to 400 mg 3 times/day)

    (i) Side effects include local irritation and dryness

iv. Vitamin E

    (a) 400 mg/day orally

    (b) Relief of mastalgia and generalized symptoms of PMS

v. Calcium

    (a) 1000 mg/day orally

    (b) May relieve several premenstrual symptoms, water retention, and dysmenorrhea

vi. Magnesium

    (a) 360 mg magnesium pyrrolidone carboxylic acid orally 3 times/day from day 15 to first day of menses

    (b) Patients with PMS may have low magnesium content in monocytes

vii. Bromocriptine

    (a) 5 mg (or as little as 1.25 mg if not tolerated) orally at night for 2 weeks preceding menses

    (b) May improve edema, breast engorgement, and tenderness

    (c) Significant side effects

viii. Yeast-based dietary supplement

    (a) Tablet combination of magnesium, pyridoxine, vitamin E, folic acid, iron, copper, and *Saccharomyces cerevisiae*

    (b) Statistically significant improvement in one double-blind placebo-controlled study in patients with mild-to-moderate PMS

d. **Surgery**

i. Oophorectomy

    (a) Drastic measure

    (b) Serious consideration for patient who is otherwise a candidate for hysterectomy

e. **Phototherapy**

i. PMS and seasonal affective disorder may be related

    (a) Disturbances in melatonin and serotonin systems influenced by photo period may cause some symptoms in both syndromes

SUGGESTED READING

1. Berger CP, Presser B: Alprazolam in the treatment of two subsamples of patients with late luteal phase dysphoric disorder: A double-blind, placebo-controlled crossover study. Obstet Gynecol 84:79–85, 1994.
2. Chuong CJ, Hsi BP: Periovulatory beta-endorphin levels in premenstrual syndrome. Obstet Gynecol 83:755–760, 1994.
3. Facchinetti F, Borella P: Oral magnesium successfully relieves premenstrual mood changes. Obstet Gynecol 78:177–181, 1991.
4. Hellberg D, Claesson B: Premenstrual tension: A placebo-controlled efficacy study with spironolactone and medroxyprogesterone acetate. Int J Gynecol Obstet 34:243–248, 1991.
5. Korzekwa MI, Steiner M: Premenstrual syndromes. Clin Obstet Gynecol 40:564–576, 1997.
6. Moline ML: Pharmacologic strategies for managing premenstrual syndrome. Clin Pharmacol 12:181–196, 1993.
7. Rubinow DR, Haban CM: Changes in plasma hormones across the menstrual cycle in patients with menstrually-related mood disorder and in control subjects. Am J Obstet Gynecol 158:5–11, 1988.
8. Thys-Jacobs S, Ceccarelli S: Calcium supplementation in premenstrual syndrome: A randomized crossover trial. J Gen Intern Med 4:183–189, 1989.
9. Wood SH, Mortola JF: Treatment of premenstrual syndrome with fluoxetine: A double-blind placebo-controlled, crossover study. Obstet Gynecol 80:339–344, 1992.
10 Yonkers KA: Antidepressants in the treatment of premenstrual dysphoric disorder. J Clin Psychiatry 58(Suppl 14):4–10, 1997.

25. Dysmenorrhea

Cynda Ann Johnson, M.D., M.B.A.

I. The Issues

Dysmenorrhea, the most common gynecologic complaint, generates innumerable telephone calls and visits to primary care physicians. It affects half of all female adolescents and is the leading cause of periodic school absenteeism. It is estimated 140 million hours of work and school are missed by women in the U.S. because of dysmenorrhea. Despite its prevalence, the physician must not adopt a laissez-faire approach to patients with dysmenorrhea, who often are incapacitated by the discomfort and frequently fear that the pain may be a manifestation of significant underlying disease. Although treatment is usually straightforward, the physician must be attuned to the patient whose symptoms do not respond to usual therapies.

II. The Theory

A. Definition

1. Dysmenorrhea is a painful, cramping sensation in the lower abdomen just before or during menses
   a. Pain is most severe on the first menstrual day
   b. Symptoms may last only a few hours—rarely more than 2 days
   c. Pain referred and distributed over the tenth thoracic to the first lumbar roots
      i. Strongest over lower abdomen and bilaterally in iliac fossae
      ii. May radiate to back and along thighs
   d. Associated symptoms
      i. Nausea most common (90% of cases)
      ii. Vomiting, diarrhea, headache, fatigue, dizziness, anxiety

2. **Primary dysmenorrhea**
   a. Rarely has onset after age 20
   b. Not associated with pelvic abnormality
   c. Associated with ovulatory cycles
   d. Pain caused by myometrial contractions
      i. Stimulated by prostaglandin $F_{2\alpha}$
      ii. Greater amount of prostaglandin $F_{2\alpha}$ during menstruation in patients with dysmenorrhea
      iii. Marked individual variation in perception of pain with contractions
      iv. More pain with dysrhythmic contractions
      v. Dyspareunia is not a feature

3. **Secondary dysmenorrhea**
   a. May occur at any age, often later in life than primary dysmenorrhea
   b. Many associations, often with organic disease
      i. Endometriosis
      ii. Uterine fibroids and adenomyosis
      iii. Cervical stenosis
      iv. Pelvic infection or adhesions
      v. Pelvic congestion syndrome
      vi. Intrauterine device
      vii. Stress and tension
      viii. Conditioned behavior
   c. Symptoms often persist longer than in primary dysmenorrhea

III. An Approach

A. History

1. Age of onset
2. Duration, timing of symptoms
3. Associated symptoms
4. Type of contraception

B. **Physical exam**
   1. Pelvic examination
C. **Drug treatment**
   1. Prostaglandin synthetase inhibitors (nonsteroidal antiinflammatory drugs [NSAIDs]) are drugs of choice to treat primary dysmenorrhea
      a. May be administered at onset of pain although thought to be more effective if administered before anticipated symptoms
      b. Fenamate family (mefenamic acid and meclofenamate) found most effective in multiple clinical trials
      c. Naproxen sodium is a popular choice—other NSAIDs approved by FDA for use in dysmenorrhea include ibuprofen and ketoprofen
      d. All NSAIDs appear to be more effective than aspirin
      e. Total blood loss decreased with use of NSAIDs—patients with heavy vaginal bleeding may continue NSAIDs for several days into the menses to decrease total flow
      f. 80% of women with dysmenorrhea get significant relief of pain and associated symptoms
   2. Other drugs
      a. Oral contraceptives provide relief in 70% of cases
      b. Calcium channel blockers such as nicardipine also reported to decrease dysmenorrhea
   3. **Failed treatment**
      a. Defined as inadequate response to 6-month trial of various NSAIDs and dosage regimens
      b. Consider secondary causes
         i. Further work-up may include: pelvic ultrasound; laparoscopy; hysteroscopy; psychological testing
         ii. Additional treatment depends on cause, degree of pain, need for contraception, age, desire for pregnancy

SUGGESTED READING

1. Alvin PE, Litt IF: Current status of the etiology and management of dysmenorrhea in adolescence. Pediatrics 70:516–525, 1982.
2. Apgar BS: Dysmenorrhea and dysfunctional uterine bleeding. Prim Care 24:161–175, 1997.
3. Cameron I: Dysfunctional bleeding. Baillieres Clin Obstet Gynaecol 3:315–327, 1989.
4. Molnår B, Baumann R: Does endometrial resection help dysmenorrhea? Acta Obstet Gynaecol Scand 76:261–265, 1997.
5. Rees MCP, DiMarzo V: Leukotriene release by endometrium and myometrium throughout the menstrual cycle in dysmenorrhoea and menorrhagia. J Endocrinol 113:291–295, 1987.

PART IV

INFERTILITY, FERTILITY, AND CONTRACEPTIVE TECHNIQUES

26. Infertility

Gary R. Newkirk, M.D.

I. **The Issues**

The major goals for evaluating the infertile couple include (1) identifying and correcting causes of infertility, (2) providing accurate information for the couple, (3) providing emotional support during and after the evaluation process, and (4) providing counseling about alternatives if pregnancy is unlikely or impossible. It is estimated that nearly 15% of couples in the United States are infertile. Infertility risk doubles for women aged 35–44 years compared with women aged 30–34 years; consequently, about one-third of women older than 35 who desire pregnancy will experience infertility. Couples seek professional help for infertility on an increasingly frequent basis. The primary care work-up of the infertile couple should be sufficient to allow diagnosis in approximately 60% of couples seeking help.

II. **The Theory**

    A. **Definition**

        1. A diagnosis of infertility is generally made when pregnancy has not occurred after 1 year of unprotected intercourse in a couple trying to conceive

    B. **Causes**

        1. There are various estimates about the frequencies of causes of infertility

        2. **Male factors**—40% of couples

            a. Disorders of spermatogenesis

            b. Obstruction of efferent ducts

            c. Disorders of sperm motility

            d. Sexual dysfunction

        3. **Female factors**—45% of couples

            a. Pelvic origin—30–50%

                i. Tubal disorders, uterine disorders, endometriosis

            b. Ovulatory origin—40%

                i. Adrenal, thyroid, pituitary disorder

            c. Cervical origin—10%

                i. Mucus problems, infectious problems

        4. **Unidentifiable factors**—15% of couples

        5. **Combined factors**—15–30% of couples

    C. **Infertility assessment tools**

        1. **Semen sample**

            a. Should be analyzed within 2 hours of ejaculation after 48 hours of ejaculatory abstinence

            b. Should be evaluated by persons experienced with fertility semen analysis

            c. If abnormality is found on the initial assessment, two additional semen analyses should be performed 2 weeks apart

            d. If abnormality persists, urologic consultation is appropriate

        2. **Ovulation** can be assessed by one or more methods:

            a. Basal body temperature (BBT)

                i. Method of recording BBT data should be explained during initial visit

            b. Serum progesterone levels

                i. Should be measured 7 days after estimated ovulation

      ii. Values consistent with ovulation vary with each laboratory, but generally values > 15 ng/ml are consistent with normal ovulatory function and levels under 5 ng/ml imply anovulation

  c. **Urinary screening of luteinizing hormone** (LH)

      i. Ovulation prediction test kits are available over the counter

      ii. Cost ranges from $30–40 per month tested

      iii. Most kits include from 5–10 urine tests per cycle

      iv. Based on serum LH surge preceding ovulation by 20–48 hours

      v. Urinary LH surge follows peak by 8–12 hours

      vi. Urine must be tested in mid-cycle as close to predicted ovulation as possible

      vii. Urine should be sampled at same time each day; some require first void, others do not.

      viii. Tests are supplied for fertility purposes, not as contraception aids

      ix. Menopause, polycystic ovary syndrome, and pregnancy may cause false-positive results

      x. Results are conflicting as to whether urinary ovulation testing improves ultimate pregnancy rates compared with other methods

  d. **Endometrial biopsy**

      i. Histologic detection of ovulation

      ii. Provides timing of progestational effect with day of cycle and can provide information about ovulation and luteal phase defects

      iii. Endometrial sampling is easily accomplished by use of small aspiration catheters (Pipelle, z-sampler). Sample 2–3 days before menses (approximately day 25 of a 28-day cycle).

3. **Postcoital testing**

  a. Evaluation of sperm–mucus interaction

  b. The couple is instructed to have intercourse after 48 hours of abstinence

  c. Pelvic examination is performed and aspirated cervical mucus is examined within 2–8 hours of intercourse

  d. Intercourse should occur within 24–48 hours of presumed ovulation as determined by methods outlined above

  e. Postcoital mucus should be examined by experienced individuals for quantity, viscosity, clarity, pH, spinnbarkeit (ability of mucus to stretch 7–10 cm between two glass slides smeared with mucus), and numbers, forms, and motility of sperm

  f. Generally, the finding of 5–10 sperm with linear motility per high power field in clear, acellular mucus with > 8-cm spinnbarkeit excludes cervical factor as major cause for infertility

4. **Hysterosalpingography** (HSP)

  a. A safe and high-yield procedure when performed in early proliferative phase of cycle (preprocedural pregnancy test usually advised)

  b. During HSP a special catheter is passed through the vagina into the endocervical canal through which contrast media is injected and fluoroscopically followed through the endometrial and fallopian tube lumen

  c. Undiagnosed pelvic mass or pelvic inflammatory disease (PID) contraindicates this procedure, as does iodine or radiocontrast dye allergy

  d. HSP can be performed during laparoscopic surgery

  e. Uterine causes for infertility include uterine abnormalities due to diethylstilbestrol (DES) (T-shaped, hypoplastic cavity), intrauterine synechiae (Asherman's syndrome), submucous or large intramural myomas, congenital anomalies, and leiomyomas

5. **Ultrasound** (transabdominal and transvaginal)

  a. Useful to help define pelvic anatomy

  b. Also documents cystic pathology, such as follicular or ovulatory cysts

6. **Laparoscopy**

  a. Indicated if HSP is contraindicated or abnormal and is also performed if historical (e.g., PID, endometriosis) or physical findings (adhesions, tubal or ovarian abnormality) implicate pelvic cause

      b. Treatment for endometriosis is discussed in separate chapter
      c. Laparoscopy is indicated if no other significant cause for infertility is identified
  7. **Laboratory tests**
      a. Fasting blood sugars, thyroid function, follicle-stimulating hormone (FSH), LH, and prolactin levels assist in the evaluation of endocrinologic factors as cause of infertility
  8. **Medication evaluation**
      a. Various medications contribute to disruption of thyroid, adrenal, or ovarian functioning in both men and women (e.g., antihypertensives, major tranquilizers, steroids)
III. **An Approach**
  A. **General comments**
    1. A timely and cost-effective approach requires initial evaluation of both male and female factors for infertility. Costs of evaluation should be discussed.
    2. An infertility evaluation entails multiple visits over a period of months
    3. Both partners should be scheduled for extended examination times
    4. The sequence in which a physician evaluates a couple's infertility varies with historical and physical findings during the initial visit
  B. **Stepwise evaluation**
    1. **Initial visit**
      a. Both partners
         i. Complete medical, family, drug, and sexual history
        ii. Complete physical examination
       iii. Laboratory examination, complete blood count, fasting blood sugar, Venereal Disease Research Laboratory (VDRL) test for syphilis, urinalysis, HIV screen
       iv. Cultures for *Chlamydia trachomatis*, *Ureaplasma urealyticum*, *Neisseria gonorrhoeae*
        v. Patient education
          (a) Alcohol, drugs, hot tubs, sexual practices, coital frequency, douching, lubricants
          (b) Explain need and method for various initial tests and data collection
             (i) Semen analysis
            (ii) Documentation of ovulation
           (iii) Postcoital test
           (iv) Evaluation of tubal patency
      b. Men
         i. Semen analysis
      c. Women
         i. Papanicolaou screening
        ii. KOH and wet mount
       iii. Utility of the following studies based on history
          (a) Thyroid function studies with history of dysthyroid symptoms
          (b) Prolactin levels in women with galactorrhea or irregular menses
          (c) Ultrasound and/or laparoscopy if pelvic exam is abnormal
          (d) Hysterosalpingogram with history of PID
          (e) If endometriosis likely, laparoscopy
          (f) Counseling with history of sexual dysfunction
       iv. Ovulatory monitoring (BBT, urinary LH) to assist in timing of tests
         v. Arrange for postcoital sample analysis with next visit
    2. **First follow-up visit**
      a. Schedule at time of midcycle/ovulation as predicted by BBT and/or urinary LH testing
      b. Review laboratory studies, semen analysis, and ovulatory monitoring data to date
      c. Obtain and analyze postcoital sample
      d. Consider and discuss need for endometrial biopsy
         i. To confirm ovulation and timing of luteal changes with day of cycle

    ii. If short luteal phase suspected (< 10 postovulation days preceding menses)

    iii. With a temperature rise that falls quickly after ovulation

    iv. If plasma progesterone level is low during luteal phase

  e. Arrange for HSP during follicular phase (day 7–9). If laparoscopy is necessary, HSP often is accomplished during laparoscopy

  3. **Second follow-up visit**

    a. Schedule during mid-luteal phase of cycle, 3 days before menses or at least 7 days after presumed ovulation

    b. Perform endometrial sampling if indicated

    c. Consider progesterone and prolactin levels if not already done

    d. Consider HSP and/or laparotomy

    e. Discuss referral to fertility specialist

C. **Management strategies for family physicians**—approach to therapy based on type of disorder

  1. **Abnormalities in male factors**

    a. Primarily evaluated by abnormal semen analysis and/or postcoital testing

    b. Education

      i. Sexual counseling

        (a) Coital frequency

          (i) Infrequent

          (ii) Poorly timed

        (b) Intercourse position

          (i) Adequate penile penetration

        (c) Masturbation

          (i) Sperm dilution

      ii. Alcohol, tobacco, drugs

        (a) Decrease sperm count

      iii. Douching, lubricants

        (a) Antisperm

        (b) Change mucus

      iv. Loose fitting clothing

        (a) Maintain ideal testicular temperature

      v. Minimize activities increasing testicular temperature

        (a) Hot tubs

        (b) Strenuous activities

        (c) Obesity

    c. Treatment of potential infection

      i. Prostatitis

      ii. Epididymitis

    d. Treatment of selected endocrinopathies

      i. Diabetes

      ii. Thyroid abnormalities

    e. Referral to urologist experienced with male infertility

      i. Varicocele surgery

      ii. Testicular biopsy

      iii. Testicular ultrasound

      iv. Hormonal therapy

        (a) Examples: testosterone, clomiphene, steroids, bromocriptine

    f. Test for sperm antibodies in semen and cervical mucus

      i. Referral usually necessary

      ii. Comanagement with therapy (e.g., corticosteroid administration) often possible

  2. **Ovarian disorders**

    a. Usually require 1 or more drug therapies

      i. Clomiphene, human chorionic gonadotropin (hCG), bromocriptine, estrogen and/or progestins, human menopausal gonadotropin (hMG), gonadotropin-releasing hormone (GnRH)

      ii. Clomiphene therapy trial

      (a) Indicated by absent or infrequent ovulation

      (b) Thyroid, pituitary, adrenal disorders must be diagnosed and managed first

      (c) Complete physical examination must be performed

      (d) With concerns about cystic ovarian conditions that may contraindicate clomiphene use, vaginal ultrasound should be performed

      (e) Endometrial biopsy may be indicated for prolonged anovulation to rule out hyperplasia

      (f) Clomiphene therapy begins with 50 mg on fifth day of cycle for duration of 5 days

      (g) Most women ovulate on day 17–20 of cycle

      (h) Intercourse should be timed accordingly

      (i) Monitor effect with BBT, postcoital checks of cervical mucus

      (j) Primary care providers experienced with its use begin clomiphene therapy and monitor effect for 3 months of therapy with above dosage. Others prefer to obtain consultation if fertility enhancing drugs are started.

      (k) Referral is often warranted if higher dosages or adjuvant drugs (e.g., hCG) required

      (l) Pelvic/vaginal ultrasound indicated for abdominal pain (implying ovarian cysts) or at least by end of 3 months of therapy

      (m) Evaluate patient for pregnancy, ovarian enlargement, or cysts every month

      (n) Referral to obstetrician/gynecologist who specializes in infertility is usually indicated before clomiphene therapy if family physician is not experienced with clomiphene or as an initial therapeutic consultation for comanagement with infertility specialist

   b. Therapy for ovulatory factors is directed toward underlying disorder, including thyroid replacement for hypothyroidism, bromocriptine for hyperprolactinemia (when pituitary macroadenoma is ruled out), or clomiphene to induce ovulation

3. **Cervical factors**

   a. Assessed initially by postcoital test

   b. Finding of leukocytes suggests cervicitis; cultures for *Neisseria gonorrhoeae*, *Ureaplasma urealyticum*, and *Chlamydia trachomatis* are useful to direct treatment.

     i. Nonmotile or non-progressively motile sperm with a "shaking" pattern suggest sperm antibodies

     ii. Timing

      (a) Inaccurate timing relative to ovulation is suggested by poor-quality cervical mucus that is abnormally thick and cloudy, and demonstrates poor spinnbarkeit

      (b) Repeat postcoital test is necessary if ovulatory timing is in question

4. **Uterine factors**

   a. Once identified, referral to infertility expert is warranted

     i. Hysteroscopy

     ii. Hysterosalpingography

      (a) May be performed by experienced family physician

     iii. Definitive surgical intervention often necessary

      (a) Polyp, fibroid, congenital anomaly/defect modification

5. **Tubal and peritoneal disorders**

   a. Broad range of disorders, including endometriosis, tubal anomalies/occlusion, pelvic adhesions

   b. Usually diagnosed by hysterosalpingogram, hysteroscopy, laparoscopy

   c. Referral necessary with comanagement of selected conditions, such as hormonal therapy for endometriosis

6. **Endometriosis**

   a. Diagnosis often requires referral for laparoscopy, hysterosalpingography

   b. Initial staging and management strategies usually require referral and comanagement

   c. Management often includes combined surgical and drug therapies

     i. Example: intra-abdominal laser therapy combined with danazol, GnRH agonists, medroxyprogesterone therapy

      ii. Combined therapy with ovulation-inducing drugs often necessary if en-
         dometriosis occurs with ovary disorder
7. **Infertility of unknown cause**
   a. Despite comprehensive evaluation 5–10% of couples have no identifiable cause
      of infertility
   b. Referral to infertility center warranted
      i. Assisted reproductive technology (ART) options are appropriate (e.g., in
         vitro fertilization, gamete intrafallopian transfer)
      ii. Supportive measures
         (a) Attitudes toward adoption and ART should be explored. Often individual
            or joint guilt about infertility can be underestimated.
         (b) Emotional support should remain part of every visit; ongoing contact
            with primary care provider is helpful.
         (c) Resolve (www.resolve.org), a national nonprofit infertility organization,
            has chapters throughout the U.S. and is an excellent resource for support
            and counseling groups. National headquarters: 5 Water Street, Arlington,
            MA 02174.

SUGGESTED READING

1. Chuang AT, Howards SS: Male infertility: Evaluation and non-surgical therapy. Urol Clin North Am
   25:703–713, 1998.
2. Collins JA: A couple with infertility. JAMA 274:1159–1164, 1995.
3. Hanson MA, Dumesic DA: Initial evaluation and treatment of infertility in a primary care setting. Mayo
   Clin Proc 73:681–685, 1998.
4. Daniluk J: Helping patients cope with infertility. Clin Obstet Gynecol 40:661–672, 1997.
5. Morell V: Basic infertility assessment. Prim Care 24:195–204, 1997.
6. Speroff L, Glass RH, Kase NG: Investigation of the infertile couple. In Speroff L, Glass RH, Kase NH
   (eds): Clinical Gynecologic Endocrinology and Infertility, 5th ed. Baltimore, Williams & Wilkins, 1994.
7. Trantham P: The infertile couple. Am Fam Physician 54:1001–1010, 1996.

27. Fertility Choices

Cynda Ann Johnson, M.D., M.B.A.

I. The Issues

The ever-increasing options for birth control methods, on one hand, and infertility intervention,
on the other, continue to expand a woman's ability to exercise fertility choices. Along with this
apparent freedom of choice is the startling statistic that 50% of pregnancies in the U.S. are unplanned; this number rises to 95% among teenage pregnancies. Over 1.3 million pregnancies
result in abortion. Yet the rate of infertility has risen to 15%. Issues surrounding fertility choices
are pervasive in the daily lives of reproductive-aged women and are a source of significant stress.
Women must decide when (if ever) to attempt to achieve pregnancy, the optimal birth control
method, how to respond to unplanned pregnancy, and the appropriate degree of intervention in
the infertile state. Studies indicate that insurance coverage, especially among Medicaid recipi-
ents, may significantly influence the choice to prevent, carry, or terminate pregnancy. The generalist physician must be prepared to assist the woman in the decision-making process and support
her choices.

II. The Theory
  A. **Fertility**
    1. In a group of fertile couples the monthly conception rate, or fecundability, is about
       20%
    2. Female fertility (actual procreation) and fecundity (capacity for procreation) de-
       crease with increasing maternal age

    a. A 1982 study in France looked at the cumulative pregnancy rate over 1 year among women undergoing artificial insemination; the results showed a cumulative pregnancy rate of 75% before age 31; 61% between ages 30 and 35; and 53% over age 35.

    b. Fertility was studied among the Hutterites, who are known to have a high rate of fertility; 11% of Hutterite women bore no children after age 34; 33% had no children after age 40; and 37% had no children after age 44.

    c. A study from the Netherlands in 1997 reported a 90% pregnancy rate from age 20–28, decreasing to 75–80% by age 35

    d. More women delay pregnancy until they are over 35 and even 40 years of age; 20% of women in the U.S. now have their first child after the age of 35.

       i. In one study of patients in a private practice, 3% of primiparas were at least 40 years of age.

    e. **Consequences of delaying pregnancy**

       i. Decreased fertility secondary to older age

       ii. Increased infertility from causes other than age, such as chronic diseases

       iii. Greater incidence of spontaneous abortion and genetic anomalies

       iv. Association between maternal age and pregnancy-induced hypertension, diabetes, abruptio placentae, placenta previa, and cesarean section

       v. Most studies show, however, that in healthy women of advanced maternal age, who are able to carry their pregnancy, neonates may be at no higher risk for adverse outcome than in younger women

B. **Prevention of pregnancy**

    1. Table 1 shows contraceptive efficacy of various forms of birth control

    2. Abstinence is an important option for many individuals

    a. Abstinence as a birth control option means avoidance of penis-in-vagina intercourse

    b. A broad range of sexual expression is possible without penis-in-vagina intercourse

    c. Insertive sex is medically inadvisable in some circumstances:

       i. Sexually transmitted diseases (STDs)

       ii. Postoperative pain

       iii. Dyspareunia

       iv. Undiagnosed postcoital bleeding

       v. Some circumstances of pregnancy and postpartum period

       vi. Immediately after myocardial infarction

       vii. Acute illness or infection

       viii. Disabling physical conditions

       ix. As a part of sex therapy

    3. See chapters on specific birth control methods for information on selecting the optimal birth control method for the individual or couple

C. **Unplanned pregnancy**

    1. Nearly one-half of all pregnancies are unplanned

    2. Among women under age 21, the abortion rate is nearly equal to the live birth rate

    3. Only 2% of unmarried women who choose to carry the pregnancy relinquish the baby for adoption

    4. Women with unintended pregnancies report higher rates of physical violence than women with intended pregnancies

D. **Abortion**

    1. Legalized in the U.S. in 1973 after the Supreme Court's decision on two landmark cases—*Roe v. Wade* and *Doe v. Bolton*

    a. The decision to perform an abortion in the first trimester of pregnancy may be made between the patient and her physician

    b. The state may regulate the abortion procedure in the second trimester in the interest of promoting the health of the pregnant woman

    c. From the time of viability of the pregnancy, the state may impose greater controls, regulating and even prohibiting abortion, except when necessary according to medical opinion for the preservation of the life or health of the pregnant woman

TABLE 1. Percentage of Women Experiencing a Contraceptive Failure during the First Year of Typical Use and the First Year of Perfect Use and the Percentage Use at the End of the First Year (United States)

Method	% of Women Experiencing an Accidental Pregnancy within the First Year of Use		% of Women Continuing Use at 1 Year
	Typical Use	Perfect Use	
Chance	85	85	
Spermicides	26	6	40
Periodic abstinence	25		63
Calendar		9	
Ovulation method		3	
Sympto-Thermal		2	
Postovulation		1	
Withdrawal	19	4	
Cap			
Parous women	40	26	42
Nulliparous women	20	9	56
Sponge			
Parous women	40	20	42
Nulliparous women	20	9	56
Diaphragm	20	6	56
Condom			
Female	21	5	56
Male	14	3	61
Pill			
Progestin-only		0.5	
Combined	5	0.1	71
IUD			
Progesterone T	2.0	1.5	81
Copper T 380A	0.8	0.6	78
LNg 20	0.1	0.1	81
Depo-Provera	0.3	0.3	70
Norplant	0.05	0.05	88
Female sterilization	0.5	0.5	100
Male sterilization	0.15	0.10	100

Adapted from Trussell J: Contraceptive efficacy. In Hatcher RA, Trussell J, Stewart F, et al (eds): Contraceptive Technology, 17th ed. New York, Ardent Media, Inc., 1998, pp 800–801.

2. In 1992 the Supreme Court ruled that states may place restrictions on abortion services, such as waiting periods and specific requirements for informed consent and parental notification
3. Legalized abortion is the most commonly performed surgical procedure in the U.S.
   a. Annual number of abortions has decreased by 15% from a high in 1990
   b. In 1995 (most recent year reported), a total of 1, 210,883 legal abortions were reported; the abortion ratio was 311 abortions per 1000 live births.
4. **Characteristics of women undergoing abortion**
   a. Women seeking abortion are more often young, white, and unmarried
   b. Most women seeking abortions are primiparas having an abortion procedure for the first time
   c. Younger women tend to obtain abortions later in gestation than older women
   d. One-half of all abortions are performed before 8 weeks of gestation; 88% before 13 weeks.
5. **Surgical methods**
   a. Suction curettage
      i. Most widely used method, accounting for 97% of abortion procedures
      ii. May be used through 14 weeks of gestation

      iii. May be done under local or general anesthesia

      iv. May be carried out in properly equipped office setting

  b. Dilation and evacuation (D&E)

      i. Optimal use from 13–16 weeks of gestation, but may be used up to 20+ weeks

      ii. Safer, faster, and less expensive than alternatives, such as medical infusion methods

      iii. May be carried out under local or general anesthesia

      iv. Requires greater cervical dilation than suction curettage

E. **Infertility**

  1. The rate of infertility (inability to conceive within 1 year) in the U.S. is increasing

  2. The infertility rate rises from 5% in the under 20 age group to 20% in the 35–39 age group

  3. Most common causes are anovulation (10–15%), pelvic factors (30–40%), male factors (30–40%)

F. **Childless marriages and couples**

  1. Couple may avoid having children

    a. Five percent of married couples choose not to have children; the term child-free marriage may be preferred.

    b. See Table 2 for reasons couples give for choosing to remain child-free

    c. In general, couples who choose not to have children can be divided into two major categories:

      i. Those who are going toward goals other than parenthood; failure to have children is secondary result.

      ii. Those who actively avoid parenthood

  2. The couple may be infertile

TABLE 2. Reasons Couples Give for Remaining Child-free

Allows lifestyle options for the future to be kept open	Older when married
Continuing love affair—relationship of the couple stronger because they only have each other	Hard to raise children today
	Lives already difficult enough
Allows time for focusing on self to "know who I am"	May have bad children
Allows self-indulgence	Never felt the need; life already full
Cheaper	Attention to zero population growth
Enjoy others' children	More interested in keeping spouse than children if spouse disinterested in reproduction
Permission for being child-free through women's movement	Already have commitments to other children— sometimes financially
Don't like saying "no" so often	
Better sex life	Belief in variety of acceptable lifestyles
Problem family backgrounds	"I don't think I would be a good parent"
More fun	Channel energy into other social concerns
More control of own time	Physician forced a decision
Time-consuming political interests	Unmarried
No assurance you will not be alone in older age	Do not like children
Fear of being walled off from other close friends	Love animals
No need to have every experience in life	Compulsive worker
Other meaning to life besides reproduction	No desire for long-term commitment
Can't have everything	Protecting children by not having them
Reproduction includes other human interactions (nurturant to whole human race)	Help raise someone else's child
	Already raised children as a child
Realization, not decision	Husband would not share responsibility
School commitments	Lesbian who does not want to impose her lifestyle on child
No desire to contribute to population overgrowth	
Quieter without children	Fear of rejection
No relief from parenthood once you start	Unsafe world

Adapted from Harper K: The Child-free Alternative. Brattleboro, Stephen Greene Press, 1980.

III. **An Approach**
  A. The generalist physician should regularly discuss fertility choices and issues with all women of reproductive age; topics and approach will vary, depending on factors such as the age of the woman, marital status, and sexual orientation.
  B. Possible topics for inclusion
    1. Range of sexual expression
    2. Relationship status
    3. Current and future pregnancy plans
    4. Contraceptive alternatives
  C. **Approach to fertility options**
    1. **Patient desiring pregnancy**
      a. See Chapter 28 (Pregnancy)
      b. Focus of history
        i. Menstrual history
        ii. Previous fertility
        iii. History of immunization or disease, including hepatitis, rubella, measles, mumps, chickenpox
        iv. History and risk of STDs
      c. Focus of physical exam—pelvic exam
      d. Other investigations as indicated
        i. Papanicolaou smear
        ii. Testing for STDs
        iii. Evidence of protection from viral infections listed above
      e. Emphasis on preconception counseling
        i. Timing and frequency of intercourse to achieve pregnancy: coital technique
        ii. Patient should begin daily vitamin containing at least 0.4 mg folic acid
    2. **Prevention of pregnancy**
      a. After complete history and physical exam, select birth control method best suited to the individual
      b. Consider the following issues
        i. Success of birth control methods used previously
        ii. Age
        iii. Pregnancy history
        iv. Expectations of compliance with method
        v. Reversibility of method
        vi. Possible future fertility
        vii. Duration of use
        viii. Need for protection from STDs
        ix. Theoretical and typical failure rate of the various methods
        x. Tolerance of possible side effects
        xi. Potential adverse effects
        xii. Medical problems
        xiii. Medications
        xiv. Drug, tobacco, alcohol use
    3. **Unplanned pregnancy**
      a. Most women with an unplanned pregnancy choose to carry the pregnancy before seeing a health care provider
        i. They need the support of their physician, whether or not their decision is favored by their usual support system
        ii. She or someone close to her may be the intended childcare provider
        iii. She may choose to have the child adopted
          (a) The adoptive process should begin immediately
          (b) A social worker or other person skilled in making arrangements should be involved
          (c) The decision to seek private or agency adoption must be made
          (d) At any point the woman may decide to withdraw from the adoptive process

b. Women in doubt about how to proceed with an unplanned pregnancy need non-judgmental counseling by their physician; a physician who is unable to provide this service should have a ready referral.
c. The woman may choose to have pregnancy termination
   i. **Preabortion evaluation**
      (a) Menstrual and obstetric history, contraceptive use, allergies, medications, other acute or chronic illness that may interfere with surgical procedure
      (b) Pelvic exam must be done immediately and not deferred until the time of termination evaluation to corroborate uterine size, menstrual history and EDC, and to assess need for STD testing
      (c) Laboratory tests should include: pregnancy test, appropriate evaluation for STDs, hemoglobin level or hematocrit, Rh antibody evaluation
   ii. The woman must have ready access to referral sources so that the procedure can be carried out in a timely fashion
   iii. A follow-up appointment should be scheduled with the primary care provider within 1 week after the termination
      (a) History should include whether antibiotic prophylaxis or Rhogam was given, and presence of fever, abdominal or pelvic pain, vaginal discharge, or continued bleeding
      (b) Pelvic exam should be performed—the uterus should be involuting and nontender
      (c) Pregnancy test should not be done because the result may still be positive
      (d) Birth control method should be chosen at the follow-up visit, if not selected at the time of the termination
   iv. Some women will return to the physician's office at a later date without termination of pregnancy
      (a) All women referred for pregnancy termination should be encouraged to return for prenatal care as soon as possible if for any reason the termination is not carried out
      (b) Reasons for not proceeding with the termination include insufficient money, decision to carry the pregnancy, and poor organizational skills resulting in the realization that the pregnancy had continued beyond the time considered reasonable for termination

4. **Infertility**
   a. Determine whether the patient meets criteria for infertility
      i. Many patients believe that they are infertile if they have not conceived in the first few months of unprotected intercourse
      ii. Review fertility awareness and methods to optimize chances for conception
      iii. Select patients in whom infertility evaluation should be undertaken sooner than the usual time frame, e.g., those with a previous history of infertility or oligomenorrhea
      iv. It is reasonable to begin an infertility evaluation in an older women, especially one over 40 years of age, after only 6 months of inability to conceive; simple evaluations can begin even sooner.
   b. Begin infertility evaluation (see Chapter 26)
      i. Many primary care physicians initiate the evaluation in their own offices
      ii. Refer to a subspecialist for more intensive evaluation
      iii. The primary care provider should be available to the patient throughout the evaluative process
         (a) Providing support for the patient during a stressful process
         (b) Discussing the process and procedures
         (c) Working with the patient to decide the depth of evaluation that should be undertaken before an alternative approach (such as adoption) is chosen
         (d) If the patient becomes pregnant, the delivering generalist may resume the patient's care

5. **Childless marriage**
    a. Role of the primary care provider
        i. Helping the couple to cope with infertility and to seek other options if desired
        ii. Regularly reevaluating the couple who choose to remain child-free, offering reliable contraception and permanent sterilization as indicated
6. **Other options**
    a. Adoption may be pursued by heterosexual or homosexual couples or single women
    b. Artificial insemination may be preferred by single women and/or lesbian couples
    c. Surrogate parenting is an option, though, with medicolegal risks and social consequences

SUGGESTED READING

1. Catanzarite V, Deutchman M, Johnson CA, Scherger JE: Pregnancy after 35: What's the real risk? Patient Care 29:41–51, 1995.
2. Chandra A, Stephen EH: Impaired fecundity in the United States: 1982–1995. Fam Plann Perspect 30:34–42, 1998.
3. Gilbert WM, Nesbitt TS: Childbearing beyond age 40: Pregnancy outcome in 24,032 cases. Obstet Gynecol 93:9–14, 1999.
4. Harper K: The Child-free Alternative. Brattleboro, Stephen Greene, 1980.
5. Hatcher RA, Trussell J, Stewart F, et al (eds): Contraceptive Technology, 17th ed. New York, Ardent Media, Inc., 1998.
6. Hollander D, Breen JL: Pregnancy in the older gravida: How old is old? Obstet Gynecol Surv 45:106–112, 1990.
7. Joyce T, Kaestner R, Kwan F: Is Medicaid pronatalist? The effect of eligibility expansions on abortions and births. Fam Plan Perspect 30:108–113, 124, 1998.
8. Koonin LM, Smith JC: Abortion surveillance—United States, 1995. MMWR 47(SS-2): 31–40, 1998.
9. Prysak M, Lorenz RP, Kisly A: Pregnancy outcome in nulliparous women 35 years and older. Obstet Gynecol 85:65–70, 1995.
10. van Balen F, Verdurmen JE: Age, the desire to have a child and cumulative pregnancy rate. Hum Reprod 12:623–627, 1997.
11. Weckstein LN: Treating the infertile woman over 40. Med Aspects Hum Sex November:22–29, 1991.

28. Pregnancy

Barbara S. Apgar, M.D., M.S.

I. The Issues

Pregnancy involves the interplay of complex hormonal and psychosocial factors. Fortunately, the majority of pregnancies achieve a successful outcome. The concept of family-centered obstetrics brings together the patient, her partner and family, and the health care provider in a unique and resourceful manner. The clinician becomes an advocate for the patient's obstetric care, and the patient assumes the responsibility of entering into this relationship in an informed position. It is a powerful bond and assumes greater prominence as issues of obstetric care begin to be scrutinized and questioned, such as the relevance of intervention strategies and measures of cost-containment. The clinician must balance the role of advocate for the patient's right to safe and effective obstetric care with the role of manager of health care dollars. The answer may lie with recent meta-analyses of evidence-based medical literature, which have resulted in new protocols and management schemes and reinvestigation of data surrounding the dictums to which clinicians have adhered for the past decade. For example, as the utility of electronic fetal monitoring and episiotomy is reexamined, a new body of literature supports the concept that low-intervention strategies produce an improved and more successful obstetric outcome in many low-risk cases. Understanding the rationale for ordering obstetric screening and diagnostic tests and for intervening when appropriate, the clinician takes on a more important role as advocate and strategist. The goal of successful maternal and fetal outcome rests largely with the knowledge of the clinician in charting the obstetric course, the patient's informed and responsible consent, and the probability that untoward and unexpected emergent events will be managed in an efficient, skilled manner. The outcome is further enhanced if the bond between patient and clinician has been encouraged and facilitated throughout both preconceptual and prenatal courses.

Family-centered obstetric care lies at the center of the balancing act between high-risk, high technologic care and the low-interventional care that the majority of patients require. The goal should not be to produce more and more high technologic equipment and protocols but to rethink the methods by which we came to our present position and to reinvent strategies that allow the patient to be part of the plan and make informed decisions. The clinician must be educated about what the literature actually presents as good, sound medical practice. The epidemic of cesarean deliveries has caused us to rethink how and why it has occurred and what can be done to lower this alarming rate of increase in surgical births. Future research should be directed toward randomized, controlled trials that answer such important questions.

II. **The Theory**
  A. **Preconceptual risk assessment**
    1. **Age risks**
       a. Risks of pregnancy at the extremes of maternal age
          i. > age 35
             (a) Genetic counseling should be offered
             (b) Risk of pregnancy loss from amniocentesis is less than or equal to risk of genetic abnormality
          ii. < age 15
             (a) Immature reproductive system
             (b) Adolescent adjustment reactions
             (c) Support system may be lacking
    2. **Ethnic populations at risk**
       a. African-American and Southeast Asian: sickle-cell disease
       b. Jewish: Tay-Sachs disease
       c. Mediterranean, Italian, Greek: beta-thalassemia
       d. Asian: alpha-thalassemia
    3. **Chronic disease risk**
       a. Medication used in chronic disease conditions may be known teratogens:
          i. Gold
          ii. Folic acid antagonists
          iii. Lithium
          iv. Isotretinoin
          v. Valproic acid
          vi. Warfarin
       b. Diabetes mellitus (uncontrolled)
          i. Increased risk of spontaneous pregnancy loss
          ii. Higher rate of anomalies in offspring
    4. **Infection risk**
       a. Rubella
          i. 15–20% of adults are not immune
          ii. Anomaly risk highest in first trimester
       b. Toxoplasmosis
          i. Current serologic antibody testing has poor predictive value
          ii. Screening in U.S. is not mandatory
       c. Cytomegalovirus (CMV)
          i. More low socioeconomic status patients are seropositive
          ii. 7% annualized rate of primary infection
       d. Hepatitis B virus (HBV)
          i. 90% of infected infants become chronic HBV carriers
          ii. More than 25% die of primary hepatocellular carcinoma or cirrhosis
          iii. Only 35–65% of HBsAg-positive women are identified by "high-risk" status
             (a) Asians or Alaskan Eskimos
             (b) Household contacts of HBsAg carriers

          (c) IV drug users

          (d) History of blood transfusions

          (e) Workers in kidney dialysis units

e. Genital herpes simplex virus (HSV)
  i. Both HSV 1 and 2 can lead to fetal and neonatal infection
      (a) Only 1 in 4 women knows she has acquired HSV
  ii. Primary disease during pregnancy (no antibodies or seroconversion)
      (a) Transmission rate of 50%
      (b) Mother and fetus may be adversely affected more than from secondary disease
      (c) 33% of neonates born to mothers with asymptomatic shedding at the onset of labor are infected
  iii. Reactivation of maternal disease during pregnancy (previous seroconversion)
      (a) Transmission rate is under 1% because of protective effect from antibodies
      (b) 3% of neonates born to mothers with asymptomatic shedding at the onset of labor are infected

f. *Chlamydia trachomatis* infection
  i. Increases the risk of intrauterine fetal death, low birth weight, and postpartum endometritis
  ii. Active maternal infection has transmission rate of 60% to newborn
      (a) Pneumonia in 16% of newborns
      (b) Conjunctivitis in 18% of newborns

g. Human papillomavirus (HPV)
  i. Condylomata may proliferate during pregnancy
      (a) Rate is higher in HIV-positive or immunocompromised women
  ii. Risk of respiratory papillomatosis (RP) is low
  iii. Smoking is important cofactor for HPV activation

h. Syphilis
  i. Congenital syphilis may cause spontaneous pregnancy loss, premature birth, congenital anomalies, or fetal death
  ii. Severity of congenital syphilis is related to the gestational age of the fetus at the time of infection
      (a) The more recent the infection, the more severe the congenital disease

i. Human immunodeficiency virus (HIV)
  i. Individuals with high-risk behavior
      (a) History of risky sexual behavior
      (b) History of IV drug use
      (c) History of blood transfusions between 1981 and 1985
  ii. Rate of transmission from HIV-infected mother to fetus is 7–71%
      (a) Prenatal, delivery or breast feeding
          (i) Greatest risk is during delivery
      (b) 25% of infants will acquire HIV from their mothers

5. **Reproductive risk**
  a. Prior obstetric history
      i. Repeated miscarriage, fetal demise, or infertility
      ii. Number of pregnancies, fetal weights, delivery types, length of labor, complications of pregnancy and delivery, anesthesia risks
      iii. Candidacy for vaginal birth after cesarean section (VBAC) and type of scar—must be determined before VBAC is attempted
  b. Menstrual history
      i. Menstrual regularity, cyclic pattern of bleeding, weight loss or gain, dysmenorrhea
          (a) Fibroids, genital tract abnormalities
      ii. Pattern of exercise or evidence of eating disorder
      iii. Knowledge of menstrual cycle and ovulation signs
  c. Sexual history
      i. Sexual dysfunction
      ii. Intimacy issues

        iii. Knowledge of sexual function

        iv. Fears and concerns

6. **Environmental risk**
   a. Occupational exposure
      i. Implicated in reproductive dysfunction
         (a) Change in spermatogenesis and oogenesis may cause infertility and pregnancy loss
      ii. Pregnancy can alter maternal and fetal susceptibility to toxins or inhaled agents
         (a) Decreased gastrointestinal transport
         (b) Increased tidal volume
      iii. Exposure
         (a) Inhalation
            (i) Paints
            (ii) Toxic fumes
            (iii) Passive smoke
         (b) Cutaneous absorption
         (c) Ingestion
         (d) Unsafe work practices
            (i) Computer terminals have not been shown to cause adverse perinatal outcome

7. **Substance abuse and illicit drug use:** goal is to decrease habit before pregnancy occurs
   a. Cigarette smoking
      i. Associated with low birth weight, stillbirth, spontaneous pregnancy loss, and sudden infant death
   b. Illicit drugs
      i. Risks
         (a) Cocaine—abruptio placenta
         (b) IV drugs—hepatitis, HIV
   c. Alcohol
      i. Safety level is unknown, but alcohol appears to be an acute fetal toxin when large amounts are consumed at one time rather than small amounts over long period of time
      ii. Associated with low birth weight, stillbirth, spontaneous pregnancy loss and fetal alcohol syndrome
      iii. Fetal alcohol syndrome is now the leading cause of mental retardation

8. **Treatment-associated risks**
   a. Previous surgery
   b. History of trauma to pelvis or back
   c. History of blood transfusion
   d. Allergies
   e. Blood type and Rh factor

9. **Preconceptual health promotion and education**
   a. Diet
      i. Folate: associated with significant decrease in risk of fetal neural tube defects
      ii. Other dietary habits
         (a) Underweight women with poor weight gain during pregnancy have higher risk of fetal and neonatal death
         (b) Obese women have higher risk of diabetes, hypertension, macrosomia, shoulder dystocia, and labor dysfunction
   b. Exercise: helpful in managing weight and stress and should be continued during pregnancy
   c. Financial and social support systems: any patient can overestimate or underestimate her social support or financial situation
      i. Unreal expectations
      ii. Denial of pregnancy

   iii. Underlying psychological condition
   iv. Embarrassment about her situation
B. **Endocrinology of pregnancy**
 1. Progesterone
  a. Function
   i. Implantation
   ii. Substrate pool for fetal adrenal gland production of glucocorticoids and min-
    eralocorticoids
  b. Production site
   i. Corpus luteum until 7th week of gestation
   ii. Placenta after 10–11th week of gestation
  c. Serum levels: maximum at term between 100–200 ng/ml
 2. Estrogen
  a. Function
   i. Possibly effective in increasing uteroplacental blood flow from combination
    of estrogens
    (a) Estriol accounts for 90% of estrogen in pregnancy
    (b) Other estrogens
     (i) Estrone
     (ii) Estradiol
   ii. Normal levels reflect fetal well-being
  b. Production site: placenta with cholesterol precursor primarily of maternal and
   some fetal origin
  c. Serum levels
   i. Primarily measured from unconjugated estriol
   ii. Less variable than total estriol levels
   iii. Clinically detectable in maternal serum at 9 weeks' gestation
   iv. Maximum at term between 11–14.5 ng/ml
 3. Human chorionic gonadotropin (hCG)
  a. Required for survival of corpus luteum
  b. May stimulate steroidogenesis in early fetal testes
C. **Prenatal evaluation**
 1. **Diagnosis of pregnancy**
  a. Absence of menses: sensitivity increased if menses have occurred regularly
  b. Other symptoms
   i. Nausea and vomiting
    (a) Occurs in up to 50% of pregnancies
    (b) May occur anytime of the day, not just morning
   ii. Mastalgia: usually apparent by 6 weeks and lasts through the first trimester
   iii. Persistent elevation of basal body temperature in luteal phase
  c. Pregnancy tests
   i. Presence of β-hCG subunit in serum or urine
    (a) A single hCG level does not predict pregnancy outcome
   ii. Serum (quantitative) β-hCG
    (a) Used for diagnosis of intrauterine pregnancy, ectopic pregnancy, sponta-
     neous pregnancy loss, and trophoblastic disease
    (b) Diagnosis by serial quantitative testing: normal pregnancy is reflected in
     a doubling of serum levels every 1.2–2.1 days
   iii. Urine
    (a) Some kits may be sensitive to as low as 10 mIU/ml
    (b) Detectable levels of home and office tests are similar
    (c) Home pregnancy tests do not need to be repeated in the office if patient
     has performed correctly
  d. Ultrasonography (USN)
   i. Valuable diagnostic tool to determine fetal viability
   ii. Transvaginal USN can detect fetal heart activity before 6 weeks' gestation
   iii. The mean gestational sac diameter is correlated with fetal heart activity

e. Progesterone levels
  i. Differ from hCG levels because they remain constant through first 9–10 weeks in normal pregnancy
  ii. After 6–8 weeks' gestation, nonviable pregnancies have significantly lower progesterone, estradiol, and hCG levels than normal pregnancies
  iii. Unlike hCG levels, a single progesterone level (< 5, > 25 ng/ml) is predictive of pregnancy outcome ($p < 0.001$)

2. **Diagnosis of abnormal pregnancy**
  a. **Ectopic pregnancy**
    i. Epidemiology
      (a) 1/66 pregnancies
      (b) Sevenfold increase in past 25 years
      (c) Risk factors
        (i) Previous history of ectopic pregnancy
        (ii) History of pelvic inflammatory disease (PID)
        (iii) Previous tubal surgery
        (iv) History of infertility
    ii. Clinical presentation
      (a) Abdominal pain 50–100%
      (b) Rebound tenderness 40–50%
      (c) Vaginal bleeding 55–84%
      (d) Adnexal mass 30–70%
      (e) Amenorrhea 60–85%
    iii. Morbidity and mortality
      (a) Third leading cause of direct maternal death
  b. **Spontaneous pregnancy loss** (miscarriage)
    i. New definitions
      (a) Anembryonic gestation (empty sac or molar pregnancy)
      (b) First trimester intrauterine fetal death
    ii. Epidemiology
      (a) Incidence varies depending on whether pregnancy was recognized or documented before clinical recognition
        (i) Overall rate of loss before 20 weeks: 2%
        (ii) Overall rate of loss up to 28 weeks: 13.4%
        (iii) Two loss periods
          • Embryonic period: 1–13 weeks
          • Fetal period: 14–20 weeks
      (b) Risks
        (i) Increased with advancing maternal age
        (ii) Increased among women with vaginal bleeding
        (iii) Increased among women with previous spontaneous pregnancy losses
        (iv) Increased adverse infant outcome if bleeding occurs in the first trimester
          • Preterm delivery
          • Delivery of low-birth-weight infant
          • Neonatal death
    iii. Etiology
      (a) Chromosomal anomalies are most common
      (b) Other causes
        (i) Insulin-dependent diabetes
        (ii) Increased caffeine use: > 163 mg/d
        (iii) Alcohol acts as acute fetal poison

3. **First prenatal visit**
  a. **History**
    i. Maternal and paternal updates from preconception counseling should be included

      (a) Obstetric history
      (b) Gynecologic history
      (c) Medical and surgical history
      (d) Genetics screening
         (i) Ethnic origin risk factors
         (ii) History of chromosomal anomalies in family
         (iii) Inherited diseases
      (e) Psychosocial situation

b. **Physical examination**
   i. Complete physical examination with vital signs
   ii. Measurement of uterine size
   iii. Measurement of pelvic anatomic relationships
   iv. Measurement of fetal heart rate if appropriate

4. **Screening tests during pregnancy**
  a. Goals of screening tests
    i. Identify patients at risk for complications
    ii. Perform tests where intervention will make a difference
    iii. Identify tests that have high cost–benefit ratio
  b. Characteristics of screening tests
    i. Generally not diagnostic
      (a) Positive screening tests lead to further testing
    ii. Specificity is not as important as sensitivity
    iii. Guidelines are generally established by consensus panel rather than from randomized controlled trials
  c. Questions to ask about a screening test
    i. Has the test demonstrated effectiveness in evidence-based medical literature trials?
    ii. Does the test actually test for the particular diagnostic category?
    iii. Is there a treatment option available?
    iv. Will the test screen women who will most benefit from the testing?
    v. Is the system able to accommodate mass screening?
  d. **Gestational diabetes mellitus** (GDM)
    i. Goal of screening
      (a) Detect any degree of glucose intolerance during pregnancy
      (b) Established diabetes should be recognized before conception
         (i) History and physical examination
         (ii) Risk factors
         (iii) Diagnosis: fasting blood sugar > 140 on 2 occasions or 200 once
    ii. No longer a clear mandate for universal screening for GDM during pregnancy
      (a) Random controlled trials do not indicate difference in outcome if diagnosed
         (i) Macrosomia is the only variable that shows a consistent improvement if GDM treated
          • < 200 grams overall
         (ii) Controversy surrounds whether GDM causes hyperbilirubinemia, hypoglycemia, hypocalcemia
         (iii) Screening should be based on the population of women at risk in the particular clinical setting
          • Adolescents—low risk
          • High prevalence of type II DM—high risk
          • GDM is so high in Native Americans that all should receive diagnostic rather than screening testing
      (b) High false-positive rate
         (i) 15% with 50-gm load
         (ii) 25% with 75-gm load
         (iii) Corrected data may increase true positives by 50%
      (c) Selective screening (24–28 weeks' gestation or earlier in high-risk women)

        (i) Age > 25–30
       (ii) > 20% of ideal body weight
     (iii) History of fetal macrosomia
     (iv) Previous GDM
      (v) First-degree relative with DM
     (vi) Unexplained fetal death or anomalies
    (vii) Hypertensive disease
   (viii) Persistent glycosuria
     (ix) Ethnic origin: Native American, Asian, Hispanic

e. **Maternal serum alpha-fetoprotein** (MSAFP)
   i. Goal of screening
     (a) Detection of open neural tube defects
        (i) Spina bifida and anencephaly: 90–95% of cases arise de novo
     (b) Detection of risk for Down syndrome and other anomalies
   ii. Interpretation of MSAFP
     (a) Major serum marker
        (i) Can be interpreted only as screening test
       (ii) Confirmation by amniotic fluid alpha-fetoprotein must be performed if MSAFP test is positive
         • Relatively high false-positive rate; 90–95% have normal amniotic fluid AFP.
         • 5–7% are positive at first screen; at repeat test, 4% remain positive.
         • USN leaves 2% with unexplained test results
     (b) Results of MSAFP
        (i) 2% require amniocentesis
         • Indicates 80–90% of anencephaly
         • Indicates 60–90% of spina bifida
   iii. Who to screen
     (a) Women whose relatives have neural tube defects
     (b) Women with diabetes
     (c) Women < age 35

f. **Triple screen** (markers)
   i. Goal
     (a) Detection of Down syndrome
        (i) Reduces numbers of amniocentesis in woman < age 35
       (ii) Can detect 89% of Down syndrome
         • 25% false-positive rate > 35 years
   ii. Who to screen
     (a) American College of Obstetricians and Gynecologists (1994) recommends triple screen for all < age 35
        (i) Not recommended for > age 35 as alternative to amniocentesis
       (ii) If requested by woman, advise of decreased ability of screening to detect Down syndrome
     (b) Lab should be able to confirm that triple test will yield a Down syndrome detection rate comparable to MSAFP alone
   iii. Interpretation
     (a) Combines AFP, estriol, and hCG
     (b) More sensitive screen for Down syndrome than MSAFP
        (i) Low MSAFP detects about 25% of Down syndrome
       (ii) Identifies those at risk > 1/190 (age 35)

g. **Infectious diseases**
   i. Rubella
     (a) Goal: prevention of fetal cellular and growth anomalies
     (b) Risks
        (i) Fetal anomaly rate of 50% in 1st trimester
       (ii) Fetal anomaly rate of 35% in 2nd trimester
      (iii) Fetal anomaly rate almost zero after 2nd trimester

    (c) Who should be screened: all reproductive age women during preconception or prenatal period

  ii. **Toxoplasmosis**

    (a) Goal: prevention of disease caused by *Toxoplasma gondii* parasites

    (b) Risks

       (i) Parasite passes transplacentally to fetus in 40% of cases

      (ii) The earlier the passage occurs, the more severe the congenital infection

         • Severe neurologic lesions in 40% of infants; hydrocephaly, microcephaly and liver dysfunction.

    (c) Avoidance of risk factors

       (i) Freezing meat and cooking until brown

      (ii) Avoiding cat excrement and changing litter

    (d) Who should be screened: no consensus except in endemic areas

       (i) *Toxoplasma* titers in selected situations

         • Universal screening results in many false + diagnoses

      (ii) If IgM rises over time or if titers > 1:512, recent infection is likely

     (iii) If IgG is high and IgM is low and unchanging, old infection is likely.

 iii. **Cytomegalovirus**

    (a) Goal: prevention of fetal infections and spontaneous pregnancy loss caused by cytomegalovirus

    (b) Populations at risk (60–70% are seropositive) where it is difficult to prevent spread of virus.

       (i) Young age and women living at home

      (ii) Health care workers in intensive care areas

    (c) Primary infection

       (i) 1% incidence with 45% transplacental transmission and 2–4% attack rate

      (ii) First half of pregnancy carries greatest risk.

     (iii) 5–10% of infections are symptomatic at birth

         • > 90% have major neurodevelopmental problems

      (iv) 95% are asymptomatic at birth

         • 20% will develop learning problems or hearing loss

      (v) Do not use IgM–specific antibodies (TORCH titers) to diagnose because 25% of primary CMV will have negative CMV IgM.

    (d) Immunity is not assured after first exposure because virus has property of latency

       (i) May reactivate at each pregnancy because antibodies are not protective, although it may modulate severity of disease

      (ii) High anti-CMV antibody correlates with high incidence of fetal infection acquired after reactivation of latent maternal infection.

    (e) Therapy: Ganciclovir eradicates viral excretion and stops or reverses injury, but CMV returns after drug is discontinued. It does not eradicate latency of CMV.

  iv. **Hepatitis B virus** (HBV)

    (a) Goal: prevention of acute and chronic liver disease

    (b) Risks

       (i) Sexual transmission of virus by contacts

      (ii) Parenteral drug abusers

    (c) Who should be screened

       (i) All pregnant women should be screened

         • Routine prenatal screening is the only strategy that will control perinatal transmission of HBV

         • Offering screening to only those who report high-risk behavior will fail to identify 50–70% of infected women

      (ii) High-risk women should be identified and counseled at the preconceptual visit

   v. **Herpes simplex virus** (HSV)
- (a) Goal: prevention of neonatal HSV infection
- (b) Risks
  - (i) Sexual transmission of virus by contacts
    - Advise condom use with infected partners
- (c) Who should be screened: women with lesions during pregnancy
  - (i) Serologic titers for HSV are not useful predictors of immunity because many have been exposed to HSV-1
  - (ii) Culture of actual lesions is best when lesion is in vesicular stage
- (d) Treatment
  - (i) Cesarean section for women with active HSV at the onset of labor
  - (ii) Acyclovir prophylaxis in late pregnancy may be more cost-effective than cesarean section. It shows no increase in number or birth defects, but is not FDA-approved for prevention of HSV in newborns.

   vi. *Chlamydia trachomatis*
- (a) Goal: prevention of intra-amniotic and postpartum infections, neonatal pneumonia, and conjunctivitis
- (b) Risks: sexual transmission by contacts
- (c) Who should be screened
  - (i) High-risk groups (adolescents, unmarried women, women with multiple sexual partners, and women with history of other STDs)
  - (ii) Chlamydia culture or PCR analysis
  - (iii) Gonorrhea assay should also be performed
- (d) Treatment
  - (i) Amoxicillin (500 mg po tid for 7 days) is more effective than erythromycin and has fewer side effects
  - (ii) Azithromycin, clindamycin, and erythromycin are equal in effectiveness

   vii. **Human papillomavirus** (HPV)
- (a) Goal: prevention of sexual transmission of HPV
  - (i) Avoidance of infected partner is the only way to prevent transmission
  - (ii) Condom use does not prevent transmission of HPV to infant
  - (iii) Cesarean birth does not completely prevent respiratory papillomatosis in infant
- (b) Risks
  - (i) Smoking acts as a cofactor for the virus. Smoking cessation strategy should be recommended.
  - (ii) Immune deficiency
- (c) Who should be screened: no screening test for HPV is available
  - (i) Papanicolaou smear sampling on annual basis and at the first prenatal visit should be performed

   viii. **Human immunodeficiency virus** (HIV)
- (a) Goals
  - (i) Reduce the vertical transmission of HIV from mother to fetus at time of delivery
  - (ii) Identify HIV-infected pregnant woman so that zidovudine can be given
    - Decreases the rate of transmission from mother to infant up to 75%
- (b) Risks for vertical transmission
  - (i) Advanced maternal age
  - (ii) Low CD4 cell counts
  - (iii) Maternal fever
  - (iv) Premature rupture of membranes (> 4 hours prior to delivery)
  - (v) Increased exposure of fetus to maternal blood
    - Scalp electrodes
    - Vaginal delivery
- (c) Risk factors
  - (i) Intravenous drug users

    (ii) High-risk sexual behavior

    (iii) Recipients of blood transfusions before 1985

  (d) Who should be screened

    (i) HIV testing should be offered during the premarriage evaluation in addition to risk prevention counseling

    (ii) Pregnant women may be required by law to sign that they consent to or decline HIV testing during pregnancy

  (e) Management

    (i) Zidovudine 100 mg po 5× per day from 14–34 weeks gestation

    (ii) Zidovudine IV 1mg/kg/hr during labor until cord clamped

    (iii) Zidovudine syrup, 2mg/kg every 6 hours for 6 weeks to newborn

ix. Group B streptococci (GBS)

  (a) Goals: prevention of GBS sepsis of neonate

    (i) 20–25% of pregnant women are colonized and GBS transmitted through hematogenous or epithelial route

    (ii) Most common cause of neonatal sepsis and meningitis

    (iii) Mortality rate up to 15% in premies

     • Attack rate 0.5–25% with known maternal risk factors

  (b) Risk factors

    (i) Prematurity

    (ii) Prolonged or premature rupture of membranes ($\geq$ 18 hrs)

    (iii) Maternal fever

    (iv) Previous affected infant

    (v) GBS bacteriuria

  (c) Who should be screened: universal screening is controversial

    (i) Cannot eradicate rectal colonization therefore antenatal treatment is ineffective except for those with GBS asymptomatic bacteriuria

    (ii) Does not predict colonization at term if cultures done at 28 weeks

    (iii) Organism is fastidious

     • Requires Todd-Hewitt broth

     • Rapid strep tests are too insensitive

     • Culture rectum and lower vagina

  (d) Management

    (i) Screening at 35–37 weeks and treating all GBS+ carriers during labor

     • IV penicillin G (5 million units stat then 2.5 million units q 4 hours until delivery)

     • IV clindamycin (900 mg q 8 hours until delivery)

    (ii) Treating on the basis of risk factors at the time of labor

x. Syphilis

  (a) Goals: prevention of congenital syphilis and identification of disease in mother

    (i) Rate of congenital syphilis is increasing in high-risk populations

    (ii) The earlier the disease in pregnancy, the worse the outcome

    (iii) The earlier the treatment, the better the outcome

    (iv) Treatment is always penicillin for all stages of syphilis. If allergic, desensitization.

     • < 20 weeks' gestation—98% cure

     • Treatment > 10 weeks before delivery often inadequate

    (v) Pregnancy may suppress response to disease so higher level of suspicion is required

    (vi) Identification of positive mother who is at higher risk of coexisting HIV infection

  (b) Risk of congenital transmission

    (i) Primary and secondary disease—nearly 100%

    (ii) Latent disease—40%

  (c) Who should be screened

(i) All women should be screened at first prenatal visit
  - Positive Venereal Disease Research Laboratory test (VDRL) or RPR should be confirmed with fluorescent treponemal antibody, absorbed test (FTA-ABS)
  - False-positive VDRL may occur in pregnancy

(ii) Rescreen high-risk pregnant women
  - At 28 weeks' gestation; allows 10 weeks until delivery.
  - During labor if high risk

(iii) Infant should not leave nursery without mother's serologic status being known

(iv) Treatment is based on maternal status
  - Cord blood is unreliable
  - FTA-ABS 19S-IgM takes weeks to perform

xi. **Asymptomatic bacteriuria** (ASB)
  (a) Goals: prevention of pyelonephritis and premature onset of labor
  (b) Significance
    (i) Presence of significant growth of single species in absence of symptoms
      - 100,000 colonies on clean catch
      - Most common organism is *Escherichia coli* (80%)
      - Other organisms include GBS and other gram-negative bacteria
    (ii) Any growth of single organism on catheter or suprapubic specimen
    (iii) Requires urine culture
      - Sensitivity of dipstick is low
  (c) Incidence
    (i) 4–7% of all pregnant women
    (ii) 12% of diabetics
    (iii) 19% of women with previous urinary tract infection
  (d) Treatment
    (i) Significant effect on decreasing risk of pyelonephritis and preterm delivery
    (ii) No significant effect on persistent bacteriuria
  (e) Who should be screened
    (i) All pregnant women should be screened
    (ii) Screen women with ASB during pregnancy in postpartum period to detect persistent bacteriuria
      - 20–55% have anatomic urinary anomalies

III. **An Approach**
  A. **Preconceptual counseling**
    1. Definition and scope of the counseling
      a. Obstetric risk assessment, health promotion, education and therapeutic intervention before pregnancy
      b. Concerns and counseling opportunities
        i. Medical diseases
        ii. Psychosocial issues
        iii. Environmental and occupational hazards
      c. Counseling should include:
        i. Identification of risk factors that influence pregnancy outcome
        ii. Assessment of couple's readiness for children and financial resources
        iii. Education about expectations of pregnancy
        iv. Performance of health maintenance examination if appropriate
        v. Performance of appropriate laboratory testing
    2. **Specific counseling strategies**
      a. Age-related risks (< 15 and > 35)
        i. Appropriate genetic counseling and referral to specialist if necessary
        ii. Ordering of antenatal testing specifically to assess fetal well-being
        iii. Identification of specific diseases and psychosocial issues peculiar to each extreme of age

b. Ethnic populations at risk
    i. African-American: sickle cell anemia screen
    ii. Jewish: Tay-Sachs screen for each partner
    iii. Mediterranean, Italian, Greek, or Asian: hemoglobin electrophoresis
c. Chronic disease states
    i. Medications
       (a) Use of databases that allow access of known and potential risks
    ii. Diabetes mellitus
       (a) Blood glucose, glycosylated hemoglobin
       (b) Diabetes education
          (i) Ophthalmologic examination
          (ii) Proper use of insulin and home monitoring
          (iii) Reproductive risk if diabetes not controlled
d. Obstetric
    i. Repeated pregnancy loss
       (a) Search for specific causes
       (b) Avoidance of alcohol, tobacco, drugs
    ii. Infertility
       (a) Charting of basal body temperature to determine ovulatory status
       (b) Sperm analysis
e. Menstrual
    i. Charting of consecutive cycle intervals
    ii. Treatment of specific causes
       (a) Anovulation, oligoovulation
       (b) Treatment of androgenic disorders
          (i) Hirsutism, alopecia, acne
    iii. Laboratory tests: thyroid-stimulating hormone, prolactin, follicle-stimulating hormone, luteinizing hormone, testosterone, and dehydroepiandrosterone sulfate, as appropriate
f. Contraception
    i. Wait to attempt conception until off hormonal contraception for 1–2 cycles
    ii. Return to fertility may be prolonged after Depo-Provera use
    iii. Wait to attempt conception until after first menses following removal of IUD
g. Sexual dysfunction
    i. Explore intimacy issues and knowledge about sex
    ii. Referral to specialist if necessary
h. Occupational
    i. Survey of chemicals or inhalants in workplace
       (a) Lead, benzene, allergens, asbestos
    ii. Survey of safety conditions
    iii. Investigate need for job transfer to decrease risk
       (a) Letter to employer about need for transfer because of specific medical condition
i. Illicit drugs, alcohol, and tobacco
    i. Both partners should be counseled
       (a) Illicit drug use may lead to violence and physical abuse during pregnancy
          (i) Drug screen in selected individuals
       (b) Smoking risk is associated with number of cigarettes smoked per day
          (i) Risk of passive smoke
          (ii) Encourage smoking cessation strategies
       (c) Alcohol may act as an acute fetal poison
          (i) No amount of alcohol is "safe," and total abstinence is recommended during pregnancy
j. **Preconceptual health promotion and education**
    i. Diet
       (a) Folate
          (i) Prevention of first occurrence of neural tube defects

　　　• CDC recommends 400 µg of folic acid/day for all women of child-
　　　　bearing age
　　(ii) Prevention of recurrent neural tube defects
　　　　• 4 mg/day from at least 1 month before conception through the first
　　　　　3 months of pregnancy
　ii. Other dietary habits
　　(a) Educate about good eating habits before pregnancy
　　(b) Discourage weight loss during the pregnancy
　　(c) Assess amount of iron, protein, and calcium in diet
　　　　(i) Ferrous sulfate, 300 mg orally 3 times/day if anemia present
　　(d) Complete blood count, cholesterol, thyroid function tests
　iii. Exercise
　　(a) Exercise prescription should be given to sedentary women
　　(b) Reasonable exercise regimens can be continued in pregnancy
　　(c) Extremes of exercise or physical work should be avoided during pregnancy
　iv. Financial and social support
　　(a) Expectations of impact of new infant on family system
　　　　(i) Emotional support
　　　　(ii) Financial support
　　　　(iii) Housing and food resources

SUGGESTED READINGS

1. Alger LS, Lovchik JC: Comparative efficacy of clindamycin versus erythromycin in eradication of ante-natal Chlamydia trachomatis. Am J Obstet Gynecol 165:375–381, 1991.
2. American Academy of Pediatrics Committee on Pediatric AIDS: Recommendations for the evaluation and treatment of HIV-exposed infants. Pediatrics 99:909–917, 1997.
3. Amstey MS, Gibbs RS: Is penicillin G a better choice than ampicillin for prophylaxis of neonatal group B streptococcal infections? Obstet Gynecol 84:1058, 1994.
4. Apgar BS, Green LA: Preventing group B streptococcal sepsis in the newborn [editorial]. Am Fam Physician 49:315–318, 1994.
5. Apgar BS, Zoschnick L: Triage of the abnormal Papanicolaou smear in pregnancy. Primary Care Clin North Am 25:483–501, 1998.
6. Bader TJ, Macones GA, Asch DA: Prenatal screening for toxoplasmosis. Obstet Gynecol 90:457–464, 1997.
7. Brown ZA, Benedetti JK, Watts H, et al: A comparison between detailed and simple histories in the diag-nosis of genital herpes complicating pregnancy. Am J Obstet Gynecol 172:1299–1303, 1995.
8. Brown ZA, Selke S, Zeh J, et al: The acquisition of herpes simplex during pregnancy. N Engl J Med 337:509–515, 1997.
9. Bush MR, Rosa C: Azithromycin and erythromycin in the treatment of cervical chlamydial infection during pregnancy. Obstet Gynecol 84:61–63, 1994.
10. Centers for Disease Control and Prevention: Prevention of perinatal group B streptococcal disease: A public health perspective. MMWR 45(RR-7):1–24, 1996.
11. Cnattingius S, Bergstron R, Lipworth L, Kramer MS: Prepregnancy weight and the risk of adverse preg-nancy outcomes. N Engl J Med 338:147–152, 1998.
12. Connor EM, Sperling RS, Gelber R, et al: Reduction of maternal–infant transmission of human immun-odeficiency virus type 1 with zidovudine treatment: Pediatric AIDS Clinical Trials Group Protocol 076 Study Group. N Engl J Med 331:1173–1180, 1994.
13. Committee on Obstetric Practice, American College of Obstetricians and Gynecologists: Prevention of early-onset group B streptococcal disease in newborns. Int J Gynaecol Obstet 54:197–205, 1996.
14. Cone RW, Hobson AC, Brown Z, et al: Frequent detection of genital herpes simplex virus DNA by poly-merase chain reaction among pregnant women. JAMA 272:792–796, 1994.
15. Daly S: Minimum effective dose of folic acid for food fortification to prevent neural tube defects. Lancet 350:1666–1669, 1997.
16. Eng CM: Prenatal genetic carrier testing using triple disease screening. JAMA 278:1268–1272, 1997.
17. Fargason CA Jr, Peralta-Carcelen M, Rouse DJ, et al: The pediatric costs of strategies for minimizing the risk of early-onset group B streptococcal disease. Obstet Gynecol 90:347–352, 1997.
18. Gibbs RS, McDuffie RS, McNabb F, et al: Neonatal group B streptococcal sepsis during 2 years of a uni-versal screening program. Obstet Gynecol 84:496–500, 1994.
19. Haddad J, Langer B, Astruc D, et al: Oral acyclovir and recurrent genital herpes during late pregnancy. Obstet Gynecol 82:102–104, 1993.

20. Hagay ZJ, Biran G, Or-Noy A, et al: Congenital cytomegalovirus infection: A long-standing problem still seeking a solution. Am J Obstet Gynecol 174:241–245, 1996.

21. Hensleigh PA, Andrews WW, Brown Z, et al: Genital herpes during pregnancy: Inability to distinguish primary and recurrent infections clinically. Obstet Gynecol 89:891–895, 1997.

22. Jonna S, Collins M, Abedin M, et al: Postneonatal screening for congenital syphilis. J Fam Pract 41:286–288, 1995.

23. Keenan C: Prevention of group B streptococcal infection. Am Fam Physician 57:2713–2720, 1998.

24. Lambert G, Thea DM, Pliner V, et al: Effect of maternal CD4 cell count, acquired immunodeficiency syndrome, and viral load on disease progression in infants with perinatally acquired human immunodeficiency virus type 1. J Pediatr 130:890–897, 1997.

25. McFarlin BL, Bottoms SF, Dock BS, Isada NB: Epidemic syphilis: Maternal factors associated with congenital infection. Am J Obstet Gynecol 170:535–540, 1994.

26. Minkoff H, Burns DN, Landesman S, et al: The relationship of the duration of ruptured membranes to vertical transmission of human immunodeficiency virus. Am J Obstet Gynecol 173:585–589, 1995.

27. Mohle-Boetani JC, Schuchat A, Plikaytis BD, et al: Comparison of prevention strategies for neonatal group B streptococcal infection: A population-based economic analysis. JAMA 270:1442–1448, 1993.

28. Musher DM, Hamill RJ, Baughn RE: Effect of human immunodeficiency virus (HIV) infection on the course of syphilis and on the response to treatment. Ann Intern Med 113:872–881, 1990.

29. Ohlsson A, Myhr TL: Intrapartum chemoprophylaxis of perinatal group B streptococcal infections: A critical review of randomized controlled trials. Am J Obstet Gynecol 170: 910–917, 1994.

30. Randolph AG, Washington AE, Prober CG: Cesarean delivery for women presenting with genital herpes lesions. JAMA 270:77–82, 1993.

31. Randolph AG, Washington AE, Prober CG: Cesarean delivery for women presenting with genital herpes lesions: Efficacy, risks, and costs. JAMA 270:77, 1993.

32. Rawstron SA, Bromberg K: Failure of recommended maternal therapy to prevent congenital syphilis. Sex Transm Dis 18:102–106, 1991.

33. Roberts SW, Cox SM, Dax J, et al: Genital herpes during pregnancy: No lesions, no cesarean. Obstet Gynecol 85:261–264, 1995.

34. Rolfs RT, Hoesoef MR, Hendershot EF, et al: A randomized trial of enhanced therapy for early syphilis in patients with and without human immunodeficiency virus infection. N Engl J Med 337:307–314, 1997.

35. Rouse DJ, Andrews WW, Goldenberg RL, Owen J: Screening and treatment of asymptomatic bacteriuria of pregnancy to prevent pyelonephritis: A cost-effectiveness and cost-benefit analysis. Obstet Gynecol 86:119–123, 1995.

36. Rouse D, Goldenberg R, Cliver S, et al: Strategies for the prevention of early-onset neonatal group B streptococcal sepsis: A decision analysis. Obstet Gynecol 83:483–494, 1994.

37. Scott LL, Sanchez PJ, Jackson GL, et al: Acyclovir suppression to prevent cesarean delivery after first-episode genital herpes. Obstet Gynecol 87:69–73, 1996.

38. Silverman NS, Sullivan M, Hochman M, et al: A randomized prospective trial comparing amoxicillin and erythromycin for the treatment of Chlamydia trachomatis in pregnancy. Am J Obstet Gynecol 170:829–832, 1994.

39. Turrentine MA, Newton ER: Amoxicillin or erythromycin for the treatment of antenatal chlamydial infection: A meta-analysis. Obstet Gynecol 86:1021–1025, 1995.

40. Van de Perre P: Postnatal transmission of human immunodeficiency virus type 1: The breast-feeding dilemma. Am J Obstet Gynecol 173:483–487, 1995.

41. Whitney CG, Pikaytis BD, Gozansky WS, et al: Prevention practices for perinatal group B streptococcal disease: A multi-state surveillance analysis: Neonatal group B streptococcal disease study group. Obstet Gynecol 89:28–32, 1997.

42. Wong S, Remington JS: Toxoplasmosis in pregnancy. Clin Infect Dis 18:853–861, 1994.

43. Zenker PN, Berman SM: Congenital syphilis: Trends and recommendations for evaluation and management. Pediatr Infect Dis J 10:516–522, 1991.

29. Natural Family Planning

Jane L. Murray, M.D.

I. The Issues

Religious and cultural concerns, as well as various medical contraindications, may make the use of chemical or barrier contraception techniques unacceptable to many women. Older methods, such as coitus interruptus and the rhythm method, have been largely replaced by newer natural family planning (NFP) techniques. NFP is used by many couples around the world to achieve pregnancy by timing intercourse to coincide with ovulation and optimal female fertility. When used to avoid pregnancy, NFP is sometimes referred to as periodic abstinence. The ovulation or Billing's method of NFP uses observation of cervical mucus production combined with symptom charting and temperature measurement; it is more reliable than the older calendar rhythm method in predicting ovulation and fertility. Coitus interruptus was used for many years by people unable to use other methods; it is far less effective than newer methods of NFP.

While only approximately 4% of American women use NFP to avoid pregnancy, recent data suggest that over 20% would be very interested in using the method if they were more knowledgeable about it. Many couples find the freedom from drugs, naturalness, effectiveness and enhanced self-awareness involved in NFP result in high satisfaction levels with the method.

II. The Theory

A. Mechanism of action

1. Observation of cervical mucus reveals certain characteristics through menstrual cycle
   a. When estrogen levels are high, just before ovulation, cervical mucus arranges itself into parallel strands forming open channels for sperm to enter and easily penetrate the mucus to unite with viable ovum
   b. Mucus during preovulation is viscous, clear, and stretchy
   c. During postovulatory portion of menstrual cycle, when progesterone levels rise, cervical mucus becomes drier, stickier, and cloudier
   d. Drier mucus prevents penetration of sperm into cervical canal and therefore assists in providing natural contraceptive barrier
2. By observing and recording characteristics of cervical mucus through several menstrual cycles, woman becomes aware of her peak or fertile times (mucus is maximally stretchable and clear) and dry or infertile times
3. Ovarian ultrasonography shows that cervical mucus characteristics identify timing of ovulation with precision
4. Coitus interruptus involves removal of penis from vagina before ejaculation
5. Older calendar rhythm method of contraception involves recording timing of menses, estimating fertile days at midcycle, and avoiding intercourse during times of presumed fertility

B. Efficacy

1. Coitus interruptus efficacy in preventing pregnancy is approximately 81% because viable sperm can be present in preejaculate fluid
2. Overall effectiveness rate for rhythm method is 80–91% because of month-to-month variability in actual ovulation cycle
3. Literature on efficacy of NFP in avoiding pregnancy is controversial and depends heavily on motivation of patients studied
   a. NFP requires substantial commitment of time, energy, and patience and cooperative partner to be most effective
   b. Perfect use efficacy is reported at 97% or higher
   c. Actual use effectiveness rates are similar to those for barrier methods: 75–80%
4. Appropriate instruction in NFP is necessary to avoid pregnancy
   a. Certified NFP teachers offer courses and private counseling which take place in multiple sessions over several months to a year

153

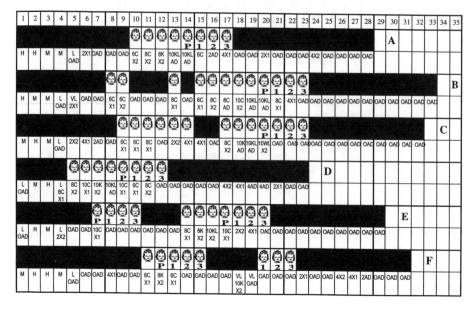

FIGURE 1. Vaginal discharge recording system. Always record the presence or absence of mucus during the light and very light days of the menstrual flow. In addition, record how often during the day you see the most fertile sign of the day and record it in the following fashion: X1 = Seen only once that day; X2 = Seen twice that day; X3 = Seen three times that day; AD = Seen all day.

H = Heavy flow	0 = Dry	B = Brown bleeding
M = Moderate flow	2 = Damp w/o lubrication	C = Cloudy (white)
L = Light flow	2W = Wet w/o lubrication	C/K = Cloudy/clear
VL = Very light flow	4 = Shiny w/o lubrication	G = Gummy (gluey)
(spotting)	6 = Sticky (¼ inch)	K = Clear
	8 = Tacky (½–¾ inch)	L = Lubricative
	10 = Stretchy (1 inch or more)	P = Pasty (creamy)
	10DL = Damp with lubrication	Y = Yellow (even pale yellow)
	10SL = Shiny with lubrication	
	10WL = Wet with lubrication	

    b. Satisfactory instruction usually cannot take place in physician's office in context of routine visits

C. **Description**
1. NFP is based on observation of three fertility signs: cervical mucus, basal body temperature, and cervix changes
2. Couples are shown how to check for viscosity, color, clarity, and consistency of cervical mucus in regular examination of vaginal discharge
3. Findings are charted daily on special grid (Fig. 1)
4. Body temperature can be checked daily
   a. Shows slight dip on day of ovulation
   b. Abrupt rise thereafter
5. Cervical os opens slightly on days just before and during ovulation

D. **Advantages**
1. Greatest advantage is that NFP requires no chemical, hormonal, surgical, or other invasive or potentially toxic or harmful intervention
2. No side effects
3. Supported by Catholic Church and thus available to millions of women worldwide who otherwise have few birth control options
4. Women learn great deal about fertility and their own body

5. Involves male partner in fertility awareness process and often enhances communication within intimate relationship
6. Predicting fertility with irregular cycles is enhanced when woman is aware of her hormonal status, as reflected in cervical mucus changes

E. **Disadvantages and cautions**
   1. Greatest disadvantage is significant time commitment necessary to learn, practice, interpret, and refine technique
   2. Requires timing of intercourse to avoid fertile periods and may inhibit spontaneity
   3. Billing's method also may result in fairly high number of days per cycle in which intercourse is to be avoided
   4. If used without complete understanding of principles of cervical mucus changes in predicting fertility or without careful charting of daily findings, NFP is associated with significant pregnancy rate
   5. Patients who have serious contraindication to pregnancy should not be advised to follow NFP method

F. **Cost**
   1. Costs associated with NFP involve instruction in method
   2. Some Catholic organizations (e.g., churches, hospitals) may provide group classes for free or nominal charge
   3. Individual sessions with certified NFP teacher may cost $10–$25 per session
   4. Some organizations and private teachers offer full series of classes, individual counseling, and follow-up for 1 year for fees ranging from $75–$500

III. **An Approach**

A. **Patient selection**
   1. Highly motivated patients in stable relationship with agreeable partner who do not wish to (or cannot) use other methods of contraception may be excellent candidates
   2. Instruction by qualified teachers requires series of class sessions and individual counseling and follow-up; method is time-consuming.
   3. Woman must be willing to observe vaginal secretions daily and be conscientious about recording all results and symptoms

B. **Instruction**
   1. Billings, Creighton, and Sympto-Thermal methods are similar techniques taught in series of four 2-hour courses spaced 1 month apart
   2. 3–5 couples usually participate together
   3. Experienced and certified teachers are necessary to ensure complete instruction
   4. Follow-up sessions and individual private counseling are usually recommended

C. **Resources** for further information and lists of trained instructors
   1. American Academy of Natural Family Planning: (314) 569-6495
   2. Creighton Model Natural Family Planning System: (402) 390-6600:
   3. Natural Family Planning Center of Washington, DC: (301) 897-9323 or (888) 637-6371
   4. Couple to Couple League (513) 471-2000

SUGGESTED READING

1. France M, France J, Townsend K: Natural family planning in New Zealand: A study of continuation rates and characteristics of users. Adv Contracept 13:191–198, 1997
2. Hilgers TW: The Ovulation Method of Natural Family Planning. Omaha, Pope Paul VI Institute Press, 1992.
3. Howie PW: Natural regulation of fertility. Br Med Bull 49:182–199, 1993.
4. Ryder REJ: "Natural family planning": Effective birth control supported by the Catholic Church. BMJ 307:723–726, 1993.
5. Stanford JB, Lemaire JC, Thurman PB: Women's interest in natural family planning. J Fam Pract 46:65–711, 1998.

30. Vaginal Barrier Contraceptive Methods

Cynda Ann Johnson, M.D., M.B.A.

I. **The Issues**

The vaginal barrier contraceptive methods include both the oldest and the newest options in contraception. Vaginal sponges, in the form of natural sea sponges, have been used since antiquity. Their recent history is checkered—the FDA approved the Today sponge in 1983, but it was withdrawn from the U.S. market in 1995 because the manufacturer was unwilling to invest in needed modernization of equipment. Diaphragm technology has changed little in 60 years. The cervical cap has changed from the silver or copper devices used earlier in this century to impermeable plastic and, most recently, latex. Finally, the first female condom was approved for over-the-counter sale in 1993, but sales have been sparse. All vaginal barrier methods have four important characteristics in common: (1) their use is controlled by the woman; (2) they provide a barrier to entry of sperm through the cervical canal; (3) they decrease the overall incidence of sexually transmitted diseases (STDs); and (4) they can be used as an adjunct to other forms of contraception to enhance their effect on either contraception or STD protection. The combination of such effects makes the vaginal barrier methods powerful options among the choices of contraceptive techniques, and their use, either alone or in combination, should be carefully considered.

II. **The Theory**
   A. **Mechanism of action**
      1. Physical barrier
         a. Female condom lines vagina and partially shields perineum
         b. Sponge, cervical cap, and diaphragm shield cervix
      2. Chemical to kill sperm
         a. Sponge is impregnated with spermicide that absorbs and traps sperm as well as kills them
         b. Cervical cap and diaphragm hold spermicide in place against cervix
   B. **Efficacy**
      1. For nulliparous women, all provide similar contraceptive efficacy during typical use (approximately 20% failure rate)
      2. For parous women, diaphragm and female condom are considerably more effective than sponge and cervical cap (approximately 20% vs. 40% failure rate, respectively)
   C. **Description of devices**
      1. **Female condom** (Reality) (Fig. 1)
         a. Thin (0.05 mm) polyurethane sheath
            i. 7.8 cm in diameter
            ii. 17 cm in length
            iii. Stronger than latex; less likely to tear or break.
            iv. Prelubricated inside with silicone-based lubricant
         b. Contains two flexible polyurethane rings in soft, loose-fitting sheath
            i. One ring lies inside at closed end of sheath, serving as insertion mechanism and internal anchor
            ii. Second ring forms external open edge and remains outside vagina after insertion
      2. **Contraceptive sponge** (discontinued in U.S. in 1995)
         a. Small, pillow-shaped polyurethane sponge
         b. Concave dimple on one side fits over cervix decreasing chance of dislodgment during intercourse
         c. Other side incorporates woven polyester loop to facilitate removal
         d. Sponge sold in Canada contains benzalkonium chloride, sodium cholate and nonoxynol-9
      3. **Diaphragm**
         a. Dome-shaped rubber cap with flexible rim

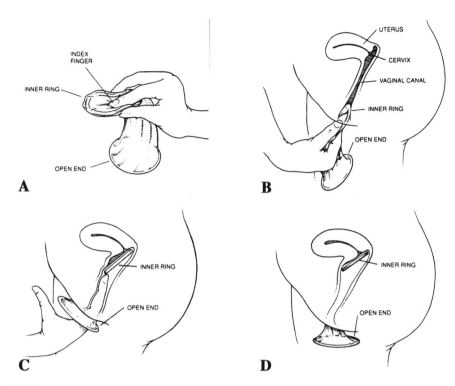

FIGURE 1.   Female condom insertion and positioning. *A*, Inner ring is squeezed for insertion. *B*, Sheath is inserted, similarly to a diaphragm. *C*, Inner ring is pushed up as far as it can go with index finger. *D*, Vaginal pouch in place. (Source: Wisconsin Pharmacal Company, 1992.)

      b. Spermicidal jelly or cream is applied inside dome and around rim before insertion

      c. Inserted so that posterior rim rests in posterior fornix and anterior rim fits snugly behind pubic bone, dome of diaphragm covers cervix

      d. Sizes from 50–100 (diameter in mm)

      e. **Spring types**

         i. **Arcing spring**

           (a) Sturdy, firm spring

           (b) More difficult to fold for insertion but springs open to original shape in vagina, facilitating correct insertion

           (c) Can be used with maximal number of anatomic types, including some patients with lax vaginal muscular and mild uterine prolapse, less prominent cervix, and spacious anterior vaginal vault

           (d) Available products: Allflex Diaphragm (Ortho)—folds at any point; Koroflex Diaphragm—folds at two points only; Ramses Bendex Diaphragm—folds at two points only.

        ii. **Flat spring**

           (a) Thin rim

           (b) Gentle spring strength

           (c) Comfortable even for women with very firm vaginal muscle tone

           (d) Can be used in women with narrow, straight vaginal vault

           (e) Does not spring as reliably to original shape in vault as other springs and may be more easily misplaced

           (f) Available product: Ortho-White Diaphragm

        iii. **Coil spring**

           (a) Sturdy construction

   (b) Compromise between features of flat and arcing springs
   (c) Suitable for women with average muscle tone and average pubic arch depth
   (d) Less likely to be felt by wearer and partner than arcing spring but easier to insert correctly than flat spring
   (e) Available products: Koromex Diaphragm; Ortho Diaphragm (coil spring); Ramses Flexible Cushioned Diaphragm (coil spring).
 f. **Wide-seal diaphragm with flexible flange** attached to inner edge of rim
   i. Available with arcing or coil spring
   ii. Disadvantage: not available from retail pharmacies; must be purchased by physician for sale to patient.
   iii. Available products: Milex Wide-seal arcing diaphragm; Milex Wide-seal Omniflex coil spring diaphragm.
 g. Plastic diaphragm introducer
   i. Available for use with coil or flat spring
   ii. Not needed by most patients
   iii. May be useful for patients with handicaps that make positioning difficult
4. **Cervical cap** (Prentif Cavity Rim Cervical Cap)
 a. Deep, soft rubber cup with round, firm rim
 b. Dome should be filled one-third full with spermicide before insertion
 c. Groove along inner circumference of rim improves seal between inner rim of cap and surface of cervix
 d. Should fit with rim snugly around base of cervix, close to junction between cervix and vaginal fornices
 e. Available in internal rim diameter sizes of 22, 25, 28, and 31 mm

D. **Advantages**
 1. **Of vaginal barrier methods as group**
  a. No systemic side effects
  b. No interference with menstrual cycle
  c. Involvement of partner not required, but partner may assist
  d. Can be used immediately
  e. Immediately effective
  f. Reduced risk of gonorrhea, chlamydia, trichomonas
  g. No negative effect on resulting pregnancy if method fails
  h. Can be used to augment other forms of birth control
 2. **Of specific methods**
  a. **Female condom**
   i. Impenetrable to human immunodeficiency virus
   ii. Over-the-counter purchase
  b. **Sponge**
   i. Continuous protection for 24 hours
   ii. Over-the-counter purchase (when available)
  c. **Diaphragm**
   i. 50% decreased incidence of pelvic inflammatory disease compared with nonusers of contraception
   ii. Decreased tubal infertility
   iii. Decreased risk of cervical neoplasia (relative risk = 0.3–0.7 compared with nonusers)
  d. **Cervical cap**
   i. Continuous protection for 48 hours without additional spermicide
   ii. Can be fitted without regard to change in vaginal size due to intercourse or alterations in body weight
   iii. Can be used in patients with some degree of uterovaginal prolapse and poor muscle tone
E. **Disadvantages and cautions**
 1. **Of vaginal barrier methods as group**
  a. Possible allergy to device
  b. Risk of toxic shock (unlikely with female condom)

    c. Devices difficult for some individuals to place correctly

    d. May interrupt spontaneity of love-making

    e. High rate of contraceptive failure

    f. Possible discomfort in patient or partner

    g. Possibility of dislodgment

    h. Difficult to remove (except female condom)

    i. Must be used at every instance of vaginal intercourse for optimal contraceptive effect

  2. **Of specific methods**

    a. **Female condom**

      i. Anchoring ring visible outside of labia

      ii. May make undesirable sound

      iii. Cannot be used with male condom

    b. **Sponge** (discontinued by manufacturer)

      i. Should not be used during menses

      ii. May cause vaginal dryness as result of uptake of vaginal moisture

    c. **Diaphragm**

      i. Must be fitted by health care provider

      ii. Some anatomic types not conducive to fitting and retaining placement

      iii. Rim of diaphragm may be felt by partner

      iv. Increased incidence of urinary tract infections

      v. Possible increased incidence of bacterial vaginosis

      vi. Possible increased incidence of vaginal candidiasis

    d. **Cervical cap**

      i. Possible odor problem with prolonged use

      ii. Must be fitted by health care provider

      iii. Limited size options

      iv. Cannot be used in patients with cervical asymmetry or cervix that is too long or flat

      v. Contraindicated in patients with vaginal or cervical infection

      vi. Contraindicated in known or suspected cervical or uterine malignancy

      vii. Should not be used during menses

      viii. Evidence of increased incidence of abnormal Papanicolaou smear found in earlier studies but not substantiated in more recent research

F. **Cost**

  1. Female condom—$2.50 each, single use

  2. Sponge (discontinued in U.S.)

    a. Available in Canada

    b. May be ordered legally through website: www.birthcontrol.com

    c. Small quantities for personal use only; $7.50–9.00 for box of 4.

  3. Cervical cap or diaphragm

    a. $50–100 for office visit and fitting charge

    b. Approximately $30 for cap or diaphragm

    c. Recommend replacement every 2 years for diaphragm and yearly for cap: immediate replacement if torn

    d. Additional cost for spermicidal cream or gel at $0.25 per application

III. **An Approach**

A. **Patient selection**

  1. Characteristics associated with higher than average risk of failure (though in counseling some patients may readily accept risk of method failure)

    a. Frequent intercourse (> 3 times/week)

    b. Age < 25 years

    c. Personal style or sexual patterns that make consistent use difficult

    d. Previous contraceptive failure (any method)

    e. Intention to delay rather than prevent pregnancy

    f. Ambivalent feelings (on part of patient or partner) about desirability of becoming pregnant

2. Vaginal barrier methods used alone are not good choice for women who need excellent contraceptive effect and/or optimal protection from STDs
3. Vaginal barrier methods used alone are good choice for women:
   a. At low risk for STDs
   b. Who are motivated to use method optimally
   c. Who want reasonable control over fertility but would accept pregnancy if method failed
   d. Engaging infrequently in vaginal intercourse
   e. Who are breastfeeding or perimenopausal, when fertility is already decreased
4. Vaginal barrier methods used in combination are good choice:
   a. Women who want added protection and/or female-controlled method
   b. As short-term adjunct while becoming established on another form of birth control
   c. For remainder of cycle of oral contraceptives if pills have been taken imperfectly
   d. During menses (diaphragm and female condom) on esthetic basis

B. **Proper use**
   1. **General instructions**
      a. Use at every instance of vaginal intercourse
      b. Wash hands with soap and water before insertion and removal
      c. Partner may check placement of device
      d. Sponge, diaphragm, and cervical cap should remain in place at least 6 hours after intercourse
      e. Oil-based lubricants should not be used
      f. Douching after intercourse is not recommended
   2. **Female condom**
      a. Insertion—follow directions on package insert (see Fig. 1)
         i. Hold pouch with open end hanging down
         ii. Spread labia with one hand
         iii. Thumb and middle finger of other hand can be used to squeeze inner ring into narrow oval for insertion; use index finger as guide.
         iv. Inner ring and pouch are pushed deep into vagina with outer ring resting against outer lips
      b. Removal—immediately after intercourse
      c. Repeated intercourse—use new female condom
      d. Maximal duration of protection—8 hours
      e. Longest wear recommended—8 hours
   3. **Sponge**
      a. Preparation—remove sponge from package and moisten with two tablespoons of clean water and squeeze once
      b. Insertion—along back wall of vagina; push dimple against cervix.
      c. Check placement—should cover cervix
      d. Removal—by grasping loop; remove all pieces from vagina if sponge falls apart.
      e. Repeated intercourse—leave sponge in place
      f. Maximal duration of protection—24 hours
      g. Longest wear recommended—30 hours
   4. **Diaphragm**
      a. Preparation—squeeze quarter's worth of spermicidal jelly into dome and spread additional spermicide around rim. Efficacy decreased when spermicide not used though newer form of spermicide-free diaphragm being investigated
      b. Insertion
         i. Insert folded diaphragm with one hand while spreading labia with other
         ii. May lie down, squat, or raise one foot as on stool
      c. Check placement
         i. Front rim behind symphysis
         ii. Back rim behind cervix
         iii. Dome covering cervix

   d. Removal
      i. Using forefinger or middle finger, hook bent finger over anterior rim
      ii. Motion for removal is down first, then out
   e. Repeated intercourse
      i. Fill plastic applicator with spermicide and insert into vagina
      ii. Also prudent to add applicator of spermicide if intercourse is delayed more than 1 hour after initial insertion
   f. Maximal duration of protection—6 hours
   g. Longest wear recommended—24 hours
   h. Care of diaphragm
      i. Wash diaphragm, spermicide applicator, and inserter with plain soap and water
      ii. Check diaphragm for holes or leaks
      iii. Dry gently
      iv. Place diaphragm in case

5. **Cervical cap**
   a. Preparation—fill dome one-third full with spermicide
   b. Insertion
      i. Patient must be able to identify cervix (consistency and approximate size of end of nose)
      ii. Position may be lying, squatting, or with one foot propped up
      iii. Spread labia with one hand and insert folded cap (opposite rims together) into vagina
      iv. Slide cap into vagina along back wall until cervix is identified, then press rim of cap around entire cervix
   c. Check placement
      i. Press dome against cervix
      ii. Sweep finger around cervix, making sure no portion is uncovered
   d. Removal
      i. Locate cap rim and press until suction is broken
      ii. Tilt cap off cervix
      iii. Hook finger around rim and pull it sideways out of vagina
   e. Repeated intercourse
      i. Leave cap in place
      ii. Applicator of spermicide may be inserted directly into vagina
   f. Maximal duration of protection—8 hours
   g. Longest wear recommended—48 hours
   h. Care of cervical cap: wash cap with plain soap and water, check for leaks or tears, dry gently, place in case

SUGGESTED READING

1. Bounds W, Guillebaud J: The diaphragm with and without spermicide. A randomized, comparative efficacy trial. J Reprod Med 40:764–774, 1995.
2. Cohall AT, Cullins VE, Darney PD, Nelson AL: Contraception in the 1990s: New methods and approaches. Patient Care 15(Suppl):1–12, 1993.
3. Fihn SD, Latham RH, Roberts P, et al: Association between diaphragm use and urinary tract infection. JAMA 254:240–245, 1985.
4. Hatcher RA, Trussell J, Stewart F, et al (eds): Contraceptive Technology, 17th ed. New York, Ardent Media Inc., 1998.
5. Heath CB: Helping patients choose appropriate contraception. Am Fam Physician 48:1115–1124, 1993.
6. Hooton TM, Fihn SD, Johnson C, et al: Association between bacterial vaginosis and acute cystitis in women using diaphragms. Arch Intern Med 149:1932–1936, 1989.
7. Hooton TM, Hillier S, Johnson C, et al: *Escherichia coli* bacteriuria and contraceptive method. JAMA 265:64–69, 1991.
8. Kirkman R, Chantler E: Contraception and the prevention of sexually transmitted diseases. Br Med Bull 49:171–191, 1993.
9. McCabe E, Golub S: Making the female condom a "reality" for adolescents. J Pediatr Adolesc Gynecol 10:15–23, 1997.

10. Rosenberg MJ, Davidson AJ, Chen JH, et al: Barrier contraceptives and sexually transmitted diseases in women: A comparison of female-dependent methods and condoms. Am J Public Health 82:669–674, 1992.

31. Vaginal Spermicides

Cynda Ann Johnson, M.D., M.B.A.

I. The Issues
Free of risks associated with hormonal contraception, inexpensive, and available over the counter vaginal spermicides are used as a single contraceptive agent or as an adjunct to vaginal barrier methods and condoms. The vaginal spermicides also have protective properties against the spread of sexually transmitted diseases (STDs). The increasing number of available brands in several different vehicles attests to the secure role of vaginal spermicides in the growing contraceptive market.

II. The Theory
A. Mechanism of action
1. All contain sperm-killing chemical
   a. Nonoxynol-9—active agent in most spermicides (surfactant that destroys sperm cell membrane)
   b. Octoxynol—only other agent available in U.S

B. Efficacy
1. Studies show range of failure rates from <5–50%
2. Efficacy generally comparable to vaginal barrier methods

C. Description of products
1. **Foam**
   a. May be used alone or with diaphragm or condom
   b. Contraceptive effect is immediate; remains effective for at least 1 hour.
   c. Also acts as partial lubricant
2. **Creams and gels**
   a. Options for use
      i. May be used alone but usually marketed for use with diaphragm; gel is preferred by most women.
      ii. May be used with cervical cap
      iii. Some gels marketed as tasteless
      iv. Viscous gel acts as lubricant and as additional barrier method
   b. Contraceptive effect is immediate
      i. Remains effective for at least 1 hour when used alone
      ii. Remains effective for 6–8 hours when used with diaphragm or cervical cap
3. **Suppositories**
   a. May be used alone or with condom
   b. Contraceptive effect begins 10–15 minutes after insertion
   c. Penile penetration before complete dissolution and disbursement of contraceptive results in discomfort for both partners
   d. Remains effective for only 1 hour
4. **Film**
   a. May be used alone or with diaphragm or condom
   b. Contraceptive effect begins 15 minutes after insertion
   c. Remains effective for only 1 hour

D. Advantages
1. Available over the counter
2. No systemic side effects

3. No interference with menstrual cycle
4. No effect on pregnancy if method fails (previous concerns about teratogenicity of vaginal spermicides were unfounded)
5. Controlled by woman
6. Effective soon or immediately after insertion
7. May be used to augment other forms of birth control
8. Some protective effect against STDs, especially gonorrhea, chlamydia, genital herpes
9. Possible protection against sexual transmission of hepatitis B
10. Decreased risk from cervical cancer
11. May be used as lubricant
12. May be used as emergency or back-up measure if another method fails
13. May be used when breastfeeding
14. May be used intermittently
15. Less precise insertion required than with vaginal barrier methods
E. **Disadvantages and cautions**
    1. Incomplete protection from STDs
    2. Effect on spread of human immunodeficiency virus unclear; some studies show increased transmission.
    3. Possible allergy to spermicidal agent or ingredients in base; vaginal suppositories seem more likely to cause burning sensation in some women.
    4. Inability to use agent correctly
    5. May interrupt spontaneity of love-making
    6. Relatively high rate of contraceptive failure
    7. Must be used at every instance of vaginal intercourse for optimal contraceptive effect
    8. May be considered messy
F. **Cost**
    1. Suppositories—$4 for 12 suppositories
    2. Tube of gel or container of cream—$12
    3. Film—$9.25 for 12 sheets
    4. Cost per single episode of intercourse from $0.35 to $1.30 (for one single-use packet of gel)

III. **An Approach**
A. **Patient selection** (similar to vaginal barrier methods)
    1. Spermicides used alone are not good choice for women who need:
        a. Excellent contraceptive effect
        b. Optimal protection from STDs
    2. Spermicides used alone are good choice for women:
        a. Who want over-the-counter contraception
        b. Who want least expensive form of contraception
        c. At low risk for STDs
        d. Motivated to use method optimally
        e. Who want reasonable control over fertility but would accept pregnancy if method failed
        f. Engaging infrequently in vaginal intercourse
        g. Who are breastfeeding or perimenopausal, when fertility is already decreased
    3. Spermicides used in combination are good choice for women:
        a. Who want added protection and/or female-controlled method in addition to condom
        b. As short-term adjunct while becoming established on another form of birth control
        c. For remainder of cycle of oral contraceptives if pills have been taken imperfectly
B. **Proper use**
    1. Patient or partner should wash hands with soap and water before use
    2. Insertion
        a. Patient should follow instructions included in package of spermicide
        b. Goal is to have spermicide deep in vagina near cervix
    3. Repeated intercourse—requires new application of spermicide
    4. After intercourse—leave spermicide in place for at least 6 hours

SUGGESTED READING

1. Kirkman R, Chantler E: Contraception and the prevention of sexually transmitted diseases. Br Med Bull 49:171–181, 1993.
2. Rosenberg MJ, Davidson AJ, Chen JH, et al: Barrier contraceptives and sexually transmitted diseases in women: A comparison of female-dependent methods and condoms. Am J Public Health 82:669–674, 1992.
3. Shapiro S, Stone D, Heinonen OP, et al: Birth defects and vaginal spermicides. JAMA 247:2381–2384, 1982.
4. Whaley KJ, Barratt RA, Zeitlin L, et al: Nonoxynol-9 protects mice against vaginal transmission of genital herpes infections. J Infect Dis 168:1009–1011, 1993.
5. Wittkowski KM, Susser E: The protective effect of condoms and nonoxynol-9 against HIV infection. Am J Public Health 88:590–596, 1998.

32. Condoms

Cynda Ann Johnson, M.D., M.B.A.

I. **The Issues**
The issue with condoms becomes not "Should I use a condom?" but "Can I really afford not to use a condom?" The condom remains an effective form of contraception, and it also limits the spread of sexually transmitted diseases (STDs) far better than any other device or substance used alone. When counseling about birth control options, the physician should not assume knowledge and/or use of the condom but must repeatedly point out its important role in addition to other chosen birth control methods. Furthermore, the physician should not assume that certain types of patients are not at risk for STDs but give all patients the benefit of counseling about the proper use of condoms.

II. **The Theory**
A. **Mechanism of action**
1. Placed over erect penis, the condom acts as mechanical barrier to contact of semen with any surface outside condom
2. Some have spermicide (chemical that kills sperm) on inside and/or outside condom but there is little evidence these are more effective at preventing pregnancy
B. **Efficacy**
1. Failure rates are less than those quoted for vaginal barrier methods or spermicides
2. Failure rate is approximately 3% per year for perfect user and 14% per year for typical user
C. **Description**
1. Manufactured from latex (rubber), processed collagenous tissue from intestinal cecum of lambs (skin or natural membrane condoms), polyurethane, or plastic
   a. Latex condoms are superior to skin condoms in protection from STDs because small pores in natural condoms have been shown to permit passage of hepatitis B virus, herpes simplex virus, and human immunodeficiency virus (HIV)
   b. The first polyurethane male condom has been marketed in the U.S. since mid-1997 for the latex-sensitive person. These condoms are thinner and stronger and may enhance sensitivity
   c. Plastic condoms, manufactured from a plastic material used in non-allergenic examination gloves, have received FDA approval and will be marketed soon
   d. Both polyurethane and plastic condoms are expected to be effective for the prevention of STDs
2. Over 100 different brands, varying in size, shape, thickness, presence of lubricants or spermicides, texture, reservoir tips, color, scent
3. Continuing development of both materials and marketing to enhance acceptability

D. **Advantages**
1. Best overall choice of contraception for prevention of STDs, including gonorrhea, ureaplasma, HSV, HIV
2. STD protection during anal or oral intercourse
3. Prevention of infertility through protection from STDs
4. Hygienic
    a. Prevents contact of genital lesions and discharges between partners
    b. Prevents postcoital discharge of semen from vagina
5. Prevention of sperm allergy and antibodies
    a. Local allergy
    b. Sperm antibodies may be factor in infertility
6. Erection enhancement
    a. Decreased penile sensitivity may maintain erection longer and aid in prevention of premature ejaculation
7. Small package fits easily in purse or pocket
8. Available over the counter
9. Relatively inexpensive; free in some settings.
10. No systemic side effects
11. No interference with menstrual cycle
12. Involvement of partner not required but may assist with placement if desired
13. Evidence of male's involvement in contraceptive effort
14. Can be used to enhance effect of other methods
15. Can be used intermittently
16. Effective immediately after placement
17. No negative effect on resulting pregnancy if method fails
18. Good record of pregnancy prevention

E. **Disadvantages and cautions**
1. Allergy to latex in 1–3% of population
2. Male control issues—unwillingness to use condom
3. Unwillingness of female to request male usage of condom
4. Male perception of reduced sensitivity in glans penis
5. Interruption of spontaneity of lovemaking
6. Breakage or slippage of condom in 1–2% during vaginal intercourse
7. Oil-based lubricants are contraindicated with latex—disrupt integrity of condom and predispose to breakage
8. Must be used with every act of intercourse for optimal contraceptive effects and STD prevention

F. **Cost**
1. Average cost is $0.50 ($.30–$1.10) per condom
2. One of least expensive forms of birth control

III. **An Approach**
A. **Patient selection**
1. Male condom is good contraceptive choice for nearly all couples
2. Should be used along with another contraceptive method for couples requiring superb contraception

B. **Proper use**
1. Condom should be unrolled onto erect penis before it comes into contact with woman's genital area
2. Consider use during oral or anal sex
3. ½ inch empty space should be left at tip of condom
4. If additional lubrication is necessary, it must be water-based; spermicidal agents also may be used.
5. Condom should removed soon after ejaculation while penis is still erect
6. Rim of condom should be held close to base of penis to prevent slippage or spillage until male has moved well away form women's genitals
7. Condom may then be slid off penis but must be held carefully to avoid spilling semen

C. **Condom breakage and slippage**
   1. Rates of both breakage and slippage average 2%
      a. Groups experiencing higher rates include black males, men in low-income brackets, men using condoms infrequently, men engaging in high-risk sexual behaviors, including multiple partners and anal intercourse
   2. If condom breaks or slips off while still in contact with partner's genitals:
      a. Insert spermicidal agent into vagina
         i. Wash off vagina with soap and water if spermicide is not available
      b. Wash penis with soap and water

SUGGESTED READING

1. Roddy RE, Cordero M: A randomised controlled trial comparing nonoxynol-9 lubricated condoms with silicone-lubricated condoms for prophylaxis. Sex Transm Inf 74:116–119, 1998.
2. Rosenberg MJ, Waugh MS: Latex condom breakage and slippage in a controlled clinical trial. Contraception 56:17–21, 1997.

33. Intrauterine Devices

Cynda Ann Johnson, M.D., M.B.A.

I. **The Issues**
When economic pressures from high-cost litigation resulted in mass removal of intrauterine devices (IUDs) from the market in the mid 1980s only the progesterone-T (Progestasert) IUD remained available. In 1988, the copper-T 380A (Paragard) became available in the United States. It is expected that the extensively studied, low-risk, low-side-effect levonorgestrel IUD will join the others soon. To protect patients as well as themselves, the manufacturers now accompany IUDs with extensive information materials and strict patient selection criteria. The improved side-effect profile, increased number of years that some IUDs may be allowed to remain in place, excellent cost-effectiveness over time, and disenchantment with other forms of contraception are slowly beginning to increase the popularity of IUDs, but it is doubtful that they will regain the peak of their popularity in the 1960s and 1970s, when 10% of women in the U.S. using contraception had an IUD.

II. **The Theory**
   A. **Mechanism of action**
      1. Complete mechanism not understood
      2. Hostile uterine environment created by IUD, not allowing implantation of fertilized egg, is a concept that does not appear valid
      3. Prevention of fertilization by sperm is major mechanism of action
         a. Sperm immobilized; IUD interferes with migration of sperm to fallopian tubes.
         b. IUD speeds transport of ovum through fallopian tubes, not allowing time for fertilization
   B. **Efficacy**
      1. Typical failure rate for copper-containing IUD is 0.8% in first year
      2. Typical failure rate for progesterone-containing IUD is 2% in first year
      3. Excellent efficacy rate, but higher failure rate than more recently introduced products, including injectable and implantable progestins
      4. Fewer failures with careful insertion techniques in women qualifying for IUD
   C. **Description of products** (Fig. 1)
      1. **Copper IUD**
         a. "T" is made of polyethylene
         b. Barium sulfate is added to make IUD radiopaque for ease of locating IUD if string from vagina is missing

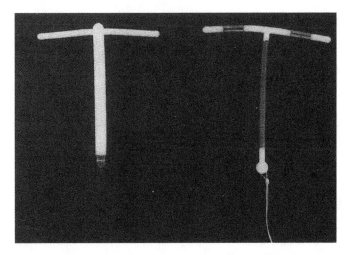

FIGURE 1. Intrauterine devices currently being marketed in the United States. *Left*, progesterone-releasing IUD; *right*, copper T380A. (From Herbst AL, Mishell DR, Stenchever MA, Droegemueller W: Comprehensive Gynecology, 2nd ed. St. Louis, Mosby–Year Book, 1992, with permission.)

    c. Fine copper wire is wound around stem and midportion of both arms of "T"
    d. Single-filament polyethylene clear or white string is tied through small hole at bottom of "T," creating effect of double string
    e. Visible string in vagina provides examiner with clue as to type of IUD in place
  2. **Progesterone-containing IUD**
    a. "T" is made of ethylene vinyl acetate copolymer
    b. Reservoir in vertical stem of "T" contains: 38 mg of progesterone (releasing 65 µg/day of progesterone); barium sulfate; silicon oil base.
    c. Double string through hole in base of "T" is blue-black in color
D. **Advantages**
  1. Of IUDs as group
    a. Provide excellent contraception
    b. Do not require compliance on part of user
    c. May be used in lactating women
    d. May be used in patients for whom systemic hormonal contraception causes unwanted side effects or is contraindicated
    e. Decreased risk of ectopic pregnancy compared to nonusers of contraception
  2. Of specific devices
    a. Copper IUD
      i. Cost-effective if left in place at least 2 years
      ii. May be left in place for 2 years
    b. Progesterone IUD
      i. May decrease dysmenorrhea and uterine blood flow by as much as 40%
E. **Disadvantages and cautions**
  1. **Of IUDs as group**
    a. Medicolegal concerns, especially for nulliparous patients
    b. Do not provide protection from sexually transmitted diseases (STDs)
    c. Cannot be used in patients with history of pelvic inflammatory disease (PID) or high risk for any STD
    d. Should not be used in patients with multiple sexual partners
    e. Increase in menstrual disorders
      i. Dysmenorrhea
      ii. Increased bleeding or spotting results in request for removal in 10–15% of patients

      f. Increased risk of PID, especially during early postinsertion period; transient bacteremia within 4–6 minutes after insertion in 13% of patients in one study.

      g. May enhance risk of contracting human immunodeficiency virus

      h. Risk of expulsion is 2–10% in first year

      i. Women with valvular heart disease may be more susceptible to subacute bacterial endocarditis with IUD in place

      j. High ectopic pregnancy rate (5%) in patients who become pregnant with IUD in place

      k. Increased difficulty with insertion and increased rate of expulsion in patients with anatomic abnormalities of uterus

      l. Increased rate of tubal infertility
         i. Especially in former users of Dalkon shield
         ii. Not in parous women over 25 years of age in monogamous relationship
         iii. Not in patients using copper-containing IUDs

  2. **Of specific devices**
    a. **Copper-containing IUD**
      i. Width of crossbar on "T" may make insertion difficult, even in multiparous women
      ii. Allergy to copper
    b. **Progesterone-containing IUD**
      i. Yearly insertion places patient at higher risk for PID
      ii. 6–10-fold ectopic pregnancy rate in patients who become pregnant compared with copper-containing IUD

F. **Cost**
  1. $200–300 total cost for IUD and placement
  2. May be even higher in private settings

III. **An Approach**
  A. **Patient selection**
    1. IUDs are good contraceptive choice for women who:
      a. Are at low risk for STDs
      b. Are multiparous
      c. Have been in mutually monogamous relationship for more than 6 months
      d. Want long-term, reversible contraception
      e. Have completed their families but do not desire permanent sterilization
      f. Are unreliable in use of oral contraception or barrier methods
    2. IUDs are not good contraceptive choice for women with:
      a. High risk for STDs
      b. Heavy, painful menstrual periods (although progesterone-containing IUDs may be tried in such women)
      c. Anemia
      d. Anatomic abnormalities of uterus, including fibroids
      e. Prior problems with IUDs, including pregnancy and expulsion
      f. Valvular heart disease
      g. History of ectopic pregnancy
      h. Abnormal Papanicolaou smear

  B. **Proper use**
    1. Timing of insertion
      a. Any time during menstrual cycle
      b. Must have assurance that patient is not pregnant; although best assurance is normal menses, infection and expulsion rates may be higher when IUD is inserted during menstrual period.
    2. Prophylactic antibiotics—no consensus on this issue
    3. Indications for patient follow-up
      a. Yearly exam, including Papanicolaou smear
      b. Menstrual disorder
      c. Missing string or string too long or too short
      d. Pelvic or abdominal pain

e. Abnormal vaginal discharge or odor
f. IUD expulsion
g. Late period and possible pregnancy

C. **Other IUDs**

1. Lippes loop
   a. Not available in U.S. since 1985
   b. All plastic, inert material
   c. No removal date
   d. Patients presenting with Lippes Loop
      i. Some have forgotten about it or assume that it has fallen out
      ii. Presence suspected by string—string may be one of several colors, single or double
      iii. No indication for removal if patient desires to keep it
      iv. Radiograph if patient suspects she has Lippes Loop, but string not present
2. IUDs used in other countries
   a. Various dates of expiration
   b. Radiograph may aid in determination of IUD type and therefore appropriate action
   c. Ring-type IUD
      i. Used in China
      ii. Most commonly used IUD in the world
      iii. Various shapes and styles of stainless steel rings
      iv. Usually stringless
         (a) Meant to be left in place indefinitely
         (b) Usually requires surgical procedure for removal

SUGGESTED READING

1. Burkman RT: Modern trends in contraception. Obstet Gynecol Clin North Am 17:759–774, 1990.
2. Cohall AT, Cullins VE, Darney PD, Nelson AL: Contraception in the 1990s: New methods and approaches. Patient Care 15(Suppl):1–12, 1993.
3. Ortiz ME, Croxatto HB: Mechanisms of action of intrauterine devices. Obstet Gynecol 51:842–851, 1996.
4. Pollack AE, Girvin S: When should an IUD be removed and replaced. Med Aspects Hum Sex 26:46–58, 1992.
5. Skjeldestad FE: How effectively do copper intrauterine devices prevent ectopic pregnancy? Acta Obstet Gynecol Scand 76:684–690, 1997.
6. Toivonen J: Intrauterine contraceptive device and pelvic inflammatory disease. Ann Med 25:171–173, 1993.
7. United Nations Development Programme: Long-term reversible contraception: Twelve years of experience with the Tcu380A and Tcu220C. Contraception 56:341–352, 1997.

34. Levonorgestrel Implants (Norplant)

Cynda Ann Johnson, M.D., M.B.A.

I. **The Issues**

Thoughtful preparation preceded the release of Norplant in the U.S. The first clinical research with progestin-releasing capsules was carried out in the late 1960s, and women in many countries had been using Norplant successfully before it was marketed in the U.S. in 1990. The demonstration kit contains nearly all materials, information, and instructions that clinicians need to add Norplant insertion to their practice. Even so, for the first several years after its introduction into the market, health care providers were encouraged to learn Norplant insertion techniques from certified trainers, with the understanding that the manufacturers would support formally trained providers in the event of malpractice litigation. Norplant, however, has not been the answer to the need for ideal, long-term reversible contraception. As suspected by generalists who have dealt with contraceptive issues, American women are generally intolerant of the prolonged, irregular bleeding patterns so common in Norplant users. Less expected was the difficulty in removing the implants, which has led to the majority of threats of malpractice. Clearly, Norplant has a role, but that role is still being defined. A two-capsule system may soon replace the six-capsule system. That improvement, plus further research into a different hormone or delivery system that will minimize menstrual irregularities, should result in increased acceptance of this long-awaited contraceptive.

II. **The Theory**
   A. **Mechanism of action**
      1. Levonorgestrel depresses pituitary gonadotropin peaks and ovarian response; ovulation is suppressed in majority of cycles.
      2. Levonorgestrel alters cervical mucus which becomes scanty and viscous resulting in poor sperm penetration
      3. Interruption of early pregnancy is not mechanism of action
   B. **Efficacy**
      1. Published failure rates vary from 0.04–0.4 pregnancies per hundred women in first year of use
      2. Increased failure rate is 3.7% at 5 years of use
      3. Increased failure rate in obese women (Table 1), but prevention of pregnancy still greater in women with levonorgestrel implants than for most other forms of reversible contraception
      4. Depth of preinsertion evaluation to rule out pregnancy is variable; higher pregnancy rates in patients in whom pregnancy testing not carried out and/or implants placed at nonspecific time in cycle.
      5. Rapidly increasing failure rate in sixth year mandates capsule removal
   C. **Description**
      1. Norplant System consists of 6 flexible, closed capsules made of Silastic (silicone polymer)
      2. Each capsule is 34 mm in length, 2.4 mm in diameter
      3. Each capsule contains 36 mg of crystalline levonorgestrel
      4. Levonorgestrel diffuses through capsule
         a. Amount of steroid diffused from capsule is related to surface area of capsule
         b. Rate of diffusion is related to thickness and density of capsule
         c. Duration of release is related to amount of steroid in capsule
      5. Dose of levonorgestrel supplied per day depends on length of time capsules have been in place
         a. 85 µg/day during first few weeks of use
         b. Amount declines to 50 µg/day by 9 months after insertion
         c. 35 µg/day released at 18 months
         d. 30 µg/day released in fifth year of use
         e. Rate of release between years 2–5 is fairly constant, resulting in blood level of 0.4 mg/ml

TABLE 1. Pregnancy Rates per 100 Woman-Years by Year and Weight Group

Weight Group (kg)	Year of Use				
	1	2	3	4	5
< 50	0.2	0.1	0.1	0.2	0.3
50–59	0.1	0.1	0.2	0.5	0.6
60–69	0.0	0.1	0.4	0.9	0.8
≥ 70	0.3	0.0	0.7	0.7	3.0
P within year	NS	NS	< .05	< .05	< .05

NS = not significant.
From Su-Juan G, Ming-Kuan D, Ling-De, et al: A 5-year evaluation of Norplant contraceptive implants in China. Obstet Gynecol 83:673–678, 1994, with permission.

       f. Rapid decline in blood level after removal of implants
          i. Mean plasma half-life after removal is 40 hours
          ii. Levonorgestrel is not detectable in blood stream after 5 days to 2 weeks

D. **Advantages**
  1. No estrogen side effects
  2. Rapidly reversible
  3. Decreased incidence of anemia
  4. Decreased incidence of dysmenorrhea
  5. Long-term contraception
  6. Does not require compliant patient
  7. Low risk of ectopic pregnancy (1.3 per 1000 women-years)
  8. Not coitus-dependent
  9. No interference with breastfeeding
  10. Does not appear to have negative effect on serum lipid concentrations
  11. Cost-effective with long-term use
  12. Rapid recovery of fertility

E. **Disadvantages and cautions**
  1. Not cost-effective for short-term use
  2. Requires surgical insertion and removal
  3. Removal can be difficult
  4. Decreased effectiveness in patients on antiseizure medication
  5. No protection from STDs

F. **Side effects**
  1. Irregular menstrual bleeding
    a. Majority of users have irregular bleeding at least for first year; more than one-third continue to have irregular bleeding over remainder of 5 years.
    b. Total number of bleeding and spotting days per month decreases from 13 to 9 from first to twelfth months (average of 5.4 days/month in control cycles)
    c. Over 5 years, about 20% of women have implants removed because of bleeding problems
    d. 10% or less have amenorrhea
    e. Total blood loss is slightly less for users of levonorgestrel implants than for controls
  2. Other side effects
    a. See Chapter 121 for most frequent side effects in one series
    b. See Table 2 for principal medical conditions other than menstrual irregularities leading to removal

G. **Cost**
  1. Approximate cost for kit is $375
    a. Health care provider may purchase kits up front but in most settings practitioner does not wish to incur initial cost
    b. Patient may arrange to buy kit or it is covered by insurance
      i. Most insurance plans, including Medicaid, cover cost of kit
      ii. Norplant Foundation provides free Norplant kits for indigent patients who do not qualify for Medicaid
  2. Additional cost for counseling, history and physical exam, Papanicolaou smear, and pregnancy testing ranges from $200 or less up to $700
  3. Charge for removal of implants is usually separate, in range of $100–$200
  4. In cases of very difficult removal, further charge for radiograph or ultrasound to localize implant may be incurred

III. **An Approach**
A. **Patient selection**
  1. Levonorgestrel implants are good contraceptive choice for women who:
    a. Believe they do not want to bear any or more children but do not wish to undergo permanent sterilization. Desire permanent sterilization but are Medicaid recipients under the age of 21
    b. Are approaching menopause

TABLE 2.   Principal Medical Conditions Other than Menstrual Problems Leading to Removal

Condition	Event (n)	Incidence per 10,000 yr
Headache	49	10.9
Myoma	38	8.5
Dizziness	35	8.0
Weight gain	35	7.8
Acute hepatitis	30	6.7
Ovarian cyst	24	5.4
Hypertension	20	4.5
Low platelet count	17	3.8
Breast hyperplasia	12	2.7
Hyperthyroidism	10	2.2
Arm/hand numbness or limited mobility	10	2.2
Pigmentation problem	9	2.0
Breast masses	8	1.8
Pulmonary tuberculosis	8	1.8
Chronic hepatitis	7	1.6
Pain, discomfort at implant site	7	1.6

From Su-Juan G, Ming-Kuan D, Ling-De Z, et al: A 5-year evaluation of Norplant contraceptive implants in China. Obstet Gynecol 83:673–678, 1994, with permission. (10,718 women participated in the study, accounting for 44,954 years of use of the Norplant system.)

    c. Are over 35 and smoke
    d. Want long-term birth spacing
    e. Have difficulty with compliance in using birth control
    f. Have had estrogen side effects when taking combined oral contraceptives or should otherwise avoid estrogen use
    g. Are breastfeeding
    h. Are not candidates for IUD
    i. Want long-term but rapidly reversible contraception at any stage of reproductive lives
    j. Are taking teratogenic medications
    k. Have had unplanned pregnancies
  2. Levonorgestrel implants (used alone) are not good contraceptive choice for women who:
    a. Are taking antiseizure medications
    b. Need protection from STDs
    c. Have been intolerant of progestin side effects in other forms of contraception
    d. Are suspected to be intolerant of irregular vaginal bleeding
    e. Are considering pregnancy in near future
    f. Have history of migraines or severe headaches (these women may be tried on progesterone-only pill to determine if headaches worsen or improve)
    g. Are at risk for subacute bacterial endocarditis
    h. Have history of cardiovascular disease
       i. This recommendation based on older data with higher-dose combined oral contraceptives
      ii. Patients with cardiovascular disease in whom pregnancy is contraindicated may find levonorgestrel implants to be good contraceptive choice if they are not interested in permanent sterilization
    i. May be allergic to progestational agents
    j. Have severe acne or are concerned that acne may increase (progesterone-only pill may be tried first)
B. Counseling
  1. User acceptance of any contraceptive method is related to quality of preuse counseling
  2. Especially important for levonorgestrel implants; user depends on health care provider for initiation and discontinuation of method.

TABLE 3. Instructions for Care after Insertion of Norplant

1. Leave the outer bandage in place for 24 hours and keep the area dry. After removing the outer bandage, leave the adhesive strip in place until it falls off. Feel free to shower or bathe as usual.

2. Heavy lifting or strenuous exercise of the arm containing the implants should be avoided for the first 24 hours after insertion. You may resume your other daily activities immediately.

3. Bruising around the implants is normal and will usually resolve within 5 to 7 days after insertion. If you experience minor discomfort, Tylenol or Advil may be helpful.

4. If you develop severe pain or redness over the implants or near the incision, heavy bleeding from the wound, fever (greater than 101 degrees), or notice the tip of an implant is visible at the incision, contact your health care provider immediately. (This may even happen some months after the implants have been placed.)

5. After insertion, you may notice a change in your menstrual bleeding pattern. This is common and does not indicate a problem. If you experience heavy bleeding or are concerned about your bleeding, please call your health care provider.

6. If you have a medical problem related to Norplant, contact your primary care provider.

    3. Sample counseling protocol
       a. Carried out by nurse practitioner, nurse, or assistant
       b. Required for all prospective implant patients
       c. Preceded by primary care provider who carries out appropriate history, physical exam, and laboratory investigations
       d. One-hour session includes group (30–45 minutes) followed by individual counseling
       e. Content
          i. Discussion of contraceptive choices
         ii. Specific information about levonorgestrel implants
            (a) Effectiveness, advantages and disadvantages
            (b) Appropriate candidates for method
            (c) Contraindications, reversibility
            (d) Discussion of insertion procedure, viewing kit; handling sample implants, viewing video.
            (e) Discussion of postinsertion care (Table 3)
            (f) Side effects, including warning signs of possible problems
            (g) Scheduling insertion and reviewing checklist (Fig. 1)
  C. **Insertion**—see Chapter 121
  D. **Managing bleeding problems**
    1. Goal is to help patients continue method for 1 year, after which irregular bleeding often decreases
    2. All management choices provide only short-term relief

☐ 1. Documented history and physical examination, including a pelvic examination, Papanicolaou smear, and breast examination, within the past 6 months. (The patient must have had an initial visit with her physician.)

☐ 2. Patient has viewed the preinsertion video and has had a chance to ask questions.

☐ 3. Patient packets have been given.

☐ 4. Patient has signed the risk and benefit sheet and signed a standard consent form.

☐ 5. Patient has been given an insertion date correlated with the first 7 days of her menstrual cycle.

Insertion Day

☐ 1. Serum pregnancy test done and results on chart.

☐ 2. Blood pressure and history recorded by nurse.

☐ 3. Postinsertion care sheet is given to the patient.

FIGURE 1. Norplant checklist.

3. Medication options to manage polymenorrhea
   a. Nonsteroidal antiinflammatory medications can be used although caution regarding gastric side effects
   b. Combined oral contraceptives are easy to use, if not otherwise contraindicated, but they contain progestins, which may be counterproductive
   c. Low-dose oral estrogens may be used if estrogen not contraindicated
   d. Conjugated estrogen, 0.625–1.25 mg can be prescribed for 10–21 days or in 21-day cycles (with 7 days off) for several months
      i. Withdrawal bleeding results, but pattern, at least, is regular

SUGGESTED READING

1. Darney PD: Hormonal implants: Contraception for a new century. Am J Obstet Gynecol 170:1536–1543, 1994.
2. Díaz S, Croxatto HB: Clinical assessment of treatments for prolonged bleeding in users of Norplant™ implants. Contraception 42:97–109, 1990.
3. Fleming D, Davie J: Continuation rates of long-acting methods of contraception: A comparative study of Norplant® implants and intrauterine devices. Contraception 57:19–21, 1998.
4. Kaeser L: Public funding and policies for provision of the contraceptive implant, fiscal year 1992. Fam Plann Perspect 26:11–16, 1994.
5. Shoupe D, Mishell DR Jr: The significance of bleeding patterns in Norplant implant users. Obstet Gynecol 77:256–260, 1991.
6. Sivin I, Stern J: Rates and outcomes of planned pregnancy after use of Norplant capsules. Norplant II rods, or levonorgestrel-releasing or copper TCu 380Ag intrauterine contraceptive devices. Am J Obstet Gynecol 166:1208–1213, 1992.
7. Su-Juan G, Ming-Kuan D: A 5-year evaluation of Norplant contraceptive implants in China. Obstet Gynecol 83:673–678, 1994.

35. Depot Medroxyprogesterone Acetate

Cynda Ann Johnson, M.D., M.B.A.

I. The Issues

On October 29, 1992, depot medroxyprogesterone acetate (DMPA, Depo-Provera), a long-acting, injectable progestin, was approved by the Food and Drug Administration (FDA) for use as first-line contraception. Until then it had been approved in the U.S. only for treatment of endometrial and renal cancers. Ninety other countries had already supported the use of DMPA, with a patient experience of 30,000,000 women. In 1973 and 1975 the Fertility and Maternal Health Drugs Advisory Board had recommended approval, but their recommendations were overruled by the FDA, which cited a 1972 study in which beagle dogs had developed breast tumors while receiving DMPA as part of a drug study. In its approval statement, the FDA acknowledged that the beagle dog study was not relevant to humans. The World Health Organization (WHO) study in 1991 determined that risks of cancer associated with use of DMPA are no greater than those associated with use of oral contraceptives. The relative risk of breast cancer for all ages with any use was 1.2. Other safety concerns focused on bone density and low-birth-weight infants. A study at Auckland Hospital in New Zealand compared women who had been using DMPA for at least 5 years with two control groups—premenopausal and postmenopausal women. Bone density was 7.5% lower at the femoral neck in DMPA users than in premenopausal controls. No additional loss was seen with longer use, and bone density increased when DMPA was discontinued (up 3% after 1 year and 6% after 2 years). Postmenopausal controls had greater bone loss then DMPA users. The investigators concluded that the overall risk/benefit balance was not seriously affected by osteoporosis. A study in Thailand of pregnancies estimated to have occurred within the first 4 weeks after DMPA injection revealed a twofold increase in low birth weight. The risk of low birth weight diminished as the time between injection and conception increased.

The investigators concluded that the attributable risk of DMPA to low birth weight was small, especially if the injection was given appropriately within 5 days of the onset of the last regular menstrual period.

As a decade since FDA approval approaches, DMPA has a confirmed niche in the armamentarium of hormonal treatment options. Cancer concerns have been put to rest; no new studies cite increases in low-birth-weight babies born to mothers who had used DMPA; but the possibility of decreased bone density after prolonged use remains. Clinicians should follow the literature, adjusting their practices to include bone density measurements, serum estradiol measurements, addition of estrogen, and/or time-limited usage as indicated.

II. **The Theory**
  A. **Mechanism of action**
    1. Primary mechanism
      a. Circulating levels of progestin are adequate to block luteinizing hormone (LH) surge and suppress ovulation
    2. Secondary mechanisms
      a. Thickening of cervical mucus creates barrier to sperm penetration
      b. Altered endometrium decreases ability of ovum to implant
  B. **Efficacy**
    1. Failure rate of only 0.3%/year with perfect use (i.e., every 12 week injection)
  C. **Description of product**
    1. Delivered as microcrystals suspended in aqueous solution
    2. Microcrystals dissolve slowly, releasing active progestin
  D. **Advantages**
    1. Exceptional contraceptive control
    2. Lack of interference with intercourse
    3. Long-acting
    4. Fewer compliance concerns than with many methods
    5. No estrogen-related side effects
      a. Safe for patients with history of thromboembolism
      b. May be used in women over 35 who smoke
    6. Cost-effective ($25–30 every 3 months)
    7. Reduced risk of endometrial cancer and possibly ovarian cancer
    8. Positive effect on endometriosis
    9. Suppression of cyclic mastalgia
    10. No significant drug interactions
    11. Fewer seizures in seizure-prone patients
    12. **Advantages in special populations**
      a. **Sickle-cell patients**—DMPA may inhibit intravascular sickling and increase red blood cell survival
      b. **Breastfeeding mothers**—DMPA may increase quantity and protein content of breast milk
  E. **Disadvantages and cautions**
    1. Requires return visit and repeat injection every 12 weeks
    2. No immediate restoration of fertility with discontinuation
    3. Modest negative effect on serum lipids
      a. While HDL may fall slightly, there seems to be no concomitant rise in LDL; any negative effect difficult to determine.
    4. Possible increase in incidence of cervical cancer
      a. Relative risk is 1.1–1.2 compared with controls
      b. Patients should have yearly Papanicolaou smears
    5. Inconsistent data regarding decrease in bone density with long-term use; if patient is perimenopausal or has risk for osteoporosis, may warrant measurement.
  F. **Contraindications**
    1. Known or suspected pregnancy
      a. Theoretical and medicolegal consideration even though current data show no increased risk for birth defects caused by hormones during pregnancy
    2. Unexplained abnormal vaginal bleeding

a. DMPA may mask serious or treatable diagnosis

b. Withhold DMPA until diagnosis is made

3. Known or suspected malignancy of breast

4. Allergy to DMPA

5. Acute liver disease not considered a contraindication

G. **Side effects**

1. **Irregular bleeding**

a. Expected in all patients

b. Irregular menstrual periods often with bleeding 7 days or more in first few months of use

c. Menstrual bleeding decreases over time

i. Amenorrhea common after 9–12 months of use

ii. 50% are amenorrheic within 1 year

d. Abnormal bleeding pattern is most common reason for discontinuance

i. 13% discontinue at 12 months for irregular or increased bleeding; another 13% discontinue at 12 months for amenorrhea.

2. **Weight gain**

a. Related to increased body fat rather than fluid retention

b. Results of initial studies

i. 60% gain weight during first 6 months

ii. Average weight gain is 5 pounds at 1 year, 15–16 pounds at 3 years, remaining constant thereafter

3. **Infertility**

a. After one 150-mg injection, mean interval before return of ovulation is 4.5 months

b. Thereafter, delay to conception is approximately 9 months after most recent DMPA injection; unaffected by duration of use.

c. 70% conceive within 12 months after discontinuation and over 85% by 24 months

d. No evidence supports permanent infertility

4. Headaches—17% of users

5. Nausea

6. Dizziness

7. Breast tenderness—3% of users

8. Psychological effects, including loss of libido (5%), depression, nervousness (11%), fatigue

9. Acne

10. Hair loss or growth

H. **Cost**

1. 150 mg vial of DMPA costs about $30 with injection fee additional in most settings

2. Follow up of abnormal bleeding another cost in substantial percentage of women

III. **An Approach**

A. **Patient selection**

1. **Good method** for women who:

a. Failed other forms of contraception

b. Have history of estrogen side effects

c. Want long-term, reversible contraception

d. Have difficulty with compliance

e. Have dysfunctional uterine bleeding

f. Have uterine fibroids

g. Are breastfeeding

h. Are immediately postpartum

i. Have endometriosis

j. Have significant dysmenorrhea

k. Are mentally retarded (only with careful counseling and when completely voluntary)

l. **Have special medical problems**

i. Hemoglobinopathy

ii. Hepatic disease (still listed in package insert as contraindication)

       iii. Infection with human immunodeficiency virus
       iv. Hypertension
       v. Prior thromboembolism (still listed in package insert as contraindication)
       vi. Renal disease
       vii. Valvular heart disease
       viii. Vascular disease
       ix. Psychosis
          (a) But may increase certain symptoms in some women
          (b) Delayed reversibility is potential problem
       x. Seizure disorder
    m. Who should not become pregnant because of potential fetal risk due to use of:
       i. Intravenous drugs
       ii. Anticonvulsant medications
       iii. Chemotherapeutic agents
       iv. Isotretinoin
       v. Other teratogenic drugs
  2. **Suboptimal choice** for women with:
    a. Such difficulty with compliance that they cannot seek injection in timely fashion
    b. History of significant progestational side effects
    c. Desire for rapidly reversible contraception
    d. Desire to become pregnant in near future
    e. Fear of intramuscular injections
    f. Intolerance of unpredictable bleeding patterns or amenorrhea
B. **Counseling**
  1. Successful use depends on careful patient selection and thorough counseling:
    a. Potential for weight gain
    b. Probability of irregular menstrual bleeding
    c. Amenorrhea (not harmful)
    d. Importance of timeliness of injections
    e. Lack of protection from STDs
  2. Obtain consent (example of consent form shown in Fig. 1)
C. **Administration**
  1. **Initial dose**
    a. Administer within 5 days of beginning of regular menstrual period
      i. Effective immediately with no back-up method needed

Date _____

Time _____

After discussing the various other options for birth control with Dr. _____, I prefer to use depot medroxyprogesterone acetate (DMPA, Depo-Provera). I understand the risks and side effects, but believe it is the best choice for me at this time.

Today I will receive _____ mg of depot medroxyprogesterone acetate by intramuscular injection. I realize that I must return to the _____, in _____ weeks for my next injection and that failure to do so may result in inadequate contraception by this method. Thereafter, I will be instructed in the frequency of repeat injections, but realize that injections of the medication will be necessary at least every three months as long as depot medroxyprogesterone acetate is my contraception of choice. I accept a continued risk of pregnancy of 0.4%, even though I receive all injections as instructed. I understand that when I stop receiving injections of depot medroxyprogesterone acetate, the time it takes for my fertility to return to its previous level is unpredictable, but may be as long as nine months after my last injection.

_____   _____
Signature of witness   Signature of patient

FIGURE 1.   Consent for administration of depot medroxyprogesterone acetate.

    b. Administration at other times in cycle should be discouraged when at all possible
        i. Occasionally necessary for high-risk patients but causes concern about reliable timing for administration of follow-up injections
        ii. Pregnancy test (preferably serum) before injection
        iii. Continue back-up method for 7 days
    c. For postpartum patients
        i. May administer before hospital discharge or within 5 days of delivery
        ii. Manufacturer suggests withholding DMPA in lactating women until 6 weeks postpartum
            (a) No data indicate adverse effect on quality or quantity of breast milk
            (b) Many experts freely administer DMPA to women initiating breastfeeding
        iii. DMPA may slow uterine involution and increase lochia
            (a) Use caution with postpartum women who are significantly anemic
    d. For postabortion patients
        i. Safe; should be administered as soon as possible.

2. **Follow-up dosing**
    a. Ask patient to return in 12 weeks for repeat injection
    b. Contraceptive levels of progestogen probably maintained for up to 4 months
    c. Reinjection within 13 weeks of previous dose or pregnancy test is desirable
    d. Visits with health care provider generally increase cost
        i. Health care provider should see patient before each injection to assess side effects and bleeding pattern until she is using method successfully
        ii. Further follow-up visits at least annually
        iii. Patient should be encouraged to call if concerning side effects appear

3. **Dosing amounts**
    a. 150 mg administered intramuscularly, regardless of patient's weight
    b. 150 mg/ml solution recommended for contraception
        i. High-strength (400 mg/ml) solution not approved for contraceptive use at usual dosage solution every 3 months
        ii. High-strength solution more painful and has not yet been studied for reliability of contraceptive effect

4. **Site of injection**
    a. Inject in deltoid or gluteal muscles
    b. Injection site should not be rubbed
        i. Spreads medication over larger area
        ii. Speeds uptake of drug
        iii. Shortens duration of efficacy

5. **Treatment of patients with dysfunctional uterine bleeding** (DUB)
    a. Frequently obese patients with anovulation
    b. Also effective for patients with ovulatory DUB whose abnormal bleeding is hard to control
    c. Larger doses of progestin usually required
    d. Perform endometrial biopsy to confirm anovulation and estrogen excess
    e. Alternate regimen
        i. 150–300 mg initially (higher doses are for more obese women with heavy bleeding)
        ii. Second dose 1 month later
        iii. Third dose 2 months after second dose
        iv. Some patients require injection every 2 months
        v. Very obese patients with chronic anovulation have required as much as 400–600 mg
        vi. If bleeding is difficult to control, perform endometrial biopsy to determine status of endometrium
            (a) Proliferative phase endometrium indicates that additional progestin is necessary to counteract elevated estrogen status
            (b) Progesterone effect indicates that amount of progestin is adequate or excessive and another reason for continued bleeding needs to be sought

SUGGESTED READING

1. Bonhomme MG, Potts DM, Fortney JA, Allen MY: Safety of depot medroxyprogesterone acetate. Lancet 338:942, 1991.
2. Cohall AT, Cullins VE, Darney PD, Nelson AL: Contraception in the 1990s: New methods and approaches. Patient Care 15(Suppl):1–12, 1993.
3. Euhus DM, Uyehara C: Influence of parenteral progesterones on the prevalence and severity of mastalgia in premenopausal women: A multi-institutional cross sectional study. J Am Coll Surg 184:596–604, 1997.
4. Garza-Flores J, De la Cruz DL, de Bourges VV, et al: Long-term effects of depot-medroxyprogesterone acetate on lipoprotein metabolism. Contraception 44:61–71, 1991.
5. Grimes DA (ed): Depot medroxyprogesterone acetate: An overview of DMPA and its FDA approval. Contracep Rep 3:1–6, 1992.
6. Kaunitz AM: Long-acting injectable contraception with depot medroxyprogesterone acetate. Am J Obstet Gynecol 170:1543–1549, 1994.
7. Naessen T, Olsson SE: Differential effects on bone density of progestogen-only methods for contraception in premenopausal women. Contraception 52:35–39, 1995.
8. Petta CA, Faundes A: Timing of onset of contraceptive effectiveness in Depo-Provera users: Part I. Changes in cervical mucus. Fertil Steril 69:252–257, 1998.
9. WHO Collaborative Study of neoplasia and steroid contraception: Breast cancer and depot-medroxyprogesterone acetate: A multinational study. Lancet 338:833–838, 1991.

36. Progesterone-only Pills

Cynda Ann Johnson, M.D., M.B.A.

I. The Issues

The progesterone-only pill, sometimes called the minipill, has not been a popular choice for contraception. Many physicians do not even consider progesterone-only pills when describing the range of birth control options to a patient. However, in certain patients progesterone-only hormonal contraception is desirable, but their needs for contraception may be short term; others may find injectable and implantable agents unacceptable. For such women, the minipill provides the optimal contraceptive choice.

II. The Theory

A. **Mechanism of action**
   1. Irregular inhibition of ovulation
   2. Other progestin effects
      a. Thickened cervical mucus and decreased mucus volume result in poor sperm penetration
      b. Atrophic endometrium
      c. Premature luteolysis

B. **Efficacy**
   1. Failure rate is about 3% for typical user
   2. Failure rate is probably highest in patients who ovulate regularly on minipill; these women have greatest satisfaction rates, however, because of regular menses.
   3. Failure rate is lowest for patients in whom ovulation is consistently inhibited, resulting in infrequent, irregular bleeding; reasonable satisfaction to many patients though irregularity may cause concern about possibility of pregnancy.
   4. Most patients ovulate irregularly, resulting in irregular, unpredictable cycles and least patient satisfaction

C. **Description of products**
   1. All brands are not available at most pharmacies
   2. Physician should become knowledgeable about a few available products and prescribe primarily these

3. Older studies showed more progesterone side effects with levonorgestrel than norethindrone

D. **Advantages**
1. No estrogen side effects
2. No pill break; all pills in packet are identical.
3. Decreased total menstrual blood flow
4. Decreased dysmenorrhea
5. No interference with breastfeeding and volume of breast milk
6. Compares favorably with combined oral contraceptives (most comparisons carried out with older, higher-dosage combined oral contraceptives)
   a. No increased risk of cardiovascular disease
   b. Lower incidence of headaches
   c. Lower incidence of blood pressure elevation
   d. Less breast tenderness
   e. Less interference with psychological functioning (e.g., depression)
7. Reasonable option for short-term contraception

E. **Disadvantages and cautions**
1. Fewer noncontraceptive benefits than with combined oral contraceptives (OCs)
2. Requires reliable patient; pill must be taken daily.
3. Breakthrough and irregular bleeding expected
4. Little protection from sexually transmitted diseases (STDs)
5. Possible increased incidence of ovarian cysts compared with users of combined OCs
6. Effectiveness may be decreased in users of antiseizure medications and other medications that induce hepatic enzymes

F. **Cost**
1. Similar to combined oral contraceptives
2. $100–$300/year
3. Lower costs with generic brands and at family planning clinics
4. Cost-effective when compared with subdermal implants if these are removed within first few years after placement

III. **An Approach**

A. **Patient selection**
1. **Best candidates are breastfeeding women**
   a. No interference with volume of breast milk compared with combined oral contraceptives
   b. Relatively short-term need
   c. Increased effectiveness (probably in part because patients are already relatively infertile while breastfeeding)
   d. Most breastfeeding women have infrequent periods and ovulation, resulting in less breakthrough bleeding on minipill
2. Consider minipill for patients who want to take pill but have estrogen side effects on combined oral OCs, especially women:
   a. With elevated blood pressure, particularly if blood pressure was documented to rise after placement on combined OCs
   b. With migraine headaches or headaches that began or increased after beginning combined OCs
   c. Who become nauseated on combined OCs
   d. With breast tenderness on combined OCs
3. Women over 35 who smoke but prefer to take OCs
4. Consider using minipill for several months before placing subdermal implants; prescribe levonorgestrel (Ovrette), which is same hormonal agent as in subdermal implants.
   a. Appropriate candidates are women who are likely to be intolerant of irregular cycles or women who have had difficulty with side effects of combined OCs
   b. Inappropriate to use minipill to simulate expected bleeding pattern before placing subdermal implants because mechanism of release and absorption of levonorgestrel are different in two products

B. **Proper use**
1. Most successful in women who are excellent candidates and have been carefully counseled on expected side effects
2. Transition to minipill is most easily made by starting first packet within 5 days of regular menstrual period; back-up method is not essential after first month.
3. Pill should be taken every day at 24-hour intervals
   a. Sperm penetration increases rapidly with increased interval of dosing
   b. Back-up method of contraception should be used if interval between pills > 27 hours
4. **Result of missing pill** is more difficult to determine clinically than with combined OCs
   a. Bleeding pattern is usually irregular
   b. Determining when to order pregnancy test is more difficult
   c. With missed pill, it is advisable to add back-up, usually barrier method
      i. Continue back-up method for at least 2 days
      ii. Missed pill should be taken by patient immediately when remembered
   d. If 2 days of pills are missed
      i. Patient should take 2 pills for 2 days in row
      ii. Back-up method should be started immediately and continued for remainder of cycle
      iii. Patient should be suspicious of signs or symptoms of pregnancy

SUGGESTED READING

1. Heath CB: Helping patients choose appropriate contraception. Am Fam Physician 48:1115–1124, 1993.
2. McCann MF, Potter LS: Progestin-only contraception: A comprehensive review. Contraception 50:S1–S195, 1994.
3. Sheth A, Jain U, Sharma S, et al: A randomized, double-blind study of two combined and two progesterone-only oral contraceptives. Contraception 25:243–252, 1982.
4. Vessey MP, Lawless M, Yeates D, McPherson K: Progestin-only oral contraception: Findings in a large prospective study with special reference to effectiveness. Br J Fam Plann 10:117–121, 1985.

37. Combined Oral Contraceptives—The Pill

Cynda Ann Johnson, M.D., M.B.A.

I. The Issues

The pill—these two words embody a concept of contraception known to most sexually aware people in the U.S. With more than 35 options for combined oral contraceptives currently available, such medications have continued to be extensively studied and refined since their release by the Food and Drug Administration in 1960. Interest in the estrogen component of the pill has resulted in continued lowering of the estrogen content to a level that minimizes adverse effects while preserving contraceptive effect. The outcome is a combined oral contraceptive (OC) that can be used by a broader group of patients and continued by many until menopause. Current research emphasizes the progestin component of the pill as the optimal type and dosage regimen are sought. The pill is the number-one form of reversible contraception in the U.S. Despite newer options in birth control, none is likely to usurp its position at the top. Yet many unintended pregnancies occur in women taking combined oral contraception. Only a few such pregnancies are due to failure of the contraceptive method; most are due to noncompliance in daily use of the pill. Primary care physicians have continued opportunity to help women to choose a birth control method or to assess the appropriateness of their current methods. Physicians should choose pill candidates carefully and educate women in the use of the pill as well as problem-solving techniques. The result will be a more informed group of consumers and fewer untoward outcomes.

II. **The Theory**
   A. **Mechanism of action**
      1. Inhibition of ovulation
         a. Pulsatile release of luteinizing hormone (LH) is maintained during OC use, although follicle-stimulating hormone (FSH) is suppressed
         b. After a 7-day pill-free interval, normal early follicular-phase pulse pattern is found, even in long-term pill users
      2. Alteration of ovum transport
      3. Changes in uterine environment
         a. Altered uterine secretions leading to regions of edema and abnormal cellularity
         b. Atrophied endometrial bed hampering implantation
      4. Alterations in cervical mucus and capacitation (activation of enzymes) that inhibit sperm transport
      5. Acceleration of luteolysis (degeneration of corpus luteum)
   B. **Efficacy**
      1. Failure rate is about 3% for typical user and 0.1% with perfect use
      2. Pills with only 20 μg ethinyl estradiol have slightly higher rate of failure, even with perfect use (0.8%)
      3. Perfect use requires that pills be taken at same time every day, with adherence to specific instructions when patient experiences vomiting or diarrhea or takes competing medications
      4. High rate of discontinuance
         a. Only 50–75% of women who start pill are still using it after 1 year
         b. Most women discontinue the pill for nonmedical reasons
         c. Unintended pregnancies occur because many women who discontinue the pill do not immediately begin an alternate form of contraception
   C. **Description of products**
      1. Table 1 lists the composition of OCs currently available in U.S.
      2. Pills are available in monophasic, biphasic, and triphasic cycles, depending on variations in composition of active pills within packet
         a. Bi- and triphasic options were developed primarily in effort to address problems with midcycle spotting while keeping estrogen dose low
      3. Packets contain 21 pills with pharmacologic activity
         a. 28-day packets contain 7 placebo pills; users take 1 pill/day.
         b. 21-day packets do not contain placebo pills; users take 7-day pill break after completion of cycle.
      4. **Estrogen component**
         a. Ethinyl estradiol (EE) and mestranol are the only two estrogens found in currently used OCs
            i. Mestranol is converted to pharmacologically active EE by the liver
            ii. Mestranol has 67% of pharmacologic activity of EE giving mestranol 50 μg the same estrogenic content as EE 30–35 μg
            iii. Many contraindications, cautions, and reported side effects of OCs were based on effects of higher-dose pills and have decreased significantly with pills below 50 μg
            iv. EE has strong estrogenic activity compared with estrogens used for hormone replacement in menopause; thus, literature on side effects and complications experienced with OCs should not be extrapolated to hormone use in menopause.
      5. **Progestin component**
         a. Several different progestins are used in OCs available in U.S.
         b. Comparing different progestins for biologic activity is difficult; different biologic tests give variable results in term of progestational, androgenic, and endometrial potency (all are aspects of activity of progestins).
         c. Newer progestins
            i. Norgestimate, desogestrel, gestodene (awaiting approval in U.S.)
            ii. New progestins result in higher HDL cholesterol and lower LDL cholesterol

TABLE 1. Composition of Combined Oral Contraceptives

Name	Progestin	mg	Estrogen	µg
Monophasic				
Alesse	Levonorgestrel	0.1	Ethinyl estradiol	20
Brevicon	Norethindrone	0.5	Ethinyl estradiol	35
Demulen	Ethynodiol diacetate	1.0	Ethinyl estradiol	50
Demulen 1/35	Ethynodiol diacetate	1.0	Ethinyl estradiol	35
Desogen	Desogestrel	0.15	Ethinyl estradiol	30
Genora 1/35	Norethindrone	1.0	Ethinyl estradiol	35
Genora 1/50	Norethindrone	1.0	Mestranol	50
Levlen	Levonorgestrel	0.15	Ethinyl estradiol	30
Loestrin 1.5/30	Norethindrone acetate	1.5	Ethinyl estradiol	30
Loestrin 1/20	Norethindrone acetate	1.0	Ethinyl estradiol	20
Lo/Ovral	Norgestrel	0.3	Ethinyl estradiol	30
Modicon	Norethindrone	0.5	Ethinyl estradiol	35
Nelova 1/35/E	Norethindrone	1.0	Ethinyl estradiol	35
Nelova 0.5/35E	Norethindrone	0.5	Ethinyl estradiol	35
Nordette	Levonorgestrel	0.15	Ethinyl estradiol	30
Norethin 1/35E	Norethindrone	1.0	Ethinyl estradiol	35
Norethin 1/50M	Norethindrone	1.0	Mestranol	50
Norinyl 1/35	Norethindrone	1.0	Ethinyl estradiol	35
Norinyl 1/50	Norethindrone	1.0	Mestranol	50
Norlestrin 1/50	Norethindrone acetate	1.0	Ethinyl estradiol	50
Ortho-Cept	Desogestrel	0.15	Ethinyl estradiol	30
Ortho-Cyclen	Norgestimate	0.25	Ethinyl estradiol	35
Ortho-Novum 1/35	Norethindrone	1.0	Ethinyl estradiol	35
Ortho-Novum 1/50	Norethindrone	1.0	Mestranol	50
Ovcon 35	Norethindrone	0.4	Ethinyl estradiol	35
Ovcon 50	Norethindrone	1.0	Mestranol	50
Ovral	Norgestrel	0.5	Ethinyl estradiol	50
Zovia 1/35 E	Ethynodiol diacetate	1	Ethinyl estradiol	35
Zovia 1/50 E	Ethynodiol diacetate	1	Ethinyl estradiol	50
Multiphasic*				
Estrostep	Norethindrone acetate	1 (21)	Ethinyl estradiol	20 (5)
				30 (7)
				35 (9)
Jenest	Norethindrone	0.5 (7)	Ethinyl estradiol	35 (21)
		1.0 (14)		
Mircette	Desogestrel	0.15 (21)	Ethinyl estradiol	20 (21)
		0 (7)		0 (2)
				10 (5)
Ortho-Novum 7/7/7	Norethindrone	0.5 (7)	Ethinyl estradiol	35 (21)
		0.75 (7)		
		1.0 (7)		
Ortho-Novum 10/11	Norethindrone	0.5 (10)	Ethinyl estradiol	35 (21)
		1.0 (11)		
Ortho Tri-Cyclen	Norgestimate	0.180 (7)	Ethinyl estradiol	35 (21)
		0.215 (7)		
		0.250 (7)		
Tri-Levlen	Levonorgestrel	0.05 (6)	Ethinyl estradiol	30 (6)
		0.075 (5)		40 (5)
		0.125 (10)		30 (10)
Tri-Norinyl	Norethindrone	0.5 (7)	Ethinyl estradiol	35 (21)
		1.0 (9)		
		0.5 (5)		
Triphasil	Levonorgestrel	0.05 (6)	Ethinyl estradiol	30 (6)
		0.075 (5)		40 (5)
		0.125 (10)		30 (10)

* Multiphasic product: number in parentheses indicates days of each phase. Also available with added iron: Loestrin, Estrostep.

          iii. Lower free testosterone levels, higher sex hormone-binding globulin levels, greater affinity to progesterone-binding sites gives fewer androgenic side effects

          iv. Fewer amenorrheic cycles—withdrawal bleeding occurs at least every 2 months in all women using pills with newer progestins

          v. Several WHO collaborative studies show increased risk of venous thromboembolism in patients using OCs containing desogestrel or gestodene than in patients using levonorgestrel-containing OCs though these studies need to be confirmed in additional studies

             (a) Any overall risk increase due to venous thromboembolism is offset by decline in risk of myocardial infarction

D. **Possible side effects** of OCs relative to hormone content
   1. **Estrogen excess**
      a. Increase in breast size, cervical ectropion, dysmenorrhea, increased menstrual bleeding, mucorrhea, growth of uterine fibroids, chloasma, thromboembolic phenomena, capillary fragility, telangiectasias, hepatocellular adenomas, rise in cholesterol concentration in gallbladder bile
   2. **Estrogen deficiency**
      a. Absence of withdrawal bleeding, bleeding and spotting early in pill cycle, continuous spotting, pelvic relaxation symptoms, atrophic vaginitis, vasomotor symptoms, nervousness
   3. **Progestin excess**
      a. Cervicitis, appetite increase, depression, fatigue, decreased libido, neurodermatitis, weight gain (noncyclic), leg vein dilation
   4. **Progestin excess** (from androgenic effect)
      a. Acne, cholestatic jaundice, hirsutism, increased libido, oily skin and scalp, rash and pruritus, edema, increased LDL cholesterol, decreased HDL cholesterol, decreased carbohydrate tolerance
   5. **Progestin deficiency**
      a. Breakthrough in second half of cycle, delayed withdrawal bleeding, dysmenorrhea, heavy flow
   6. **Combination symptoms**
      a. Estrogen excess or progestin deficiency
         i. Bloating, dizziness, syncope, edema, headache (cyclic), irritability, leg cramps, nausea, vomiting, visual changes, weight gain (cyclic)
      b. Progestin excess or estrogen excess
         i. Breast tenderness, headaches, hypertension, myocardial infarction

E. **Advantages of OCs**
   1. Highly efficacious
   2. Option throughout reproductive years
   3. Reversibility—baseline pregnancy rate with in 3 months after discontinuing OCs
   4. Beneficial effects on menstrual cycle
      a. 60% less blood loss compared with natural cycle
      b. Decreased dysmenorrhea
   5. Decreased incidence of pelvic inflammatory disease
   6. Decreased incidence of ovarian cancer—up to 80% decrease in long-term users
   7. Decreased incidence of endometrial cancer—up to 60% in long-term users
   8. Decreased risk for benign breast disease
   9. Lower incidence of ectopic pregnancy
   10. Improvement in acne
   11. Not coitus-dependent
   12. Decreased incidence of osteoporosis
   13. Treatment and prevention of endometriosis

F. **Disadvantages and cautions**
   1. Pill must be taken every day
   2. Many potential side effects (see above)
      a. Some side effects diminish or resolve after few cycles while others persist

3. Medication interaction
   a. OCs interact with other drugs, producing various adverse effects
   b. Antibiotics, especially with long-term use, may decrease contraceptive effect
   c. Antiseizure drugs decrease contraceptive effect (exception is valproic acid)
4. Should not be used in lactating women because of potential decrease in milk production
5. No protection against sexually transmitted diseases (STDs)

G. **Medical contraindications**
   1. Lower-dose pills result in fewer contraindications
   2. Thrombophlebitis—the pill may be used in women with thromboembolism from trauma if OCs are otherwise optimal choice.
   3. Coronary artery disease
   4. Breast cancer
   5. Estrogen-dependent neoplasia
   6. Pregnancy—fortunately the current literature does not demonstrate increase in birth defects in women who mistakenly took birth control pills during pregnancy
   7. Hepatitis
      a. OCs should not be used during bout of acute hepatitis
      b. Whether OCs should be used in women with abnormal liver function tests remains controversial
   8. Women over 35 years of age who smoke 15 or more cigarettes/day
      a. Such women have increased risk of cardiovascular complications on OCs
      b. Because the amount of smoking may be variable, most clinicians do not prescribe OCs for any woman over 35 who admits to smoking cigarettes
   9. Undiagnosed vaginal bleeding—the underlying cause of bleeding should be investigated before manipulating the pattern of bleeding with OCs.

H. **Medical conditions of potential concern**
   1. Hypertension
      a. Women under 35 years of age with controlled hypertension may use OCs
      b. Women over 35 years of age with hypertension are at greater risk from cardiovascular disease
      c. Women whose blood pressure increases after beginning OCs should use another form of contraception
   2. Sickle-cell or sickle-C disease
      a. Sickle-cell trait is definitely not a contraindication to use of OCs
      b. Women with sickle-cell or sickle-C disease have an increased risk of thromboembolism, but no evidence suggests a further increased risk with use of low-dose OCs
   3. Migraine headaches—use OCs with caution
      a. Continue pill if headaches improve
      b. Discontinue pill if headaches worsen
      c. If headaches are stable, reevaluate the optimal form of birth control for patient
      d. Avoid use of OCs if headaches are associated with neurologic impairment
   4. Diabetes mellitus—use OCs with caution in diabetic women who smoke
   5. Active gallbladder disease—OCs may accelerate development of gallbladder disease in predisposed women
   6. Gilbert's disease (congenital unconjugated hyperbilirubinemia)—monitor for increased hyperbilirubinemia

I. **Controversial effects**
   1. Breast cancer
      a. Women older than 55 who were previous users of OCs are probably not more likely than never-users to develop breast cancer
      b. Younger women who have used OCs may have an increased risk of developing of breast cancer before age 35
   2. Cervical cancer—the literature is divided about whether OCs are risk factor
   3. Cancer of liver—some studies show increased risk for hepatocellular cancers in ever-users of OCs
   4. Functional ovarian cysts
      a. Higher-dose OCs markedly decrease risk of functional ovarian cysts

        b. Recent studies have evaluated whether multiphasic OCs increase rather than decrease risk
           i. Low-dose OCs probably reduce risk compared with nonusers but protective effect is significantly less than with higher-dose OCs
    5. Lactation
        a. Use of OCs in nursing women should not be considered before lactation is well established, at least 8 weeks after delivery
        b. Hormonal content of OCs consumed by breastfeeding women does not have negative effect on nursing infant
        c. OCs may decrease supply of breastmilk
        d. Duration of nursing is overall less in women on OCs than in women on progestin-only pills or nonhormonal forms of contraception
  J. Cost of combined OCs is $100–$300/year, excluding charge for office visits

III. **An Approach**
  A. **Patient selection**
    1. Combined OCs are a good choice for women who:
        a. Can remember to take pill every day
        b. Want to space children
        c. Have endometriosis
        d. Need short- or long-term reversible contraception
        e. Have acne
        f. Are postpartum or postabortion
        g. Have heavy and/or painful menses
        h. Have a family history of ovarian cancer
        i. Have used OCs correctly in past
        j. Have recurrent ovarian cysts (consider 50-μg pill)
        k. Are anovulatory or have irregular periods
    2. Combined OCs are not good choice for women who:
        a. Have other evidence of poor compliance
        b. Have previously become pregnant while apparently using OCs
        c. Are taking long-term antibiotics, antiseizure medications, high-dose vitamin C (> 1 gm/day), or other medications known to interfere with effectiveness of OCs
        d. Are over 35 and smoke cigarettes
    3. Patient beliefs about OCs
        a. In one study, 80–95% of educated women were unaware of many health benefits of OCs; 49% believed substantial risks were involved.
        b. Physicians should emphasize health benefits of OCs and attempt to dispel common misconceptions
  B. **Use of OCs**
    1. **Before prescribing OCs**
        a. History and physical exam (with emphasis on weight, blood pressure, breast exam, and pelvic exam with Papanicolaou smear) to determine presence of absolute or relative contraindications to use of OCs
        b. Mammography as indicated for age and risk
        c. Laboratory tests
            i. Lipid profile in all women in whom individual risk is not known or who have a family history of hyperlipidemia or first-degree relative with history of myocardial infarction before age 50
              (a) Recheck yearly for women over 35 or otherwise at risk
          ii. Fasting blood sugar initially and yearly for all women over 35 or otherwise at risk for cardiovascular disease
         iii. Alternate approach
              (a) Kjos et al. found no significant adverse metabolic markers in women older than 35 who were long-term users of OCs
              (b) Results of study did not support routine lipid and diabetes screening before initiating or during use of low-dose OCs

2. **Choice of pill**
   a. Most patients should be started on < 50-µg pill
      i. Clinicians should be familiar with several lower-dose pills to find combination that seems well tolerated in most patients
      ii. Triphasic pills or OCs with newer progestins combine acceptably lower hormone content with minimal breakthrough bleeding
      iii. Women who have successfully used < 50-µg pill in past may be started on same pill
      iv. Women on 50-µg pills should be prescribed lower-dose pill unless there is specific reason for maintaining higher dose; many women who previously were switched to higher-dose pills because of intermenstrual spotting do equally well on triphasic pill or newer pill.
   b. Avoid generic pills, which may be marketed with only 75% bioavailability of hormone content
   c. Possible indications for 50-µg pill
      i. Women on medications known to decrease effectiveness of OCs
         (a) Other options for birth control should be carefully explored
         (b) If the decision is to use OCs despite competing drug, intermenstrual spotting may be an indication of decreased pill activity and mandates change to different form of birth control
         (c) Decreasing pill-free interval is more likely to maintain ovarian suppression and enhance efficacy of pill in such women

3. **Instructions for starting pill**
   a. Schedule options for starting OCs
      i. Immediately after abortion at 12 or fewer weeks gestation
      ii. 1 week after abortion or miscarriage at 13–28 weeks gestation
      iii. On first day of menstrual period
      iv. On first Sunday after menstrual period begins
         (a) Some brands of OCs have schedule preset to this regimen
         (b) Menstrual flow usually subsides for the weekend before beginning the next pill pack (whether this is advantageous depends on woman's lifestyle)
      v. Immediately (early pregnancy must be ruled out)
      vi. Postpartum period—begin OCs 2 weeks after delivery to avoid problems with hypercoagulability
      vii. Although back-up method is not essential for woman choosing first three schedules, it is safest approach for women beginning OCs; back-up should be continued for at least 7 days.
   b. Pill should be taken at same time every day; suggest associating pill ingestion with another activity usually carried out at about same time each day, such as brushing teeth or taking out contact lenses.
   c. Only 3-month supply of OCs should be given initially, with follow-up visit scheduled before last pack is finished
      i. Interval history at follow-up visit should include questions about possible side effects of the OCs, pattern of vaginal bleeding, and success in taking pill reliably
      ii. Blood pressure should be taken and weight checked
      iii. Lipid profile should be repeated in women in whom initial level was borderline or elevated

4. **Counseling issues**
   a. Encourage all patients not to smoke; women taking OCs have another important reason not to smoke.
   b. Encourage women at risk for STDs to use condoms in addition to OCs
   c. Determine with patient what her back-up method of birth control will be; this method should be readily available.
   d. Patient should keep an additional pill pack with her at all times if she leaves her primary pack at home
   e. Problems during first 3 cycles of OCs

      i. Intermenstrual spotting is not uncommon
        (a) In general, pill should be continued
        (b) Switching pills in first few months usually ends in frustration for patient and doctor and mistaken assumption that there are multiple pill types which patient cannot take successfully
        (c) Pills must be continued in order arranged in pack, regardless of point in cycle when spotting occurs
  f. Nausea and/or vomiting after taking pill
      i. Pill should be taken at night
      ii. Pill may be taken with food
      iii. Symptoms frequently resolve
      iv. Back-up method should be used
      v. Consider diagnosis of pregnancy
  g. Missed pills
      i. 1 missed pill
        (a) Should be taken as soon as remembered
        (b) Back-up form of birth control is not essential, but may be used for 7 days for added protection
      ii. 2 missed pills
        (a) Both missed pills should be taken as soon as remembered
        (b) Back-up method should be used for 7 additional days
      iii. 3 missed pills
        (a) Discard current pill pack and begin new pack as though it were initial start
        (b) Use back-up method for 7 days
  h. Gastroenteritis—use back-up method for remainder of cycle
  i. Missed period
      i. If no pills were missed
        (a) Physician should be contacted
        (b) Follow-up depends on whether the patient has experienced previous episodes of absent menses and degree of concern about pregnancy
        (c) Next pill pack should be started at usual time
      ii. If 1 or more pills were missed
        (a) Physician should be contacted
        (b) Pregnancy testing and other appropriate follow-up
  j. Perceived problems
      i. Unless patient believes that problem is serious and pill-related, she should call for advice before stopping pill
        (a) Many patients become pregnant when stopping pill temporarily because of possible side effects
        (b) Potentially serious symptoms include severe headaches, chest pain, eye or speech problems (any neurologic symptoms), and severe calf or thigh pain

C. **Changing pills**
  1. Pill changes should be made on the basis of the cause of presumed side effects
  2. Symptoms of estrogen excess
    a. Choose pill with lower estrogen
    b. Pill with relatively high dose of progestin may counteract symptoms
  3. Symptoms of estrogen deficiency are uncommon
    a. Patients with nervousness and presumed vasomotor symptoms may have another cause for such symptoms
    b. Atrophic vaginitis is rare in patients on OCs
    c. Spotting in first half of cycle may be corrected with another pill, which simply has different progestin or different (usually higher) estrogen/progestin ratio
    d. Triphasil/Tri-Levlen OCs have 40 µg of EE in midcycle and may be used to correct midcycle spotting
    e. Absence of withdrawal bleeding does not need to be corrected if patient is determined not to be pregnant and is not overly anxious about absence of menses

D. **Special considerations**
   1. Intermenstrual spotting in patient who has been free of spotting on OCs may have a chlamydial or other vaginal infection
   2. Scheduled surgery
      a. Patient on low-dose pills may continue to take them
      b. If patient is NPO after surgery, arrangements for restarting pill depend on number of pills missed
   3. Increased blood pressure
      a. If blood pressure increases after starting OCs, pill should be discontinued
      b. Blood pressure will return to normal within few months if elevation was truly pill-induced
      c. Patients whose blood pressure increased on combined OCs may still be candidates for progestin-only contraception, in which amount of progestin absorbed daily is much lower than for combined OCs
   4. Women over 50
      a. Risk of cardiovascular disease is increased
      b. Consider changing from OCs to hormone replacement therapy
      c. Determine whether patient is menopausal
         i. If FSH level is > 30 pg/ml during pill-free week, patient is probably menopausal
         ii. If FSH level is not elevated to menopausal levels, patient should use another form of birth control in addition to hormone replacement drugs
   5. Short course of antibiotic therapy—using a back-up method is encouraged
   6. Manipulating menstrual cycle
      a. Patient may discontinue pill packet before last contraceptive pill to manipulate time of menses
      b. Manipulating time of menses by increasing number of pills in cycle is more difficult
         i. Spotting is more likely with added pills
         ii. Monophasic pills are more easily manipulated in this manner
   7. Desire for pregnancy
      a. Stop the pill
      b. Barrier method of birth control may be used for next few months until regular cycling is established; this aids in dating resulting pregnancy.
      c. Conception at any time after stopping OCs is not associated with adverse effects
   8. Galactorrhea
      a. May result from suppression of prolactin-inhibiting factor by OCs
      b. May be most noticeable in pill-free week
      c. Work-up should include careful exam, mammograms if indicated, test of discharge for occult blood and prolactin level
         i. If work-up is negative and prolactin level is normal, patient may continue OCs if desired; if OCs are discontinued, galactorrhea should resolve by 3–6 months.
         ii. If work-up is negative but prolactin level is elevated, patient should discontinue OCs
            (a) Prolactin level should return to normal within 3 months if elevation was secondary to OCs
            (b) OCs may be restarted if level normalizes
            (c) Further work-up is indicated if level remains elevated
   9. Symptoms during the pill-free week (dysmenorrhea, menorrhagia, menstrual migraines)
      a. At least one study supports using active pills only for up to 12 weeks, thus delaying these symptoms
      b. Mircette, a newer OC which has 21 days of active pills followed by 2 days of placebo and 5 days of estrogen-only pills, may also be used to decrease these symptoms

SUGGESTED READING

1. Connell EB: Rational use of oral contraceptives in the perimenopausal woman. J Reprod Med 38:1036–1040, 1993.
2. DeCherney AH, Speroff L [chairmen of symposia]: Next generation of contraception: Oral contraceptives in the 1990s. Am J Obstet Gynecol 167:1159–1202, 1992.
3. Erwin PC: To use or not to use combined hormonal oral contraceptives during lactation. Fam Plann Perspect 26:26–33, 1994.
4. Hatcher RA, Trussell J, Stewart F, et al (eds): Contraceptive Technology, 17th ed. New York, Adrian Media, Inc., 1998.
5. Jick SS, Walker AM, Jick H: Oral contraceptives and endometrial cancer. Obstet Gynecol 82:931–935, 1993.
6. Kjos SL, Gregory K, Henry OA, Collins C: Evaluation of routine diabetes and lipid screening after age 35 in candidates for or current users of oral contraceptives. Obstet Gynecol 82:925–930, 1993.
7. Kubba A, Guillebaud J: Combined oral contraceptives: Acceptability and effective use. Br Med Bull 49:140–157, 1993.
8. Martinelli I, Sacchi E, Landi G, et al: High risk of cerebral vein thrombosis in carriers of a prothrombin gene mutation and in users of oral contraceptives. N Engl J Med 338:1793–1797, 1998.
9. Rosenberg L, Palmer JR, Zauber AG, et al: A case-control of oral contraceptive use and invasive epithelial ovarian cancer. Am J Epidemiol 139:654–661, 1994.
10. Speroff L: Mircette: A novel oral contraceptive. Am J Obstet Gynecol 179:S1–S2, 1998
11. Speroff L, DeCherney A: Evaluation of a new generation of oral contraceptives. Obstet Gynecol 81:1034–1047, 1993.
12. Stenchever MA: Risks of oral contraceptives use in women over 35. J Reprod Med 38(Suppl): 1030–1035, 1993.
13. Sulak PJ, Cressman BE: Extending the duration of active oral contraceptive pills to manage hormone withdrawal symptoms. Obstet Gynecol 89:179–183, 1997.
14. WHO Collaborative Study of Cardiovascular Disease and Steroid Hormone Contraception: Effect of different progestagens in low oestrogen oral contraceptives on venous thromboembolic disease. Lancet 346:1582–1588, 1995.

38. Tubal Ligation

Gary R. Newkirk, M.D.

I. **The Issues**
Voluntary sterilization remains the most widely used contraceptive method in the United States. Nearly 20% of married women have undergone tubal ligation. Minilaparotomy and laparoscopy are abdominal approaches considered to be safe, quick, and readily available. In particular, the minilaparotomy tubal ligation uses readily available surgical equipment, is technically less demanding, and can be applied to both interval and postpartum circumstances. Thus it is the method of choice for many family physicians. Family physicians who are skilled with basic surgical techniques are in an ideal position to discuss and perform permanent sterilization procedures for both men and women.

II. **The Theory**
  A. **Mechanism of action**
    1. Permanent disruption of both fallopian tubes to prevent ovum fertilization by sperm
  B. **Efficacy**
    1. Less then 1 pregnancy per 100 women per year
    2. Slightly higher failure rates if performed immediately after delivery or abortion
  C. **Description of techniques** (see Table 1 for advantages and disadvantages)
    1. Techniques
      a. Minilaparotomy
        i. Involves small abdominal incision, usually < 5 cm (2 in)
        ii. Segment of the tube is removed

TABLE 1. Minilaparotomy vs. Laparoscopy: Advantages and Disadvantages

Advantages	Disadvantages
Minilaparotomy	
Easy to learn	Takes longer than laparoscopy
Requires only basic surgical training and skill	Difficult in obese women and women with pelvic
Instruments are inexpensive	scarring or adhesions
Most complications are minor	Scar slightly larger
Useful as postpartum or interval method	More abdominal incision pain
	High rate of wound infections
Laparoscopy	
Very low complication rate	Complications may be serious
Quick, 10–15-minute procedure	Requires abdominal insufflation with added risk
Very small incision	More difficult to learn; specialized training for
Laparoscope can be used for other diagnostic	physician and staff
and therapeutic purposes	Expensive equipment requiring maintenance and repair
Less painful	Not recommended in immediate postpartum period

From Leskin L, Rinehart W: Female Sterilization. Population Reports 13(9), Series C, May 1985, with permission.

  b. Laparoscopy
    i. Involves inserting into abdomen telescope-like instrument through which fallopian tubes can be identified and clips, rings, or electrocautery can be applied
    ii. Tubal reversal success rates are highest with either clips or rings and lowest with electrocautery or methods removing tubal segments
 2. Timing
  a. Interval tubal ligation
    i. Tubal ligation performed at times other than immediate postpartum period
  b. Postpartum tubal ligation
    i. Tubal ligation within 72 hours of delivery
D. **Indications**
 1. Desire for permanent sterilization
 2. Medical conditions for which pregnancy places mother at significant risk for irreversible morbidity or death
 3. Known, severe inheritable genetic disease in which childbearing is not desired
E. **Contraindications**
 1. Absolute
  a. Active peritoneal infections
  b. Severe chronic heart, lung, or metabolic disease
    i. Abdominal insufflation (laparoscopy) and head-down (Trendelenburg) position may cause acute cardiopulmonary decompensation
  c. Any unstable medical condition
  d. Inability to tolerate adequate anesthesia
  e. Lack of informed consent
 2. Relative
  a. Prior significant pelvic or abdominal infection
    i. May make minilaparotomy and/or laparoscopy more difficult
    ii. Laparotomy may be necessary
  b. Severe obesity, especially with history of pelvic or abdominal infection
  c. Inability to provide sterile operative setting or manage anesthesia and complications of anesthesia
  d. Surgical risk
    i. Increased with heart disease, irregular pulse, hypertension, pelvic masses, uncontrolled diabetes, bleeding disorders, severe nutritional deficiencies, severe anemia, and umbilical or hiatal hernia
    ii. Risks of future pregnancies must be balanced with risks of permanent sterilization procedures
  e. Patient unsure of desire for permanent sterilization

F. **Risks of procedure**
1. Death rates
    a. Female sterilization results in very few deaths
    b. Most are related to anesthetic overdose or drug reaction, infection, or hemorrhage
    c. Mortality rates after sterilization are far lower than with childbirth
2. Major complications
    a. Occur in < 2% of all procedures
    b. 0.3% require 3 or more nights in hospital
    c. Laparotomy needed in 0.02–1.2% (in large studies) to resolve complications
    d. Delayed complications requiring readmission to hospital occur in < 1% of procedures
    e. Minilaparotomy and laparoscopy have similar rates of major complications
    f. Major complications of laparoscopy include unique problems related to insertion of instrument and gas insufflation of abdomen
        i. Gas embolism, subcutaneous emphysema, cardiac arrest, vessel or organ laceration
        ii. Open laparoscopy may make some of these complications less likely
3. Minor complications
    a. Minilaparotomy compared with laparoscopy
        i. Appears to have higher rate of minor complications (12% vs. 7%)
        ii. Longer average operating time
        iii. Convalescence slightly longer
        iv. Associated with more pain
    b. Other minor complications of minilaparotomy
        i. Wound infections
        ii. Slight blood loss
        iii. Uterine perforation by uterine manipulation instruments
        iv. Bladder injury
        v. Most are immediately recognized and managed intraoperatively
    c. Laparoscopy
        i. Very high rates of complications have been reported with laparoscopy in inexperienced hands
        ii. Chest and shoulder pain are common after laparoscopy secondary to trapped gas after insufflation of abdomen
    d. Postprocedural pain
        i. Most pain can be managed with oral agents
        ii. Narcotics are rarely necessary after third postoperative day
4. Long-term complications
    a. No compelling evidence that female sterilization causes long-term complications
    b. Menstrual cycles do not change as result of sterilization, but preoperative abnormalities are likely to persist
    c. Sterilized women do not appear to have different rates of pelvic inflammatory disease, cervicitis, hysterectomy, dilation and curettage
    d. Sterilized women are no more likely to experience severe psychiatric problems than unsterilized women
G. **Risks for regret**
1. 1–2% of all women with tubal ligation seek reversal of sterilization ("tubal regret")
2. 90% of women give remarriage as reason for desiring reversal
3. Only 30–70% of these women are candidates for reversal surgery
4. Risk factors for regret
    a. Marital disharmony at time of sterilization
    b. Age under 30 at time of sterilization
    c. Religious, socioeconomic, and educational background do not correlate well with regret, nor do parity and number of live children
    d. Regret may be slightly more prevalent after postpartum sterilization procedures
    e. Regret is more likely when tubal ligation chosen on basis of financial difficulties, health, or emotional problems

        f. Women with identified risks should not necessarily be denied surgery, but prudent physicians will counsel them that they fall into high-risk category

  H. **Tubal reversal**
1. Pregnancy occurs in about 50% of women undergoing surgery for reversal
2. Most "reversible" techniques
   a. Techniques that do not use electrocautery
   b. Techniques in which smallest segment of tube was removed from within isthmic portion of tube
   c. Techniques in which < 3 cm of tube was damaged or removed

  I. **Cost**
1. Varies with method
2. Includes both physician and hospital charges
3. Regional variation in fees common
4. Postpartum procedure using same spinal (e.g., epidural anesthesia during labor)
   a. Physician fee: $800–$1200
   b. Hospital fee: $1400–$2400
5. Interval tubal ligation, minilaparotomy
   a. Physician fee: $800–$1200
   b. Hospital day surgery: $2000
6. Laparoscopy interval tubal ligation
   a. Same as 5 above
7. At time of cesarean section
   a. Physician fee: $0–300
   b. Hospital fee: $1400

III. **An Approach**
  A. **Patient selection and issues for counseling**
1. Contraception among married women in U.S. aged 35–44 years
   a. Nearly 40% rely on permanent sterilization for birth control
   b. Oral contraceptives account for 14%
   c. Vasectomy accounts for 10%
2. Federally funded sterilization programs require
   a. Patient age of 21 years or older
   b. Mental competence
   c. Mandatory wait of 30 days after signing consent (or 72 hours in event of preterm delivery)
   d. Use of government-published patient education booklet with consent form
3. Methods for performing female sterilization include laparotomy, minilaparotomy, laparoscopy, vaginal approaches, and transcervical methods (Table 2)
   a. Minilaparotomy and laparoscopy
      i. Abdominal approaches
      ii. Easiest to learn
      iii. Currently recommended methods in U.S.
      iv. Highly effective
         (a) Pregnancy rates after 1 year are usually < 1 per 100 women
         (b) Common reasons for failure relate to pregnancy already existing at time of operation, surgical error in identifying fallopian tube, spontaneous reanastomosis of severed tube, or fistula formation allowing sperm and/or egg passage
   b. Minilaparotomy is safest sterilization method in postpartum period
      i. Complication approaches that of interval sterilization
   c. Laparoscopy is not as safe during immediate postpartum period as at other times
   d. Postpartum and postabortion sterilizations appear to be somewhat less effective than interval sterilization
   e. Postpartum sterilization accounts for 50% of all female sterilizations
4. Major factors related to development of complications include operator's experience with tubal sterilization, patient obesity, prior pelvic or abdominal surgery or other medical problems, diabetes mellitus, heart disease, asthma, bronchitis, or emphysema

TABLE 2. Common Tubal Ligation Methods

Open procedures: Minilaparotomy ligation techniques	
Pomeroy technique	The most common surgery performed for both interval and postpartum tubal ligations. Absorbable catgut sutures are used to tie the base of a loop of midportion (ampullary) tube. The ligated loop of tube is then removed. As the suture absorbs, the ends pull apart and are obstructed by the healing/scarring process. From 3–6 cm of tube is destroyed.
Parkland technique	A small length of tube is separated from the mesosalpinx, ligated at each end about 2 cm apart, and the free segment between the ligatures is removed.
Irving technique	A very effective yet more difficult method that cannot easily be reversed. The tube is cut and the uterine end buried beneath the peritoneum within the wall of the uterus. The remaining end is buried within the mesosalpinx.
Uchida technique	A technically demanding yet very effective method becoming more popular in the U.S. The tube is severed and the uterine end buried within the mesosalpinx.
Fimbriectomy	Accomplished by complete removal of the fimbriated end of the tube. The procedure appears to have a higher pregnancy rate, and reversal is unlikely.
Laparoscopy	
Open vs. closed laparoscopy: occlusion	A small incision is made within or just below the umbilicus to allow passage of a special cannula around which the skin makes an airtight seal. The cannula allows insufflation of the abdomen and the passage of the laparo-scope and instruments to allow occlusion of the tubes. This procedure is considered safer than traditional closed laparoscopy, especially in women with prior pelvic or abdominal surgery or infection. With the closed laparoscopic procedure, the laparoscope is inserted blindly through the abdominal wall.
Clips	By means of laparoscopic guidance, clips are applied to occlude the tubal lumen. Hulka (spring-loaded) and Filshie (titanium/silicone rubber) are commonly used. Clips destroy < 1 cm of tissue, and reversals are considered much easier.
Electrocoagulation	A bipolar probe is passed through a small segment of tube to cauterize and obstruct the lumen.
Tubal ring	A small silastic ring is stretched and placed over a loop of fallopian tube and then released. The tube is blocked by compression. Usually a 2–3-cm segment of the tube is involved. Reversal is more successful than with electrocauterization and either Irving or Uchida techniques.

From Chi IC, Gates D, Thapa S: Performing tubal sterilizations during a woman's postpartum hospitalization: A review of the United States and international experience. Obstet Gynecol Surv 47:71–79, 1992, with permission.

    5. Thoroughly discuss alternatives:
       a. Lowest-dose oral contraceptives can be used until menopause in nonsmoking women without contraindications
       b. Progestin-only pills can be used until menopause in women with estrogen-related contraindications
       c. Copper IUD can be left in place for 10 years
       d. Injection contraception every three months
       e. Subdermal contraceptive implants can last up to 5 years
  B. **Preoperative visit**
    1. Requires at least limited visit, preferably within 10 days (some hospitals require < 5 days) of anticipated surgery
    2. Preoperative evaluation and counseling for female permanent sterilization warrant focused attention; counseling should not be hurried or "tacked on" to end of acute illness visit.
    3. Specific time should be scheduled to discuss contraceptive options, risks, technique, and follow-up demands of sterilization surgery
    4. Written materials are advisable
    5. Many insurance carriers require preauthorization

6. If federal funding is to be used, be mindful of mandatory 30-day wait and age requirements
7. In monogamous relationship, meet with partner to address his concerns; partner written consent is not mandatory, but explore reasons if he is not supportive.
8. Complete medical history should be reviewed
   a. Prior pelvic or abdominal surgery or infection
   b. Drug allergies/intolerances
   c. History of heart disease (shortness of breath on exertion), diabetes, bleeding disorder, endometriosis, dysfunctional uterine bleeding
   d. Papanicolaou smear history
   e. Prior anesthesia complications
   f. Review need for other surgery at time of tubal ligation (e.g., dilatation and curettage, breast biopsy, studies to evaluate urinary incontinence, treatment of cervical disease)
9. Discuss anticipated anesthesia
10. Other topics for review
    a. Anticipated postoperative morbidities (pain, limited lifting)
    b. Risk factors for regret
    c. Review current contraceptive methods—is pregnancy a possibility at time of surgery?
    d. Can smoking patients quit at least several days before surgery?

C. **Preoperative examination**
   1. Focus on heart, lungs, breast, and abdomen
   2. During pelvic examination assess presence of vulvar, vaginal, or cervical pathology; perform cultures (gonorrhea, chlamydia) as necessary.
   3. Assess degree of uterine prolapse, urinary incontinence; have patient bear down and cough.
   4. Perform bimanual examination to assess uterine size, shape, and tenderness and mobility—can uterus be easily brought out of pelvis, or is it frozen in particular direction?
   5. Palpate ovaries for enlargement; pay particular attention to uterine mobility.
   6. Estimate degree of abdominal wall obesity
   7. Illustrate to patient location and size of anticipated abdominal incision and ultimate scarring

D. **Laboratory tests**
   1. Typically, hospitals require hemoglobin and urinalysis as minimal tests for general anesthesia
   2. Perform pregnancy testing if there is any question about this possibility
   3. In patients with clinical evidence of cervicitis or pelvic inflammation, culture and treat accordingly
      a. Schedule surgery when treatment and clinical response have been adequate

E. **Preanesthesia counseling**
   1. Many hospital day surgery or outpatient surgery services offer preanesthesia counseling
   2. Patient can meet with intake nurse and/or anesthetist to discuss issues, such as anesthesia, risks, time to present to hospital, requirements for no oral ingestion
   3. Should be used whenever available; in many hospitals, a requirement.

F. **Special considerations**
   1. Call hospital surgery personnel with special requests for anticipated surgery
   2. Apprise of special instrumentation

G. **Checklist for tubal ligation**
   1. Patient counseling should include alternative methods, risks of surgery, failure rates, regret assessment
   2. Operative and sterilization permits must be signed and witnessed (30-day waiting period for federally funded procedures)
   3. Preoperative physical examination within 5–10 days of procedure; contraindications to anesthesia and surgery clarified.
   4. Preoperative hemoglobin (or hematocrit), urinalysis, pregnancy test performed; results reviewed before surgery.

5. Patient ingests nothing by mouth 8 hours before surgery
6. Preanesthesia counseling by anesthesia personnel; general anesthesia should be available.
7. Newborn examined and found to be healthy for postpartum sterilization

H. **Follow-up visit**
1. Patient should be seen in office at any time complication occurs or at least within 7–14 days
2. Tubal pathology report should be reviewed suggested reading
3. Final healed scar make take up to one year to blend and reach baseline status
4. Education that pregnancy, including ectopic pregnancy can occur until menopause after tubal ligation.

SUGGESTED READING

1. Association of Voluntary Surgical Contraception: http://www.AVSC/org/ (Excellent patient information.)
2. Carignan CS: Tubal sterilization: Implications of the CREST Study. The Female Patient 22:45–51, 1997.
3. Chi IC, Gates D, Thapa S: Performing tubal sterilizations during a woman's postpartum hospitalization: A review of the United States and international experiences. Obstet Gynecol Surv 47:71–79, 1992.
4. Chi IC, Potts M, Wilkens L: Rare events associated with tubal sterilizations: An international experience. Obstet Gynecol Surv 41:7–19, 1986.
5. Hatcher RA, Trussell J, Stewart F, et al (eds): Contraceptive Technology, 17th ed. New York, Ardent Media, Inc., 1998.
6. McGonigle KF, Huggins GR: Tubal sterilization: Epidemiology of regret. OB/GYN Oct:15–24, 1990.
7. Pati S, Carignan C, Pollack AE: What's new with female sterilization: An update. Contemp OB/GYN June:91–117, 1998.
8. Peterson HB, Xia Z, Hughes JM, et al: The risk of pregnancy after tubal sterilization: Findings from the U.S. Collaborative Review of Sterilization. Am J Obstet Gynecol 174:1161–1170, 1996.
9. Sterilization. ACOG Technical Bulletin, Number 222, April 1996.

39. Emergency Contraception

Gary R. Newkirk, M.D.

I. **The Issues**
Nearly one-half of all pregnancies in the U.S. in 1995 (over 3.5 million) were unintended. As many as three-fourths of first coitus experiences occur without contraception. Conception rates may be as high as 30% if two episodes of unprotected intercourse occur within 2 days. Nearly one-half of women with unintended pregnancies said that they would have considered emergency contraception if they had known it was available. Currently, over one-half of all elective terminations of pregnancy could be prevented if emergency contraception were available on a widespread basis. In the U.S. elective termination has become the most common surgical procedure. With effective emergency contraception, abortions could be reduced by as much as 800,000 procedures per year. The Food and Drug Administration (FDA) has issued a statement supporting the use of certain oral contraceptives in specific doses for emergency contraception. Emergency contraception is a component of contraception that demands physician and public education and media publicity. Preven™ (Gynetics) is now approved by the FDA as an emergency contraceptive kit.

II. **The Theory**
A. **Definitions:** emergency contraception, intraception, postcoital contraception, and "morning after" are equivalent terms referring to prevention of pregnancy after unprotected intercourse
1. Both the National Institutes of Health and the American College of Obstetricians and Gynecologists define pregnancy as beginning with implantation. According to this definition, the prevention of pregnancy before implantation is contraception and not abortion.

B. **Proposed interventions**
 1. Initial research demonstrated effectiveness of high doses of estrogen in preventing ovum implantation
  a. High rate of gastrointestinal side effects, primarily nausea and vomiting
 2. Subsequent hormonal regimens used combination oral contraceptives, initially Ovral[TM]
  a. Lower hormone doses (Ovral = ethinyl estradiol, 50 μg, and norgestrel, 0.5 mg)
  b. Fewer side effects
  c. Protocols now expanded to use essentially all major brands of combined oral contraceptives
  d. Protocols developed for progestin-only pills as well (Table 1)
 3. Insertion of copper intrauterine device (IUD) noted to be highly effective when inserted up to 7 days after intercourse
C. **Exact mechanism of action unknown**
 1. Oral contraceptives
  a. Depend on day of cycle and how soon after exposure therapy is started
  b. Probably interfere with implantation, cervical mucus changes, tubal motility changes, interfere with corpus luteum development
 2. IUD
  a. Thought to prevent implantation
  b. Possible effect of copper on tubal function
D. **Effectiveness**
 1. Combined oral contraceptives
  a. Depend on how soon therapy is started after coitus: the sooner, the better
  b. 3% failure rate per event of unprotected intercourse
  c. Must be started within 72 hours of exposure; protocols for longer periods under investigation.
 2. Copper IUD
  a. 0.1% failure rate
  b. May be inserted up to 5–7 days after coitus
E. **Cost**
 1. One pack of oral contraceptives, which provides sufficient medication for 5 episodes of emergency contraception, costs $20–30
 2. IUD costs approximately $175–300
 3. Provider visit, initial pregnancy test
  a. Estimated costs: $30–60 for visit
  b. $10–25 for pregnancy test

TABLE 1. Yuzpe Method Equivalent Doses[1]

Brand Name	Formulation	No. of Pills With Each Dose[4]
Ovral[TM]	0.05 mg ethinyl estradiol	2
	0.50 mg norgestrel	
Lo-Ovral[TM]	0.03 mg ethinyl estradiol	4
	0.30 mg norgestrel	
Nordette[TM]	0.03 mg ethinyl estradiol	4
	0.15 mg levonorgestrel	
Triphasil[TM]	0.3 mg ethinyl estradiol	4
(yellow pills only)	0.4 mg levonorgestrel	
Progestin-only Protocol[2]		
Ovrette	0.075 mg norgestrel	20
Preven[TM] kit[3]	0.05 mg ethinyl estradiol	2
	0.25 mg levonorgestrel	
	(packaged with pregnancy test)	

[1]Virtually any combined OCP can be used (see references)
[2]Other options may be available
[3]Only FDA-approved postcoital prevention
[4]Dose repeated in 12 hours after first dose

F. **Indication:** desire to prevent pregnancy in multiple settings:1
   1. Intercourse without contraception
   2. Missed multiple birth control pills with intercourse
   3. Broken or leaky condom
   4. Ejaculation on external genitalia
   5. IUD expelled
   6. Sexual assault
G. **Contraindications**
   1. Currently pregnant
   2. Significant contraindications to estrogens or progestins
      a. IUD insertion can be considered
   3. Contraindications to IUD
H. **Precautions**
   1. Undiagnosed vaginal bleeding
   2. Impaired liver, kidney, or heart function
   3. Significant precaution related to routine use of oral contraceptives
   4. Women who cannot take estrogens can use progestin-only protocols
   5. For use of IUD
      a. Risk of sexually transmitted disease (STD), rape, nulligravida, no desire for long-term use of IUD
III. **An Approach**
   A. **Patient education**
      1. Offered at time of contraception counseling
      2. Counsel teens, male and female, at time of clinical encounters (e.g., sports exams)
      3. Discuss with receptionists and personnel in charge of phone triage for patients
   B. **Facilitate institution of therapy as soon as possible**
      1. Established patient
         a. Review chart for potential adverse effects
         b. Arrange for pregnancy test
         c. Office visit desirable, but may not be mandatory
      2. New patient
         a. Arrange for provider visit
         b. Review history
            i. Medical history, most recent menstrual period, previous cycle length, estimated ovulation time, number of hours since unprotected sex
      3. Discuss patient's feelings about continuing pregnancy if pregnancy is not prevented
         a. No evidence that pregnancy will be harmed, but no absolute guarantee that it will not
      4. Clarify patient's risks for oral contraceptives or IUD
      5. Check vital signs, perform pregnancy test
      6. Discuss follow-up in 2–3 weeks
      7. Discuss further contraceptive needs
      8. Pelvic exam, cultures with possibility of STD exposure
         a. Mandatory with rapes
   C. **Prescribe therapy**
      1. Ovral, 2 tablets immediately and in 12 hours or insert IUD
      2. For nausea or vomiting
         a. Dimenhydrinate (Dramamine), 50-mg tablet every 4–6 hours
         b. Promethazine hydrochloride (Phenergan), 25-mg tablet every 12 hours, or 25-mg rectal suppository every 12 hours
   D. Instructions to patients
      1. For Ovral use
         a. Take first dose as soon as possible
            i. With food reduces nausea
         b. If patient vomits within 1 hour, call office; may need to repeat first dose.
         c. Watch for warning signs of hormone complications
            i. Chest pain, shortness of breath, calf pain, severe headaches, weakness, numbness, blurred vision, loss of vision, jaundice, abdominal pain

2. Return to clinic in 2–3 weeks
   a. Pregnancy test
   b. Repeat cultures for rape victims
3. Discuss future contraception
4. Review STD risk, consider HIV screening

SUGGESTED READING

1. American College of Obstetricians and Gynecologists. Emergency Oral Contraception. Washington, DC, ACOG Practice Patterns, 1996.
2. Huges EC (ed): Committee on Terminology, The American College of Obstetricians and Gynecologists: Obstetric-Gynecologic Terminology. Philadelphia, FA Davis Company, 1972.
3. Internet resource: Emergency contraception. http://opr.princeton.edu/ec/ec.html. An excellent source for providers, continually updated and well-linked.
4. Glasier A: Emergency postcoital contraception. New Engl J Med 337:1058–1064,1997.
5. Speroff L, Darney P: A Clinical Guide for Contraception. Baltimore, Williams & Wilkins, 1992, pp 113–116.
6. Trussell J, Koenig J, Ellertson C, Stewart F: Preventing unintended pregnancy: The cost-effectiveness of three methods of emergency contraception. Am J Public Health 87:932–937, 1997.
7. Trussell J, Stewart F, Guest F, Hatcher R: Emergency contraceptive pills: A simple proposal to reduce unintended pregnancies. Fam Plann Perspect 24:269–273, 1992.
8. Yuzpe AA, Thurlow MA, Ramzy I, et al: Postcoital contraception: A pilot study. J Reprod Med 13:53, 1994.

PART V

GYNECOLOGIC INFECTIONS AND SEXUALLY TRANSMISSIBLE DISEASES

40. Syphilis

Cynda Ann Johnson, M.D., M.B.A.

I. **The Issues**
Twenty years ago a test for syphilis was still a part of routine admitting laboratory tests in many hospitals. Most positive results were from old, previously treated (with arsenic in some cases) disease or from false-positives. Routine syphilis testing dropped, but the communicable disease climate changed and the incidence of syphilis began to rise, peaking in 1990. Primary care physicians must consider syphilis testing in high-risk women and women with compatible symptoms. Unfortunately, in many generalist offices, syphilis testing is omitted. Perhaps because most specimens for other sexually transmitted diseases (STDs) are collected during the pelvic examination, remembering to order a blood test is more difficult. When considering an STD, think syphilis.

II. **The Theory**
  A. Causative organism
     1. Syphilis is caused by *Treponema pallidum*, a strict anaerobic spirochete
     2. Organism cannot be grown in laboratory *in vitro*
  B. **Transmission**
     1. Spirochete is transmitted during sexual contact through abraded areas in skin (often microabrasions) or mucosal surface
     2. Risk of infection to partners of people with syphilis is about 30%
     3. Women appear to be at higher risk for contracting syphilis than men engaged in same high-risk behaviors
     4. Individuals harboring spirochete are capable of transmitting disease for about 1 year
     5. Spirochete is also transmitted across placenta to produce chronic infection in fetus
        a. Clinical disease is not evident before 18 weeks of gestation (with case reports of disease in first trimester)
  C. **Incidence**
     1. Syphilis in the U.S. was almost epidemic during 1986–1990, but since then incidence has declined > 80%.
     2. More common in non-Hispanic blacks than any other racial/ethnic group and is concentrated in southern U.S.
     3. Current incidence is 3.2 cases per 100,000 population
  D. **Spectrum of clinical disease**
     1. **Primary syphilis**
        a. Chancre
           i. Painless, red, round, firm ulcer with granular base and well-formed raised edges
           ii. Develops at site of inoculation—commonly forchette, cervix, anus, labia, nipples
           iii. Usually appears at about 3 weeks but may develop any time between 10–90 days after exposure
           iv. Chancre heals spontaneously in 3–8 weeks
        b. Regional adenopathy is present during primary episode
     2. **Secondary syphilis**
        a. Disease disseminates after several weeks

201

      b. By 6 weeks after first manifestation of primary syphilis, evidence of secondary syphilis appears

      c. Systemic symptoms include low-grade fever, headache, sore throat, malaise

      d. Dermatologic manifestations

          i. Frequently pruritic

          ii. Diffuse and symmetric rash, often maculopapular

          iii. Characterized by location on palms and soles

          iv. Syphilis was called "the great imitator" because of variety of skin manifestations

      e. Genital manifestations

          i. Moist cutaneous external lesions called condyloma lata; must be differentiated from condyloma acuminata, which are characteristic lesions of human papillomavirus

          ii. Mucus patches resemble lesions of genital herpes

          iii. Genital lesions are highly infectious

      f. Other manifestations include generalized adenopathy, hepatitis, nephrosis, alopecia

      g. Untreated lesions resolve in 3–12 weeks

  3. Latent stages

      a. Early latent

          i. Less than 1 year from onset of disease

          ii. One-fourth of patients have clinical recurrence with manifestations similar to those of secondary syphilis

          iii. Patient is infectious during this stage

      b. Late latent

          i. More than 1 year from onset of disease

          ii. Patient is not infectious by sexual contact but may transmit spirochete transplacentally

          iii. Patient is at greater risk of tertiary syphilis or neurosyphilis at this stage

  4. Tertiary (late) syphilis

      a. One-third of untreated patients progress from late latent stage to tertiary syphilis

      b. Results in progressive damage to central nervous system, cardiovascular system, musculoskeletal system, and involvement of various organ systems with gummas

  5. Neurosyphilis

      a. Patients with neurologic disease are usually placed in separate category because central nervous system disease may actually occur at any stage of syphilis

  6. Congenital syphilis

      a. May result in stillbirth, neonatal death, or prematurity

      b. Early manifestations include maculopapular skin rash, lesions of the oropharynx (mucus patches), iritis, chorioretinitis, hepatosplenomegaly, lymphadenopathy

      c. If early congenital syphilis is left untreated, late congenital syphilis develops, characterized by Hutchinson's teeth, saddle nose, saber shins, mental retardation, eighth nerve deafness

III. **An Approach**

  A. **Diagnosis**

    1. **Whom to test**

      a. Any patient with clinical manifestations that may be part of any stage of syphilis

      b. Any patient with another STD or at high risk for contracting STD (U.S. Preventive Services Task Force recommendation)

      c. Users of crack cocaine

      d. Prison inmates

      e. Pregnant women

          i. All pregnant women at first prenatal visit, optimally in first trimester (U.S. Preventive Services Task Force recommendation)

          ii. Women at high risk for STDs should be retested in third trimester

          iii. Many states require repeat testing at time of delivery

    2. **How to test**

      a. **Dark-field examination**

          i. Demonstrates *T. pallidum* on fresh specimen from lesion of infected patient

      ii. Applicable only for primary and secondary syphilis

      iii. Collecting specimen

         (a) Clean lesion with normal saline, dry with cotton gauze, minimize bleeding

         (b) Apply pressure to lesion to express clear fluid, which is applied to microscope slide

         (c) Place coverslip over slide and seal edges with petroleum jelly

         (d) Specimen should be evaluated promptly but only limited number of facilities may have ability to carry out dark-field examinations

   b. **Serologic testing**

      i. Nonspecific tests for reagin-type antibodies

         (a) Venereal Disease Research Laboratory (VDRL) and rapid plasma reagin (RPR) tests

         (b) May be negative when chancre first appears but becomes positive in 100% of cases by 4–6 weeks

         (c) Continues to be positive during secondary and latent stages

         (d) Use for screening and to follow response to therapy

         (e) Titer of 1:16 or greater is usually associated with active syphilis; fourfold changes in titers are considered significant, but same serologic test must be performed

         (f) Cord blood tests positive in infected newborns and by passive transfer of maternal antibodies in uninfected infant

            (i) Since symptoms not usual at birth, follow titers monthly or treat for syphilis

         (g) False-positives in 1% of patients (usually transient) with viral infections, autoimmune disease, IV drug use, pregnancy

      ii. Specific antitreponemal antibody tests

         (a) Microhemagglutination assay for antibodies to *T. pallidum* (MHA–TP) and fluorescent treponemal antibody–absorption (FTA–ABS)

         (b) Use to confirm positive nonspecific test

         (c) Result reported as reactive or nonreactive

         (d) In general, test remains positive even after treatment though test may revert to negative within 2–3 years in up to 25% of patients who are treated early in course of disease

      iii. New rapid tests are being developed but have not replaced standard tests noted above

3. **Reinfection or persistence of active syphilis**

   a. Follow titer of nonspecific test (e.g., VDRL)

   b. Successful therapy

      i. Early syphilis—titer decreases and becomes negligible in 6–12 months

      ii. Late syphilis (> 1 year's duration)—titer becomes negligible in 12–18 months

      iii. Rising titer indicates need for further work-up for untreated neurosyphilis

4. **Diagnosis of neurosyphilis**

   a. Indications for spinal tap

      i. Consider for any patient who is asymptomatic but has positive serologic diagnosis of syphilis

      ii. Any patient with syphilis who has evidence of neurologic involvement

      iii. Any patient with late latent syphilis who:

         (a) Failed treatment

         (b) Will not be treated with penicillin

         (c) Has serum RPR or VDRL titer equal to or greater than 1:32

         (d) Has other evidence of late syphilis

         (e) Has positive test for human immunodeficiency virus (HIV)

      iv. No need for spinal tap in patients with early syphilis who do not have neurologic findings

      v. If spinal tap is not performed on high-risk individuals, they should be treated with protocols for patients with neurosyphilis

    b. Results of spinal tap in patients with neurosyphilis
- i. Pleocytosis, elevated protein concentrations, reactive VDRL (cannot perform RPR on spinal fluid); leukocyte count elevated to > 5 white blood cells (WBCs)/mm^3
- ii. Positive VDRL in CSF should be considered diagnostic of neurosyphilis (if specimen was not contaminated by blood), but it may be negative when neurosyphilis is present
- iii. Positive FTA–ABS is less specific but more sensitive test in CSF
- iv. Falling WBC count is sensitive measure of successful therapy

B. Treatment

1. Whom to treat
    a. All patients with syphilis documented by dark-field exam or treponemal antibody test
    b. Previously treated patients with 4-fold rise in quantitative nontreponemal test
    c. Patients in whom diagnosis cannot be ruled out

2. How to treat
    a. Penicillin
- i. Parenteral penicillin G is preferred treatment for all stages of syphilis
- ii. Specific preparation and length of treatment depend on stage of disease and manifestations
- iii. Parenteral penicillin G is only therapy with documented efficacy for syphilis during pregnancy
  - (a) Pregnant women with history of penicillin allergy should be skin-tested
  - (b) Carry out desensitization to penicillin if skin test positive

    b. Recommended regimens for patients with primary or secondary syphilis
- i. Benzathine penicillin G, 2.4 million U intramuscularly in single dose
- ii. Nonpregnant penicillin-allergic patients
  - (a) Doxycycline, 100 mg orally 2 times/day for 2 weeks
  - (b) Tetracycline, 500 mg orally 4 times/day for 2 weeks
- iii. Other regimens are less effective
- iv. Single-dose ceftriaxone is effective only for treating incubating syphilis
- v. Follow-up consists of clinical and serologic evaluation at 3 and 6 months
  - (a) Patients with fourfold increase in titer of nontreponemal test have either failed treatment or are reinfected
    - (i) Test for HIV infection
    - (ii) Perform spinal tap unless reinfection likely
    - (iii) Re-treat with regimen for late latent syphilis

    c. Recommended regimens for patient with latent syphilis
- i. Early latent syphilis—benzathine penicillin G, 2.4 million U intramuscularly in single dose
- ii. Late latent syphilis or latent syphilis of unknown duration—benzathine penicillin G, 2.4 million U/week intramuscularly for 3 weeks
- iii. Penicillin-allergic patients
  - (a) As in primary syphilis, but treat patient with late latent syphilis for 4 weeks
- iv. Follow-up consists of clinical and serologic evaluation at 6 and 12 months
  - (a) If fourfold increase in titer or failure of high titer (1:32 or more) to decrease fourfold, evaluate patient for neurosyphilis and retreat

    d. Recommended regimens for late (tertiary) syphilis
- i. Same as for late latent syphilis
- ii. Follow-up recommendations are not clear

    e. Recommended regimens for neurosyphilis
- i. Aqueous crystalline penicillin 12–24 million U daily, administered as 2–4 million U intravenously every 4 hours for 10–14 days
- ii. Alternative regimen for patients in whom compliance with therapy can be assured is procaine penicillin 2–4 million U intramuscularly daily, plus 500 mg probenecid 4 times daily, for 10–14 days

      iii. Follow-up

         (a) Repeat evaluation of CSF if pleocytosis was present initially every 6 months until cell count is normal

         (b) Cell count should decrease by 6 months and be normal by 2 years or patient should be retreated

   f. Special recommendations for treatment and follow-up apply to pregnant women and patients infected with HIV

   g. Jarisch-Herxheimer reaction

      i. Acute febrile reaction within 24 hours of treatment for syphilis; common among patients treated for early syphilis

      ii. Antipyretics may be used; no specific therapy

      iii. Patients should be warned of this reaction

   h. Consultation is recommended in difficult cases (pregnancy, neurosyphilis, HIV-infection), in patients with complicated disease or poor response to treatment, or whenever serologic results of serologic tests are confusing

C. Other management considerations

  1. **Evaluation and treatment of sex partners**

   a. At-risk partners

      i. Sexual contact with patient during following periods before treatment

         (a) Primary syphilis—3 months plus duration of symptoms

         (b) Secondary syphilis—6 months plus duration of symptoms

         (c) Early latent syphilis—1 year

      ii. Long-term partners of patients with late syphilis

   b. Persons sexually exposed to patient within 90 days of treatment for primary, secondary, or early latent syphilis should be treated even if results of serologic tests are negative

   c. Persons sexually exposed to patient > 90 days before treatment for primary, secondary, or early latent syphilis should be treated if serologic test results are not immediately available or if opportunity for follow-up is uncertain

  2. **HIV infection**

   a. All patients with syphilis should have test for HIV infection

   b. Serologic tests may be unreliable and unpredictable in some HIV-infected patients

   c. Consider diagnosis of syphilis in HIV-infected person with neurologic symptoms

SUGGESTED READING

1. Centers for Disease Control and Prevention: Primary and secondary syphilis—United States, 1997. MMWR 47:493–497, 1998.
2. Centers for Disease Control and Prevention: 1998 Guidelines for treatment of sexually transmitted diseases. MMWR 47(RR-1):28–40, 1998.
3. Finelli L, Budd J, Spitalny KC: Early syphilis: Relationship to sex, drugs, and changes in high-risk behavior from 1987–1990. Sex Transm Dis 20:89–95, 1993.
4. Goldmeier D, Hay P: A review and update on adult syphilis, with particular reference to its treatment. Int J STD AIDS 4:70–82, 1993.
5. U.S. Preventive Services Task Force: Guide to Clinical Preventive Services, 2nd ed. Alexandria, VA, International Medical Publishing, 1996, pp 287–292.
6. Young H, Moyes A: A new recombinant antigen latex agglutination test (Syphilis Fast) for the rapid serological diagnosis of syphilis. Int J STD AIDS 9:196–200, 1998.

41. Gonorrhea

Cynda Ann Johnson, M.D., M.B.A.

I. The Issues

Resistance is the continued battle in the control of gonorrhea. In 1980, nearly all gonorrhea organisms were sensitive to penicillin. An era of increasing resistance has followed—to penicillin and ampicillin, tetracycline, and spectinomycin. Recently strains of gonorrhea found in Asia have shown decreased susceptibility to ciprofloxacin. The bacteria remain sensitive to ceftriaxone, but this drug is expensive and requires an injection. The primary care provider's role in this battle is to control the disease on the front line—through patient education, screening of high-risk individuals, and prompt treatment of patients and contacts.

II. The Theory

A. **Causative organism**—*Neisseria gonorrhoeae*
   1. Gram-negative, intracellular diplococcus
   2. Fastidious organism, requiring 2–10% CO_2 environment
   3. Thrives in columnar or transitional but not squamous epithelium

B. **Transmission**
   1. Sexual transmission is most common
      a. Incubation period is 3–5 days
      b. Female has 80–90% chance of contracting gonorrhea after single sexual encounter with infected male, whereas male has only 25% chance of acquiring infection from single encounter with infected female
   2. May be acquired by neonate during birth process
   3. Conjunctiva may also be infected from amniotic fluid at delivery, via contaminated hands, or from accidental inoculation in laboratory

C. **Incidence and prevalence**
   1. Epidemic peaked in 1975 but number of cases began to increase again in 1985; now a 71% decrease to about 124 cases per 100,000 population
   2. Rates in blacks 35 times higher than whites: among women, ages 15–19 have highest rate (among men, ages 20–24 have highest rate); highest prevalence in southern U.S.
   3. Other risks include: low level of education; casual sexual contact; greater number of contacts per year; nonuse of condoms; prior history of gonorrhea or chlamydia

D. **Spectrum of clinical disease**
   1. Symptoms of gonorrhea depend of site of infection; mucopurulent discharge is common but the majority of women remain asymptomatic
   2. Endocervix is most common site of primary infection
   3. Other primary sites of infection
      a. Urethra (may have discharge, dysuria or urinary frequency), Bartholin's glands, and Skene's glands
      b. Oropharynx; symptoms include mild sore throat and erythema of pharynx with rare occurrence of oral ulcerative lesions and pharyngeal exudate
      c. Anorectal region; symptoms range from mild pruritus and mucoid discharge to severe proctitis
      d. Conjunctiva; purulent conjunctivitis with extensive inflammation rare in adults
   4. Syndromes of secondary infection
      a. Upper tract disease
         i. Up to 20% of infected women develop pelvic inflammatory disease (PID)
         ii. Delay of treatment from first symptom (usually lower abdominal pain) increases rate of infertility
         iii. Infection usually ascends during menstrual period, with symptoms thereafter
         iv. Contiguous spread via posterior peritoneal gutters may lead to perihepatitis
      b. Disseminated gonococcal infection
         i. Bacteremia with fever, chills, skin lesions

      (a) Embolic lesions appear as small vesicles that become pustules and develop hemorrhagic base; center becomes necrotic
         (i) Most common sites are volar aspects of upper extremities
         (ii) Lesions resolve spontaneously without scarring
      (b) Joint symptoms
      (c) May progress to meningitis or endocarditis
      (d) Half of patients have positive blood cultures
    ii. Septic arthritis at ankles, knees and wrists with purulent synovial effusion
      (a) Joint fluid tests positive for gonococcal organisms
      (b) Blood cultures often negative at this stage

III. An Approach

A. Whom to screen

1. Any women with characteristic symptoms
2. High-risk women at annual pelvic exam (U.S. Preventive Services Task Force recommendation)
   a. History of sexually transmitted disease (STD) or PID
   b. Partner with known STD or characteristic symptoms
   c. Multiple sexual partners (more than two in previous year)
   d. Commercial sex workers
   e. Any patient who fits criteria for chlamydia screening (see Chapter 44)
3. All pregnant women
   a. Rescreen very-high-risk women at second prenatal visit if first culture was negative and in third trimester

B. How to test

1. **Gram stain**
   a. Only in symptomatic cases
   b. Sensitivity is only 60% in women
   c. Sample from endocervix should be rolled in thin layer onto microscope slide
   d. Positive result is evidence of intrapolymorphonuclear, gram-negative diplococci
2. **Culture**
   a. Standard of care for testing women
   b. Collecting specimen
      i. Endocervix
      ii. Other sites of possible infection (review sexual practices with patient) including anus, oropharynx, urethra (in women who have had hysterectomy)
      iii. Insert dry, cotton-tipped swab into orifice, move it from side to side for 15–30 seconds
      iv. Plate immediately onto Thayer-Martin media with appropriate addition of CO_2, depending on system and transport mechanism
      v. Sensitivity is 90% for culture of single specimen with careful collection and processing techniques
      vi. Fermentation testing for speciation may be necessary on pharyngeal specimens (other species of *Neisseria* are normal mouth flora) or in low-risk patient with positive culture
      vii. Gram stains positive for gram-negative intracellular diplococci should be confirmed by culture
3. **Nonculture tests**
   a. Recently marketed DNA tests (e.g., GenProbe) allow cost-effective testing for both gonorrhea and chlamydia on single specimen with good sensitivity and specificity
   b. Rectal and pharyngeal gonorrhea can also be detected accurately with DNA tests
   c. Tests using urine sample or vaginal swab will allow testing without use of speculum.

C. Therapy

1. **Recommended regimens for uncomplicated gonococcal infections** (cervix, urethra, rectal)
   a. First-choice agents

       i. Ceftriaxone, 125 mg intramuscularly in single dose
      ii. Cefixime, 400 mg orally in single dose
    iii. Ciprofloxacin, 500 mg orally in single dose
    iv. Ofloxacin, 400 mg orally in single dose
     v. Azithromycin 2 g orally in single dose (CDC cautions that this is expensive and associated with GI upset but has advantage of efficacy against both gonorrhea and chlamydia)

  b. Regimen effective against chlamydia should be added
  c. Cure > 95% of cases of anal and genital infection
  d. If pharyngeal infection is likely, ceftriaxone, ciprofloxacin or ofloxacin should be used (> 90% of cases are cured)
  e. Pregnant patients should be treated with cephalosporin; those who cannot tolerate cephalosporin should be treated with spectinomycin, 2 g intramuscularly in single dose
  f. Infants born to infected mothers should be treated with single dose of ceftriaxone
  g. Patients with gonorrhea should be tested for syphilis—regimens that include ceftriaxone, doxycycline, or erythromycin cure incubating syphilis
  h. Alternative regimens
      i. Spectinomycin, other injectable or oral cephalosporins, other quinolones
     ii. If any of these is used (usually because of availability or treatment of another condition), specifics of prescribing and sites of infection susceptible to agent should be reviewed

2. **Recommended regimens for disseminated gonococcal infection**
  a. Hospitalization
  b. Ceftriaxone, 1 g intramuscularly or intravenously every 24 hours
  c. Patients allergic to beta-lactam drugs—spectinomycin, 2 g intramuscularly every 12 hours
  d. Continue parenteral treatment until 24–48 hours after improvement; complete therapy with oral antibiotic for total duration of at least 7 days
      i. Cefixime 400 mg orally 2 times/day
     ii. Ciprofloxacin, 500 mg orally 2 times/day
    iii. Ofloxacin 400 mg orally 2 times/day

3. **Recommended regimens for gonococcal meningitis and endocarditis**
  a. Hospitalization
  b. Ceftriaxone, 1–2 g intravenously every 12 hours
  c. Continue therapy for 10–14 days in patients with meningitis
  d. Continue therapy for at least 4 weeks in patients with endocarditis

4. **Recommended regimens for adults with gonococcal conjunctivitis**
  a. Ceftriaxone, 1 g intramuscularly in single dose
  b. Lavage eye with saline solution 1 time

5. **Treatment of sexual partners**
  a. Include partners of patients with disease at any site
  b. Evaluate and treat for gonorrhea and chlamydia
  c. Partners of symptomatic patients—if last sexual contact was within 30 days of onset of symptoms
  d. Partners of asymptomatic patients—if last sexual contact was within 60 days of diagnosis
  e. Most recent sexual contact should be evaluated and treated regardless of time of exposure
  f. Patient should avoid sex until she and her partners have completed therapy and are free of symptoms

D. **Follow-up testing**
  1. Test of cure is recommended in following situations
    a. Pregnancy
    b. Patient or partner not symptom-free
      i. Repeat culture for gonorrhea with antibiotic sensitivity testing
  2. Report positive tests according to state regulations

SUGGESTED READING

1. Blake DR, Duggan A: Evaluation of vaginal infections in adolescent women: Can it be done without a speculum? Pediatrics 103:939–944, 1998.
2. Centers for Disease Control and Prevention: 1998 Guidelines for treatment of sexually transmitted diseases. MMWR 47(RR-1):59–70, 1998.
3. Jephcott AE: Microbiological diagnosis of gonorrhoea. Genitourin Med 73:245–252, 1997.
4. Lind I: Antimicrobial resistance in *Neisseria gonorrhoeae*. Clin Infect Dis 24:S93–S97, 1997.
5. Mertz KJ, Levine WC: Screening women for gonorrhea: Demographic screening criteria for general clinical use. Am J Public Health 87:1535–1538, 1997.
6. Phillips RS, Hanff PA, Wertheimer A, Aronson MD: Gonorrhea in women seen for routine gynecologic care: Criteria for testing. Am J Med 85:177–182, 1988.
7. U.S. Preventive Services Task Force: Guide to Clinical Preventive Services, 2nd ed. Alexandria, VA, International Medical Publishing, 1996, pp 293–302.
8. Washington AE, Browner WS, Korenbrot CC: Cost-effectiveness of combined treatment for endocervical gonorrhea: Considering coinfection with Chlamydia trachomatis. JAMA 257:2056–2060, 1987.
9. Young H, Anderson J: Non-cultural detection of rectal and pharyngeal gonorrhoea by the GenProbe PACE 2 assay. Genitourin Med 73:59–62, 1997.

42. Genital Herpes

Cynda Ann Johnson, M.D., M.B.A.

I. The Issues

A woman presented to the office with florid primary genital herpes, proved by culture. Individually presenting themselves as monogamous, husband and wife were angry at each other and defied their primary care physician to explain how she had acquired the infection. Exhaustive questioning and review of the facts finally revealed that the husband had a painful, vesicular lesion on the tip of his nose shortly before his wife broke out with herpetic lesions. The couple had engaged in oral-genital sex while the lesion was present. Both parties were contrite and forgiving and thanked the physician profusely for saving their marriage.

II. The Theory

A. **Causative organism:** herpes simplex virus (HSV)
   1. Contains inner core of double-stranded DNA surrounded by glycoprotein envelope
      a. HSV-2 is cause of most genital herpes infections
      b. HSV-1, commonly found on mouth, causes 15% of genital herpes infections
   2. Latency
      a. After virus invades host, it is able to enter sensory nerve terminals, move up to sensory sacral ganglia that supply skin and mucosa of affected site, and remain in latent state without apparent cell damage
      b. Various triggers, known and unknown in each individual, cause virus to be reactivated to replicate viral components

B. **Transmission**
   1. By close physical contact, usually sexual
      a. Incubation period is 1–45 days (average: 5.8)
      b. Chance of women developing genital herpes if exposed to infected man is 80–90%
      c. Condoms used at every episode of intercourse are relatively effective in controlling spread
      d. Persons with active lesions should abstain from sexual activity

C. **Incidence and prevalence**
   1. Half a million cases diagnosed annually with prevalence of approximately 30 million cases
   2. High rate of asymptomatic infection

a. Nearly two-thirds of HSV-2–seropositive individuals have no history of symptomatic genital herpes; 80% of these still shed the virus

b. 20% of people in U.S. over age 30 are seropositive

c. 50% of women with history of gonorrhea or syphilis are seropositive

D. **Spectrum of clinical disease**

1. **Primary genital herpes** (no previous antibodies to HSV-1 or HSV-2)

a. Two-thirds of patients have systemic symptoms, including fever, headache, pharyngitis, malaise, myalgias, backache

   i. Cerebrospinal fluid sample may be positive for aseptic meningitis in up to one-third of patients

   ii. Other neurologic symptoms include urinary retention, constipation, paresthesias, lower extremity weakness

   iii. Symptoms usually begin within 1 week of exposure, peak within 4 days and subside over next week

b. Genital lesions

   i. Local prodrome is itching, erythema, pain, preceding appearance of lesions by 1–2 days

   ii. Small painful vesicles or pustules distributed over labia majora and minora and mons pubis and occasionally in vagina

   iii. Vaginal discharge in 75% of patients

   iv. 80% have dysuria

   v. Cervical involvement such as friability or vesiculation in 90%

   vi. Lesions continue to appear for 4–10 days; individual lesions coalesce into large wet ulcers that persist for 1–2 weeks, then crust and heal without scarring

   vii. Extragenital cutaneous lesions occur commonly on hips and buttocks

   viii. Tender inguinal adenopathy appears during second and third weeks and is last symptom to resolve

2. **First episode of nonprimary genital herpes**

a. Initial clinical episode in patients with previously circulating antibodies to HSV-1 or HSV-2

b. Symptoms are characteristic of recurrent disease

3. **Recurrent genital herpes**

a. 70–90% of people infected with HSV-2 have recurrence compared with 15–25% of people with HSV-1

b. Recurrences are most frequent soon after primary infection

c. Known triggers for recurrence include menses, trauma to area, altered immune status, and emotional stress

d. Symptoms of recurrent disease are generally milder

   i. Few have constitutional symptoms

   ii. May have prodrome ranging from tingling to severe pain lasting hours to few days

   iii. Distribution and numbers of lesions are more limited

   iv. Lesions erupt over 3 days and resolve over 7–10 days

   v. Virus is generally shed for about 4 days

4. **Genital herpes and pregnancy**

a. Goal is to prevent neonatal HSV, which is associated with high morbidity and mortality

b. Neonatal infection may manifest as mucocutaneous disease (least severe), encephalitis, and/or disseminated disease

c. Neonatal HSV is usually acquired by exposure to virus in maternal genital tract during delivery

d. Infants born to mothers with primary HSV are at greater risk of developing infection (> 40%) than are infants born to mothers with recurrent infection (< 5%)

e. Study of infants exposed to HSV-2 at birth indicated that infants at greatest risk were those lacking specific maternal antibody to gG-2, and that anti–gG-2 appeared to be protective

f. Most women who infect their infants have no history of genital herpes

    E. **Differential diagnosis** includes syphilis, chancroid, lymphogranuloma venereum, granuloma inguinale

III. **An Approach**

    A. **Diagnosis**

      1. **Whom to test**

        a. Patients with genital herpes suspected on clinical grounds

          i. Confirm diagnosis on at least one occasion

            (a) Only patients with confirmed genital herpes should be given antiviral agents

            (b) Positive laboratory diagnosis aids in dealing with psychosocial aspects

        b. **Pregnant women**

          i. Seek consultation

          ii. No schema of antepartum screening is of value for predicting infection of neonate at delivery

          iii. Cesarean section is indicated if lesions are present at time of labor or if membranes are ruptured (at term); question remains if cesarean section is ever indicated in recurrent infection

        c. Patients at risk

          i. Risk profile is less clear-cut than in other STDs

          ii. Screening for asymptomatic patients is not indicated

      2. **How to test**

        a. **Tzanck smear**

          i. For immediate diagnosis

          ii. Collect the specimen by unroofing a vesicular lesion, gently scraping the base of lesion with blunt scalpel (#21), transferring the specimen onto glass slide and fixing immediately

          iii. Positive smear shows characteristic multinucleated giant cells

          iv. Sensitivity of Tzanck smear is 85–95% with 95% specificity

        b. **Pap smear**

          i. Specimen taken from mucous membranes

          ii. Sensitivity is only 60–70% with 95% specificity

        c. **Culture**

          i. Confirmatory test of choice

          ii. Expensive and time-consuming

          iii. Collect the specimen by unroofing a vesicular lesion (or sampling from open ulcer), rubbing the base of lesion vigorously (but gently) with cotton or Dacron-tipped swab and placing the swab immediately into transport media, following guidelines for transport and storage

          iv. Virus detected in 90% of vesicles, 70% of ulcers, and 25% of crusted lesions

          v. Results usually available in 3 days, but most laboratories wait 7 days before determining culture to be negative

        d. **Other detection methods**

          i. Immunologic, electron-microscopic, and DNA hybridization method

          ii. Rapid monoclonal antibody, using either immunoperoxidase staining or direct immunofluorescence, may become test of choice

    B. **Therapy**

      1. **Antiviral drugs**

        a. Do not eradicate the latent virus

        b. Do not affect subsequent risk, frequency, or severity of recurrences after administration is discontinued

        c. Topical use less effective

        d. Patients with human immunodeficiency virus (HIV) and other immunocompromised patients may require higher doses and longer courses of acyclovir or other agents

      2. **First clinical episode** of genital herpes—use regimens for 7–10 days or until clinically resolved

        a. Acyclovir, 200 mg orally 5 times/day

        b. Acyclovir 400 mg orally 3 times/day

    c. Famciclovir 250 mg orally 3 times/day
    d. Valacyclovir 1 g orally 2 times/day
3. **Recurrent disease**
    a. Not routinely indicated in immunocompetent patients
    b. If used, institute treatment during prodrome or within 2 days of onset of lesions for maximal benefit
    c. Recommended regimens—treat for 5 days
       i. Acyclovir, 400 mg orally 3 times/day
      ii. Acyclovir, 200 mg orally 5 times/day
     iii. Acyclovir, 800 mg orally 2 times/day
     iv. Famciclovir 125 mg orally 2 times/day
      v. Valacyclovir 500 mg orally 2 times/day
4. Daily suppressive therapy for patients with frequent recurrences (6 or more per year) reduces recurrence rate by 75%
    a. Does not totally eliminate viral shedding or potential of transmission
    b. Discontinue after 1 year and reassess rate of recurrent disease
    c. **Recommended regimen**
       i. Acyclovir, 400 mg orally 2 times/day
      ii. Famciclovir 250 mg orally 2 times/day
     iii. Valacyclovir 250 mg orally 2 times/day
     iv. Valacyclovir 500 mg orally once daily (less effective than other regimens in patients with > 10 episodes/year)
    d. Safety and efficacy documented with daily use of acyclovir for up to 6 years; with famciclovir and valacyclovir for 1 year
5. **Pregnant women**
    a. First clinical episode may be treated with any regimen of acyclovir recommended for first clinical episode in nonpregnant patient
6. Safety of famciclovir and valacyclovir in pregnancy not established

SUGGESTED READING

1. Centers for Disease Control and Prevention: 1998 Guidelines for treatment of sexually transmitted diseases. MMWR 47(RR-1):20–26, 1998.
2. Dwyer DE, Cunningham AL: Herpes simplex virus infection in pregnancy. Baillieres Clin Obstet Gynaecol 7:75–105, 1993.
3. Forsgren M, Malm G: Herpes simplex virus and pregnancy. Scand J Infect Dis 100(Suppl): S14–S19, 1996.
4. Maccato ML, Kaufman RH: Herpes genitalis. Dermatol Clin 10:415–421, 1992.
5. Prober CG: Herpetic vaginitis in 1993. Clin Obstet Gynecol 36:117–187, 1993.
6. Smith MA, Singer C: Sexually transmitted viruses other than HIV and papillomavirus. Urol Clin North Am 19:47–62, 1992.
7. Whitley RJ, Kimberlin DW: Treatment of viral infections during pregnancy and the neonatal period. Clin Perinatol 24:267–283, 1997.

43. Trichomonas Infection

Cynda Ann Johnson, M.D., M.B.A.

I. The Issues

Two issues often plague the generalist caring for women with trichomonas infection. The first is mode of transmission. Is trichomonas always sexually transmitted? Most authoritative texts admit that fomite transmission exists but caution that it is rare. The generalist, however, often encounters cases in which sexual transmission seems highly unlikely. A common scenario is an elderly woman who has not been sexually active for many years. Was the infection sexually transmitted many years ago, remaining asymptomatic? It seems doubtful. The second issue is the

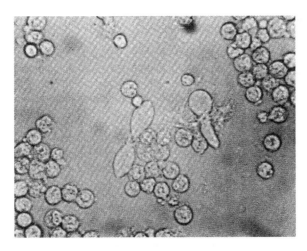

FIGURE 1. Trichomonads in wet mount prepared with physiologic saline. (From Gardner HL: Trichomoniasis. In Gardner HL, Kaufman RH (eds): Benign Diseases of the Vulva and Vagina, 2nd ed. St. Louis, Mosby–Year Book, 1981, with permission.)

pregnant patient with trichomonas infection. Increasing evidence indicates trichomoniasis may be associated with adverse effects in pregnancy and should be treated. Since initial warnings of the teratogenicity of metronidazole in pregnancy, clinicians have been reluctant to treat pregnant patients, particularly in the first trimester, although study after study reports no harmful effects. The primary health care provider must take a stand on both issues: in the first situation the provider should give appropriate support and not dogmatically tell her that she "must have gotten the trichomonas through sexual transmission," and in the second case the provider should have the grounding in science to choose to medicate the patient appropriately.

II. **The Theory**

A. **Causative organism:** *Trichomonas vaginalis* (Fig. 1)
   1. Anaerobic, flagellated, motile protozoan
   2. Slightly larger than white blood cell
   3. Thrives best in pH of 5.0–7.5

B. **Transmission**
   1. Sexual exposure
   2. Rarely, as described above, via fomites such as washcloths or from infested reservoirs such as hot tubs

C. **Clinical manifestations**
   1. Primarily infects vagina, but also cervix, Bartholin's glands, periurethral glands, urethra, and bladder
   2. Symptoms
      a. Many infections are asymptomatic
         i. Women may have chronic trichomonas infection that continues to be asymptomatic because of frequent douching or even oral contraceptives, which may keep number of organisms at low level
         ii. Asymptomatic women usually have lower vaginal pH than women with acute, symptomatic disease
      b. Symptomatic patients
         i. Profuse, frothy, yellow to green malodorous vaginal discharge—though considerable variability in character of discharge
         ii. Pruritus
         iii. Vaginal burning
         iv. Vulvar edema, erythema
         v. Red stippled, "strawberry" vagina or cervix (well-visualized on colposcopic examination)

D. **Pregnancy**
1. Association between trichomonas vaginitis and adverse pregnancy outcomes includes: premature rupture of membranes and preterm labor
2. Test high-risk patients in pregnancy
    i. Women with symptoms
    ii. Women with history of STD

III. **An Approach**
A. **Diagnosis**
1. No single method is perfect
2. Suggested by clinical picture
3. Confirmation by microscopic visualization of motile organism on wet drop examination
    a. Most common method of diagnosis; standard of care
    b. Diagnosis can be made by visualization of single motile organism
    c. When heavy infiltration of polymorphonuclear cells is present, trichomonads may be obscured
4. Visualization on urinalysis
5. Detection on Papanicolaou smear
    a. False-positive results because diagnosis is made by observing suspicious but nonviable organisms
    b. Positive predictive value of only 40% in average population
6. Culture
    a. Feinberg-Whittington or Diamond's culture medium
        i. Available only in select laboratories
        ii. Results not available for 2–7 days
        iii. Probably underused
            (a) Order in controversial cases
            (b) As follow-up to unexpected positive Papanicolaou smear
            (c) Combination of culture and wet mount results in greatest diagnostic accuracy
    b. Monoclonal antibody staining of direct specimens
        i. Not commonly available
        ii. False-positives with dead organisms possible

B. **Therapy**
1. **Metronidazole** is only medication available in U.S. to treat trichomonas infection
    a. Side effects include metallic aftertaste, nausea, vertigo, headache, rash, abdominal pain
    b. Potential disulfiram (Antabuse)-type reaction causing severe systemic symptoms
        i. Avoid alcohol until 24 hours after completion of therapy
2. **Recommended regimen**
    a. 2 g orally in single dose (dividing dose over 24 hours is less effective)
    b. Alternative regimen—500 mg twice a day for 7 days
    c. 95% cure rate for either regimen
    d. Metronidazole gel is not indicated for treatment of trichomoniasis
3. **Treatment in pregnancy**
    a. Recommended treatment is metronidazole 2 g orally as single dose
    b. Based on current literature, treat with metronidazole any symptomatic patient in first trimester and all infected patients in second and third trimester
    c. Clotrimazole or Betadine douching may afford symptomatic relief
4. **Avoid sexual contact** between patient and partners until both have completed therapy and are asymptomatic
5. **Test for cure** if symptoms persist after completion of therapy and in all pregnant patients
6. **Resistant strains**
    a. Although the most common reason for "resistant" trichomonas is actually reinfection, rarely a strain of trichomonas with decreased susceptibility is encountered
    b. Retreat patient, using alternative regimen, regardless of which regimen was used initially

c. Continued resistance
   i. Treat with 2 g orally in single dose daily for 3–5 days though neurotoxicity more likely in high-dose therapy
   ii. Seek consultation
     (a) Culture and sensitivity testing are indicated but not widely available
   iii. Other medications
     (a) Tinidazole, available in Europe, is indicated for treatment of trichomonas infection
     (b) Intravaginal nonoxynol-9 was effective in 1 case report
     (c) Other possibilities include mebendazole, furazolidone, anisomycin

SUGGESTED READING

1. Centers for Disease Control and Prevention: 1998 Guidelines for treatment of sexually transmitted diseases. MMWR 47(RR-1):74–75, 1998.
2. Krieger JN, Tam MR, Stevens CE, et al: Diagnosis of trichomoniasis: Comparison of conventional wet-mount examination with cytologic studies, cultures, and monoclonal antibody staining of direct specimens. JAMA 259:1223–1227, 1988.
3. Livengood CH III, Lossick JG: Resolution of resistant vaginal trichomoniasis associated with the use of intravaginal nonoxynol-9. Obstet Gynecol 78:954–956, 1991.
4. Weinberger MW, Harger JH: Accuracy of the Papanicolaou smear in the diagnosis of asymptomatic infection with *Trichomonas vaginalis*. Obstet Gynecol 82:425–429, 1993.

44. Chlamydial Infection

Cynda Ann Johnson, M.D., M.B.A.

I. **The Issues**
Chlamydial infection is the most common sexually transmitted disease (STD) in the United States. Despite recent downward trends in frequency of diagnosis at family planning clinics, over 4 million cases of chlamydial infection are diagnosed each year. The spectrum of disease is broad. Morbidity and, in some settings, mortality are significant, yet many patients remain asymptomatic. The economic impact on society is huge ($2.5 billion annually). Such issues as parameters for screening, accurate and cost-effective diagnosis, identification of partners, and optimal treatment regimens remain under intense investigation. The primary care provider has an important role in implementation of resulting protocols and in educating patients.

II. **The Theory**
  A. **Causative organism:** *Chlamydia trachomatis*
    1. Classified as bacterium
    2. Obligate intracellular parasite that infects columnar epithelium
  B. **Transmission**
    1. Sexual contact is primary mode of transmission for oculogenital strains
    2. Condoms prevent transmission
    3. May be transmitted to neonate during passage through birth canal
    4. Serotypes causing trachoma show high rates of child-to-child and intrafamilial passage
  C. **Occurrence**
    1. Approximately 4 million cases each year (1996 data); 4–9% of persons in primary care populations
  D. **Spectrum of clinical disease**
    1. Symptoms of chlamydial infection depend on site; vaginal discharge and dysuria are most common
    2. Endocervix is the most common site of infection within female genital tract
    3. Urethra and rectum are other sites of initial infection

4. Upper tract infection
   a. Represents ascending infection
   b. Symptoms include lower abdominal pain and menstrual abnormalities
   c. Up to 50% of cases of pelvic inflammatory disease (PID) are caused by chlamydia in some studies
   d. Significant factor among causes of infertility and ectopic pregnancies
5. Pregnancy
   a. Transmission to infant occurs in up to 70% of untreated pregnant women
E. **Comparison with gonorrheal cervicitis**
   1. Frequently found in association with gonorrhea
   2. Together represent cause of most cases of mucopurulent cervicitis
   3. Chlamydia is asymptomatic 5 times more often than gonorrhea
   4. Chlamydia has longer incubation period (6–14 days) than gonorrhea (3–5 days)

III. **An Approach**
A. **Diagnosis**
   1. **Whom to test**
      a. Any woman with mucopurulent cervical discharge
      b. Any woman with symptoms characteristic of chlamydial infection at any site
      c. Screen asymptomatic women with any of following characteristics
         i. All sexually active women aged < 20 years
            (a) Chlamydia test at each pelvic examination unless single mutually monogamous partner since most recent test
         ii. Annual screening of women aged 20–24 years who meet one of the following criteria and women > 24 years who meet both
            (a) Inconsistent use of barrier contraception
            (b) New sex partner or more than 1 sex partner during previous 3 months
         iii. Pregnant women with history of STD
            (a) Rescreen high-risk women in third trimester
      d. Consider screening patients with following characteristics
         i. All women under age 25 years
         ii. Unmarried sexually active women
         iii. Sexual partner with another partner in past 3 months
         iv. Sexual partner with symptom characteristic of chlamydia
         v. Use of oral contraceptives—especially if unexpected intermenstrual spotting
         vi. History of STD
         vii. Spontaneous or voluntary termination of pregnancy
         viii. Abnormal vaginal bleeding
         ix. Papanicolaou smear showing inflammation
         x. Evidence of cervicitis
   2. **How to test**
      a. **Cell culture**
         i. Advantages
            (a) Most specific (100%) with acceptable sensitivity (70–90%)
            (b) Detects infection even when only small numbers of organisms are present
         ii. Disadvantages
            (a) Method is technically difficult; specific transport and storage criteria
            (b) Requires 3–7 days to obtain result
            (c) Detects only viable organisms
         iii. Indications for use
            (a) Prepubertal girls
            (b) For urethral and rectal specimens
            (c) To verify positive nonculture test with potential for adverse psychosocial consequences or in population of low prevalence
            (d) To verify negative nonculture test
      b. **Nonculture tests**
         i. Advantages

(a) Sensitivity of tests in 70–90% range

(b) Results available sooner than for culture

(c) Less influenced by transport, storage factors

ii. Disadvantages

(a) Most are less than 99% specific—results in false-positives in low-risk population

iii. Direct fluorescent antibody tests

(a) Results within 7 days

(b) Processing time is 30–40 minutes

iv. Nucleic acid hybridization tests (DNA probe)

(a) Results within 7 days

(b) Some also allow testing for gonorrhea with single specimen

v. Enzyme immunoassay

(a) Storage time according to manufacturer's directions

(b) Standard tests require 3–4 hours processing time

(c) Rapid chlamydia tests

(i) Developed for office-based testing

(ii) Packaged as single units

(iii) Do not require expensive or sophisticated equipment

(iv) Performance characteristics still being evaluated

(v) Processing time within 30 minutes

c. **Collecting specimens**

i. Obtain specimens for chlamydia tests after other tests, including Papanicolaou smear

ii. Remove remaining secretions and discharge from cervical os with sponge or swab stick

iii. For nonculture test, use swab supplied or specified by manufacturer to collect specimen

iv. For culture test, do not use swab with wooden shaft, which may be toxic to chlamydia organisms; consider use of brush, which may increase sensitivity of test

v. Insert sampler 1–2 cm into canal, specifically beyond squamocolumnar junction

vi. Rotate sampler against endocervix for 10–30 seconds

vii. Withdraw sampler without touching any vaginal surfaces and place it in appropriate transport medium

B. **Therapy**

1. **Recommended regimens for lower tract disease**

a. Azithromycin, 1 g orally in single dose

b. Doxycycline, 100 mg orally 2 times/day for 7 days

2. **Alternative regimens**

a. Erythromycin base, 500 mg orally 4 times/day for 7 days

b. Erythromycin ethylsuccinate, 800 mg orally 4 times/day for 7 days

c. Ofloxacin, 300 mg orally 2 times/day for 7 days (for women > 18 year old)

3. **Treatment in pregnancy**—any approved regimen of erythromycin or azithromycin noted above

4. **Treatment of infants**

a. Infants born to mothers with chlamydial infection should receive erythromycin 24 hours after birth

b. Continue treatment for 10 days

5. **Treatment of sexual partners**

a. Partners of symptomatic patients—evaluate and treat all persons who had sexual contact with patient within 30 days of onset of patient's symptoms

b. Partners of asymptomatic patients—evaluate and treat all persons who had sexual contact with patient within 60 days of diagnosis

c. Most recent sexual contact should be evaluated and treated regardless of time of exposure

d. Patient should avoid sex until she and her partners have completed therapy and are free of symptoms

C. **Follow-up testing**
   1. Test of cure is reasonable in the following situations
      a. Pregnancy
      b. Patient or partner not symptom-free
   2. Do not retest until 3 weeks or more after completion of therapy
      a. Culture test may be falsely negative before that time because of small numbers of organisms
      b. Nonculture test may be falsely positive because of continued excretion of dead organisms
D. **Report positive tests** according to state regulations

SUGGESTED READING

1. Bush MR, Rosa C: Azithromycin and erythromycin in the treatment of cervical chlamydial infection during pregnancy. Obstet Gynecol 84:61–63, 1994.
2. Centers for Disease Control and Prevention: 1998 Guidelines for treatment of sexually transmitted diseases. MMWR 47(RR-1):53–59, 1998.
3. Krettek JE, Arkin SI, Chaisilwattana P, Monif GRG: *Chlamydia trachomatis* in patients who used oral contraceptives and had intermenstrual spotting. Obstet Gynecol 81:728–731, 1993.
4. Majeroni BA: Chlamydial cervicitis: Complications and new treatment options. Am Fam Physician 49:1825–1829, 1994.
5. Phillips RS, Aronson MD, Taylor WC, Safran C: Should tests for *Chlamydia trachomatis* cervical infection be done during routine gynecologic visits? An analysis of the costs of alternative strategies. Ann Intern Med 107:188–194, 1987.
6. Sellors JW, Pickard L, Gafni A, et al: Effectiveness and efficiency of selective vs. universal screening for chlamydial infection in sexually active young women. Arch Intern Med 152:1837–1844, 1992.
7. U.S. Preventive Services Task Force: Guide to Clinical Preventive Services, 2nd ed. Alexandria, VA, International Medical Publishing, 1996, pp 325–334.

45. Bacterial Vaginosis

Cynda Ann Johnson, M.D., M.B.A.

I. **The Issues**

Bacterial vaginosis (BV) is the most prevalent form of vaginitis in the U.S., accounting for over 10 million patient visits per year. It is also, arguably, the least understood vaginitis. As understanding of BV has evolved, so has its name. First known as nonspecific vaginitis as early as 1894, it was consecutively attributed to *Haemophilus vaginalis*, *Corynebacterium vaginalis*, and *Gardnerella vaginalis* (to keep up with the naming of ostensible offending organisms). As it is becoming clear that there is no single offending organism and that the condition may not be actual infection as judged by usual criteria, the term to refer to the condition is once again changing—first to anaerobic vaginosis and most recently to bacterial vaginosis. Other puzzling issues include whether or not BV is a sexually transmissible disease, the impact of BV on morbidity, the most reliable diagnostic criteria, and appropriate treatment regimens. Primary care physicians must educate patients about this enigmatic disorder and keep current on the basics of diagnosis and treatment.

II. **The Theory**
   A. **Normal vaginal milieu**
      1. pH: 3.8–4.2
      2. Acidophilic lactobacilli are predominant organisms in normal vaginal flora
         a. Produce lactic acid which results in pH of 3.8–4.2
            i. Inhibits growth of *Gardnerella vaginalis* and anaerobes
         b. Interfere with bacterial adherence to epithelial cells (called "clue" cells)
         c. Inhibit overgrowth of *Candida* species

      d. Hydrogen peroxide-producing strains of lactobacilli
         i. Significant bactericidal action against anaerobes and *Gardnerella vaginalis*
B. **Alterations in normal vaginal milieu results in BV**
   1. Causes of pH increases includes menstruation, hormonal changes and vaginal intercourse
   2. Loss of lactobacilli, especially hydrogen peroxide-producing strains, results in further increase in pH and overgrowth of other bacteria
     a. Bacterial concentrations 100–1000-fold of: anaerobes; *Bacteroides (Prevotella)* sp.; *Peptostreptococcus* sp.; *Eubacterium* sp.; *Mobiluncus* sp.; facultative anaerobes; *Gardnerella vaginalis; Mycoplasma hominis*
   3. Foul-smelling vaginal odor from increased numbers of anaerobic bacteria
     a. Anaerobic metabolism produces amines while the elevated pH volatizes amines, releasing "fishy" odor
   4. Increased numbers of *Candida* species due to increasing pH
C. **BV is "vaginosis," not "vaginitis"**—that is, number of bacteria increase without inflammation (no increase in white blood cells)
D. **Risk factors:** presence of other sexually transmitted diseases (STDs), multiple sexual partners, longer history of coital experience; possible risk factor—presence of intrauterine device
E. **Symptoms:** discharge, vaginal odor, occasionally worse after intercourse; 50% of patients are asymptomatic
F. **Vaginal discharge** (see Table 1 for comparison with other vaginal infections)
G. **Associated complications** with relative risks (rr)
   1. Not pregnancy-related
     a. Pelvic inflammatory disease (PID), rr = 9.2
     b. Postabortal PID, rr = 3.0
     c. Post-hysterectomy infections, rr = 3.2–4.3
   2. Pregnancy-related
     a. Preterm delivery, rr = 1.4–3.8
     b. Premature rupture of membranes, rr = 2.4
     c. Amniotic fluid infection, rr = 1.5–2.7
     d. Chorioamnionitis, rr = 2.6
     e. Postpartum endometritis, rr = 2.2–5.8
H. **Can BV be transmitted sexually?**
   1. Arguments for sexual transmission
     a. Consistent association of BV with multiple sexual partners
     b. Decreased prevalence in monogamous couples

TABLE 1. Differential Diagnosis of Vaginal Infections

Diagnostic Criteria	Syndrome			
	Normal	Bacterial Vaginosis	Candidal Vulvovaginitis	Trichomonal Vaginitis
Vaginal pH	3.8–4.2	> 4.5	≤ 4.5 (usually)	> 4.5
Discharge	White, clear, flocculent	Thin, homogeneous, white to gray, adherent, often increased	White, curdy, like cottage cheese, sometimes increased	Yellow to green, frothy, adherent, increased
Amine odor (KOH) "whiff" test	Absent	Present (fishy)	Absent	Fishy when present
Microscopic	Lactobacilli	Clue cells, coccoid bacteria, no WBCs	Mycelia, budding yeast, pseudohyphae with KOH preparation	Trichomonads, WBCs > 10/hpf
Main patient complaints	None	Discharge, bad odor—possibly worse after intercourse	Itching/burning, discharge	Frothy discharge, bad odor, vulvar pruritus, dysuria

KOH = potassium hydroxide, WBC = white blood cells.
From Bacterial Vaginosis: Diagnosis and Treatment. Elk Grove Village, IL, Curatek Pharmaceuticals, 1993, with permission.

      c. Rare in virgins; occasional infection probably from gastrointestinal tract

      d. Protective effect of condoms

   2. Arguments against sexual transmission

      a. Failure to demonstrate benefits in treating male partner

      b. No disease state in males, i.e., bacteria do not persist in males

      c. Bacterial vaginosis found in virginal women

III. **An Approach**

A. **Diagnosis**

1. **Clinical diagnosis** (3 of 4 criteria required)
   a. 20% or more of vaginal epithelial cells as clue cells
   b. pH > 4.5 (sample pooled vaginal discharge or vaginal wall—avoid cervix which usually has higher pH)
   c. Positive KOH "whiff" test
   d. Homogeneous discharge
2. **Culture diagnosis**
   a. Unreliable, has no role
   b. *Gardnerella vaginalis* found in up to 60% of cultures from asymptomatic women
3. **Papanicolaou (Pap) smear**
   a. Clue cells on Pap smear: 90% sensitive, 97% specific
   b. *Gardnerella vaginalis* on Pap smear: 25% sensitive, 58% specific
4. **Gram stain of vaginal discharge**
   a. May be best single diagnostic test for BV
   b. Requires experience to interpret accurately
   c. Reveals relative concentration of morphotypes characteristic of BV
   d. Clue cells identifiable
   e. Few white blood cells
5. **Research methods** (few of which are relevant to clinical practice)
   a. Thin-layer chromatography (which demonstrates increased diamines in vaginal fluid)
   b. Gas-liquid chromatography (which gives a pattern characteristic of relevant organic acids)
   c. Proline aminopeptidase determination
   d. Qualitative cultures
   e. DNA probes

B. **Treatment**

1. **Goals of treatment**
   a. Principal goal: to relieve symptoms of infection
   b. Increasing evidence for treatment to prevent secondary complications of BV (see above)
2. **Medication options**
   a. Primary therapy—nonpregnant women
      i. Metronidazole, 500 mg, orally, twice a day for 7 days (cure rate 95%)
   b. Alternative regimens—nonpregnant women
      i. Metronidazole, 2 g orally in a single dose (84% cure rate)
      ii. Clindamycin cream, 2%, 1 applicatorful (5 gm) intravaginally at bedtime for 7 days
      iii. Metronidazole gel, 0.75%, 1 applicatorful (5 gm) intravaginally, twice daily, for 5 days
      iv. Clindamycin, 300 mg orally twice daily for 7 days
   c. Primary therapy—pregnant women
      i. Metronidazole 250 mg orally 3 times/day for 7 days
   d. Alternative therapy—pregnant women
      i. Metronidazole 2 g orally as single dose
      ii. Clindamycin 300 mg orally 2 times/day for 7 days
      iii. Metronidazole gel 0.75%, 1 applicator full intravaginally 2 times/day for 5 days
3. **Metronidazole**—special concerns
   a. Must avoid alcohol during treatment and for 24 hours thereafter (disulfiram-like reaction because metronidazole blocks alcohol metabolism)

    b. Metal taste in mouth, especially in longer courses of treatment

    c. Prolongs prothrombin time in patients taking warfarin

    d. Significant gastrointestinal upset in many patients; worse with single dose therapy

    e. Intravaginal metronidazole

        i. Mean peak serum concentration only 2% compared with that of 500-mg oral dose

4. **Pregnancy**—special concerns

    a. Treatment of high-risk pregnant women who are asymptomatic might reduce risk of premature delivery

        i. Screen and treat all high-risk patients in second trimester

        ii. Do not use intravaginal metronidazole or intravaginal clindamycin in high-risk obstetrical patients, especially with a history of previous premature delivery

    b. Low-risk pregnant women who are symptomatic with BV should be treated as outlined above

5. **Follow-up visits** not necessary if symptoms resolve

6. **Recurrent disease**

    a. Consider other vaginal/cervical infection

    b. Repeat first-line regimen or try alternative regimens

    c. No long-term maintenance regimen with any therapeutic agent is currently available

    d. If several recurrences, suggest repeat examination after therapy to document cure

    e. Treatment of partner is option if several recurrences, but efficacy not proved

    f. Recurrence may be relapse rather than reinfection

        i. Many asymptomatic "cured" women continue to have abnormalities in vagina flora

          (a) Most common is slightly elevated pH (4.5–4.6) caused by continued unbalance in vaginal flora

             (i) Break cycle of recurrence by lowering pH of vagina with Acijel, acidifying clear gel

             (ii) Prescribe one applicator intravaginally twice daily to break cycle of recurrence

             (iii) If no recurrence of BV, decrease frequency of use

             (iv) Most patients can be maintained on 2 doses a week

             (v) Over several months, Acijel may be discontinued as cycle of recurrence is broken and normal vaginal milieu has been restored

    g. Remaining questions

        i. Would more prolonged therapy result in lower recurrence rate with fewer residual abnormalities?

        ii. Is 2% clindamycin applied intravaginally associated with high recurrence rate?

        iii. Should patients with recurrent BV receive maintenance therapy?

        iv. Should steps be taken to maintain a normal pH?

SUGGESTED READING

1. Centers for Disease Control and Prevention: Guidelines for treatment of sexually transmitted diseases. MMWR 47 (RR-1):70–74, 1998.
2. Colli E, Landoni M: Treatment of male partners and recurrence of bacterial vaginosis: A randomised trial. Genitourin Med 73:267–70, 1997.
3. Davis JD, Connor EE: Correlation between cervical cytologic results and Gram stain as diagnostic tests for bacterial vaginosis. Am J Obstet Gynecol 177:532–535, 1997.
4. Kurki T, Sivonen A: Bacterial vaginosis in early pregnancy and pregnancy outcome. Obstet Gynecol 80:173–177, 1992.
5. Nilsson U, Hellberg D: Sexual behavior risk factors associated with bacterial vaginosis and *Chlamydia trachomatis* infection. Sex Transm Dis 24:241–146, 1997.
6. Schmitt C, Sobel JD: Bacterial vaginosis: Treatment with clindamycin cream versus oral metronidazole. Obstet Gynecol 79:1020–1023, 1992.
7. Shoubnikova M, Hellberg D: Contraceptive use in women with bacterial vaginosis. Contraception 55:355–358, 1997.

46. Vulvovaginal Candidiasis

Cynda Ann Johnson, M.D., M.B.A.

I. **The Issues**

Although second in frequency of the vulvovaginitides (bacterial vaginosis is first), vulvovaginal candidiasis is certainly first in the minds of our patients. Issues of recurrence, potentially intense symptoms, over-the-counter treatments, and newer oral therapy put this condition on the forefront of the popular press. Standard treatment regimens are not curative in many cases—in others, the patient has another condition altogether. The astute generalist is sensitive to the women who comes into the office already exasperated, is aware of methods of investigation to clarify the diagnosis, and has experience with multiple treatment options to provide welcomed, individualized care and a successful medical outcome.

II. **The Theory**

  A. **Causative organism:** yeast

   1. Most common species is *Candida albicans*, which accounts for 65–95% of all isolates
   2. Many other *Candida* species have similar sensitivities to antifungal agents
   3. *Candida glabrata*
      a. Previously known as *C. torulopsis*
      b. Causes 5–10% of all vaginal yeast infections
      c. Relatively resistant to many common antifungal agents
   4. Other fungal infections infrequently manifesting as vulvitis
      a. *Trichophyton rubrum* (tinea cruris)
      b. *Pityrosporum orbiculare* (pityriasis versicolor)

  B. **Transmission**

   1. Most commonly candidal organisms gain access to vaginal lumen and secretions from adjacent perianal areas
   2. Sexual transmission may be factor in 20% of cases
      a. Evidence supporting sexual transmission of yeast infections
         i. Nearly 10% of men examined after sexual contact with women harboring yeast infections developed mycotic balanitis
         ii. Fourfold increase in yeast colonization in male partners of infected women
         iii. Isolation of same strains in infected couples
      b. Evidence against sexual transmission
         i. No direct association between yeast infection and other sexually transmitted diseases (STDs)
         ii. No difference in yeast isolation rates in STD vs. non-STD populations
         iii. Routine treatment of male partner does not affect cure or recurrence rates in female

  C. **Prevalence**

   1. *Candida* can be isolated in as many as 25% of asymptomatic women
   2. Acute infections associated with presence of large number of organisms
   3. 75% of women have at least one symptomatic episode during lifetime; nearly half have two or more episodes
   4. < 5% have recurrent disease
   5. 20–30% of patients with *Candida* infection have dual or multiple pathogens

  D. **Factors predisposing to candidal overgrowth**

   1. Reproductive age group
   2. Frequent intercourse
   3. Pregnancy (up to 20% affected in late pregnancy)
   4. High blood glucose levels
   5. Use of antibiotics, especially broad-spectrum
   6. Use of corticosteroids, especially in high doses
   7. Depressed cell-mediated immunity

8. High-dose oral contraceptives (possibly)
9. High-carbohydrate diets (possibly)
10. Tight-fitting jeans or underwear implicated
E. **Theoretical factors predisposing to recurrent, chronic disease**
1. Lower antibody titers to *Candida* (although no level of antibody predictably prevents repeat infection)
2. Lack of cellular immune response to *Candida* antigen
3. Intracellular phase of *Candida*
4. Acquired acute hypersensitivity reaction to *Candida* antigen
a. Patients present with severe vulvar manifestations with minimal exudative vaginal discharge and few organisms
b. Elevated titers of antigen-specific IgE in vagina
c. Small studies show reduction in frequency of recurrent episodes of vaginitis using *Candida* antigen for desensitization
F. **Clinical manifestations**
1. Asymptomatic in many cases
2. Vulvar pruritus—90% of symptomatic patients
3. Vulvar erythema
4. Vulvar burning
5. Edema of labia minora
6. Vulvar excoriations (from scratching)
7. Vaginal soreness, irritation
8. Dyspareunia
9. Redness of vaginal tissues
10. Vaginal pH = 4.0–4.7
11. External dysuria
12. Vaginal discharge
a. Classic—thick, like cottage cheese (20%)
b. Adherent to vaginal and vulvar tissues
13. Minimal odor
14. Normal cervix
15. Presence of second infection in 20%
16. Symptoms exacerbated in premenstrual week but improve with onset of menstrual flow
III. **An Approach**
A. **Diagnosis**
1. **Characteristic symptoms**
a. Healthy, low-risk patients may be encouraged to self-treat with over-the-counter (OTC) antifungal preparation in acute situation, avoiding physician and laboratory charges
2. **Vaginal secretion testing**
a. 10% KOH preparation reveals mycelia, pseudohyphae, spores
b. Predominance of lactobacilli compared with other causes of vaginitis, especially bacterial vaginosis
c. No pseudohyphae seen in *C. glabrata* infection
d. Positive vaginal secretion testing and characteristic clinical manifestations are adequate for diagnosis in most cases
3. **Gram stain**—may be positive when wet mount is negative due to excessive cellular debris
4. **Papanicolaou smear**—sensitivity only 50%
5. **Culture**
a. Sabouraud's or other fungal culture media
b. Routine culture: nearly half of positive results are in asymptomatic patients
c. Helpful in cases apparently resistant to treatment
i. Confirms non–*C. albicans* species, especially *C. glabrata*
d. Culture of vaginal discharge should be done before dismissing *Candida* as diagnosis in symptomatic patient
e. May be useful in recurrent infections

B. **Therapy**
1. Asymptomatic women with yeast found on laboratory exam need not be treated routinely
   a. Finding should be reported to patient
   b. Offer her option of treatment
   c. Consider treatment of immunosuppressed patients
2. Test of cure not indicated routinely in asymptomatic patients after course of therapy
3. Intravaginal formulations of azoles are drugs of choice
   a. **Recommended regimens**
      i. Butoconazole 2% cream, 5 g intravaginally for 3 days (available OTC)
      ii. Clotrimazole
          (a) 1% cream, 5 g intravaginally for 7–14 days (OTC)
          (b) 100-mg vaginal tablet for 7 days (OTC)
          (c) 100-mg vaginal tablet, 2 tablets for 3 days
          (d) 500-mg vaginal tablet, single dose
      iii. Miconazole
          (a) 2% cream, 5 g intravaginally for 7 days (OTC)
          (b) 200-mg vaginal suppository, 1 suppository for 3 days
          (c) 100-mg vaginal suppository, 1 suppository for 7 days (OTC)
      iv. Tioconazole, 6.5% ointment, 5 g intravaginally, single application (OTC)
      v. Terconazole
          (a) 0.4% cream, 5 g intravaginally for 7 days
          (b) 0.8% cream, 5 g intravaginally for 3 days
          (c) 80-mg suppository, 1 suppository for 3 days
      vi. Fluconazole 150 mg orally (one dose)
      vii. Nystatin 100,000 unit vaginal tablet daily for 14 days (only non-azole recommended for primary therapy)
   b. Vaginal azole preparations are oil-based and may weaken latex condoms and diaphragms; nystatin is not oil-based
   c. All azoles are more effective than nystatin
      i. 80–90% cure rates for one course of therapy
   d. Use additional azole cream twice daily externally to treat local symptoms
   e. Azoles may be used in pregnant women
   f. Terconazole is marketed for use in non–*C. albicans*-resistant strains
   g. Suppositories may fall out, especially in multiparous women
   h. Over-the-counter preparations may be more expensive than prescription-only formulations
   i. Reserve single-dose therapy for mild cases
   j. Short-course therapy offers better compliance, but patient needs to be instructed that symptoms may not resolve until few days after administration of medication has been completed
   k. If symptoms persist after course of over-the-counter medication or recur within 2 months, patient should seek medical care
      i. Careful history to determine frequency and compliance with OTC therapy
      ii. Because patient has already self-medicated, confirmatory test should be performed
      iii. Combination of oral and vaginal therapy is usually curative while providing quicker symptomatic relief than oral alone
   l. Women who get symptomatic yeast infections when placed on antibiotics may begin treatment at first sign of symptoms
      i. Consider single oral azole weekly for duration of antibiotic therapy or titrate antibiotic to low enough dose that yeast vaginitis does not occur
   m. Vaginal preparations may cause intense burning
      i. Usually after several courses of treatment or during severe infection
      ii. Possibly hypersensitivity reaction; may signal onset of allergy to preparation
      iii. Combination of local application of steroids and oral azole usually results in comfort and cure

4. **Recurrent, resistant disease**
   a. Review risk factors; modify if possible
   b. Confirm by culture
   c. Old preparations are very effective for resistant infections
      i. Gentian violet 1%, applied intravaginally and on vulva with gauze sponge or sponge stick
         (a) Single treatment usually effective
         (b) Twice weekly for 2 weeks as alternative
         (c) Gentian violet tampons inserted daily for 6–8 hours for most resistant cases
      ii. Boric acid, 600-mg vaginal capsules
         (a) Daily for 2 weeks (98% cure rate)
         (b) Twice daily for 2 weeks, if still symptomatic
         (c) Repeat process if microscopic examination of vaginal discharge reveals evidence of continued yeast infection
         (d) If still abnormal, prescribe 1 suppository daily during menstruation for 4 months
   d. Multiple treatment regimens have been tried for recurrent disease
      i. Monthly administration of 500-mg suppository of clotrimazole
      ii. 2-week course of oral azole
      iii. Low-dose oral azole chronically (expensive)
         (a) Monitor for side effects (e.g., liver enzyme abnormalities)
      iv. Premenstrual administration of oral or vaginal preparation
      v. Weekly boric acid capsules
      vi. Consider simultaneous course of treatment for sexual partner
      vii. Daily ingestion of *Lactobacillus acidophilus*–containing yogurt appears to decrease both candidal colonization and infection in women with recurrent candidiasis
      viii. Hyposensitization to *Candida* antigen (research technique)

SUGGESTED READING

1. Centers for Disease Control and Prevention: Guidelines for treatment of sexually transmitted diseases. MMWR 47(RR-1):70–74, 1998.
2. Hilton E, Isenberg HD, Alperstein P, et al: Ingestion of yogurt containing *Lactobacillus acidophilus* as prophylaxis for candidal vaginitis. Ann Intern Med 116:353–357, 1992.
3. Jovanovic R, Congema E, Nguyen H: Antifungal agents vs. boric acid for treating chronic mycotic vulvovaginitis. Reprod Med 36:593, 1991.
4. Oriel JD, Partridge BM, Denny MJ, Coleman JC: Genital yeast infections. BMJ 4:761, 1972.
5. Palacios HJ: Hypersensitivity as a cause of dermatologic and vaginal moniliasis resistant to topical therapy. Ann Allergy 37:110–115, 1976.
6. Sobel JD: Epidemiology and pathogenesis of recurrent vulvovaginal candidiasis. Am J Obstet Gynecol 152:924–935, 1985.
7. Sobel JD: Recurrent vulvovaginal candidiasis: A prospective study of the efficacy of maintenance ketoconazole therapy. N Engl J Med 315:1445–1458, 1986.
8. Sobel JD: Vulvovaginitis. Dermatol Clin 10:339–359, 1992.
9. Spinillo A, Pizzoli G, Colonna L, et al: Epidemiologic characteristics of women with idiopathic recurrent vulvovaginal candidiasis. Obstet Gynecol 81:721–727, 1993.
10. White DJ, Johnson EM, Warnock DW: Management of persistent vulvovaginal candidosis due to azole-resistant *Candida glabrata*. Genitourin Med 69:112–114, 1993.

47. Human Papillomavirus Infection

Barbara S. Apgar, M.D., M.S.

I. The Issues

The discovery of the association between human papillomavirus (HPV) and cervical cancer has sparked discussion and debate among clinicians and researchers. The biology of the virus, the risk factors involved in the manifestation of the disease, and the cofactors that alter the host immune response are being actively studied as a means of understanding the oncogenic progression of the virus. The clinical spectrum of HPV-associated disease is highly variable. In clinical practice, emphasis has been placed on a particular subset of patients whose viral expression involves persistence or progression of the virus. As the epidemiology of HPV has been further elucidated, the other subset of patients with no clinical expression of the virus but evidence of the presence of molecular HPV DNA is also receiving attention. Current data support the hypothesis that the spectrum of cervical disease referred to as cervical intraepithelial neoplasia (CIN) comprises histologically distinct entities: low-grade CIN and high-grade CIN. HPV-associated disease alternates between periods of active expression and periods of latency that may be controlled by the strength of the immune system and cofactors that act to promote or discourage viral expression. If HPV-associated disease is to be managed in an intelligent and rational manner, the clinician must understand the unique characteristics of the virus in relation to other sexually transmitted diseases. The patient also must understand the natural history of the virus and the proper method of follow-up. Inherent in this is the understanding of the relation of the virus to high-risk behaviors such as multiple sexual partners and smoking. Patient education is important to avoid unreasonable expectations.

II. The Theory

A. Structure of HPV

1. Papillomaviruses are subgroup of papovaviruses
   a. Very small, nonenveloped DNA viruses
2. Each papillomavirus type is specific for:
   a. Single species (human, bovine, etc.)
   b. Type of epithelium (squamous, columnar)
   c. Anatomic location (skin, lower genital tract, etc.)
3. HPV DNA is cut into open reading frames (ORFs) or sequences of coding for proteins and signals for governing their formation; viral ORFs are divided into:
   a. **Early (E) region** (transcribed early in viral life cycle)
      i. Establishes and maintains viral control over infected cells and initiates viral DNA replication
   b. **Late (L) region**
      i. Involved in capsid (coat of virus) synthesis and virion (coat + DNA) assembly
      ii. Encodes for viral structural proteins that are produced late in viral life cycle when infectious virus is produced
      iii. Transcription from this region appears to be governed by regulators produced only by differentiated cells of intermediate and superficial layers of squamous epithelium
   c. **Upstream regulatory regions (URRs)**
      i. Non-coding region of viral genome important in regulating viral replication and transcription of sequences in early region

B. Types of HPV

1. Large number of distinct HPV types that display significant differences in DNA sequence
2. Specific HPV DNA type is maintained from primary clinical expression to recurrent cancer
   a. May indicate possible persistence of HPV-associated disease or may represent failure to eradicate virus from host tissue

      i. Incubation period after infection with HPV has been theoretically estimated to be 20–50 years in some patients with invasive disease, indicating persistence of the virus in this situation

3. Virus is classified as specific HPV type
   a. Viral types are numbered in order of discovery
   b. > 70 genotypes of HPV have been identified, of which about 30 infect cervix.
      i. Affinity for epidermal or mucosal sources

4. Classification schemes are divided into risk of oncogenic transformation (low, intermediate, high) of host tissue
   a. Invasive cervical neoplasm is much less common than its precursor lesion, squamous intraepithelial lesion (SIL) which is confined to width of epithelium
      i. Over 90% of invasive disease specimens demonstrate presence of HPV DNA
      ii. Preservation in cervical cancer of HPV types identical to high-grade squamous intraepithelial lesion (HGSIL) further supports role of HPV in producing malignant state
         (a) Suggests that high-risk viral types integrated into genome do not regress
         (b) Integration of multiple oncogenic HPV types may confer higher risk of recurrence
      iii. Invasive cervical cancers that are HPV-negative are rare and poorly understood
         (a) May contain HPV types not yet determined or be etiologically distinct group
         (b) May be due to failure of current and old methods of HPV DNA typing to detect low viral copy numbers in invasive cancer

5. **Categorization of viral subtypes by risk**
   a. **Low-risk viral types**
      i. HPV types 6/11, 42, 43, and 44 show no association with invasive cancer
      ii. High rate of regression, low rate of progression
   b. **Intermediate-risk viral types**
      i. HPV types 31, 33, 35, 51, and 52
      ii. Underrepresented in invasive cancers and thus designated as intermediate-risk status
      iii. Do not regress as readily as low-risk viral types
   c. **High-risk viral types**
      i. HPV types 16, 18, 45, and 56 are associated with invasive cancer
         (a) Found in 77.4% of HGSILs and 84.3% of invasive cancers
         (b) If persistent high-grade HPV types are present for many years, risk of eventually showing signs of more serious disease is greater
      ii. Type 16 specifically
         (a) Found commonly in both HGSIL and invasive cancer
         (b) Detected in 47.1% of invasive cancers, 47.1% of HGSILs and 16.2% of LGSILs (low-grade squamous intraepithelial lesions) and 1.5% of cytologically normal women
         (c) HPV 16 in cervical neoplastic tissue also has been found in recurrent disease specimens from same patient
      iii. Type 18
         (a) Detected 2.6 times more commonly in invasive cancer that occurred within 1 year of normal cytologic smear
         (b) Found in adenocarcinomas of the endocervix (glandular neoplasia)

C. **Biology of HPV**
   1. Biologic behavior of HPV is defined in terms of three phases
      a. Replication
         i. Parallels normal mitotic division of host cell
      b. Clinical expression
         i. Highly variable in presentation
         ii. Majority of infected individuals never fully manifest clinical disease by complete viral expression
      c. Latent HPV DNA in absence of clinical expression
         i. Depends on strength of host immune system

2. **Biologic spectrum of HPV**
   a. Viral genome must be transported through superficial and intermediate layers of genital epithelium to nucleus of basal cells, where it is translated and transcribed
   b. Two types of viral-specific proteins are produced
      i. Transforming proteins induce certain host cell functions
      ii. Regulatory proteins control expression of virus
   c. Four phases involved:
      i. **Inoculation phase**
         (a) During sexual intercourse, inoculation occurs at sites of microtrauma throughout lower genital system
         (b) HPV virion (DNA plus its coat or capsid) penetrates to basal layer of epithelium, where it crosses cell membrane
         (c) Virion must shed its coat to cross cell membrane
      ii. **Incubation phase**
         (a) Viral genome (HPV DNA) crosses host cell membrane by means of specific receptors and is rapidly transported to cell nucleus
         (b) Once inside nucleus, virus exists as self-replicating extrachromosomal particle termed an episome
            (i) HPV in precancerous cervical lesions occurs as episomal particle, retaining biologic independence and not joining with host DNA to create permanent mutation
            (ii) Explains regression potential
            (iii) Virus remains in episomal state if cells in basal layer of epithelium remain undifferentiated
            (iv) As episome replicates, it continues to produce additional viral DNA that infects neighboring cells
            (v) Each of episomal viral genomes has capacity to replicate with each mitosis, thus replicating exact viral copy numbers that remain stable over time
         (c) Incubation phase lasts from 6 weeks to 8 months, during which large areas of genital epithelia are colonized or infected with HPV DNA
            (i) This is latent or dormant phase when HPV infection is not clinically apparent
            (ii) No complete virions or completely intact viruses exist
            (iii) Because complete virion must be present to be infectious, it is postulated that HPV cannot be transmitted during latent phase
      iii. **Active expression phase**
         (a) According to host immune system, latent virus may proceed to active expression phase
         (b) Basal layer of epithelium exhibits alterations in cellular growth, intermediate layers exhibit increased viral replication, and mature layers exhibit viral cytopathic effect called koilocytosis or "hollow cells"
            (i) Koilocytes are characterized by chromatin clumping, nuclear atypia, and formation of cytoplasmic vacuolization that appears as perinuclear halo or clearing
            (ii) Koilocytes cannot undergo malignant transformation because viral cytopathic effect occurs only in terminally differentiated cells that are dying or already dead
         (c) Nuclear atypia and enlargement are more specific than koilocytosis and 100% sensitive for predicting HPV infection
            (i) Koilocytosis resulting from HPV infection must demonstrate nuclear enlargement and atypia
            (ii) These features distinguish it from other processes, such as trichomoniasis or estrogen deficiency, that may exhibit nuclear vacuolization without nuclear atypia of squamous cells
         (d) Epithelial and capillary growth can occur during active expression phase

        (e) Virus has now progressed from episomal to productive form dependent on viral–host interaction

            (i) Viral DNA replication occurs independently of host DNA synthesis and occurs primarily in intermediate and superficial layers of squamous epithelium. Large amounts of HPV DNA result in infectious virions.

            (ii) As HPV-infected cells move toward surface, viral capsid proteins are produced, and complete virion is again assembled, thus producing characteristic HPV-cytopathic effects (koilocytosis)

        (f) Clinical manifestations of virus are highly variable during this phase

            (i) Condylomata

            (ii) SIL (low- and high-grade)

    iv. **Host containment phase**

        (a) Characterized by activation of host immune response

        (b) If immunity is impaired, clinical expression of HPV may continue

            (i) Lesions may be treated during this phase

            (ii) Although clinical manifestations may disappear, virus is not destroyed

        (c) If immune system is activated to produce response, viral changes may regress and return to latent or dormant phase

        (d) According to competency of immune system, individual may remain in long-term clinical remission or continue to exhibit sustained or persistent HPV-associated disease or demonstrate recurrences after disease-free interval

        (e) Individuals who show persistence or reactivation of previously inactive disease are most likely to undergo progression of virus

D. **Prevalence of HPV**

    1. HPV DNA has been detected in cytologically normal cervical samples in approximately 6 % of women presenting for routine gynecologic care

      a. Prognostically, about 28 % of HPV-positive women with normal Pap smears develop histologically confirmed CIN.

      b. HPV DNA is rare in postmenopausal women without recent history of abnormal Papanicolaou smear

    2. HPV DNA is very low or zero in virginal women

    3. HPV DNA in pregnant women without history of abnormal cytology have same prevalence as nonpregnant women

    4. Correlation with age

      a. HPV prevalence among cytologically normal women peaks among sexually active women in their 20s and then decreases substantially

        i. Correlates with age of onset of sexual intercourse

        ii. Strongest predictor of HPV positivity—number of sexual partners in last year—tends to increase with age

        iii. Older women may have fewer sexual partners and be exposed to fewer HPV types

      b. Major determinant of severity of HPV cervical precursor lesion is age

        i. Low-grade disease is most common in women in their 20s and represents a transient condition in most

        ii. More than 50% of young women who developed CIN 2–3 did so within 24 months of initial detection of a positive HPV test

        iii. High-grade disease is most common in women in their 30s and 40s

        iv. HPV DNA among women with cervical cancer remains high, regardless of age

        v. Point prevalence of early cytopathic effects (koilocytosis) of HPV infection, marked by types 6 and 11, also declines with age

E. **Cofactors and risks**

    1. HPV may not be sufficient in and of itself to cause malignant transformation

      a. Time interval between inoculation of HPV and occurrence of neoplasia may be several decades

      b. Prevalence of HPV is higher than lifelong risk of developing cervical cancer

2. **Sexual behavior**
   a. Cervical cancer does not occur in women who have never been sexually active
   b. First coitus is independent factor in assessing cancer risk
      i. If primary cause of cervical cancer is HPV, age of first coitus is at least measure of age at first exposure to oncogenic agent
      ii. Not only increases risk of SIL but also associated with both low and high grades of SIL
      iii. Critical age of first coitus seems to vary
         (a) Risk before age of 18 years is particularly damaging to immature squamous epithelium
      iv. Difference of only few years in age at which exposure begins can result in substantial change of risk in later life
   c. Role of male partner
      i. Sexual intercourse may be vehicle for transmitting carcinogenic factor responsible for development of cervical neoplasia
      ii. Mere number of sexual contacts of husband appears to increase risk to his partner only if he has acquired HPV through intercourse
      iii. Subsequent wives of husbands whose previous wives had cervical cancer are at increased risk of cervical cancer
      iv. Male partners of women with cervical cancer have higher number of female partners than male partners of women without cervical cancer
      v. Countries where male sexual promiscuity and use of prostitutes are accepted but wives are expected to be monogamous have high incidence of cervical cancer in wives
      vi. Male's history of multiple sexual partners is associated with increased risk of cancer in his monogamous partner
      vii. HPV acts differently than other STDs in relation to male factor
         (a) It cannot be assumed that condom use protects against HPV spread because HPV is located throughout lower genital system and condoms do not prevent scrotal to vulvar transmission
         (b) It cannot be assumed that if one partner is treated for HPV, the other partner will get better faster or be cured of HPV-associated disease
         (c) It cannot be assumed that HPV disease expression indicates recent exposure
      viii. Role of androscopy
         (a) Not recommended as routine screening test for genital warts in men
            (i) Magnification may be helpful in treating condyloma on male genitalia
         (b) Used to survey male genitalia if atypical condylomata are present
         (c) Treatment of clinical or subclinical condylomata in male has not been shown to decrease viral transmission to female partner

3. **Smoking**
   a. Cigarette smoking is risk factor for CIN 1–3 and invasive cancer
      i. Independent of other risk factors for cervical cancer
      ii. Cumulative risk with increasing smoking exposure
      iii. Risk remains after adjustment for age at first intercourse and number of sexual partners
   b. There is stepwise dose-response relationship between risk and number of cigarettes smoked
      i. Risk is greatest in women < 30 years of age
      ii. Combined risk of smoking and exposure to passive smoke is greater than for either risk alone
   c. Mechanism
      i. Cigarette smoking may act as cofactor that interacts with HPV to initiate carcinogenesis
         (a) Depends on state of Langerhans cells in cervical epithelium
         (b) Women with HPV-associated disease demonstrate fewer Langerhans cells on histologic evaluation than women with normal cervical epithelia

      ii. Constituents of cigarette smoke can be transmitted through blood to distant tissues and organs and have been detected in cervical epithelia of smokers

      iii. Tobacco smoke contains mutagens and carcinogens that may act as initiators, cofactors, or promoters in cervix

      iv. Plasma levels of beta carotene are decreased in cigarette smokers with normal cervical cytology and are further decreased in smokers with CIN

  4. **Hormonal influence**

    a. Pregnancy

      i. Temporary immunosuppression during pregnancy may allow HPV-positive cell to escape from regular immune surveillance

    b. Steroid hormones

      i. Mechanism

        (a) May have promoting effect in inducing expression of viral oncoproteins

        (b) May involve presence and expression of glucocorticoid-responsive element in non-coding region of HPV type 16

        (c) May induce HPV 16 gene expression in cervical keratinocytes directly through 3 hormone response elements in regulatory region of viral genome

        (d) May act by increasing susceptibility of cervical cells to HPV infection

      ii. Oral contraceptive pills (OCPs)

        (a) Possible association between OCPs and HPV has been subject of numerous studies; data continue to be controversial and conflicting because of bias and confounding factors

        (b) Link between OCPs and adenocarcinoma is being investigated.

  5. **Dietary factors**

    a. Folate

      i. Folate nutritional status interacts strongly with established risk factors for SIL such as smoking and OCP use

      ii. Normal levels of folate appear to protect against SIL

      iii. Lowest rate of HPV-16 infection is observed in women with highest levels of red blood folate

      iv. After viral genome has been incorporated into host DNA, folic acid supplements have little or no effect on course of HPV infection

  6. **Immune suppression**

    a. Human immunodeficiency virus (HIV)

      i. SIL occurs more frequently and is more serious in women with HIV infection

        (a) HIV-infected women who are immunocompromised have more advanced SIL, larger cervical lesions, and more associated vulvovaginal condylomata than HIV-negative women

        (b) High rates of persistent and recurrent SIL after standard therapies

        (c) HIV-positive women with CD4 T-cell counts $< 500/mm^3$ have higher rates of recurrence

      ii. Approximately 50% of symptomatic HIV-positive women exhibit SIL on cytology

        (a) HIV prevalence in women with cytologic characteristics of SIL is about 13%

        (b) Papanicolaou smears are adequate for initial evaluation in HIV-infected women

        (c) Severity of SIL does not appear to be associated with age

III. **An Approach**

  A. **Observation of HPV-associated cervical lesions**

    1. Low-grade squamous intraepithelial lesions (LGSILs)

      a. Because LGSILs have high rate of spontaneous regression, observation is acceptable strategy with following exceptions

        i. Patients with poor compliance history

        ii. Immunocompromised patients

      b. National Cancer Institute (NCI) guidelines recommend repeat cytologic testing as alternative to immediate colposcopy
         i. Some clinicians may elect to perform colposcopy after LGSIL is discovered and, if LGSIL is confirmed by biopsy, then follow with cytology and/or cytology and colposcopy
         ii. No definite guidelines on how long to continue to follow patients with LGSIL before considering treatment however treatment should be considered if LGSIL has persisted for 1–2 years
  2. High-grade squamous intraepithelial lesions (HGSILs)
      a. Observation is not recommended for HGSILs
      b. Considered definite cancer precursor; spontaneous regression rate is minimal

B. Cryotherapy of cervical lesions
  1. Indications for use of cryotherapy on cervical transformation zone
      a. All grades of SIL if involvement < 2 quadrants on ectocervix
      b. Criteria for ablative therapy must be met (see Chapter 115)
  2. Cure rates
      a. Diminish as size of lesion increases, especially if > 2 quadrants are involved
      b. May approach 95% if criteria for ablative therapy are followed
      c. After retreatment, cure rates may approach 98%
      d. Lesions at the 3- and 9-o'clock positions have higher degree of inadequate tissue necrosis from cryotherapy because of increased blood supply to these areas from uterine arteries
  3. Treatment guidelines
      a. Cryoprobe should cover entire transformation zone, not just lesion
      b. Double freeze technique is best to obtain adequate cryonecrosis in the 3 and 9 o'clock positions
      c. Destruction to depth of 5–7 mm should eradicate involved gland crypts in over 90% of cases
      d. 5-mm depth of destruction is recommended as appropriate therapy
  4. Follow-up visits
      a. 4, 8, 12, 18, and 24 months after treatment
      b. Visits should include cytologic screening and colposcopy
      c. Most treatment failures are detected within first year after treatment
         i. Failures should be retreated with loop electrosurgical excision

C. Loop electrosurgical excision procedure (LEEP) of cervical lesions
  1. Indications for use of LEEP on cervical transformation zone
      a. All grades of SIL
  2. Cure rates
      a. Over 90% for all grades of SIL
      b. Unlike ablative techniques, LEEP provides specimen for histologic analysis
  3. Treatment guidelines
      a. LEEP is outpatient procedure performed under local anesthesia
      b. Safety for clinician and patient is especially important when electrosurgical equipment is used
         i. Insulated instruments, grounding pad, and smoke evacuator are standard equipment
         ii. Clinician must be aware of power requirements associated with individual electrosurgical unit (ESU)
      c. Standard loop of 2.0 cm × 0.8 cm is capable of excising most transformation zones and allows adequate depth of excision without excessive removal of stromal tissue
         i. Cutting too deep invites excessive blood loss and poor repair
  4. Management of complications
      a. Postoperative stenosis is rare except in postmenopausal patients if the entire excised bed is not fulgurated
      b. Postoperative infection is rare; if it occurs, broad-spectrum antibiotics should be administered

    c. Postoperative bleeding should be managed by fulguration followed by packing of crater with Monsel's paste

    d. Long-term fertility and pregnancy rates after LEEP are unknown, but short-term rates demonstrate no adverse effects

  5. Follow-up visits

    a. Since entire transformation zone is excised, patient can be returned to cytologic surveillance faster than with ablative techniques

    b. Cytology and/or colposcopy at 6 and 12 months

    c. If follow-up visits are normal, patient returns to annual cytologic screening

D. **Laser ablation** of HPV-associated cervical disease

  1. Indications

    a. All grades of SIL

  2. Treatment guidelines

    a. Initial and maintenance costs of laser equipment are high

    b. Laser is ideal treatment for large cervical lesions

      i. 20% of lesions in adolescents extend onto fornix or into vagina

    c. Can be performed in office under local anesthesia

  3. Complications

    a. Postoperative bleeding is most common complication

  4. Follow-up visits

    a. Same as for cryotherapy of cervix

E. **Conization of cervix**

  1. Should be performed in following situations

    a. Colposcopic examination is unsatisfactory

    b. Squamous lesion is deeper than 1 cm in endocervix

    c. Absence of cytologic, colposcopic, and histologic correlation

SUGGESTED READING

1. Azocar J, Abad SMJ, Acosta H, et al: Prevalence of cervical dysplasia and HPV infection according to sexual behavior. Int J Cancer 45:622–625, 1990.
2. Basu J, Palan PR, Vermund SH, et al: Plasma ascorbic acid and beta-carotene levels in women evaluated for HPV infection, smoking and cervix dysplasia. Cancer Detect Prev 15:165–170, 1991.
3. Bauer HM, Ting Y, Greer CE, et al: Genital human papillomavirus infection in female university students as determined by a PCR-based method. JAMA 265:474–477, 1991.
4. Brinton LA: Oral contraceptives and cervical neoplasia. Contraception 43:581–595, 1991.
5. Brisson J: Determinants of persistent detection of human papillomavirus DNA in the uterine cervix. J Infect Dis 173:794–799, 1996.
6. Burnett AF, Grendys EC, Willet GD, et al: Preservation of multiple oncogenic human papillomavirus types in recurrence of early-stage cervical cancers. Am J Obstet Gynecol 170:1230–1233, 1993.
7. Butterworth CE, Hatch KD, Soong SJ, et al: Oral folic acid supplementation for cervical dysplasia: A clinical intervention trial. Am J Obstet Gynecol 166:803–809, 1992.
8. Edebiri AA: Cervical intraepithelial neoplasia: The role of age at first coitus in its etiology. J Reprod Med 35:256–259, 1990.
9. Evander M: Human papillomavirus infection is transient in young women: A population-based cohort study. J Infect Dis 171:1026–1030, 1995.
10. Fruchter RC, Maiman M, Sillman FH, et al: Characteristics of cervical intraepithelial neoplasia in women infected with the human immunodeficiency virus. Am J Obstet Gynecol 171:531–537, 1994.
11. Henry MJ, Stanley MW, Cruikshank S, et al: Association of human immunodeficiency virus–induced immunosuppression with human papillomavirus infection and cervical intraepithelial neoplasia. Am J Obstet Gynecol 160:352–353, 1989.
12. Ho GYF, Burk RD, Klein S, et al: Persistent genital human papillomavirus infection as a risk factor for persistent dysplasia. J Natl Cancer Inst 87:1365–1371, 1995.
13. Kjaer SK, De Villiers EM, Dahl C, et al: Case-control study of risk factors for cervical neoplasia in Denmark. I: Role of the "male factor" in women with one lifetime sexual partner. Int J Cancer 48:39–44, 1991.
14. Kiviat NB, Koutsky LA: Do your current cervical cancer control strategies still make sense? J Natl Cancer Inst 88:3–4, 1996.
15. Koutsky LA, Holmes KK, Critchlow CW, et al: A cohort study of the risk of cervical intraepithelial neoplasias grade 2 or 3 in relation to papillomavirus infection. N Engl J Med 327:1272–1278, 1992.
16. Krebs HB: Treatment of vaginal intraepithelial neoplasia with laser and topical 5-fluorouracil. Obstet Gynecol 73:657–660, 1989.

17. Lorincz AT, Temple GF, Kurman RJ, et al: Oncogenic association of specific human papillomavirus types with cervical neoplasia. J Natl Cancer Inst 79:671–677, 1987.
18. Lorincz AT, Reid R, Jenson AB, et al: Human papillomavirus infection of the cervix: Relative risk associations of 15 common anogenital types. Obstet Gynecol 79:328–337, 1992.
19. Maiman M, Fruchter RG, Serur E, et al: Human immunodeficiency virus infection and cervical neoplasia. Gynecol Oncol 38:377–382, 1990.
20. Matorras R, Ariceta JM, Rementeria A, et al: Human immunodeficiency virus-induced immunosuppression: A risk factor for human papillomavirus infection. Am J Obstet Gynecol 164:442–444, 1991.
21. Melkert PW, Hopman E, van den Brule AJ: Prevalence of HPV in cytomorphologically normal cervical smears, as determined by the polymerase chain reaction is age dependent. Int J Cancer 53:919–922, 1993.
22. Moscicki AB, Palefsky J, Smith G, et al: Variability of human papillomavirus DNA testing in a longitudinal cohort of young women. Obstet Gynecol 82:578–585, 1993.
23. Nasiell K, Roger V, Nasiell M: Behavior of mild cervical dysplasia during long-term follow-up. Obstet Gynecol 67:665–668, 1986.
24. Nuovo GJ, Pedemonte BM: Human papillomavirus types and recurrent cervical warts. JAMA 263:1223–1226, 1990.
25. Palan PR, Romney SL, Mikhail M, et al: Decreased plasma beta-carotene levels in women with uterine cervical dysplasias and cancer. J Natl Cancer Inst 80:454–455, 1988.
26. Parazzini F, La Vecchia, Negri E, et al: Risk factors for cervical intraepithelial neoplasia. Cancer 69:2276–2282, 1992.
27. Pater A, Bayatpour M, Pater MM: Oncogenic transformation by human papillomavirus type 16 deoxyribonucleic acid in the presence of progesterone or progestins from oral contraceptives. Am J Obstet Gynecol 162:1099–1103, 1990.
28. Reid R, Greenberg M, Jenson AB, et al: Sexually transmitted papillomaviral infections. I. The anatomic distribution and pathologic grade of neoplastic lesions associated with different viral types. Am J Obstet Gynecol 156:212–222, 1987.
29. Remmink A, Helmerhorst T, Walboomers JM, et al: HPV in follow-up of patients with cytomorphologically abnormal cervical smears: A prospective nonintervention study. Int J Cancer 61:1–5, 1995.
30. Riou G, Favre M, Jeannel D, et al: Association between poor prognosis in early-stage invasive cervical carcinomas and non-detection of HPV DNA. Lancet 335:1171–1175, 1990.
31. Shen LH, Rushing L, McLachlin CM, et al: Prevalence and histologic significance of cervical human papillomavirus DNA detected in women at low and high risk for cervical neoplasia. Obstet Gynecol 86:499–503, 1995.
32. Schiffman MH: Recent progress in defining the epidemiology of human papillomavirus infection and cervical neoplasia. J Natl Cancer Inst 84:394–398, 1992.
33. Wright TC, Sun XW, Koulos J: Comparison of management algorithms for the evaluation of women with low-grade cytologic abnormalities. Obstet Gynecol 85:202–210, 1995.

48. Lymphogranuloma Venereum

Mark Larson, M.D.

I. The Issues

Lymphogranuloma venereum (LGV) is a rare disease in the United States. The number of reported cases per year is less than 1000. LGV, however, is endemic in Western New Guinea, India, Australia, and the Caribbean. It tends to occur in travelers to endemic areas and their sexual contacts. LGV should be considered in the differential diagnosis of genital ulcer disease and inguinal lymphadenopathy. Because of the small size of the ulcerative lesions, LGV probably poses less of a theoretical risk for human immunodeficiency virus (HIV) transmission than other causes of genital ulcer disease.

II. The Theory

A. **Causative organism:** invasive serovars L1, L2, or L3 of *C. trachomatis*
  1. Classified as bacterium
  2. Obligate intracellular pathogen
B. **Transmission**—primarily through sexual contact

C. **Prevalence**—endemic in tropical regions, travelers to endemic areas
D. **Spectrum of clinical disease**
1. Primary stage
   a. Incubation period: 3 days–3 weeks
   b. Small painless vesicle or nonindurated ulcer or papule on the penis, labia, or vagina
   c. Often unnoticed
2. Secondary stage
   a. Infection spreads via the regional lymphatics
   b. Unilateral or bilateral bubo (tender, firm lymph node collection)
      i. Most common presentation among heterosexual men
      ii. Lymph nodes above and below the inguinal ligament (groove sign)
      iii. 20% have enlarged femoral lymph nodes
      iv. Sinus tract formation
   c. Proctocolitis
      i. Common in women and homosexual men.
   d. Systemic symptoms (hematogenous spread)
3. Tertiary or anorectogenital stage
   a. Inguinal lymphadenopathy resolves after 2–3 months if left untreated
   b. Elephantiasis of penis and scrotum rarely occurs
   c. Rectal stricture, fistulas, perirectal abscesses
III. **An Approach**
A. **Diagnosis**
1. History and clinical presentation
2. Rule out other sexually transmitted diseases (STDs)
3. Culture for *C. trachomatis*
   a. Aspirate lymph node through intact skin to prevent sinus tract formation.
4. Complement fixation (CF) test
   a. CF titer > 1:64 is diagnostic
5. Microimmunofluorescence (micro-IF)
   a. Not readily available
B. **Therapy**
1. Recommended: doxycycline, 100 mg orally twice daily for 21 days
2. Alternatives
   a. Erythromycin, 500 mg orally 4 times/day for 21 days
   b. Sulfisoxazole, 500 mg orally 4 times/day for 21 days
3. Treatment in pregnancy: erythromycin
4. Management of sex partners
   a. Evaluate and treat all persons who have had sexual contact with patient within 30 days before onset of symptoms
C. **Follow-up testing**
1. Treat until resolution of signs and symptoms
2. Consider testing for other STDs

SUGGESTED READING

1. Centers for Disease Control and Prevention: 1998 Guidelines for treatment of sexually transmitted disease. MMWR 47(RR-1):27–28, 1998.
2. Goens JL, Schwartz RA, De Wolf K: Mucocutaneous manifestations of chancroid, lymphogranuloma venereum and granuloma inguinale. Am Fam Physician 49:415–425, 1994.
3. Joseph AK, Rosen T: Laboratory techniques used in the diagnosis of chancroid, granuloma inguinale, and lymphogranuloma venereum. Dermatol Clin 12:1–8, 1994.
4. O'Farrell N, Hooden AA, Coetzee KD, Van den Ende J: Genital ulcer disease: Accuracy of clinical diagnosis and strategies to improve control in Durban, South Africa. Genitourin Med 70:7–11, 1994.

49. Granuloma Inguinale

Mark Larson, M.D.

I. **The Issues**

Granuloma inguinale (donovanosis) is an uncommon cause of genital ulcer disease in the United States. It is, however, quite common in tropical and semitropical regions of the world. It occurs in several stages. Because of various morphologies and sites of infection, clinical diagnosis is difficult. It should be considered in the differential diagnosis of painless genital ulcer disease. It is of significance because genital ulcer disease is a well-established risk factor for human immunodeficiency virus (HIV) transmission.

II. **The Theory**
  A. **Causative organism:** *Calymmatobacterium granulomatis*, intracellular gram-negative rod
  B. **Transmission**—primarily through sexual contact
  C. **Prevalence**—endemic in tropical and subtropical regions
  D. **Spectrum of clinical disease**
      1. Painless, irregular, clean-based, granulomatous genital ulcer
      2. Incubation period: 8–80 days
      3. Nodular or hypertrophic
      4. Mutilating, ulcerodestructive process
      5. No enlarged lymph nodes
      6. Untreated disease may result in lymphatic obstruction

III. **An Approach**
  A. **Diagnosis**
      1. History and clinical presentation
      2. Rule out other sexually transmitted diseases (STDs)
      3. Punch biopsy of peripheral granulation tissue.
          a. Wright-Giemsa stain
          b. Intracytoplasmic inclusion bodies (Donovan bodies) within histiocytes
          c. Short, pleomorphic gram-negative rods with bipolar staining
          d. Leishmaniasis, rhinoscleroma, and histoplasmosis have smaller inclusions
      4. Serum complement fixing antibodies
      5. Positive skin reaction to intradermal Donovan antigen
  B. **Therapy**
      1. Continue treatment until all lesions have completely healed, for a minimum of 3 weeks
      2. Recommended
          a. Trimethoprim-sulfamethoxazole, 160/800 mg orally twice daily
             or
          b. Doxycycline, 100 mg orally twice daily
      3. Alternatives
          a. Ciprofloxacin, 750 mg orally twice daily
          b. Erythromycin, 500 mg orally 4 times/day
      4. Add aminoglycoside if lesions are not responding
      5. Treatment in pregnancy: erythromycin
      6. Management of sex partners
          a. Evaluate and treat all persons who have had sexual contact with patient within 60 days before onset of symptoms and have signs and symptoms of disease.

SUGGESTED READING

1. Centers for Disease Control and Prevention: 1998 Guidelines for treatment of sexually transmitted disease. MMWR 47(RR-1):26–27, 1998.
2. Goens JL, Schwartz RA, De Wolf K: Mucocutaneous manifestations of chancroid, lymphogranuloma venereum, and granuloma inguinale. Am Fam Physician 49:415–425, 1994.

3. Joseph AK, Rosen T: Laboratory techniques used in the diagnosis of chancroid, granuloma inguinale, and lymphogranuloma venereum. Dermatol Clin 12:1–8, 1994.
4. O'Farrell N, Hooden AA, Coetzee KD, Van den Ende J: Genital ulcer disease: Accuracy of clinical diagnosis and strategies to improve control in Durban, South Africa. Genitourin Med 70:7–11, 1994.
5. Rauman C, Sarma PS, Ghorpade A, Das M: Treatment of donovanosis with norfloxacin. Int J Dermatol 29:298–299, 1990.

50. Chancroid

Mark Larson, M.D.

I. The Issues

Chancroid is a cause of painful genital ulcer disease (GUD). It is endemic in many areas of the United States and the world. In some parts of the world it is the most common cause of GUD. It is important because genital ulcers, especially those caused by Haemophilus ducreyi, enhance transmission of human immunodeficiency virus (HIV). The recent rise in syphilis and chancroid in the U.S. is associated with drug use, urban poverty, and prostitution.

II. The Theory

  A. **Causative organism:** *Haemophilus ducreyi*, gram-negative streptobacillus

  B. **Transmission**—sexual

  C. **Prevalence**

    1. Endemic

      a. Tropical and semitropical regions

      b. Southern Florida and New York City

    2. Uncommon in other areas of U.S.

    3. Underreported because of difficulty of culture

III. An Approach

  A. **History**

    1. GUD

      a. Cofactor for HIV transmission

      b. Particular attenuation with chancroid infection

      c. 10% coinfected with *Treponema pallidum* or HSV

    2. Incubation period: 4–5 days

  B. **Physical exam**

    1. Painful genital ulcer

      a. Tender inguinal lymphadenopathy

      b. Deep ulcer with soft consistency

    2. Lesions resolve

    3. Lymphatic blockage may occur

  C. **Diagnosis**

    1. Culture for *Haemophilus ducreyi*

      a. Special culture media, difficult

      b. Gram-negative streptobacillus in chains/clusters

        i. "School of fish" appearance

    2. Probable diagnosis

      a. Painful genital ulcer(s) with tender inguinal lymphadenopathy

      b. No evidence of *T. pallidum*

      c. No evidence of HSV

  D. **Therapy**

    1. Recommended regimen

      a. Azithromycin, 1 g orally × 1

      b. Ceftriaxone, 250 mg intramuscularly × 1

      c. Erythromycin base, 500 mg orally 4 times/day for 7 days

    d. Ciprofloxacin, 500 mg orally twice daily for 3 days
        i. Contraindicated for pregnant and lactating women and for children < 17 years old

E. **Follow-up**
1. Reexamine in 3–7 days
    a. Ulcers should show improvement
2. If no improvement, consider:
    a. Correct diagnosis?
    b. Coinfection
        i. Other STD
        ii. HIV
    c. Noncompliance?
    d. Resistant *H. ducreyi*?
        i. Consider *in vitro* testing
    e. Consider needle aspiration of lymphadenopathy
3. Test for HIV and syphilis at diagnosis and at 3 months

F. **Sexual contacts**
1. Sexual contacts within 10 days before onset of symptoms should be examined and treated

G. **Pregnancy**
1. Safety of azithromycin not established

H. **HIV-positive patients**
1. Follow closely
2. Longer course of therapy
3. Healing may be slower
4. Increased frequency of coexistent HSV
5. Suggest 7-day erythromycin therapy

SUGGESTED READING

1. Centers for Disease Control and Prevention: 1998 Guidelines for treatment of sexually transmitted disease. MMWR 47(RR-1):27–28, 1998.
2. Goens JL, Schwartz RA, De Wolf K: Mucocutaneous manifestations of chancroid, lymphogranuloma venereum and granuloma inguinale. Am Fam Physician 49:415–425, 1994.
3. Joseph AK, Rosen T: Laboratory techniques used in the diagnosis of chancroid, granuloma inguinale, and lymphogranuloma venereum. Dermatol Clin 12:1–8, 1994.
4. Levine WC, Berg AO, Johnson RE, et al: Development of sexually transmitted diseases treatment guidelines. Sex Transm Dis 21(Suppl 2):S96–S101, 1994.
5. Martin DH, Di Carlo RP: Recent changes in the epidemiology of genital ulcer disease in the United States. The crack cocaine connection. Sex Transm Dis 21(Suppl 2):S76–S80, 1994.
6. O'Farrell N, Hooden AA, Coetzee KD, Van den Ende J: Genital ulcer disease: Accuracy of clinical diagnosis and strategies to improve control in Durban, South Africa. Genitourin Med 70:7–11, 1994.
7. Perine PL: Sexually transmitted diseases in the tropics. Med J Aust 160:358–366, 1994.
8. Roggen EL, Hoofd G, Van Dyck E, Piot P: Enzyme immunoassays (EIAs) for the detection of anti-*Haemophilus ducreyi* serum IgA, IgG, and IgM antibodies. Sex Transm Dis 21:36–42, 1994.
9. Thomas DL, Quinn TC: Serologic testing for sexually transmitted diseases. Infect Dis Clin North Am 7:793–824, 1993.

51. Scabies

Mark Larson, M.D.

I. The Issues

Scabies has been known as a cause of pruritic rash since Biblical times. It is caused by a mite with 8 short legs that can move at a rate of 25 mm/minute. It survives solely in human skin, burrowing in the stratum corneum. The predominant symptom is pruritus. The body mounts a cell-mediated and humoral immune hypersensitivity response to the mite's saliva and feces. Initially the response takes 4–6 weeks but occurs within 24 hours in subsequent infections. The papular, pruritic eruption is of immune origin and bears no relation to location of the mites; it may cause burrows, vesicles, and chronic nodules. Norwegian (crusted) scabies may occur when the immune response is impaired (e.g., by human immunodeficiency virus [HIV]).

II. The Theory

A. **Causative organism:** *Sarcoptes scabiei*

B. **Transmission**
1. Direct contact
2. Fomite
   a. Mites < 2 days off host
3. Crowded conditions
4. Nosocomial
5. Secondary attack rate 38% among household contacts

C. **Prevalence**
1. Incidence of 2–5%
2. Seen often in immigrant children
3. 300 million cases/year worldwide
4. Most common in people younger than 40 years

D. **Spectrum of clinical disease**
1. Intense pruritus
   a. Worse at night or after hot shower
2. Symmetric, papulovesicular lesions, 2–3 mm in diameter, accompanied by macules, pustules, scaly plaques
3. 3–15-mm burrows
4. Location
   a. Flexor surfaces of wrists and dorsal surfaces of interdigital spaces in two-thirds of patients
   b. Breasts, periumbilicus, belt line, buttocks, thighs, penis, scrotum, elbows, feet, ankles, anterior axillary folds
   c. Infants and children
      i. Any skin surface
      ii. Often bullous
5. Norwegian scabies
   a. Highly infectious
   b. No itching
6. Zoonotic scabies
   a. Shorter incubation period
   b. Self-limited, will not live in human skin
   c. Papulovesicular, erythematous, pruritic
   d. Bleeding from excoriated lesions

III. An Approach

A. **Diagnosis**
1. High index of suspicion
   a. Often rash is not characteristic
   b. Trial of therapy may be warranted

2. Definitive diagnosis
   a. Observation of mites, scybala, or eggs
   b. Epidermal shave biopsy or scraping
      i. Sterile mineral oil at edge of suspected burrow
      ii. Scrape with no. 15 blade
      iii. Examine microscopically
3. Probable diagnosis
   a. Burrows
      i. Web spaces
      ii. Ink test: apply, penetrate burrows
      iii. Liquid tetracycline followed by alcohol results in yellow-gray fluorescence with Wood's lamp
B. **Therapy**
   1. **Recommended**
      a. Permethrin cream 5% (Nix)
         i. Applied to all areas of body from neck down and washed off after 8–14 hours
   2. **Alternative**
      a. Lindane 1% (Kwell)
         i. Apply 1 oz of lotion or 30 g of cream to entire body except face and scalp for 8 hours; wash off thoroughly; reapply to hands if washed
         ii. Low incidence of side effects, which include neurotoxicity, seizures, aplastic anemia
         iii. Should not be used following bath, in persons with extensive dermatitis, pregnant or lactating women, or children younger than 2 years
         iv. Resistance has developed in some areas
      b. Sulfur (6%)
         i. Apply thinly to all areas for 3 nights. Wash between applications.
      c. Ivermectin
         i. Single oral dose 200 µg/kg or 0.8% topical
         ii. No controlled clinical trials.
   3. **Other management**
      a. Wash clothing and bed linens in hot water or remove from body contact at least 72 hours; fumigation not necessary
      b. Pruritus: Calamine lotion, antihistamines, short course of steroids
      c. Secondary bacterial superinfection: topical or systemic antibiotics
      d. Consider simultaneous treatment of entire populations in closed communities (e.g., nursing homes) to control infection
      e. Sexual contacts should be examined and treated
C. **Follow-up**
   1. Pruritus may continue for weeks
   2. Consider retreatment with other regimen
D. **Pregnancy, infants and young children**
   1. Permethrin
E. **HIV-infected patients**
   1. Same treatment as for other persons
   2. Increased risk for Norwegian scabies

SUGGESTED READING

1. Centers for Disease Control and Prevention: 1998 Guidelines for treatment of sexually transmitted disease. MMWR 47(RR-1):106–108, 1998.
2. Billstein SA, Mattaliano VJ: The "nuisance" sexually transmitted diseases: Molluscum contagiosum, scabies, and crab lice. Med Clin 74:1487–1505, 1990.
3. Commens CA: We can get rid of scabies: New treatment available soon. Med J Aust 161:317–318, 1994.
4. Fraser J: Permethrin: A top-end viewpoint and experience. Med J Aust 160:806, 1994.
5. Lawrence GW, Sheridan JW, Speare R: We can get rid of scabies: New treatment available soon. Med J Aust 161:232, 1994.

6. Mellanby K: Scabies. London, Oxford University Press, 1943.
7. Schlesinger I, Oelrich M, Tyring SK: Crusted (Norwegian) scabies in patients with AIDS: The range of clinical presentations. South Med J 87:352–356, 1994.
8. Spielman A, Wachtel M: Insects and mites. In Gorbach SL, Bartlett JG, Blacklow NR (eds): Infectious Diseases. Philadelphia, W.B. Saunders, 1992, pp 2037–2039.

52. Molluscum Contagiosum

Mark Larson, M.D.

I. **The Issues**

Molluscum contagiosum is a self-limited cutaneous disease occurring mostly in children and young adults. Humans are believed to be the only hosts for the molluscum contagiosum virus (MCV). Adults with molluscum contagiosum and their partners should be evaluated for other sexually transmitted diseases (STDs). Although molluscum contagiosum in children is usually transmitted nonsexually, the index of suspicion for sexual abuse should be high.

II. **The Theory**
   A. **Causative organism:** MCV
      1. Double-stranded DNA virus
      2. Family: Poxviridae
      3. Intracellular parasite that infects epidermal cells
      4. Two strains: MCV1 and MCV2
   B. **Transmission**
      1. Children: usually nonsexually via direct skin contact
      2. Adults: sexual or nonsexual contact
   C. **Prevalence**
      1. Occurs worldwide
      2. More common in tropical and subtropical regions
      3. Disease of children and young adults
   D. **Spectrum of clinical disease**
      1. Self-limited, benign cutaneous infection
      2. Waxy, smooth spherical papules; umbilicated apex contains central plug
      3. Usually asymptomatic
      4. Molluscum dermatitis: inflammatory reaction in 10% of patients
      5. Location
         a. Children: trunk and extremities
         b. Adults: lower abdominal wall, inner thighs, pubic area, genitalia

III. **An Approach**
   A. **Diagnosis**
      1. Clinical diagnosis
      2. Biopsy: molluscum bodies (cytoplasmic inclusions)
      3. Differential diagnosis: varicella, milia, Darier's disease, lichen planus, histiocytoma, basal cell epithelioma, warts, keratocanthomas, subepidermal fibrosis, dermatitis herpetiformis
   B. **Therapy**
      1. Evaluate adults for other STDs
      2. Watchful waiting is indicated
         a. Lesions may resolve spontaneously after few months
         b. If lesions do not resolve, treatment may be indicated
         c. All active treatments leave scarring
            i. Patients must give informed consent
      3. Lesion removal
         a. Curettage or electrodessication

b. Entire lesion is easier to remove with electrodessication
c. Destruction of base required to remove all infected tissue
    i. Cryotherapy, phenol, silver nitrate, TCA, podophyllum, Condylox, canthari-
       dine, and Retin-A all can be used to destroy base
4. Counseling
    a. Lesions occur secondary to close contact
    b. Usually an STD in young adults

SUGGESTED READING

1. Billstein SA, Mattaliano VJ: The "nuisance" sexually transmitted diseases: Molluscum contagiosum, scabies, and crab lice. Med Clin 74:1487–1505, 1990.
2. Brown ST, Nalley JF, Kraus SJ: Molluscum contagiosum. Sex Transm Dis 8:227–234, 1981.
3. Feldman YM, Nikitas JA: Sexually transmitted molluscum contagiosum. Dermatol Clin 1:103–110, 1983.
4. Margolis S: Genital warts and molluscum contagiosum. Urol Clin North Am 11:163–170, 1984.
5. Postlethwaite R: Molluscum contagiosum: A review. Arch Environ Health 21:432–452, 1970.
6. Smith MA, Singer C: Sexually transmitted viruses other than HIV and papillomavirus. Urol Clin North
   Am 19:47–62, 1992.

53. Pediculosis Pubis

Mark Larson, M.D.

I. **The Issues**

Pediculosis pubis (crab louse) is one of three species of lice that infest humans. The infection can
be intensely uncomfortable, but rarely has long-term sequelae.

II. **The Theory**
   A. **Causative organism:** *Pediculosis pubis* (crab louse)
      1. 1-mm long, with 3 pairs of large legs and crab-like appearance
      2. Claws of pubic lice match diameter of pubic and axillary hair; thus they are found in
         other areas of body
      3. Survival of louse depends on human blood
   B. **Transmission**
      1. Person to person through intimate contact
      2. Fomite transmission less common because of shorter life span (24 hours) and de-
         creased movement compared with other species of lice
   C. **Prevalence**
      1. 3 million cases/year in U.S.
      2. Highest incidence: single persons 15–25 years old
   D. **Spectrum of clinical disease**
      1. May be asymptomatic
      2. Allergic sensitization occurs within 5 days
         a. Pruritus
         b. Scratching, erythema, irritation
         c. Mild fever, malaise, irritability
         d. Immunity
         e. Superinfection
      3. Lice on pubic hair
III. **An Approach**
   A. **Diagnosis**
      1. Careful history
      2. Consider lice infestation
      3. Examine for lice and nits
      4. Verify microscopically

B. **Therapy**
   1. All drugs listed are relatively effective; choice depends on availability and cost
      b. Permethrin 1% creme rinse (Nix)
         i. Apply to affected areas; wash off after 10 minutes
         ii. Less potential toxicity.
      a. Lindane 1% shampoo (Kwell)
         i. Apply to affected areas; wash off after 4 minutes
         ii. Not recommended for pregnant, lactating women or children under 2 years
         iii. Least expensive
         iv. Toxicity (seizure, aplastic anemia) not noted with 4-minute treatment
      c. Pyrethrins with piperonyl butoxide (Rid, Triple X, A-200, Pyrinate shampoo, BARC)
         i. Apply to affected areas; wash off after 10 minutes
   2. **Pregnancy:** permethrin or pyrethrins with piperonyl butoxide
   3. Eyebrows: Apply occlusive petroleum jelly twice daily for 10 days
   4. Bedding and clothing: Wash in hot water
      a. Nonwashable items: Insecticides that contain pyrethrin-piperonyl butoxide
   5. Treat sexual partners within last month
   6. HIV infection: same treatment
C. **Follow-up**
   1. Evaluate after 1 week if symptoms persist
   2. Retreat with alternative regimen
   3. Consider testing for other STDs
   4. Consider sexual abuse

SUGGESTED READING

1. Centers for Disease Control and Prevention: 1998 Guidelines for treatment of sexually transmitted disease. MMWR 47(RR-1):105–106, 1998.
2. Billstein SA, Mattaliano VJ: The "nuisance" sexually transmitted diseases: Molluscum contagiosum, scabies, and crab lice. Med Clin 74:1487–1505, 1990.
3. Imandeh NG: Prevalence of *Pthirus pubis* (Anoplura, Pediculidae) among sex workers in urban Jos, Nigeria. Appl Parasitol 34:275–277, 1993.
4. Klaus S, Shvil Y, Mumcuoglu KY: Generalized infestation of a 3½-year-old girl with the pubic louse. Pediatr Dermatol 11:261–128, 1994.

54. Human Immunodeficiency Virus Disease

Bruce E. Johnson, M.D.

I. **The Issues**

The pervasive spread of disease caused by the human immunodeficiency virus (HIV) can be viewed only as a distressing and depressing tragedy. Originally identified in 1981, infection with this virus now ranks as one of the major worldwide public health challenges for the foreseeable future. In this country, especially worrisome is the pattern of disease in women. Demographics document increasing incidence in women, especially black and Hispanic women. Treatment of HIV disease has made incredible strides in recent years, with deaths from AIDS down discernibly. Even so, prevention remains the cornerstone to any future impact on overall disease load and current trends do not hold great optimism for long-term reduction in new infection. Women are involved in a key role for prevention of transmission of disease to the next generation. The issues involved in HIV infection and AIDS are voluminous; this chapter focuses on issues frequently encountered by the primary care practitioner. Details of therapy for HIV infection itself, as well as complicating diseases, is changing rapidly and becoming more complex. This chapter will outline important issues for the generalist who chooses to remain

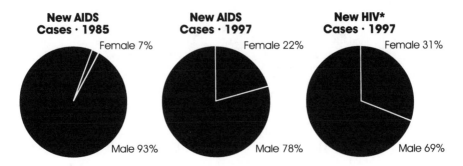

FIGURE 1.   Women are increasingly affected by HIV/AIDS.

involved in the care of HIV-positive patients, but also chooses to leave the details of therapy to specialist colleagues.

II. **The Theory**
   A. **Demographics** (Figs. 1 and 2)
      1. Nationwide, rise in new cases of AIDS in both sexes has moderated, with substantial decline in new cases among homosexual men
      2. Subgroups, however, demonstrate persistent increase incidence
        a. In 1985, women accounted for only 7% of all new cases of HIV; now, the 120,000–160,000 women with HIV account for 22% of all new cases
          i. In 1997, women registered a 3% increase in new cases, while men showed a 3% decline
        b. Increased cases among heterosexual women, especially among black and Hispanic women who account for 75% of all females with HIV
      3. As of December 1997, CDC identified > 640,000 cases of AIDS
        a. Fatalities number > 390,000
        b. For many subgroups, e.g., teenagers and young adults, AIDS is the single most important cause of death after accidents
      4. Important not to lose sight of dramatic fall in AIDS deaths attributed to introduction of multidrug antiretroviral therapy
        a. Since 1996, deaths from AIDS have fallen by 25%
   B. **Microbiology of HIV**
      1. RNA retrovirus

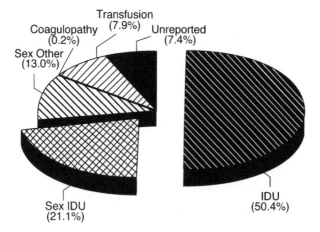

FIGURE 2.   AIDS in women by exposure category. IDU = intravenous drug user. (From Centers for Disease Control and Prevention, January 1992.)

     a. Gains entry to cell through CD4 receptor on T-cell, transcribes genomic RNA into DNA, and integrates into DNA of host cell (process called reverse transcription)

     b. Remains as provirus for life of host cell

        i. Signal for active replication unclear but latent period can last greater than 10 years

     c. Replicates within cell, using host resources

        i. Uses host cell DNA as template to form RNA virus

     d. Cell death occurs after budding of huge numbers of HIV disrupts cell membrane, releasing RNA virus into blood

  2. Preference for human T-cells

     a. Remains dormant in T-cells, often those in lymph nodes

        i. Multiple signals to begin replication include mitogens, antigens, cytokines, and stimulating factors

     b. T-cells circulate in blood and can be measured

        i. Measurement of T-cells with CD4 receptors on surface referred to as CD4 count

     c. Disease becomes more symptomatic as population of CD4 T-cells drops

        i. T-cells important to cell-mediated immunity; as number of T-cells drops, opportunistic infections more likely

       ii. CD4 count can have direct relation to risk of infection

C. **Disease exposure**

  1. Most women infected from one of two sources (Fig. 2)

     a. Sex with HIV-positive man (partner or sex for money)

     b. Intravenous drug use

        i. Multiple use of needles

       ii. Sex for money to support drug habit

     c. Other exposure to HIV widely publicized but less common

        i. Health care workers, emergency care workers, lab workers, casual contacts

     d. Virtually no transmission through nation's blood supply since 1985

  2. HIV found in many body fluids

     a. Blood, semen, vaginal secretions, breast milk

     b. Detected in tears and saliva, but transmission through these routes is rare

  3. Transmission of HIV easier from male to female than from female to male

     a. Suspect that microabrasions with vaginal intercourse provide entry to HIV present in semen

     b. Anal intercourse likely to produce abrasions

     c. Vaginal/cervical disease (e.g., cervicitis) or inflammation also provides site of entry

        i. Frequent finding with multiple sexual partners

       ii. Explains association between HIV disease and syphilis, genital ulcers, and other mucosa-damaging conditions

  4. IV drug use in minority communities related to rise of HIV positivity in minority women

     a. Both as IVDUs themselves and as sexual partners to HIV-positive IVDU men

D. **Natural history of disease**

  1. After exposure, person may be asymptomatic, or develop acute illness

     a. Acute illness occurs 1–6 weeks after infection presenting as "viral infection" with fever, arthralgia, myalgia, rash, diarrhea, aseptic meningitis, night sweats, oral or genital ulcers

     b. Recovery expected; patient enters asymptomatic phase

     c. High index of suspicion in patients at risk for HIV

        i. One site for identification of HIV carriers is in STD clinics as the practices leading to STDs are the same high-risk practices as HIV

  2. Asymptomatic phase lasts up to 8–10 years

     a. Evidence of deterioration of immune status may be seen within 3 years, characteristically by fall in CD4 count

  3. Complex of symptoms presages AIDS in untreated women

      a. Typically occurs as CD4 count drops below 200

      b. May be constitutional (e.g., unexplained fever, weight loss, fatigue, rash, diarrhea)

  4. AIDS-defining disease includes infection with parasite (e.g., *Pneumocystis*), virus (e.g., cytomegalovirus), fungus (e.g., *Cryptococcus*), mycobacterium, or neoplasm (e.g., Kaposi's sarcoma) in HIV-positive person

      a. Of particular import are specific diseases in women

         i. Recurrent candidal or other vaginal infections

         ii. Cervical cancer

  5. Early infections frequently treatable, especially if CD4 count > 200

      a. With CD4 count < 50, debilitating infections (e.g., fungal and mycobacterial) ensue

  6. Entire focus of disease has changed in past decade with multidrug therapies

      a. Life expectancy prolonged, especially asymptomatic phase

  7. Progression of disease, characterized by wasting, fever, fatigue, skin rashes, diarrhea, and neurologic disease, including progressive dementia

E. Prevention

  1. Must focus on education and counseling, especially for following target groups

      a. Women in low socioeconomic groups

      b. Women with multiple sexual partners

      c. Adolescents and young adult women

      d. Women who engage in sex trade

      e. IVDUs

  2. Reduction of risk factors

  3. Safe sexual practices

  4. Intervention in IV drug use practices

  5. Use of barrier methods to prevent transmission

  6. Continued surveillance of blood supply

      a. Early in epidemic, detection not available

      b. Some infections from tainted blood, especially in hemophilia, surgeries with high blood usage (e.g., cardiac surgery)

  7. Prevention practices by health care workers, emergency care personnel, lab workers

F. Treatment (Table 1)

  1. **Non-nucleoside reverse transcriptase inhibitors**

      a. Inhibit action of reverse transcriptase, which converts single-stranded RNA to double-stranded DNA

  2. **Nucleoside reverse transcriptase inhibitors**

      a. Similar action but at the next step from the non-nucleoside reverse transcriptase inhibitors

  3. **Protease inhibitors**

      a. Prevents packaging of newly manufactured viral protein into infectious virions

  4. These three antiretroviral agents have revolutionized therapy of HIV disease such that goal realistically can be to suppress viral RNA production to undetectable levels

  5. Unfortunately, women often have poorer prognosis, even with treatment, than men

      a. May be related to other pressures, especially care for children, or self-denial

      b. With family/home concerns, have trouble coordinating care, following treatment regimen, obtaining social services

TABLE 1. Antiretroviral Drugs (available in early 1998)

Non-nucleoside reverse transcriptase inhibitors (NNRTIs)	Protease inhibitors
Nevirapine (Viramune)	Saquinavir (Fortovase)
Delavirdine mesylate (Rescriptor)	Ritonavir (Norvir)
Nucleoside reverse transcriptase inhibitors (NRTIs)	Indinavir sulfate (Crixivan)
Zidovudine (AZT) (Retrovir)	Nelfinavir mesylate (Viracept)
Didanosine (ddI) (Videx)	
Zalcitabine (ddC) (Hivid)	
Stavudine (d4T) (Zerit)	
Lamivudine (3TC) (Epivir)	

  6. Specific treatment regimens for antiretroviral agents, as well as therapy of opportunistic infections, beyond scope of this chapter

III. **An Approach**
  A. **Prevention**
    1. **Education**
      a. Widespread, explicit, matter of fact
        i. Education directed toward population at risk
          (a) Example of success—promotion of condom use among prostitutes
        ii. Specifically include education directed toward adolescents and women in high-risk settings
          (a) Sexually transmitted disease (STD) clinics, IVDU treatment centers, spouse abuse shelters
      b. Must be continuous and ongoing
        i. Relapse among previously compliant groups
          (a) Loss of urgency
          (b) New circumstances (e.g., new lover)
          (c) New members of population (e.g., young who have not yet been intensively educated)
    2. **Reduction of risk factors**
      a. IV drug use intervention
        i. Use of clean needles (or use of bleach)
        ii. Do not use needles of others
        iii. Assistance and treatment to stop IV drug use
      b. Avoidance of unprotected sex with HIV-positive partners
        i. Especially for sexual partners of IVDUs
          (a) Estimated HIV prevalence among IVDUs in New York is 60%
        ii. Multiple sex partners, including prostitutes
      c. Encourage abstinence among sexually inactive
      d. Safe sex for women requires use of condoms
        i. Latex condoms
          (a) Natural (sheep) condoms may allow passage of virus through sheath
        ii. Proper application of condoms
          (a) Requires forthright instruction
          (b) Applied early; remains on penis after withdrawal
          (c) Used for vaginal, oral, and anal sex
        iii. In some circles it now is considered appropriate for women to buy and carry condoms in case partner "forgets"
          (a) Advertising in women's magazines
        iv. Female condom an alternative
    3. **Identification and follow-up of contacts**
      a. Classic public health measures
        i. Unfortunately, HIV positivity not reportable disease in almost half states in U.S.; AIDS is reportable, but not positive HIV test
      b. Relatively high rate of HIV among persons with STD may make STD a marker condition, focusing testing in this group
    4. **Continued assurance of safety of blood supply**
      a. Questionnaires of donors
      b. Testing of all units for HIV antibody
    5. **Protective measures for emergency and medical personnel** in contact with potentially HIV-positive persons
      a. Gloves, special clothing, masks, facial barriers
  B. **Diagnosis and identification of HIV disease**
    1. Virus remains dormant without disease for many years; identification in asymptomatic phase depends on testing for antibody
    2. Antibody test is enzyme-linked immunosorbent assay (ELISA) directed against HIV antibody
      a. Both sensitivity and specificity > 99%

    b. Repeat ELISA test for suspected false-positives
        i. If positive again, perform Western blot
            (a) Directed against specific viral coat proteins
            (b) Considered confirmatory, with rare false-positives
    c. False-positive ELISA test may occur during other viral illnesses (e.g., herpes zoster) and after certain viral immunizations, including influenza
    d. False-negatives may occur in end-stage AIDS (body cannot produce antibody), shortly after infection (not enough time to build antibody titers), and infrequently with paraprotein diseases

3. Quantitatiave HIV RNA levels can be directly measured
    a. Two technologies—branched DNA (bDNA) and reverse transcriptase–initiated polymerase chain reaction (RT-PCR)
    b. RT-PCR levels tend to run twice bDNA
        i. Both tests accurate but must run all tests in same patient using same technique to maintain consistency
    c. As of 1998, only RT-PCR has FDA approval—most recommendations assume RT-PCR technology

4. Counseling must accompany testing
    a. Prepare to advise low-risk persons about meaning of false-positives
        i. Advise caution if result is positive
        ii. Deflect anxiety while awaiting confirmatory tests
    b. Prepare to counsel high-risk persons about positive results
        i. Explain expected steps to confirm
        ii. Natural history of disease
        iii. Potential treatments
        iv. Offer hope in face of devastating diagnosis

5. Current testing of high-risk, asymptomatic population largely voluntary
    a. Populations may be targeted but not compelled to take test
        i. Examples: STD clinics, jails and prisons, IVDU treatment centers
    b. Many states require discussion of HIV testing for all pregnant women but leave final decision regarding testing to the patient
        i. Multiple opinions favor voluntary testing for fear that some women, who believe themselves to be at high risk, will not present for prenatal care to avoid HIV test

6. Differential use of CD4 count and HIV RNA level
    a. HIV RNA level used to start, or modify, retroviral therapy
    b. CD4 count used to begin prophylaxis for opportunistic infections

7. Once CD4 count falls low enough, patient at risk for development of "defining disease" (CDC nomenclature)
    a. Defining disease usually opportunistic infection (Table 2)
        i. In certain geographic areas, defining disease may not be unusual (e.g., coccidioidomycosis in Southwest, histoplasmosis in Midwest)
    b. Persistent diarrhea, > 1 month, without other cause, may be "defining disease"
    c. Defining disease may be neoplasm
        i. Cervical cancer
        ii. Kaposi's sarcoma
        iii. Other neoplasms, such as B-cell lymphomas, typically develop late in HIV disease

TABLE 2. Microorganisms that Take Advantage of T-cell Defects

Parasites	Fungi	Bacteria	Viruses
Pneumocystis	*Candida*	*Mycobacterium tuberculosis*	Cytomegalovirus
Toxoplasma	*Cryptococcus*	*M. avium-intracellulare*	Herpes simplex virus
Cryptosporidium	*Histoplasma*	*Salmonella*	Varicella zoster virus
Isospora	*Coccidioides*		
Microspora			

    d. Defining disease may be persistence or aggressiveness of "common" female disorders

        i. Recurrent vaginal candidiasis in high-risk women

        ii. Rapidly progressive cervical cancer

        iii. Widespread, aggressive herpes genitalis

        iv. Human papillomavirus (HPV) disease with cervical dysplasia, condyloma acuminatum

    e. Presence or suspicion of defining disease must prompt testing for HIV (if not already done)

    f. Combination of HIV seropositivity and defining disease meets CDC criteria for AIDS—at this point, disease must be reported to health departments in all 50 states and true prevalence figures generated

C. **Primary care of HIV-positive patients**

  1. **Initial medical examination**

    a. **History**

        i. Constitutional symptoms such as fever, fatigue, loss of appetite, weight loss

        ii. Risky behavior (e.g., multiple partners, IV drug use, hepatitis)

        iii. Gynecologic history, including STDs, cervical disease (colposcopy, treatment)

        iv. Contraceptive practices

    b. **Physical exam**

        i. Vital signs, including weight

        ii. Skin

          (a) Rashes, infections, lesions

        iii. Eyes

          (a) CMV retinitis, AIDS microangiopathy (resembles diabetic retinopathy)

        iv. Mouth

          (a) Thrush, aphthous ulcers

        v. Lymph nodes

          (a) Large nodes or "crops" suggest active HIV replication and advancing disease

        vi. Genitalia

          (a) Vaginal discharge, ulcers, chancre, condyloma

          (b) Cervical changes (Papanicolaou smear)

          (c) Evidence of pelvic inflammatory disease

    c. **Laboratory tests**

        i. Complete blood count with differential, blood chemistry (with liver enzymes)

        ii. Urinalysis

        iii. Chest radiograph (as baseline)

        iv. Cultures for gonorrhea, chlamydia

        v. Screening tests

          (a) Venereal Disease Research Laboratory (VDRL) test for syphilis

            (i) If positive, treat with higher doses of penicillin than in immunocompetent patients

          (b) Hepatitis

            (i) A—if negative, discuss vaccine

            (ii) B and C—if negative, discuss vaccine (B only at present); if positive, patient needs further evaluation

          (c) *Toxoplasma*

            (i) Positive IgG titer may prompt prophylaxis if/when CD4 count < 200

          (d) PPD

            (i) Include anergy tests (*Candida*, mumps)

            (ii) Positive test at 5-mm induration (not 10 mm as in immunocompetent patient)

            (iii) Treat PPD-positive patients in conjunction with specialist knowledgeable of local patterns of drug resistance

        (e) CD4 count
            (i) CD4 test is subject to variability between labs and even time of day
            (ii) Standardize drawing sample for all HIV patients to same lab and same time of day
        (f) Quantitative HIV RNA test
        (g) Tests of unknown usefulness
            (i) Titers for *Cryptococcus*, skin tests for *Coccidioides*, *Histoplasma*
            (ii) Serum level of vitamins B_{12} and B_6, zinc, selenium

  d. **Immunizations**
    i. Pneumococcal vaccine, polyvalent (23 strains)
    ii. *Haemophilus influenzae* B vaccine
    iii. Yearly influenza vaccine
      (a) Though influenza usually not fatal, may be mistaken for more severe illness and provoke unnecessary testing
    iv. Hepatitis A vaccine
      (a) Nonimmune sexually active patient
    v. Hepatitis B vaccine if high risk
    vi. Tetanus booster every 10 years
    vii. Controversial immunizations
      (a) Polio, diphtheria, should remain from childhood; if booster needed, proceed with killed virus vaccine
      (b) Mumps, rubella, measles
        (i) Live, attenuated virus may cause disease in immunocompromised host and usually not given unless risks for disease high

  e. **Lifestyle recommendations**
    i. Identify drug abusers and refer to drug rehabilitation center
      (a) IV use of heroin and cocaine poor prognostic factor in HIV disease
    ii. Identify alcohol abusers and refer for rehabilitation
    iii. Cessation of smoking
    iv. Safe sex habits
    v. Balanced diet
      (a) Advise against undercooked meats and fish, unwashed vegetables
    vi. Counsel about cat litter, gardening (*Toxoplasma*)
    vii. Appropriate rest
      (a) HIV/AIDS an exhausting disease
      (b) Rest crucial to well-being
    viii. Travel
      (a) Considerations include infections in foreign countries, *Coccidioides* in southwest U.S., *Histoplasma* in midwestern U.S.
    ix. Pets
      (a) Numerous infections from animals
    x. "Nutritional" or "herbal" treatments
      (a) Little or no proven benefit
      (b) Most interest focuses on vitamins B_{12} and B_6, zinc, selenium

2. **Surveillance**
  a. Periodic visits to review medical and psychosocial status
  b. Review of risk assessment
    i. Prevent "slippage," whereby HIV-positive person stops safe habits
  c. Search for constitutional symptoms
    i. Fever, sweats, weight loss often sign of advancing HIV disease
  d. Physical exam
    i. Special attention to skin, mouth, nodes, genitourinary tract
  e. Laboratory tests
    i. Complete blood count, blood chemistries
    ii. CD4 count
    iii. HIV RNA titers
  f. Review of contraceptive practices and desires

TABLE 3. Disease Occurrence in Relation to CD4 Count

CD4 Count > 200, < 500	CD4 Count < 200	CD4 Count < 50
Kaposi's sarcoma	*Pneumocystis*	*Mycobacterium avium-intracellulare*
Thrush	*Toxoplasma*	Cytomegalovirus
Oral hairy leukoplakia		Lymphoma

3. **Referral to specialist**
   a. Important task for primary care provider is to know when to refer
      i. Work in concert with knowledgeable specialist
      ii. Recommendations and treatments change rapidly and are increasingly complex—unrealistic to expect primary care provider to remain current
   b. Increasing controversy regarding initiation of antiretroviral therapy
      i. Some experts suggest waiting for signs of increasing disease such as declining CD4 count or increasing HIV RNA titers
         (a) Despite natural history of long disease-free period, critics of this course point to missed opportunity to suppress virus
      ii. Others advocate more aggressive therapy including initiation of antiretroviral therapy at time of diagnosis with goal to suppress HIV RNA titer to undetectable levels indefinitely
         (a) Critics of this course point to long-term treatment with toxic medications, problems with adherence to therapy, expense
      iii. In any case, therapy is usually started well before appearance of opportunistic infection
         (a) Therapy typically involves three drugs, at least one of which is a protease inhibitor
   c. Most important problem with more aggressive approach to antiretroviral therapy is adherence
      i. HIV drug resistance develops rapidly with virtually all but most complete adherence to drug regimen
      ii. Regimens often involve more than 20 medications taken per day, as often as every 4 hours (including during night) and either with, or avoiding, meals
      iii. Intensive education helps with patient compliance but even most motivated patient sometimes has difficulties
   d. Other circumstances which may prompt referral
      i. Positive PPD (any stage of disease)
         (a) Depending on local patterns, may involve multidrug regimens, especially for *Mycobacterium avium-intracellulare* and *M. tuberculosis*
      ii. CD4 < 200
         (a) Consider prophylaxis against *Pneumocystis*, *Toxoplasma*
      iii. Cytomegalovirus disease
         (a) Difficult to treat, especially ophthalmitis; therapy toxic
      iv. Others
         (a) Certain parasites (e.g., *Isospora*) and fungi (e.g., *Cryptococcus*) not so much cured as controlled
         (b) Malignancies (e.g., Kaposi's sarcoma, lymphoma) need specialized treatment
         (c) Aggressive cervical cancer
D. **Psychosocial support**
   1. Anxiety and depression common
      a. Treatment important and often successful
   2. Suicide more common than in similar age groups without HIV
   3. Progressive mental deterioration (AIDS dementia)
   4. Recent recognition of "survivor" or "second-life" syndrome
      a. Unexpected consequence of success of retroviral therapy
      b. Refers to patients who might have thought death imminent, but in whom therapy dramatically changes prognosis

       i. May have changed financial status, even "spent down" savings and now with few resources

      ii. May have gone through grieving process and need to begin thinking long-term once again

   c. Counseling and support groups can be helpful, along with realistic financial planning (including job search)

5. Support groups

   a. Patients appreciate support, because often they experience fear, harassment, ostracization

   b. Different types of support

      i. Community resources

      ii. Advocacy groups

         (a) Assistance with insurance, fight discrimination in housing, assist with complaints regarding employment

      iii. Patient support—group sessions with leader

      iv. Family support

      v. Home services

   c. Some communities have clearing-house offices that coordinate government and private sources of assistance

6. Spiritual issues

   a. Any person with terminal disease may search for meaning to illness

   b. Physician needs sympathetic, permissive attitude

      i. Referral to clergy if appropriate

      ii. Reminders of previous lifestyle counterproductive

7. Family support

   a. Family may have fear of disease

      i. Need specific recommendations for prevention of transmission

   b. Anticipation of complications

      i. Especially alarming are debility and need for personal care; also progressive dementia

   c. Single mothers with children

      i. May be ostracized from family

      ii. Children may be HIV-positive

      iii. Fathers unable to be located

      iv. Children face foster home and adoption

      v. Need social services before debility and dementia ensue

8. Advance directives and hospice care

   a. Should be addressed as daily activities become difficult

   b. Arrangement for community services

E. **Pregnancy**

1. High probability (> 30%) of transmission of HIV to neonate without treatment

2. Zidovudine (AZT) alone reduces risk of transmission to neonate by 70%

3. AZT alone no longer optimal therapy for prevention of disease progression in female

   a. Recommend at least three drugs even during pregnancy

   b. Certainly reduces HIV transmission, and risks to fetus low though probably not absent

4. Treatment during pregnancy still evolving and referral to specialist strongly encouraged

5. If appropriate, counseling should be offered for adoption or abortion

6. Best alternative is prevention

   a. Discuss contraception at each periodic visits

   b. Most forms of contraception effective in HIV disease, assuming correct use, but patient must be encouraged to use contraception

SUGGESTED READINGS

1. Centers for Disease Control and Prevention: Public Health Service Task Force recommendations for the use of antiretroviral drugs in pregnant women infected with HIV-1 for maternal health and for reducing perinatal HIV-1 transmission in the United States. MMWR 47(RR-2):1–31, 1998.

2. Centers for Disease Control and Prevention: Report of the NIH panel to define principles of therapy of HIV infection, and guidelines for the use of antiretroviral agents in HIV-infected adults and adolescents. MMWR 47(RR-5):1–82, 1998.
3. Jewett JF, Hecht FM: Preventive health care for adults with HIV infection. JAMA 269:1144–1153, 1993.
4. Kahn JO, Walker BD: Acute human immunodeficiency virus type 1 infection. N Engl J Med 339:33–39, 1998.
5. Minkoff HL, Augenbraun M: Antiretroviral therapy for pregnant women. Am J Obstet Gynecol 176:478–489, 1997.
6. Natchbandi IA, Longenecker JC: A decision analysis of mandatory compared with voluntary HIV testing in pregnant women. Ann Intern Med 128:760–767, 1998.
7. Rabkin JG, Ferrando S: A "second life" agenda: Psychiatric research issues raised by protease inhibitor treatments for people with the human immunodeficiency virus or the acquired immunodeficiency syndrome. Arch Gen Psychiatry 54:1049–1053, 1997.
8. Royce RA, Sena A: Sexual transmission of HIV. N Engl J Med 336:1072–1078, 1997.
9. Yerly S, Perneger TV: A critical assessment of the prognostic value of HIV-1 RNA levels and CD4 cell counts in HIV-infected patients. Arch Intern Med 158:247–252, 1998.

55. Hepatitis B and Hepatitis C

Bruce E. Johnson, M.D.

I. The Issues

Hepatitis B and hepatitis C have a special impact on women, not least because these diseases are sexually transmitted, with transmission favoring the male-to-female route. Of additional concern (although the frequency is not high) is that infection constitutes a risk for health care workers, especially nurses and laboratory technicians, who care for infected patients and who are at risk for needlesticks in the course of performing their jobs. Most importantly, pregnant women with hepatitis B or C are at risk of transmitting the virus to the fetus; for hepatitis C, fetal transmission represents a significant means of maintaining the viral pool. Although acute, symptomatic episodes of hepatitis occur, especially with hepatitis B, subacute disease is the norm; thus the initial presentation often is with signs and symptoms of chronic hepatitis. Diagnosis and treatment at any stage is not simple. Chronic hepatitis is difficult to treat; therapy tends to be toxic and only occasionally successful. The greatest effect on epidemiology will be in prevention, for which there are promising options. Although they are very different viruses, the diseases produced by the hepatitis B (HBV) and hepatitis C (HCV) virus are similar enough that they are considered simultaneously in this chapter. Specific differences between the viruses and their diseases are noted.

II. The Theory

A. Epidemiology

1. Differences in prevalence between developed and developing countries
   a. Prevalence high for both viruses in sub-Saharan Africa and Far East, especially Indochina
   b. More than 200 million carriers for HBV worldwide
   c. Total number of HCV carriers worldwide not known, may exceed HBV
2. **HBV carriers** (representing possible infectivity) infrequent in general U.S. population
   a. Prevalence 0.1–0.5% in U.S.
      i. Prevalence up to 5–20% in certain Far East or tropical countries
   b. Some subgroups, however, have increased rates
      i. Up to 30% in patients with certain diseases (e.g., polyarteritis nodosa, HIV, chronic renal disease on hemodialysis) and injection drug users
   c. Other groups with serologic evidence of virus have common denominator of exposure to infected carriers
      i. Hemophiliacs (multiple blood product transfusion)
      ii. Sexual partners of acutely infected persons

       iii. Sexually promiscuous persons (especially prostitutes and homosexual men)
       iv. Residents and staff of large, crowded institutions (e.g., facilities for mentally retarded, prisons)
  d. Up to 250,000 new cases of HBV in U.S. each year
       i. 6000/year die of sequelae of chronic HBV disease
       ii. Up to 5% of entire U.S. population will get acute HBV at some time in life; vast majority clears virus from blood and becomes noninfective

3. **HCV prevalence less clear**
  a. 4 million Americans with HCV (prevalence 1.6%) with up to 3.2% African Americans and 2.1% Hispanics
       i. Among women screened at pregnancy, prevalence up to 1.8% in some locales
  b. Estimated 30,000 new cases/year (down from 150,000/year in 1989)
  c. Among injection drug users seroprevalence up to 60%
  d. HCV implicated in up to 12,000 deaths/year and likely to rise (due to rise in incidence until a decade ago)
  e. Cirrhosis/liver failure from HCV now most common reason for liver transplantation

4. **Transmission**
  a. **Blood-borne transmission**
       i. Blood transfusion highly infective
         (a) Current screening for antibodies against HBV and HCV in U.S. virtually eliminates this source
         (b) In past HCV accounted for 90% of posttransfusion hepatitis; now less than 1% (< 1/100,000 units transfused)
       ii. Whole blood, red cells, single-donor platelets, plasma now virtually free from virus; pooled blood products also very safe (despite problems in past)
         (a) U.S. blood supply exceptionally safe, but supply in developing countries more problematic
       iii. Products such as albumin and hyperimmune globulin are safe since both HBV and HCV inactivated by cleansing methods (e.g., heating to 60°C or cold ethanol extraction)
       iv. Injection drug users at high risk
       v. Case reports of transmission associated with tattooing, but mostly in Far East, not U.S.
  b. **Sexual transmission**
       i. Transmission via sexual intercourse higher for HBV than HCV
       ii. Not as likely as through blood interchange
       iii. Both HBV and HCV associated with multiple sexual partners, receptive anal intercourse, and intercourse with injection drug user
         (a) Intercourse accounts for < 29% of source identification for HCV
         (b) Incidence rises with duration of sexual exposure to HCV-positive partner (e.g., length of marriage)
         (c) Transmission almost always male-to-female
         (d) Poor transmission due to low circulating levels of HCV (compared with HBV); long-term, multiple exposures needed for infection
       iv. HCV infection seen frequently in association with HBV antibodies; also high prevalence in HIV-infected patients
         (a) Probably reflects lifestyle (e.g., injection drug use) rather than codependent transmission
  c. **Occupational exposure**
       i. Transmission of both HBV and HCV through human bites and saliva; isolated reports of HBV (not HCV) through contact with tears, secretions, body fluids (ascitic, pleural)
       ii. Primary concern is needlestick
         (a) Nurses (particularly dialysis nurses), laboratory technicians, blood bank workers

    (b) Higher for HBV because of higher number of infectious units per milliliter blood

    (c) Likelihood of development of HBV after one needlestick > 10%; for HCV, < 10%

  iii. Appropriate precautions among police, firemen, ambulance workers

    (a) Gloves, masks when dealing with unruly persons with unknown HBV, HCV, HIV status

  d. **Maternal–fetal transmission** (vertical transmission)

    i. Most likely source of transmission in sub-Saharan Africa and Far East

    ii. Likelihood of HBV transmission depends on e antigen (see below)

      (a) HBV antigen and e antigen (denotes significant infectivity) result in 90% infection rate in fetus

      (b) HBV without e antigen results in only 10–15% rate of fetal infection

    iii. Newborn infrequently become clinically ill with HBV but likelihood of carrier state

      (a) Fetal studies suggest intrauterine infection in only 10% of cases, conclude that over 75% occur during vaginal birth

    iv. Transmission of HCV from mother to child as low as 5%

      (a) Rate increases with level RNA particles in mother's blood; if HCV RNA > 1,000,000 units/ml, up to 18% transmission

    v. Breast milk poor to nonexistent risk for both HBV and HCV

  e. Considerable effort in U.S. to account for all modes of transmission

    i. With investigation, most exposure can be detected for HBV

    ii. However, with HCV, exposure via blood transfusion or injection drug use, sexual or occupational exposure, or maternal–fetal transmission accounts for only 80–90% of cases—remainder unknown

      (a) Sexual transmission assumed, but doubt remains

  f. Variations in prevalence, modes of transmission, social and sexual behavior, and genotypes lead to different patterns of infection worldwide

    i. In sub-Saharan Africa and Far East, maintenance of both HBV and HCV through maternal–fetal transmission

    ii. In U.S. and western Europe, maintenance largely through sexual contact, injection drug use

B. **Virology**

  1. **Hepatitis B virus**

    a. DNA virus, mostly double-stranded but with partial single-stranded genome

      i. Uses replicative strategy similar to retroviruses (e.g., HIV)

      ii. Classified as hepadnavirus (hepatotropic DNA virus)

    b. Electron microscopy demonstrates three forms

      i. Spherules and filaments (22 nm)

        (a) Identical with outer coat of HBV

      ii. Large spherical particles (42 nm)

        (a) Intact virion

    c. Serologic studies identify several antigens and antibodies originating from various parts of virion

      i. Hepatitis B surface antigen (HBsAg)—polypeptide derived from outer protein coat of virus

        (a) Multiple subtypes valuable for disease typing in epidemiology but not clinically important

      ii. Anti-HBs or HBsAb—the antibody to HBs antigen

      iii. Hepatitis B core antigen (HBcAg)—antigen associated with surface of nucleocapsid

      iv. Anti-HBc or HBcAb—the antibody to HBc antigen, often present in serum before HBcAg detectable

      v. Hepatitis B e antigen (HBeAg)—nonparticulate antigen apparently derived from internal component or degradation product of core of HBV

        (a) Associated with high infectivity

        (b) HBsAg mothers with HBeAg invariably transmit infection to fetus; without HBeAg, infection uncommon

      vi. Anti-HBe or HBeAb—antibody to HBe antigen

    d. Virus attacks hepatocytes and replicates, using reverse transcription process

      i. Generates enormous numbers of particles

        (a) Up to 10 trillion particles/ml

      ii. Produces antigens and antibodies listed above

        (a) Clearing or chronic infection (carrier state) depends on immunologic response

        (b) Progress may be followed by pattern of serologies (see below)

      iii. Rarely, virus found in other tissues; in general, disease limited to liver

2. **Hepatitis C virus**

    a. Single-stranded RNA virus with lipid envelope

    b. Approximately 50 nm in size

    c. HCV genome highly complex and variable

      i. Geographic distribution of genotypes to some degree, but considerable "mixing" throughout world

    d. HCV genome mutates frequently

      i. Important negative consequences for developing vaccine

    e. Antigens and antibodies for clinical testing focus on genome rather than protein coat

      i. Second-generation test (ELISA-II) uses antibody to several portions of genome

        (a) May take several weeks to develop titer

      ii. Recombinant immunoblot assay (RIBA3)

        (a) RIBA3 test not confined to infrequent ELISA confirmation in person with no risk factors

      iii. HDV RNA uses polymerase chain reaction (PCR) technology to amplify number of viral units in blood

        (a) Reported as units/ml

        (b) Essential test to plan and follow therapy

3. **Hepatitis D virus**

    a. Must be mentioned because of intimate association with HBV

    b. Defective RNA virus that requires HBV for encapsulation and, hence, replication

    c. Not found outside of HBV infection

    d. Often coinfects or superinfects HBV disease

    e. Strongly associated with fulminant hepatitis

    f. Mode of transmission almost always blood-borne

C. **Serologies of HBV and HCV**

1. Clinically most hepatitis infections look similar

    a. Differentiation must be made because, for example, hepatitis A is virtually always benign and self-limited, whereas infection with HCV has high likelihood of leading to chronic disease

    b. Serology essential to differentiate past, but cured, disease from carrier state in HBV (though not as helpful in HCV)

2. **Hepatitis B** (Table 1)

    a. HBsAg is first detectable marker of HBV infection

      i. Precedes symptoms, jaundice, and transaminase elevation

      ii. Titers rise early in disease and, in most cases, fall 1–2 months after jaundice, becoming undetectable beyond 6 months if disease cleared

    b. Anti-HBs titers rise after HBsAg disappears

      i. May be gap or window between detection of HBsAg and anti-HBs of several weeks to months

    c. HBcAg is protected by HBsAg protein; no HBcAg present during active HBV infection

      i. Once HBsAg has cleared, however, anti-HBc is present

      ii. Anti-HBc usually precedes anti-HBs by several weeks

TABLE 1. Interpretation of HBV Serology

	HBsAG	HBeAg	Anti-HBs	Anti-HBc	Anti-HBe	Interpretation
1.	+	+	−	±	−	Acute HBV, high infectivity
2.	−	−	+	+	+	Resolving HBV, low infectivity
3.	−	−	−	+	±	Resolving HBV, window, low infectivity
4.	+	+	−	+	−	Chronic HBV, high infectivity, carrier
5.	−	−	+	±	−	Remote HBV, resolved, low infectivity
6.	−	−	+	−	−	Immunization with HBsAg

      iii. Presence of anti-HBc in window confirms clearance of HBV infection and resolution of disease

    d. Anti-HBs persists indefinitely once HBV infection cleared; anti-HBc may persist for years but generally disappears with time

    e. Anti-HBs is protective antibody; that is, presence of anti-HBs protects against additional disease even with repeated exposure to infective virus

    f. HBeAg present during replication phase (acute phase) of disease but should disappear with resolution of disease

      i. Anti-HBe appears before HBeAg disappears and also persists indefinitely

    g. Consequently, in typical disease in which virus infects, causes disease, and is cleared, serum shows persistence of anti-HBs and anti-HBc

    h. If virus is not cleared, patient is at risk for carrier state and serology is different

      i. Carrier state defined by persistence of HBsAg, but titers vary

      ii. Value in searching for markers of viral replication (e.g., HBeAg)

        (a) Presence of HBsAg and HBeAg denotes high infectivity in chronic carrier or liver disease with high likelihood to transmit virus to fetus in pregnancy

    i. In general, presence of HBsAg and/or HBeAg is indication of chronic hepatitis; patient should be considered infectious

  3. **Hepatitis C**

    a. Clinical presentation usually different from HBV (see below); acute, symptomatic illness occurs only 10–20% of time

    b. More commonly presents as chronic hepatitis

      i. In this setting, need to differentiate from HBV, but not HAV or other viral hepatitis

    c. Usually use ELISA test to identify, while HCV RNA level used to determine viral load

    d. Level of HCV RNA correlates with infectivity

    e. Possible to have simultaneous HCV and HBV

      i. Serologies do not cross-react

      ii. Positive tests indicate presence of both viruses

D. **Pathology**

  1. **Acute hepatitis**

    a. Clinically, HBV and HCV infections are indistinguishable and typical for acute hepatitis of many causes

      i. Acute HCV recognized in only 10–20% of cases and typically mild

    b. Occasionally, in recovery may have prolonged cholestatic phase

    c. Rare occurrence of fulminant hepatitis shows massive hepatic necrosis at postmortem exam

  2. **Chronic hepatitis**

    a. Several different patterns of injury characterized as chronic hepatitis

      i. No pattern specific to HBV or HCV

      ii. Pathologic terms probably represent degrees on spectrum with merging from one pattern to next

    b. Chronic persistent hepatitis

      i. Infiltration of portal areas with mononuclear cells

      ii. No erosion of limiting plate or extension of inflammation into lobule

    iii. Minimal fibrosis but no cirrhosis (i.e., no fibrosis extending from portal area to lobule)

    iv. As long as pathology identified as chronic persistent, progression to cirrhosis is not imminent

  c. Chronic active hepatitis

    i. Although clinical features may suggest this diagnosis, liver biopsy necessary to confirm

    ii. Four important characteristics

      (a) Mononuclear and plasma cell infiltration of portal zones

      (b) Hepatocyte necrosis at edges of lobule with erosion of limiting plate (piecemeal necrosis)

      (c) Connective tissue extending from portal area into lobule

      (d) Hepatic regeneration with rosettes

    iii. Process is patchy, with interspersed regions showing little or no change

    iv. Evidence that many cases of chronic active hepatitis progress to cirrhosis

3. Immunologic manifestations

  a. Considerable evidence that some of pathologic changes in chronic hepatitis from HBV and/or HCV due to immunologic mechanisms

    i. Monocytic infiltrations are T-lymphocytes and plasma cells

    ii. Circulating autoantibodies detected in serum

      (a) Antimitochondrial, anti–smooth muscle

    iii. Other autoimmune diseases may occur or coexist, such as Coombs-positive hemolytic anemia, proliferative glomerulonephritis, cryoglobulinemia, poly-arteritis nodosa

    iv. Extrahepatic manifestations such as arthritis, rash, myalgia coincide with deposition of immune complexes and low complement levels

III. An Approach

A. Clinical manifestations

1. Acute hepatitis B and C

  a. **Acute prodrome phase**—more often HBV than HCV, but still only 30% of cases—may persist for 1–2 weeks

    i. Nausea, vomiting, fatigue, myalgia, arthralgia/frank arthritis, rash (erythematous or urticarial), photophobia, headache, anorexia

    ii. Anorexia often associated with variations in olfaction and taste

      (a) Lose appetite for alcoholic drinks

      (b) Lose desire for cigarette smoking

    iii. Onset of clinical jaundice accompanied by relief of many constitutional symptoms

    iv. Perhaps 25% HBV and 75% HCV anicteric with mild, flu-like symptoms

  b. **Characteristic physical findings**

    i. Enlarged liver with discomfort in right upper quadrant

    ii. Jaundice generally not evident until bilirubin above 2.5–3.0 mg/dl

    iii. Jaundice generally persists for 1–2 weeks but may persist for 4–6 weeks if course complicated with cholestatic phase

    iv. Most patients do not require hospitalization unless

      (a) Nausea and vomiting resulting in electrolyte imbalance and dehydration

      (b) Inability to care for self at home

      (c) Prolonged (> 16–17 s) prothrombin time (PT)

  c. **Laboratory abnormalities**

    i. Mild neutropenia/lymphopenia

      (a) May see atypical lymphocytes

    ii. PT not affected in usual cases

    iii. Transaminases (aspartate aminotransferase [ASAT] and alanine aminotransferase [ALAT]) elevated, usually within 15–60 days after exposure

    iv. Alkaline phosphatase variably increased; more so in cholestatic context

    v. Acute HBV typically demonstrates presence of HBsAg and HBeAg within weeks

      vi. HCV antibodies detected by ELISA in 2–12 weeks

        (a) HCV RNA detected earlier but usually not measured unless suspicion—and positive ELISA

2. **Chronic hepatitis B and C**

  a. Approximately 5% HBV goes on to develop chronic hepatitis; unfortunately as many as 85% HCV acute disease is not cleared and progresses to chronic hepatitis

  b. Early chronic hepatitis symptoms vague and nonspecific

    i. Most frequent presentation is well patient with mild elevation of transaminases

      (a) Initial acute hepatitis may be forgotten or subclinical

    ii. Symptomatic patient may have fatigue, anorexia, mild nausea

  c. Late chronic hepatitis demonstrates complications of cirrhosis

    i. Fatigue, malaise, anorexia, low-grade fever, jaundice

    ii. Cirrhosis

      (a) Ascites, variceal bleed, coagulopathy, encephalopathy

    iii. Extrahepatic manifestations of chronic hepatitis seen especially in women

      (a) Amenorrhea, arthralgia, acne, erythema nodosa, sicca syndrome

  d. **Physical findings**

    i. Jaundice

    ii. Early hepatomegaly; late cirrhotic, shrunken liver

    iii. Splenomegaly, ascites, abdominal vessels, other signs of portal hypertension

    iv. Extrahepatic signs of chronic liver disease

      (a) Spider angioma (especially upper chest, back), palmar erythema, asterixis, encephalopathy

  e. **Laboratory changes of chronic hepatitis**

    i. Frequent elevations of transaminases (e.g., AST > 100 IU/dl)

      (a) HBV almost invariable

      (b) HCV may have prolonged period with "normal" transaminases though by the time chronic active hepatitis is present, AST elevated

    ii. Frequent elevation of bilirubin with cirrhosis

    iii. Patient with progressive cirrhosis develops hypoalbuminemia, hypergammaglobulinemia, prolonged PT

    iv. Autoantibodies not infrequent, especially in women, including antinuclear, anti–smooth muscle, antimitochondrial

    v. Serology

      (a) Chronic hepatitis due to HBV (e.g., chronic active) almost invariably has positive HBsAg and HBeAg

        (i) Indolent chronic HBV hepatitis (e.g., chronic persistent) may have only HBsAg with anti-HBe and anti-HBc

      (b) Chronic hepatitis due to HCV shows serology positive for ELISA with variable levels of HCV RNA

B. **Differential diagnosis**

1. **Acute hepatitis**

  a. Other organisms

    i. Infectious mononucleosis (Epstein-Barr virus), cytomegalovirus, herpes simplex, coxsackievirus

    ii. Toxoplasmosis

  b. Drugs

    i. Classic examples: methyldopa, acetaminophen, halothane, isoniazid, sodium valproate, phenytoin, chlorpromazine, amiodarone, erythromycin, oral contraceptives, trimethoprim-sulfamethoxazole

  c. Alcohol

  d. Acute cholecystitis, common duct stone, ascending cholangitis

  e. In pregnancy

    i. Severe preeclampsia

    ii. Cholestatic hepatitis of pregnancy

2. **Chronic hepatitis**
   a. Chronic persistent vs. chronic active
      i. Can differentiate only with biopsy
   b. Autoimmune disease
      i. Common in women
      ii. Associated with autoimmune antibodies and symptoms of arthralgia, myalgia, skin rash, pleurisy, pericarditis
   c. Wilson's disease
   d. Alpha-1 antitrypsin deficiency
   e. Primary biliary cirrhosis
C. **Prognosis**
   1. **HBV**
      a. Most patients with acute hepatitis recover without hospitalization or complications
         i. Rare severe complications include
            (a) Fulminant hepatitis
               (i) Up to 80% mortality rate without liver transplantation
            (b) Pancreatitis, myocarditis, aplastic anemia, transverse myelitis, polyarteritis nodosa
         ii. Coinfection or superinfection with delta virus increases fatality rate (up to 2–5%)
         iii. First infection has higher fatality rate in pregnant than in nonpregnant women, though still very low (< 1%)
      b. Of patients with acute hepatitis, 90% clear virus and suffer no sequelae
         i. Serology shows anti-HBs and anti-HBc
      c. Of remaining 10%, half eventually clear virus or have no further sequelae
         i. May require months to years to become free of virus
      d. For patients who do not clear virus, several outcomes possible
         i. Chronic carrier without chronic liver disease
            (a) Varying degrees of infectivity
            (b) Risk to sexual partners, shared needles, fetus
         ii. Chronic carrier with chronic persistent hepatitis
         iii. Chronic carrier with chronic active hepatitis
            (a) High likelihood of progression to cirrhosis
   2. **HCV**
      a. Current estimate: only 15% of patients contracting acute HCV eventually clear virus
      b. Remaining cases have significant likelihood of progressing to some form of chronic liver disease
      c. Within 20 years as many as 20% of patients with chronic hepatitis develop cirrhosis
   3. **Hepatocellular carcinoma**
      a. Both HBV and HCV strongly associated with development of cancer
         i. Usually in chronic carriers or patients with cirrhosis
      b. Hepatocellular is one of most common cancers worldwide; chronic HBV and HCV carrier state most significant risk factor
      c. Unfortunately, while still not common, incidence in U.S. increasing
D. **Treatment of chronic hepatitis**
   1. **HBV**
      a. For unknown reasons, rate of spontaneous conversion from HBsAg to anti-HBs is 8–10% per year in U.S.
         i. Seen in healthier persons (i.e., not injection drug users or HIV-infected)
      b. Approved treatment with interferon-alpha
         i. Several studies suggest up to 45% of patients receiving interferon become HBeAg-negative after 1 year, though only 7% also clear HBsAg, becoming HBsAg-negative
         ii. Side effects high; interferon given by injection with frequent nausea, achiness, fatigue, fever, flu-like syndrome

(a) Side effects frequently limit dose or length of therapy ("like having the flu for a year")

c. Current investigation includes therapy with nucleoside analog lamivudine
    i. Inhibits DNA replication
    ii. Oral medication tolerated with few side effects
    iii. Trials as single agent or given with interferon

d. Patient selection important
    i. Must have biopsy-proven chronic hepatitis
       (a) Better results with chronic persistent, but chronic active often treated
       (b) Less likely to be successful in biopsy-proven cirrhosis

e. General measures important
    i. Abstain from alcohol, injection drug use, implicated medications
    ii. Appropriate diet, social support etc.

f. Therapy usually given in consultation with hepatologist
    i. Complications frequent
    ii. Treatment failure (up to 70% of those chosen for therapy) raises question of transplantation

2. **HCV**

a. Chronic carrier state and progression to chronic liver disease more likely than with HBV
    i. Progression quite variable with some developing cirrhosis early, whereas others may have only mild changes after decades

b. Only approved therapy is interferon-alpha
    i. Same side effects as noted for HBV

c. Therapy preceded by liver biopsy (showing absence of cirrhosis), transaminase levels, HCV RNA level
    i. HCV RNA > 1,000,000 units/ml associated with low likelihood of response

d. Goal of therapy is normalization of transaminases and absence of HCV RNA in blood
    i. In those cases studied with repeat liver biopsy, shows some reversal of histology

e. Trials vary dose, frequency and length of therapy
    i. Best results demonstrate transaminase improvement in 30–40% of patients, and loss of RNA in 20–30%

f. Recent trials using oral antiviral agent ribavirin—usually in combination with interferon

g. Cost of therapy high—interferon-alpha alone runs > $5000/year—plus other therapy, office visits etc.

E. **Prophylaxis and vaccination**

  1. **General measures**

    a. Medical personnel caring for patients with HBV or HCV should use appropriate precautions
       i. Extreme caution with blood drawing, IVs, invasive procedures; glove and hand washing; masks, glasses if splashing of blood or body fluids anticipated

    b. Protection of household partners
       i. Neither virus easily passed by casual contact
          (a) Most household members not at significant risk
          (b) Avoid obvious contacts (e.g., toothbrush, shared razor)

    c. Sexual contacts of HBV- and HCV-positive patients should practice safe sexual techniques
       i. Use of latex condom (male or female condom), avoid anal intercourse, avoid intercourse during menstruation
       ii. Long-standing HCV negative partner of HCV positive patient should consider using safe sex techniques—even though likelihood of transmission low (if it had not already happened, unlikely to happen in future)

  2. **Treatment of persons exposed to HBV**

    a. Sexual contact with person infected with acute hepatitis B

      i. Should treat within 14 days of exposure to patient with HBV
      ii. Give hepatitis B immunoglobulin (HBIG)
      iii. Begin vaccination process after 3 months if contact is HBsAg carrier
      iv. 3 months after HBIG, begin vaccination
      v. Suggest HCV and HIV testing
  b. Sexual contact with person infected with HCV
      i. No immunoglobulin and no vaccination
      ii. Transmission unlikely after single sexual encounter—encourage safe sex practices
  c. Needlestick
      i. Ascertain HBV status; if HBsAg-negative, observation may be adequate
      ii. For unknown status or HBsAg-positive, treat with HBIG
        (a) Recall that up to 5% of all hospital admissions are HBsAg-positive and often do not know their status

3. **Vaccination** (HBV)
  a. Vaccine available for HBV; none for HCV
  b. Before vaccinate adult, check HBV antibody status
      i. If anti-HBc positive, vaccine not needed
  c. Should be offered to high-risk adults
      i. Injection drug users, sexual contacts of HBV-positive persons, multiple sexual partners
      ii. Certain hospital personnel (e.g., dialysis and surgical nurses, floor nurses, laboratory technicians, physicians, surgeons)
      iii. Certain public servants (e.g., ambulance workers, fireman, police)
  d. Consists of three-part injection, given at 0, 1, and 6 months
  e. Pregnancy not a contraindication
      i. Currently, screening for HBV commonly performed on all pregnant women
      ii. Finding HBsAg positive is indication for vaccine—confers protection on fetus
  f. Sometimes, may choose to check whether vaccine effective by measuring anti-HBs
      i. If antibody absent, revaccinate
      ii. If antibody present, no need for "booster"
  g. Currently in U.S., recommendation for universal immunization of infants and children, which, if effective, will greatly decrease, if not eliminate, HBV in this country

SUGGESTED READING

1. Alvarez-Munoz MT, Vazquez-Rosales JG, Torres-Lopez FJ: Infection of pregnant women with hepatitis B and C viruses and risks for vertical transmission. Arch Med Res 28:415–419, 1997.
2. Centers for Disease Control and Prevention: 1998 Guidelines for Treatment of Sexually Transmitted Diseases. MMWR 47(RR-1):101–104, 1998.
3. Dusheiko GM: Treatment and prevention of chronic viral hepatitis. Pharmacol Ther 65:47–73, 1995.
4. Gross JB: Clinician's guide to hepatitis C. Mayo Clin Proc 73:355–361, 1998.
5. Hunt CM, Carson KL, Sharara AI: Hepatitis C in pregnancy. Obstet Gynecol 89:883–890, 1997.
6. Lau DR, Everhart J, Kleiner DE: Long-term follow-up of patients with chronic hepatitis B treated with interferon alpha. Gastroenterology 113:1660–1667, 1997.
7. NIH Consensus Statement On-line: Management of Hepatitis C, March 24–26, 1997.
8. Sharara AI, Hunt CM, Hamilton JD: Hepatitis C. Ann Intern Med 125:658–662, 1996.

56. Pelvic Inflammatory Disease

Gary R. Newkirk, M.D.

I. The Issues

Pelvic inflammatory disease (PID) presents as a spectrum of inflammatory disorders within the upper genital tract of women, including any combination of endometritis, salpingitis, tubo-ovarian abscess, and pelvic peritonitis. PID remains a major public health problem. Although chlamydial and gonorrheal cervicitis are reportable diseases in most states, PID is not. Each year at least 1 million women in the U.S. are diagnosed with PID, and over 200,000 are hospitalized at an estimated total cost over 5 billion dollars. At least one-fourth of women with PID suffer serious sequelae, such as infertility, ectopic pregnancy, or chronic pelvic pain, and are at risk for major abdominal surgeries, such as tubo-ovarian abscess drainage or pelvic adhesion lysis. Teenagers account for one-fifth of the total cases. Although most young patients with PID do not have a life-threatening condition, few deny that repeated PID may become "fertility-threatening."

II. The Theory

A. **Epidemiology**—risk of PID
   1. Assessing risk for PID facilitates correct diagnosis and helps identify women who need risk-reduction counseling
   2. Considerable overlap between risk for sexually transmitted disease (STD) and risk for PID (Table 1)
   3. Exact role of intrauterine device (IUD) as risk factor for PID and sequelae such as infertility is undergoing revision
      a. Most PID among users of current copper and progestational "T" IUDs in the U.S. is related to insertion process
      b. Further risk for PID correlates with risk for acquiring new STDs
   4. Health-seeking behavior of women and their sex partner(s) remains important risk factor for PID
      a. Delay of treatment of only 1 or 2 days may increase likelihood of hospitalization by nearly 10%
      b. Institution of treatment within 3 days of onset of symptoms may reduce risk of subsequent infertility and ectopic pregnancy by 3-fold

B. **Microbiology and pathophysiology**
   1. PID results from ascending infection of bacteria that have colonized endocervix
   2. PID is usually polymicrobial, including both aerobic and anaerobic bacteria
   3. Sexually transmissible organisms most frequently implicated in causing PID include *Neisseria gonorrhoeae*, *Chlamydia trachomatis*, and genital mycoplasma
   4. Approximately one-third of women with gonococcal or chlamydial cervicitis progress to PID if untreated

C. **Pathogenesis**
   1. Exact pathogenesis of PID has yet to be determined
   2. Poor correlation between cervical cultures and cultures taken from endometrium, salpinges, and abdominal spaces
   3. Anaerobic bacteria nearly always identified within intratubal, ovarian, and pelvic abscesses, yet chlamydia and gonococci are uncommon even when cervical gonorrhea or chlamydial infection is implicated as initial cause of PID

III. An Approach

A. **Diagnostic principles**
   1. Using laparoscopy as diagnostic standard, PID is correctly diagnosed on clinical and laboratory indicators in only 65% of cases
   2. No historical, physical, or laboratory findings conclusively diagnose PID
   3. Ultimate diagnosis relies on clinical judgment coupled with empiric therapeutic intervention and careful follow-up

TABLE 1. Correlation of Risks for PID and STDs

Risk Variable	Acquisition of STD	Development of PID
Age < 25 years: 75% of cases and 10-fold increased risk 3-fold increased risk of intercourse before age 15	+	+
Marital status Increased risk with single status, divorce, separation	+	+

Contraceptive practice
  Barrier
  Birth control pill
  Intrauterine device
	–
	+
	*
		–
		–
		+

Menstrual cycle Risk increases during or shortly after menses	+	+
Douching > 3 times per month	*	+
Smoking Smokers have 2-fold greater risk than nonsmokers	+	+

+ = increased risk, – = decreased risk, * = no association reported.
Adapted from Washington AE, Aral SO, Wolner-Hanssen P, et al: Assessing risk for pelvic inflammatory disease and its sequelae. JAMA 266:2581–2586, 1991.

    4. Table 2 lists differential diagnosis for PID
    5. Table 3 summarizes data about frequency of clinical findings for PID
    6. Table 4 summarizes 1998 CDC diagnostic recommendations for PID
    7. To improve diagnostic accuracy in patients with severe symptoms, confirmation of additional criteria is warranted; failure to rule out competing diagnosis, such as appendicitis or ectopic pregnancy, places patient at risk for morbidity related to delayed treatment
    8. All laboratory studies may be entirely normal and, even when abnormal, provide only supportive rather than confirmatory evidence
    9. Urethral Gram stain and cultures for gonorrhea and chlamydia in men who are partners of women undergoing evaluation for PID provide supportive evidence; if possible, partner examination should be recommended
   10. Cervical cultures positive for gonorrhea or chlamydia strongly support diagnosis of PID if found with cervical motion and/or adnexal tenderness
  B. **Diagnostic procedures**
    1. **Culdocentesis**
      a. Samples material in posterior cul-de-sac by intravaginal needle aspiration
      b. Aspirate laden with white cells with or without organisms suggests acute PID but also may be seen with other intra-abdominal infections such as appendicitis
      c. Not widely used in U.S. to diagnose PID because it provides nonspecific information and is painful
    2. **Pelvic ultrasound**, including endovaginal probe
      a. May help to assess pelvic structures, especially in patients whose abdominal tenderness or obesity precludes palpating for abnormality
      b. May also detect pelvic abscesses
      c. May help to localize pregnancy in patients with positive pregnancy test

TABLE 2. Differential Diagnosis of PID

Appendicitis	Irritable bowel syndrome	Cholecystitis
Ectopic pregnancy	Endometriosis	Nephrolithiasis
Gastroenteritis	Ovarian torsion	Somatization
Hemorrhagic ovarian cyst		

TABLE 3. Clinical Findings of Acute PID (n = 134)

Symptoms or Signs	%
Abdominal pain	100
Adnexal tenderness	90
Cervical motion tenderness	80
Vaginal discharge	73
Abdominal rebound, guarding	61
Fever	30

Adapted from Morcos R, Frost N, Hnat M, et al: Laparoscopic versus clinical diagnosis of acute pelvic inflammatory disease. J Reprod Med 38:53–56, 1993, with permission.

3. **Endometrial biopsy**
   a. Histopathologic evaluation of transcervical aspirated specimens
   b. Demonstrated diagnostic value
   c. Results may take > 24 hours
   d. At present not widely practiced in U.S. as infection often specified as contraindication to procedure
4. **Laparoscopy**
   a. Still considered best method for diagnosing PID
   b. Indicated for patients in whom diagnosis is uncertain
   c. Laparoscopic evidence of PID includes:
      i. Hyperemia of tubal surface
      ii. Edema of tubal walls
      iii. Sticky exudate on tubal surface or fimbriated ends
   d. Expensive, cumbersome, and not without risks
   e. Usually performed on hospitalized patients with suspected PID who fail to improve or in whom diagnostic confusion persists
   f. Undiagnosed pelvic mass or nonresponding pelvic abscess often warrants laparoscopic clarification
   g. Direct culture and/or diagnostic biopsies may be obtained during laparoscopy
      i. To confirm diagnosis
      ii. To identify specific pathogens
      iii. To assist in choosing appropriate antibiotics
   h. During laparoscopy surgeon also may remove free pus, aspirate pyosalpinges, and perform lysis of adhesions, all of which are thought to enhance recovery
C. **Special considerations**
   1. **PID and pregnancy**
      a. PID rarely complicates early pregnancy

TABLE 4. Diagnostic Criteria for PID

Minimal Criteria (all three required)	Additional Criteria (increase specificity)	Definitive Criteria (minimize morbidity of incorrect diagnosis in severely ill women)
Lower abdominal tenderness	Oral temperature > 38.3°C	Histopathologic evidence of endometritis on endometrial biopsy
Adnexal tenderness	Abnormal cervical or vaginal discharge	Transvaginal sonography or other imaging techniques showing thickened fluid-filled tubes or tubo-ovarian complex
Cervical motion tenderness	Elevated erythrocyte sedimentation rate	
	Elevated C-reactive protein	Laparoscopic abnormalities consistent with PID
	Laboratory documentation of cervical infection with *N. gonorrhoeae* or *C. trachomatis*	

From Centers for Disease Control and Prevention: 1998 Sexually Transmitted Diseases Treatment Guidelines. MMWR 47(RR-1):79–86, 1998, with permission.

TABLE 5.   Hospitalization for PID (CDC Recommendations)

1. The diagnosis is uncertain, and surgical emergencies such as appendicitis and ectopic pregnancy cannot be excluded.
2. Pelvic abscess is suspected.
3. The patient is pregnant.
4. The patient is an adolescent (among adolescents compliance with therapy is unpredictable).
5. The patient has HIV infection with low CD4 counts or is taking immunosuppressive therapy.
6. Severe illness or nausea and vomiting preclude outpatient management.
7. The patient is unable to follow or tolerate an outpatient regimen.
8. The patient has failed to respond clinically to outpatient therapy.
9. Clinical follow-up within 72 hours of starting antibiotic treatment cannot be arranged.

From Centers for Disease Control and Prevention: 1998 Sexually Transmitted Diseases Treatment Guidelines. MMWR 47(RR-1):79–86, 1998, with permission.

   b. Both ectopic pregnancy and PID present with considerable overlap of symptoms and signs
   c. Clinician should perform pregnancy testing on all patients presenting with PID symptoms
   d. Failure to diagnose ectopic pregnancy places patient at risk for ectopic rupture and death
   2. **HIV test counseling** should be provided for patients with either confirmed or suspected cervical gonorrhea, chlamydia, or PID
 D. **Treatment and supportive care**
   1. **Principles of treatment**
      a. Management of PID begins with low threshold for diagnosis
      b. Empiric treatment should be instituted as soon as diagnosis of PID is suspected
   2. **Hospitalization vs. outpatient treatment**
      a. Most women with PID are treated as outpatients
      b. Most authorities suggest hospitalization and parenteral therapy with doubt about compliance with recommended treatment
      c. 1998 CDC recommendations suggest criteria for hospitalization (Table 5)
   3. **Antibiotic therapy**
      a. Initiated before culture results
      b. Must include broad-spectrum coverage (aerobic, anaerobic, chlamydial) to address wide range of potential pathogens
      c. CDC's revised regimens for outpatient and inpatient treatment take into account newer antibiotics as well as emergence of resistant organisms (Tables 6 and 7)
      d. Single-drug oral regimens for outpatient treatment of PID not currently recommended
   4. **Supportive measures**
      a. Ensure adequate hydration and pain management

TABLE 6.   Outpatient Treatment of PID

Regimen A
1. Ofloxacin 400 mg orally twice a day for 14 days,
plus
2. Metronidazole 500 mg orally twice a day for 14 days

Regimen B
1. Ceftriaxone 250 mg IM once a day
or
2. Other parenteral third-generation cephalosporin (e.g., ceftizoxime or cefotaxime),
plus
Doxycycline 100 mg orally twice a day for 14 days. (Include this regimen with one of the above regimens.)

From Centers for Disease Control and Prevention: 1998 Sexually Transmitted Diseases Treatment Guidelines. MMWR 47(RR-1):79–86, 1998, with permission.

TABLE 7.   Inpatient Treatment of PID

Regimen A
1. Cefotetan, 2 gm IV every 12 hours
or
Cefoxitin 2 g IV every 6 hours,
plus
2. Doxycycline, 100 mg IV or orally every 12 hours

Regimen B
1. Clindamycin, 900 mg IV every 8 hours
plus
2. Gentamicin, loading dose IV or IM (2 mg/kg body weight) followed by maintenance dose (1.5 mg/kg) every 8 hours. Single daily dosing may be substituted.

Both regimens should be continued for at least 48 hours after the patient demonstrates substantial clinical improvement. Doxycycline, 100 mg orally 2 times/day, should be continued for a total of 14 days. If tubo-ovarian abscess is present, many health care providers use clindamycin rather than doxycycline for continued therapy. Evidence is insufficient to support the use of any single-agent regimen for inpatient treatment of PID. The CDC 1998 guidelines also suggest alternative parenteral regimens supported by limited data.

From Centers for Disease Control and Prevention: 1998 Sexually Transmitted Diseases Treatment Guidelines. MMWR 47(RR-1):79–86, 1998, with permission.

      b. All patients undergoing therapy for PID require careful follow-up
      c. Hospitalized patients should undergo daily bimanual examination to assess therapeutic effectiveness
      d. Outpatients treated for PID should be reexamined in office within 72 hours to ensure improvement and compliance with recommended therapy
        i. Improvement of abdominal, cervical motion, and adnexal tenderness as well as resolution of fever and malaise should be expected within 72 hours
        ii. Lack of significant improvement requires hospitalization, parenteral therapy, and reaffirmation of diagnosis
      e. Follow-up cultures of cervix are generally advised after antibiotic therapy completed
  E. **Sequelae** (Table 8)
  F. **Prevention**
    1. PID results from sexual exposure in great majority of cases
    2. In fewer instances, postsurgical PID is related to uterine instrumentation, such as IUD insertion, hysterosalpingography, elective abortion, or dilatation and curettage
      a. Recent evidence suggests correlation of increased post-procedure infection in women with bacterial vaginosis
      b. Some advocate treatment of this common condition before uterine instrumentation
      c. Similarly, antibiotic prophylaxis with doxycycline has been shown to decrease infection related to IUD insertion
    3. For majority of women at risk, prevention of PID parallels efforts to prevent STDs

TABLE 8.   Sequelae of PID

Condition	% Affected
Recurrent PID	20–25
Tuboovarian abscess	7–16
Chronic abdominal pain	17–18
Infertility	8 (after first episode)
	20 (after second episode)
	40 (after third episode)
Ectopic pregnancy	Increases 2–10 fold

From Centers for Disease Control and Prevention: 1998 Sexually Transmitted Diseases Treatment Guidelines. MMWR 47(RR-1):79–86, 1998, with permission.

SUGGESTED READING

 1. Centers for Disease Control and Prevention: 1998 Sexually Transmitted Diseases Treatment Guidelines. MMWR 47(RR-1):79–86, 1998.
 2. Esinger SH: Culdocentesis. J Fam Pract 13:95–101, 1981.
 3. Hillis SD, Joesoef R, Marchbanks PA, et al: Delayed care of pelvic inflammatory disease as a risk factor for impaired fertility. Am J Obstet Gynecol 168:1503–1509, 1993.
 4. McCormack WM: Pelvic inflammatory disease. N Engl J Med 330:115–119, 1994.
 5. Morcos R, Frost N, Hnat M, et al: Laparoscopic versus clinical diagnosis of acute pelvic inflammatory disease. J Reprod Med 38:53–56, 1993.
 6. Munday PE: Clinical aspects of pelvic inflammatory disease. Hum Reprod 12(Suppl):121–126, 1997.
 7. Newkirk GR: Pelvic inflammatory disease: A contemporary approach. Am Fam Physician 53:1127–1135, 1996.
 8. Quan M: Pelvic inflammatory disease: Diagnosis and management. J Am Board Fam Pract 7:110–123, 1994.
 9. Walker CK, Kahn JG, Washington AE, et al: Pelvic inflammatory disease: Meta-analysis of antimicrobial regimen efficacy. J Infect Dis 168:969–978, 1993.
10. Washington AE, Berg EO: Preventing and managing pelvic inflammatory disease: Key questions, practices, and evidence. J Fam Pract 43:283–293, 1996.
11. Washington AE, Katz P: Cost of and payment source for pelvic inflammatory disease: Trends and projections, 1983 through 2000. JAMA 266:2581–2586, 1991.

57. Bartholin's Gland Infection

Gary R. Newkirk, M.D.

I. The Issues
Infection of Bartholin's glands (the greater vestibular glands) is one of the most common causes for a tender mass at the introitus. The great majority of Bartholin's gland cysts result from simple ductal obstruction with retention of sterile mucus. Such cysts are typically unilateral and may remain minimally symptomatic. If they become large or infected, they may interfere with intercourse and vulvar hygiene and cause significant pain.

II. The Theory
A. Definition of Bartholin's glands
  1. Compound racemose glands approximately the size of a pea
  2. Embedded in erectile tissue of bulb of vestibule
  3. Drained by duct approximately 2 cm in length
  4. Opens into vestibule at junction of labium minus and hymen
B. Importance of Bartholin's glands
  1. Maintain moisture of nonkeratinized epithelium of vestibule
  2. Secretions contribute little to vaginal lubrication during intercourse
C. Causes of cysts
  1. Intraluminal expansion of trapped mucus due to blockage of major duct or one of its larger branches. Possible causes include accidental or obstetric trauma, congenital atresia, epithelial hyperplasia, infection with secondary edema.
  2. Most cysts result from simple obstruction from unknown causes, remain < 4 cm, and ar not infected
  3. Infected cysts often cause severe pain signaling infection. Most contain mixed vaginal flora with either gonorrhea or chlamydia in < 10% of cases. Prior infection with either organism may result in scarring with blockage and abscess formation.
D. Differential diagnosis
  Cysts higher in vagina are often mesonephric in origin. Epidermal cysts are more superficial in location and usually more ovoid. Hernias, hydrocele, hygromas, lipomas, and masses of accessory breast tissue usually expand downward along course of major labia.

III. **An Approach**
   A. **Diagnosis**
      Location of Bartholin's gland cysts betrays the diagnosis. Typically unilateral, < 4 cm, nontender cystic mass within inferior base of minor labium. Warmth, redness, and tenderness imply infection with abscess formation. Culture cysts' content if painful or purulent and consider therapy for gonorrhea or chlamydia if either diagnosis is suspected.
   B. **Therapy**
      1. Small nontender cysts in women under age 40 can be observed unless bothersome
      2. Acute, large, or tender cysts can be treated initially by simple incision and drainage
      3. Recurrence requires creation of tract from dilated duct to vestibule
         a. Simple incision and drainage with gauze packing relieve acute abscess pain
         b. Definitive therapy with marsupialization, excision, or Word catheter insertion often necessary (see Chapter 118)
         c. In most instances, antibiotics are not necessary unless gonorrhea or chlamydia is suspected
         d. Severe symptoms with pain, edema, or cellulitis may require therapy with antibiotics effective against streptococci and staphylocci
      4. For most Bartholin's area cysts in women over age 40 and for all cysts in postmenopausal women
         a. Complete excision under general anesthesia to rule out possibility of carcinoma. This is a fairly tedious and bloody surgery that heals slowly and referral is often warranted.

SUGGESTED READING

1. Curtis JM: Marsupialization technique for Bartholin's cyst. Aust Fam Physician 22:369, 1993.
2. Downs MC, Randall HW Jr: The ambulatory surgical management of Bartholin's duct cysts. J Emerg Med 7:623–626, 1989.
3. Heah J: Methods of treatment for cysts and abscesses of Bartholin's gland. Br J Obstet Gynaecol 95:321–322, 1988.
4. Kaufman RH, Friedrich EG (eds): Benign Diseases of the Vulva and Vagina, 3rd ed. Chicago, Year Book, 1989.
5. Sweet RL, Gibbs RS: Infectious Diseases of the Female Genital Tract, 2nd ed. Baltimore, Williams & Wilkins, 1990.
6. Word B: New instrument for office treatment of cysts and abscesses of Bartholin's gland. JAMA 190:777, 1964.

PART VI

GYNECOLOGIC PAIN AND SYMPTOMATOLOGY

58. Vulvar Symptoms

Barbara S. Apgar, M.D., M.S.

I. **The Issues**
Successful diagnosis of vulvar disease depends on the patient's perception of her problem as well as visualization of anatomic structures. Most vulvar lesions exhibit striking variation and often are multicentric. The same pathologic process may exhibit different visual patterns at a single examination or at consecutive visits. To add to the confusion, similar clinical presentations may be initiated by different pathologic conditions. An adequate and accurate interpretation can be difficult when two or more diseases present with a combination of findings, such as dystrophy, infection, or neoplasia. Often biopsy is the only answer to this dilemma. Because it is important to distinguish benign from malignant processes, the clinician must be aware of the general categories of disease that affect the vulva. Some disease processes may have been present for an extended period, and the patient may have been told that her symptoms are not physical. This approach may lead to anger, resentment, and failure to consult for another opinion. It is important to make a diagnosis, if at all possible.

II. **The Theory**
  A. **Anatomic landmarks** (Fig. 1)
   1. Examination of vulva
      a. Components of squamous epithelium
      b. Glandular structures
      c. Blood vessels in stroma that surround epithelium and glands
   2. External vulvar epithelium
      a. Modified skin exhibiting hair-bearing components
      b. Meets squamous epithelium of higher glycogen content at vulvar vestibule
      c. Vulvar vestibule
         i. Extends from exterior surface of hymen anteriorly to frenulum of clitoris, posteriorly to fourchette, and laterally to Hart's line, where nonkeratinized squamous epithelium of vestibule meets more papillated keratinized epithelium of lateral labia minora.
         ii. Within vestibule are pit-like depressions that are small gland openings and surround and sometimes extend to hymen and urethra; gland orifices extend superiorly to inferior border of clitoris
   3. Micropapillomatosis
      a. Condition in which vestibular papillae are prominent
      b. Papillae are usually small (1–3 mm) and best detected with magnification but can be seen with naked eye
         i. Papillae may be single or cover most of mucosal surface of labia minora
         ii. Visualization is enhanced with use of 3–5% vinegar or acetic acid and observing acetowhite reaction
      c. Most papillae are asymptomatic
         i. If patient experiences pain or dyspareunia, biopsy is recommended
   4. Epithelium of vestibule and gland openings
      a. Extend around hymenal ring
      b. Normally produce slightly acetowhite appearance
      c. It is not normal for acetowhite reaction to be present on hairy surface of vulva

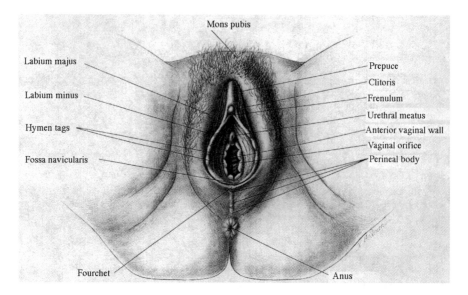

FIGURE 1. The structures of the external genitalia collectively called the vulva. (From Herbst AL, Mishell DR, Stenchever MA, Droegemueller W: Comprehensive Gynecology, 2nd ed. St. Louis, Mosby-Year Book, 1992, with permission.)

B. **Colposcopic features of vulvar tissue**
   1. **Acanthosis**
      a. Associated with both benign and malignant conditions
      b. Most common colposcopic finding on vulva
      c. Not specific for any one condition
      d. Histologic basis
         i. Nutritional support to epithelium of vulva is supplied from dermis through network of capillaries; tissue between individual papillae that supply nutrition to epithelium are called rete pegs.
         ii. Acanthosis is histologic term that denotes elongation and fusion of rete pegs
      e. Colposcopic features
         i. Decreased transmission of light into underlying stroma and acetowhite reaction
         ii. Epithelium appears thicker
         iii. Acanthotic epithelium loses tensile strength and is predisposed to fissure formation that may lead to infection
   2. **Papillosis**
      a. Characterized by abnormal upgrowth of dermal papillae, which produce wavy appearance histologically
         i. Irregular surface due to growth of papillae
            (a) As individual dermal papillae hypertrophy, they extend farther upward to superficial epithelium
         ii. Vessels may grow more prominent and enlarge and become visible with colposcope
            (a) Capillaries in elongated papillae may run tangentially to superficial epithelium, where they are visible as punctation
               (i) May or may not show acetowhite reaction
               (ii) May be associated with inflammation or neoplasia
      b. Papillae should not be confused with condylomata
   3. **Atrophy of vulva**
      a. Characterized by prominent vascular patterns because atrophic epithelium is very thin and underlying stromal vessels are easily identified

b. If atrophy is long-standing or associated with long-term topical steroids, it may display fissuring, erosion, microhemorrhages, and punctation that are easily visualized with colposcope

4. **Hyperkeratosis**
   a. Results from production of excessive surface keratin
      i. Leukoplakia or presence of visible white lesion without application of vinegar is extreme form of hyperkeratosis
   b. Identified colposcopically by attachment of keratin to surface epithelium
   c. Histology
      i. Keratinocytes can be observed in superficial layers of epithelium
   d. Differs from acanthosis by lack of abnormal epithelial thickening but may be seen in association with acanthosis

5. **Inflammation**
   a. May produce characteristic colposcopic patterns
      i. Acetowhitening, excoriation, fissuring, erythema, or abnormal vascular changes such as punctation
   b. Capillary oozing may occur in presence of inflammatory reaction
      i. Classic red lesions of vulva include those that exhibit intense inflammatory response, as in candidal vulvitis or reactive dermatitis
   c. Often not possible to identify visually the source of inflammation
      i. Cultures, wet mounts, or even vulvar biopsy may be required to determine diagnosis

III. **An Approach**
   A. **Evaluation**
      1. Vulvar lesions that do not disappear within several weeks either spontaneously or therapeutically or that tend to have chronic course must be followed closely
         a. Decisive distinctions of benign vs. malignant disease are often impossible without colposcopy or biopsy
      2. If decision is made to follow lesion with observation, baseline histologic determination should be made
         a. Subjective diagnosis without histologic confirmation of chronic or progressive lesion is not sufficient
      3. Written documentation of findings is important
      4. Biopsy of vulva (punch or excisional)
         a. Rapid and simple office procedure that is hallmark of successful management of vulvar disease
         b. Often necessary to differentiate benign and malignant conditions that cannot be determined by visual inspection alone
         c. Gross appearance of lesion not always indicative of histologic character
   B. **Non-neoplastic epithelial diseases of the vulva** (formerly termed vulvar dystrophies)
      1. International Society for the Study of Vulvar Disease proposed new classification system in 1987:
         a. Lichen sclerosus (formerly lichen sclerosus et atrophicus)
         b. Squamous cell hyperplasia (formerly hyperplastic dystrophy)
         c. Other dermatoses (e.g., lichen planus, psoriasis, seborrhea)
            i. Avoids complex terms such as leukoplakia, kraurosis vulvae, and mixed dystrophy that do not contribute to clinical understanding or treatment
            ii. Represents functional classification system acceptable to most pathologists and clinicians
      2. Characteristics of non-neoplastic epithelial vulvar lesions
         a. Presence of keratin
         b. Depigmentation
         c. Relative avascularity
            i. Vulva appears pale or white when superficial blood vessels are constricted or keratin is superimposed over vessels or vessels decrease in caliber or numbers
      3. Patient concerns

    a. Because of intense pruritus associated with dystrophic vulvar disease, some patients may become disabled because of fear of scratching in public

    b. Patient may also worry about cancer and fear that her condition is associated with poor hygiene

    c. Home remedies may add to diagnostic confusion

4. **Lichen sclerosus**

    a. Characteristics

        i. Pruritus accompanies almost all cases

        ii. May occur at either extreme of age, including childhood and can affect both genders

        iii. Familial linkages known

        iv. Long-standing lichen sclerosus may progressively destroy labia minora, resulting in introital stenosis and agglutination of labia minora to adjacent labia majora and obliteration of clitoris

        v. Edema, scarring, and agglutination of prepuce may gradually transform glans of clitoris into amorphous mass of pale tissue

        vi. Ecchymosis and superficial ulcers may occur secondary to scratching

        vii. Surface of labial tissue is usually shiny, delicate, and pale like wrinkled tissue paper

    b. Colposcopic features

        i. Grossly white lesions that may exhibit fissuring, erythema, or paleness; may resemble parchment paper

        ii. Vessels may be prominent and acanthosis may be present

        iii. Punctation usually absent

        iv. After treatment, acanthosis and prominent vessels may disappear as epithelium thickens and begins to heal

    c. Histopathologic examination

        i. Loss of rete pegs and marked thickening of epithelium

        ii. Loss of vascularity with fibrin deposition and edema in dermal layer

        iii. Below layer of edema are signs of chronic inflammation with varying amounts of subcutaneous blood in form of microhemorrhages and superficial ulceration

    d. Treatment

        i. 2% testosterone propionate in vehicle is no longer primary treatment, due to lack of efficacy and masculinization

        ii. High-potency steroids such as clobetasol are primary therapy. Response varies, and dosages have to be titrated; most patients will require long-term maintenance therapy.

        iii. Clobetasol is reported to heal deep fissures of lichen sclerosus better than testosterone without possible virilizing side effects

5. **Squamous cell hyperplasia** (replaces term hyperplastic dystrophy)

    a. Characteristics

        i. Typically occurs in adult women but not in children

        ii. Lesions are pruritic but also may exhibit intense burning

        iii. No familial inheritance

    b. Colposcopic findings

        i. Acetowhite, raised lesions with acanthosis and punctation

        ii. Coarse punctation is unusual; if present, should be biopsied

        iii. May be focal or multifocal sclerosis

        iv. Does not usually result in agglutination of labia or clitoral hood but can occur if long-standing

        v. Microhemorrhages or hypopigmentation may be present

    c. Histology

        i. Resembles lichen sclerosus with deepening and widening of rete pegs and thickening of epidermal layers

        ii. Chronic inflammatory changes with associated edema and usually some degree of hyperkeratosis are present

      d. Treatment
          i. Medium-strength topical steroids such as triamcinolone
          ii. Most lesions rapidly respond within 2–6 weeks
          iii. Long-term therapy usually not necessary
          iv. For recurrence, topical steroids can be reinitiated for short time

   6. **Lichen planus**
      a. Characteristics
          i. Common vulvar disease
          ii. Symptoms may resemble persistent vulvovaginitis
          iii. Pruritus and burning frequent especially if desquamative vaginitis present
      b. Etiology: Autoimmune cell-mediated response may be responsible
      c. Histology
          i. Characterized by thickening of granular cell layer and band-like lymphocytic and histiocytic infiltrate in upper dermis
          ii. Important to biopsy full thickness of epithelium in area where ulceration is not present
      d. Treatment
          i. No satisfactory treatment for genital lichen planus; severe disease treated with immunosuppressive agents.
          ii. Medium-strength topical steroids may be used on short-term basis (daily for 1–2 weeks) to control severe itching

   7. **Psoriasis**
      a. Characteristics: Most psoriatic lesions of vulva have sharply limited borders and dull red surface covered with scales. As scales are scratched off, punctation or microhemorrhages may be visible
      b. Histology: Superficial parakeratoses
      c. Treatment
          i. Fluorinated topical steroids may be used on intermittent basis
          ii. If plastic wrap is placed over vulva after steroid is applied, longer effect can be achieved

C. **Dark lesions of vulva**
   1. **General characteristics**
      a. Genitalia exhibit large number of melanocytes per square millimeter of skin surface; thus genital skin is usually darker than skin covering rest of body
      b. Dark lesions of vulva, whether benign or malignant, may look exactly alike; biopsy distinguishes two conditions.
          i. Melanoma accounts for < 2% of all dark lesions of vulva
      c. Dark vulvar lesions are usually small enough that punch biopsy can be performed
      d. In general, any change in color, size, or texture as well as bleeding or ulceration of dark lesions should be regarded as possible malignant change; lesions should be quickly excised for pathologic confirmation
      e. Ability of clinician to diagnose dark vulvar lesions depends on high index of suspicion and effectiveness of biopsy

   2. **Lentigo**
      a. Common vulvar lesion that first appears in adult life
      b. Characteristics
          i. Characteristic flat, circumscribed appearance
          ii. Frequently multifocal and of varying sizes
          iii. Closely resembles freckle
      c. Histology
          i. Increased melanocyte production and elongation of rete pegs
          ii. Only careful histologic study can distinguish lentigo from level 1 melanoma
      d. Yearly follow-up is recommended; lentigo should be rebiopsied if any change in original pattern occurs

   3. **Vulvar nevi**
      a. Characteristics
          i. Wide variation of depth and color

      ii. Because of potential to develop into melanoma, excisional biopsy can be both diagnostic and curative

      iii. Dysplastic and congenital nevi carry higher risk of malignant transformation

  b. Etiology

      i. Nevi arise from localized areas of undifferentiated neural crest cells

  c. Types of nevi

      i. Junctional nevus

         (a) Occurs in younger patients and usually becomes pigmented at puberty

         (b) Closely resembles lentigo

      ii. Compound nevus

         (a) Develops from junctional nevus

         (b) More raised, with less pigmentation

      iii. Intradermal nevus

         (a) Observed later in life

         (b) Paler than previously described nevi and usually more polypoid

  d. Biopsy

      i. To include all cells, biopsy sample should extend deep to dermal layer

  e. Treatment

      i. Nevi should not be treated with destructive techniques until histologic diagnosis is available

4. **Melanoma**

  a. Characteristics

      i. Accounts for 10% of all vulvar carcinomas

      ii. May occur at any age but primarily presents in postmenopausal patients

      iii. Careful attention should be directed to areas along labia majora and minora, where melanoma tends to occur most frequently

      iv. Usually no symptoms until enlarging mass is present

  b. Biopsy

      i. Large excisional biopsy should be performed that includes adequate sampling of dermis

      ii. Clinician should make accurate records regarding size of lesion, method of excision, and orientation of specimen

      iii. Cutting into lesion during biopsy does not change prognostic potential of lesion if it should prove to be melanoma

  c. Treatment: After biopsy, surgery should be performed promptly if diagnosis of melanoma is confirmed

D. **Vulvar intraepithelial neoplasia** (VIN)

1. Definitions

  a. Precancerous lesion of squamous origin that excludes Paget's disease and melanoma *in situ*

  b. International Society for the Study of Vulvar Disease in 1986 recommended terminology for VIN that deleted such confusing terms as atypia, Bowen's disease, and carcinoma *in situ*

      i. VIN was divided into three categories

         (a) VIN I—mild dysplasia

         (b) VIN II—moderate dysplasia

         (c) VIN III—severe dysplasia (carcinoma *in situ*)

2. Clinical features

  a. Multifocal nature of VIN requires careful assessment

      i. 50% of VIN lesions measure < 2.5 cm.

      ii. VIN may display varied colors (white, red, dark)

  b. The majority of VIN lesions are located on non–hair-bearing areas

  c. Approximately 50% of women with VIN present with symptoms of pruritus, irritation or a mass lesion.

3. Colposcopic findings

  a. Acetic acid may make VIN pattern easier to distinguish from other vulvar conditions, but acetowhiteness is not particularly characteristic

        i. Vulvoscopy lacks specificity and vulvar biopsy must be performed to accurately diagnose vulvar lesions.
- b. Erythema, lichenification, and hyperkeratosis may be present
- c. Punctation and vascular abnormalities are frequently seen, especially when VIN exists on mucosal surface of vulva
- d. Papule formation
  - i. Classic sign of high-grade VIN
  - ii. Papules may be pigmented or nonpigmented
    - (a) If pigmentation is present, papules may be white, red, brown, or black
- e. High-grade VIN
  - i. Tends to be sharply demarcated from surrounding skin
  - ii. Punctation and acetowhiteness may be present
- f. Low-grade VIN
  - i. Produces acetowhitening
  - ii. Border with surrounding skin is not as discrete as with higher-grade VIN
4. Age characteristics of VIN (Table 1)
  - a. Increasing prevalence in young women.
5. Histology
  - a. Intraepithelial process characterized by nuclear hyperchromasia, coarse nuclear chromatin, and disorderly mutation of keratinocytes
    - i. Cell layers are in disordered arrangement, with epithelial hyperplasia, hyperkeratosis, nuclear atypia, and bizarre mitotic figures
    - ii. Distinction between VIN I, II, or III depends on how much of epithelium is involved with abnormal features
6. Treatment
  - a. Laser or loop excision

E. **Squamous carcinoma of vulva**
1. General characteristics
  - a. Because vulva is highly vascular, potential for invasion and poor outcome is high
  - b. Invasive carcinoma is more common in elderly patients, increasing rapidly over age of 60. In this age group, any suspicious lesion should be biopsied.
2. Clinical findings
  - a. Common presenting symptom of vulvar cancer is pruritus followed by burning that is aggravated by urination
  - b. Most common sites of involvement are interlabial folds between minora and majora, posterior fourchette, and clitoris
  - c. Tumor may be exophytic, ulcerative, or infiltrative
3. Histology
  - a. Tumor exhibits parakeratotic epithelial pearls and poorly differentiated cells dispersed throughout stroma
  - b. Depth of invasion of dermis (measured in millimeters) is of great practical importance in determining prognosis
  - c. Term microinvasion is limited to lesions with invasion of < 1 mm
  - d. With deeper invasion, prognosis is worse and more radical surgery is expected

TABLE 1. Age Characteristics of Vulvar Intraepithelial Neoplasia

Incidence	Age < 40 yr	Age > 60 yr
Incidence	Increased	No change
Associated cancer	Common	Uncommon
History	Human papillomavirus	Dystrophy
Clinical findings	Pigmented, multifocal	White or red, unifocal
Etiology	Human papillomavirus	Unknown
Prognosis	May regress	May invade (10%)
Histology	Uniform cells	Not uniform

F. **Epidermal cysts of vulva**
   1. Clinical characteristics
      a. Small cystic tumors of vulva are lined by keratinized squamous epithelium
      b. Cysts contain sebaceous material with characteristic cream color and odor
      c. Cysts usually multiple; most are < 1 cm
      d. Cysts usually firm to palpation and, if squeezed, will pop and extrude sebaceous contents
   2. Treatment
      a. Large-bore needle can be inserted into cyst, but it is difficult to aspirate thick secretions
      b. If patient requests removal, its is preferable to incise cyst and gently squeeze contents
         i. Can be time-consuming
         ii. Unless cyst is infected or symptomatic, it is best left alone and patient reassured
      c. Acutely inflamed cyst should be incised and drained

G. **Acrochordon**
   1. Clinical characteristics
      a. Soft, fibroepithelial polyps that resemble skin tags
      b. May be sessile or pedunculated
      c. Gently wrinkled surface that resembles raisin
      d. Color resembles surrounding skin
   2. Treatment
      a. Acrochordons are benign, but patient may want excision for cosmetic reasons
      b. Pedicle may be tied at base before scalpel excision, or electrosurgical loop may be used to excise acrochordon at base
         i. Monsel's paste usually provides adequate hemostasis

H. **Molluscum contagiosum**—see Chapter 52

I. **Vulvar vestibulitis**
   1. Clinical characteristics
      a. Chronic syndrome characterized by severe pain produced by touching vestibule or attempting vaginal penetration
      b. Minor vestibular glands are exquisitely tender and exhibit marked erythema
      c. Minor vestibular glands are never directly involved by inflammation.
      d. Severe pain is elicited by even slight palpation of glands with cotton-tipped applicator
   2. Histology
      a. Mixed chronic inflammatory exudate
   3. Etiology
      a. Local inflammation or irritation by bacterial, fungal, or viral agents has been postulated but not proved
   4. Diagnosis can be confirmed by electromyographic reading in the presence of poor muscle recovery and reduced muscle contraction strength.
   5. Treatment
      a. No uniform response has been elicited to any specific medical therapy
      b. Short-term relief of symptoms has followed vestibular resection, but symptoms later recur in over half of patients
      c. Immunotherapy has been tried with mixed success in recalcitrant cases
      d. Because of poor outcome, referral should be made early to specialist with experience treating this frustrating disease

J. **Vulvar Paget's disease**
   1. Clinical characteristics
      a. Paget's disease is not included under the VIN classification because it originates in apocrine system, although it is considered an intraepithelial neoplasia
      b. Usually presents as vulvar pruritus in older women
      c. Gross appearance is characterized by red or tan scaly lesions
   2. Histology
      a. Paget cell is identified as large cell with large nucleus and nucleolus
      b. Paget's cell contains material with positive periodic acid-Schiff (PAS) reaction

3. Treatment
    a. Biopsy is key to successful therapy
        i. 10% of patients with vulvar Paget's disease have underlying adenocarcinoma of skin appendage etiology
        ii. Associated Paget's disease of breast must also be considered
    b. Treatment may involve wide excision or vulvectomy

SUGGESTED READING

1. Baker GE, Tyring SK: Therapeutic approaches to papillomavirus infections. Dermatol Clin North Am 15:331–340, 1997.
2. Bornstein J, Goldik Z, Stolar Z, et al: Predicting the outcome of surgical treatment of vulvar vestibulitis. Obstet Gynecol 89:695–698, 1997.
3. Colgan TJ: Vulvar intraepithelial neoplasia: A synopsis of recent developments. J Lower Genital Disease 2:31–36, 1998.
4. Elchalal U, Gilead L, Vardy D, et al: Treatment of vulvar lichen sclerosus in the elderly: An update. Obstet Gynecol Surv 50:155–162, 1995.
5. Hildesheim A, Han CL, Brinton LA, et al: Human papillomavirus type 16 and risk of preinvasive and invasive vulvar cancer: Results from a seroepidemiological case-control study. Obstet Gynecol 90:748–754, 1997.
6. Hording U, Junge J, Daugaard S, et al: Vulvar squamous cell carcinoma and papillomaviruses: Indication for two different etiologies. Gynecol Oncol 52:241–246, 1994.
7. Jones RW, Baranyai J, Stables S: Trends in squamous cell carcinoma of the vulva: The influence of vulvar intraepithelial neoplasia. Obstet Gynecol 90:448–452, 1997.
8. Kuppers V, Stiller M, Somville T, Bender HG: Risk factors for recurrent VIN: Role of multifocality and grade of disease. J Reprod Med 42:140–144, 1997.
9. Lorenz B, Kaufman RH, Kutzner SK: Lichen sclerosus: Therapy with clobetasol propionate. J Reprod Med 43:790–794, 1998.
10. Marren P, Wojnarowska F: Dermatitis of the vulva. Semin Dermatol 15:36–41, 1996.
11. Zellis S, Pincus SH: Treatment of vulvar dermatoses. Semin Dermatol 15:71–79, 1996.
12. Zorlu CG, Cobanoglu T: Medical treatment of squamous hyperplasia and lichen sclerosus of the vulva. Int J Gynaecol Obstet 51:235–238, 1995.

59. Vaginal Pain

Barbara S. Apgar, M.D., M.S.

I. The Issues

The vagina is a thin-walled, distensible fibromuscular tube that extends from the vulvar vestibule to the cervix. Diagnosis and treatment of the vagina are especially problematic. Because the vagina is a closed, topographically complex space, inspection is useless unless distention is accomplished with a vaginal speculum. The speculum examination presents a problem in itself: unless the speculum is rotated 90°, only half of the vagina is visible at any one time. The potential space of the vagina is larger in the middle and upper two-thirds than in the lower third surrounding the introitus. In most women, an axis of at least 90° is formed between the vagina and the uterus. Vaginal pain syndromes are complicated because they may involve both medical and psychological issues. Because the vagina is viewed physiologically and psychologically, problems related to medical and sexual health may be intertwined. It is important for the clinician to perform a complete vaginal examination despite the difficulty involved. The epithelium, muscular layers, blood supply, and nerves may play a role in producing the pain syndrome. If at all possible, it is important to make a diagnosis before the pain becomes chronic and more difficult to deal with.

II. The Theory

    A. **Anatomic structures:** Numerous transverse folds that form rugae help to provide for extension and distention of vagina

B. **Histology**
1. Vagina is composed of stratified squamous, nonkeratinized epithelium
2. Epithelium may become keratinized if vaginal milieu is altered. Epithelium of vagina and cervix cannot be distinguished histologically except that vagina does not have glands
   a. Because vagina contains no glands, source of vaginal secretion is not always apparent
      i. Lubrication produced as transudate from engorgement of vascular plexuses that surround vagina
      ii. This must be considered when vaginal lubrication or discharge is evaluated clinically
3. Muscular layer of vaginal mucosa allows contraction and relaxation
   a. Lower third of vagina is closely related to pelvic diaphragm
   b. Middle third is supported by levator ani muscles
   c. Vaginismus results from involuntary spasm of vaginal introital and levator ani muscles
      i. Penile penetration results in pain
      ii. May be primary or secondary
      iii. Fear of pelvic exams or use of tampons may exacerbate pain
4. Vascularity is extensively supplied from uterine artery or as branch of internal iliac artery
5. Nerve supply comes from autonomic vaginal plexus and pudendal nerve

C. **Anatomic variants**
1. **Vaginal agenesis**
   a. Pain on attempt to insert tampon or perform coitus
   b. Approximately 25% of women have short vaginal pouch
   c. Mayer-Rokitansky-Küster-Hauser syndrome
      i. Ovaries and fallopian tubes are present
      ii. Rudimentary bicornulate uterus is present
   d. Androgen insensitivity syndrome
      i. Undescended testicles and male sex ducts
      ii. Testes should be removed
   e. Exposure to diethylstilbestrol (DES)
   f. Therapy of vaginal agenesis
      i. Creation of vagina or progressive vaginal dilatation
2. **Traverse vaginal septum**
   a. Partial or complete
   b. Usually at junction of upper third and lower part of vagina
   c. Hematometrium may occur at puberty
   d. Septum is usually thick and may bleed easily with penile penetration or speculum examination
3. **Inclusion cysts**
   a. Posterior or lateral walls of lower third of vagina
   b. More common in parous women
   c. Lined by stratified squamous epithelium
   d. Contain thick, yellow, oily substance
   e. Results from small tag of vaginal epithelium buried beneath surface after gynecologic procedure
   f. Therapy: Excise if symptomatic
4. **Dysontogenetic cysts**
   a. Thin-walled, soft cysts of embryonic origin
   b. Usually in upper half of vagina
   c. Gartner's cysts
      i. Obstructed vestigial remnant of mesonephric duct
      ii. May be followed if no symptoms are present
   d. Therapy
      i. Excise for chronic mechanical obstruction
      ii. Marsupialize if acute and infected

D. **Normal vaginal secretions**
　　1. Vaginal ecosystem
　　　　a. Involves combination of hormonal, microbial, and epithelial systems
　　　　　　i. Estrogen stimulates glycogen in vaginal epithelial cells
　　　　　　ii. Glycogen is metabolized to lactic acid by lactobacilli
　　　　　　　　(a) Stimulates pH to remain about 4.0 which limits growth of pathogenic microbes
　　2. Normal vaginal secretions must be differentiated from those produced by vaginitis
　　　　a. Wet preparation
　　　　b. Culture
　　　　c. pH (normal < pH 4.5)
　　　　d. Classification of discharge
　　　　　　i. Normal vaginal secretions usually without odor, pain, or pruritus
E. **Abnormal lesions**
　　1. **Trauma**
　　　　a. Vaginal lacerations may occur from coitus, penetration injuries, foreign objects, or sexual assault
　　　　b. Most common injury: transverse tear of posterior fornix
　　　　c. Most common symptoms: pain and bleeding
　　　　d. Therapy
　　　　　　i. Prompt repair
　　　　　　ii. No place for conservative management because of secondary complications
　　2. **Vaginal intraepithelial neoplasia** (VAIN)
　　　　a. Rare condition that frequently rises from previous cervical intraepithelial neoplasia (CIN) or vulvar intraepithelial neoplasia (VIN)
　　　　　　i. Most VIN produces some pruritus, irritation or pain
　　　　b. Clinical characteristics
　　　　　　i. Most VAIN lesions are located in vaginal fornices or at apex or cuff if prior hysterectomy has been performed
　　　　　　ii. Because VAIN is usually multicentric, examination must be thorough
　　　　c. Treatment
　　　　　　i. Biopsy excision for small lesions
　　　　　　ii. Larger lesions may be treated with CO_2 laser, which facilitates control of depth of treatment
　　　　　　　　(a) 5-Fluorouracil (5-FU) has been used following CO_2 laser to eradicate small lesions
　　　　　　iii. Cryotherapy should not be performed in vagina because depth of freeze is difficult to control and rectovaginal and vesicovaginal fistulas have been reported as sequelae
　　3. **Primary invasive carcinoma**
　　　　a. Invasive carcinoma of vagina is rare as primary lesion, most cancers are metastatic
　　　　b. Lesions tend to occur high in vagina; no dominant histologic type
　　　　c. Primary presenting symptoms: vaginal bleeding and pelvic pain
　　　　d. Tumors vary in size, but most are raised, friable, granular, and Lugol's-negative
　　　　e. Early therapy with radiation is important for survival
　　4. **Exposure to diethylstilbestrol** (DES)
　　　　a. Etiology
　　　　　　i. Vagina is originally lined by cuboidal nonstratified columnar epithelium
　　　　　　ii. Eventually columnar epithelium is replaced by a core of stratified squamous epithelium
　　　　　　iii. If DES is introduced *in utero*, transformation from columnar to squamous epithelium is not completed
　　　　　　　　(a) One-third of exposed patients exhibit columnar epithelium in vagina (adenosis)
　　　　b. Symptoms
　　　　　　i. Vaginal discharge
　　　　　　ii. Postcoital bleeding
　　　　　　iii. Dyspareunia

    c. Clinical findings

       i. DES-exposed women should be examined by palpation, colposcopy, and Lugol's solution. Adenosis is Lugol's-negative.

      ii. Lesions consist of red patches that resemble columnar lakes on cervix

        (a) Adenosis has characteristic grape-like appearance but also may exhibit granularity and ulceration

        (b) Fornices should be carefully examined

    d. Histology

       i. Adenosis resembles endocervical epithelium

      ii. Lesion may contain squamous metaplasia, process whereby adenosis is converted to stratified squamous epithelium

     iii. Finding columnar epithelium or squamous metaplasia in vaginal mucosa suggests adenosis

    e. Therapy

       i. Observation for DES-exposed vaginal mucosa

      ii. Women need to be followed annually with four-quadrant cytologic smears and colposcopic examination. Annual palpation of vagina may detect small nodules developing in fornices and along vaginal wall.

    f. DES-exposed women may rarely develop clear-cell carcinoma

       i. Diagnosis and management

        (a) Most patients exhibit bleeding or vaginal discharge

        (b) Lesions are usually multiple, frequently raised, polypoid, or flat indurated plaques with ulceration

        (c) Colposcopy may reveal punctation, mosaicism, or atypical vessels

        (d) Referral and comanagement of DES abnormalities are recommended if nature of lesions is in question

  5. **Vaginal ulcers**

    a. Etiology

       i. Drying and pressure necrosis of mucosa

      ii. Tampon use, foreign objects such as pessaries, 5-FU

    b. Clinical findings include mucosal drying, peeling, layering, and ulceration

       i. Vaginal cancer must be ruled out

    c. Therapy

       i. Biopsy

      ii. Appropriate for diagnosis

III. **An Approach**

  A. **Psychological conditions**

    1. **Vaginismus**

      a. Etiology

         i. Consider sexual abuse, phobia aversion of sexuality or medical condition resulting in aversion

        ii. Lack of appropriate sex education or being told sex is "bad"

      b. Therapy

         i. Attempt to identify cause through psychotherapy

        ii. Educate patient and her sexual partner

       iii. Teach self-dilation of vagina and give patient permission to touch her genital area

       iv. Results vary, depending on how deeply anxiety and aversion are seeded

    2. **Dyspareunia**

      a. Pain during intercourse with entry (introital) or deep thrusting (vaginal)

      b. May have both psychological and medical cause

      c. Obtain history to determine type (vaginal or introital)

      d. Entrance dyspareunia

         i. The entire vulvovaginal area is painful

         (a) *Candida*, lichen sclerosus, atrophy

        ii. Pain is concentrated at the introitus

         (b) Vaginismus, inadequate lubrication

  e. Vaginal dyspareunia
    i. Estrogen deficiency, stenosis
  f. Avoid stereotyping; approach with open-minded and straightforward thinking.
    i. Use patience and logical sequence of work-up
  g. If emotional investment of patient is high, may be more difficult to treat
B. **Medical therapy**
  1. Biopsy is key to successful management of vaginal lesions
    a. Use anesthetic and pull-and-snip technique
    b. Provide hemostasis with Monsel's solution and pressure
  2. Laser—appropriate for precancerous lesions
  3. Avoid cryotherapy in vagina—cannot control depth of penetration of cryonecrosis
  4. Excision of lesions
    a. Long-handled instruments required
    b. Be cautious of lesions > 1 cm
      i. Vagina is difficult space in which to work and highly vascular

SUGGESTED READING

1. Abramov L, Wolman I, David MP: Vaginismus: An important factor in the evaluation and management of vulvar vestibulitis syndrome. Gynecol Obstet Invest 38:194–197, 1994.
2. Bornstein J, Goldik Z, Stolar Z, et al: Predicting the outcome of surgical treatment of vulvar vestibulitis. Obstet Gynecol 89:695–698, 1997.
3. Bornstein J, Zarfati D, Goldshmid N, et al: Vestibulodynia: A subset of vulvar vestibulitis or a novel syndrome? Am J Obstet Gynecol 177:1439–43, 1997.
4. Jones RW, Baranyai J, Stables S: Trends in squamous cell carcinoma of the vulva: The influence of vulvar intraepithelial neoplasia. Obstet Gynecol 90:448–452, 1997.
5. Noller KL: In utero exposure to DES: A review. The Colposcopist, Summer 1990.
6. Reid R, Omoto K, Precop S, et al: Flashlamp-excited dye laser therapy of idiopathic vulvodynia is safe, is efficacious. Am J Obstet Gynecol 172:1684–1701, 1995.
7. Schover LR, Youngs DD, Caunata R: Psychosexual aspects of the evaluation and management of vulvar vestibulitis. Am J Obstet Gynecol 167:630–636, 1992.
8. Sillman FH, Fruchter RG, Chen Y-S, et al: Vaginal intraepithelial neoplasia: Risk factors for persistence, recurrence, and invasion and its management. Am J Obstet Gynecol 176:93–99, 1997.
9. Van Lankveld JJDM, Weijenborg P, Ter Kuile MM: Psychologic profiles of and sexual function in women with vulvar vestibulitis and their partners. Obstet Gynecol 88:65–70, 1996.
10. White G, Jantos M: Sexual behavior changes with vulvar vestibulitis syndrome. J Reprod Med 43:783–789, 1998.

60. Pelvic Pain

Barbara S. Apgar, M.D., M.S.

I. The Issues

Pelvic pain is associated with actual or potential tissue damage. The perception of pain, however, is subjective. Pain that does not have a pathophysiologic cause may still be perceived as pain. It is often not possible to determine whether physical or emotional elements caused the painful event. Both acute and chronic pain may be severe. Acute pain, generally of recent and sudden onset, is associated with rebound tenderness and diminished bowel sounds. Acute pain of gynecologic origin usually presents as both abdominal and pelvic pain. Episodes of acute pelvic pain usually fall into the categories of pregnancy-related accidents, infections, mechanical occurrences, menstrual disorders, and nongynecologic disorders, such as gastrointestinal and genitourinary disease. Treatment of acute pain usually diminishes the symptoms. The symptoms may not recur once the cause of the pain is removed.

Chronic pelvic pain is noncyclic pain that lasts longer than 6 months and is not relieved by non-narcotic analgesics. Chronic pelvic pain is a nonspecific term that includes pain associated with laparoscopically evident pathology, such as endometriosis and pelvic inflammatory disease; occult pain, which usually involves nongynecologic somatic pathology, such as irritable bowel syndrome; and nonsomatic (psychogenic) pain and disorders. Whereas the management of women with laparoscopically apparent pathology seems deceptively straightforward, diagnosis of chronic pelvic pain in the absence of obvious remediable pathology (pelvalgia) is one of the most difficult diagnostic problems. Few complaints challenge the limits of professional expertise, patience, and forbearance as chronic pelvic pain. Patients are often referred to many consultants and are often angry, frustrated, and defensive.

II. **The Theory**
  A. **Anatomy**
    1. Close anatomic proximity of pelvic organs makes diagnosis of specific entities difficult
      a. Fallopian tube is one of most sensitive pelvic organs
        i. Infection of fallopian tubes along mucosal surface produces severe pain
      b. Broad ligaments are important conduits for anatomic structures
        i. Infiltration of broad ligaments with infection, cancer, or endometriosis produces pain
      c. Cardinal ligaments help to maintain anatomic position of cervix and upper vagina and provide major support of uterus and cervix
        i. Prolapse of ligament support produces pain
      d. Parametria and cul-de-sac of Douglas are important landmarks in advanced pelvic infection and cancer
        i. Cul-de-sac may be obliterated by inflammatory process associated with infection, endometriosis, or cancer
  B. **Functional pain**
    1. Etiology
      a. Pregnancy-related
        i. Spontaneous abortion; ectopic pregnancy; trophoblastic disease
      b. Adnexal disease
        i. Salpingitis; tubo-ovarian disease; endometriosis; cancer of tubes of ovary; torsion of ovary or tube; rupture of ovarian cyst
      c. Nongynecologic disease
        i. Appendicitis; renal calculi; gastrointestinal disease, such as ulcerative colitis; musculoskeletal disease, such as spinal disc herniation
    2. Character of pain
      a. Paroxysms of sharp, stabbing pain interspersed with cramping pain or no pain at all
      b. Continuous sharp and throbbing pain
      c. Usually relieved by removal of primary source
  C. **Chronic pelvic pain** (CPP)
    1. **Significance**
      a. Accounts for up to 10% of outpatient gynecologic consultations, approximately 20% of laparoscopies, and 12% of hysterectomies in U.S.
      b. Total direct and indirect costs may be conservatively estimated to exceed $2 billion annually
      c. Patients commonly describe years of disability, suffering, marital discord, and numerous unsuccessful medical evaluations
      d. 20% of women with CPP have coexistent psychological pathology
    2. **Definition**
      a. Six or more months of consistent or intermittent cyclic or acyclic pelvic pain that has necessitated at least 3 separate visits to physician without definite diagnosis
    3. **Clinical findings** (at least one)
      a. Dull or severe pain
      b. Dysmenorrhea
      c. Dyspareunia
      d. Vaginal pain
    4. **In absence of identifiable pathology** (pelvalgia)
      a. Clinical challenge

      i. Afflicted patients often distraught, angry, and demanding

      ii. Frustration usually shared by physician who is unable to find plausible cause or to effect cure but who through fear of insulting patient remains reluctant to consider psychiatric causes

      iii. Patients with pelvalgia characteristically resistant to nonsomatic explanation or treatment

          (a) As result largely of frustration, patients and physician are apt to consider "definitive" surgical therapy, consisting of removal of grossly normal uterus and adnexa

  b. **Patient with CPP and negative laparoscopy**

      i. Average estimation of normal laparoscopic findings in women with CPP is approximately 40%

      ii. Approximately 12% of hysterectomies in U.S. are done for CPP with no identifiable pathology

          (a) No study to date has documented long-term (> 1 year) efficacy of hysterectomy for CPP, particularly when grossly normal tissues are removed

          (b) Approximately 25% of patients who undergo total abdominal hysterectomy and bilateral salpingo-oophorectomy (TAH-BSO) have no significant improvement of pain

          (c) Few patients return to physician who performed procedure suggesting that hysterectomy may result in discontinuance of follow-up rather than amelioration of pain

      iii. Mean age of patients with pelvalgia is 28.6 years

      iv. CPP patients more likely to have experienced spontaneous abortion

          (a) Occult somatic pathology such as endometriosis may result from spontaneous abortion and cause CPP

          (b) Spontaneous abortion may initiate or reinforce patient's belief in intrapelvic pathology and thereby precipitate CPP

5. **Medical history**

  a. Consume 3 times as many prescription medications: narcotic and non-narcotic analgesics, anxiolytics, and sedatives

  b. Undergo cumulative major and minor surgical procedures 5 times more often

  c. Almost twice as many total sexual partners since becoming sexually active

  d. Association between CPP and prior major psychosexual trauma, including molestation, incest, and rape (48%)

      i. Suffered repeated and unreported sexual trauma and can relate onset of pelvic pain to particular assault

      ii. No studies have reached definitive conclusions about the relationship between sexual trauma and CPP

      iii. Women with CPP who admitted to sexual abuse exhibited highest degree of psychopathology with MMPI profile showing marked histrionic traits, somatic overconcern, impulsiveness, and unusual thought processes

  e. Women with CPP and no sexual abuse indicated mild depression, histrionic traits, and functional physical complaints

      i. Have difficulty forming close relationships and generally feel inadequate or dissatisfied with female roles

      ii. Tend to be emotionally insecure and immature, have strong dependency needs, and experience difficulty externalizing feelings of stress and hostility

      iii. CPP may result from patient's conversion of unacceptable problem or stress into acceptable symptom, such as pelvic pain, for which she seeks medical attention

      iv. Results of psychological testing with Minnesota Multiphasic Personality Index (MMPI) have helped to identify 3 different personality profiles, whose common feature is a tendency to develop somatic symptoms or to exaggerate existing somatic symptoms in response to stress

III. **An Approach**
   A. **Acute pelvic pain**
      1. Complete history and physical exam
         a. Character of pain
         b. Associated physical findings
         c. Emergency room visits
      2. Laboratory evaluation
         a. Human chorionic gonadotropin (hCG)
         b. Complete blood count
         c. Cultures
         d. Ultrasound
         e. Laparoscopy
      3. Treatment
         a. Referral to surgeon for evaluation of acute abdomen
         b. Antibiotic therapy for infectious etiology
         c. Conservative management only if patient is compliant and willing to attend follow-up visits
   B. **Chronic pelvic pain**
      1. Complete history and physical exam
         a. Previous work-up results
         b. Character of pain
         c. Social and sexual history
         d. Psychiatric evaluation and testing
      2. Laboratory evaluation
         a. Complete blood count
         b. Cultures
         c. Ultrasound (minimal yield)
         d. Laparoscopy
      3. Treatment of patient with CPP and laparoscopically negative evaluation
         a. Importance of psychologist as part of CPP treatment team has been well documented
            i. Immediately after gynecologic examination, patient is introduced to staff psychologist, or psychologist is called by examining physician while patient is present
            ii. Critical point in management
               (a) Having experienced pain for many years, many patients have developed pain-related behaviors integral to their personality
               (b) Patients typically reluctant to accept psychological explanation for what they are certain is physical problem
               (c) Consideration must be given to perception that psychological problems are not legitimate illnesses
               (d) Physician and psychologist together form treatment plan validating credibility of each other's management protocol
         b. Patient must not feel she is being abandoned or that family physician believes nothing is wrong with her and that "it's all in her head"
            i. Introduction is made to indicate that primary care physician is interested in determining effect of patient's chronic pain on her well-being since difficulties with work and family may be compounded by way she feels about herself
            ii. Patient should be given perception that goal is to get her in control of pain rather than letting pain control her
            iii. Patient is given opportunity to make appointment with psychologist before she leaves office
            iv. Patient is also given appointment with family physician in approximately 1 month to discuss psychiatric evaluation and management and to reinforce need for such therapy
         c. Avoidance of surgical therapy for which there is no cure.
         d. Avoidance of victimization status among enablers

SUGGESTED READING

1. Baker PK: Musculoskeletal origins of chronic pelvic pain: Diagnosis and management. Obstet Gynecol Clin North Am 20:719–742, 1993.
2. Kresch AJ, Seifer DB, Sachs LB, Barrese I: Laparoscopy in 100 women with chronic pelvic pain. Obstet Gynecol 64:672–674, 1984.
3. Ling FW, Slocumb JC: Use of trigger point injections in chronic pelvic pain. Obstet Gynecol Clin North Am 20:809–815, 1993.
4. Lipscomb GH, Ling FW: Relationship of pelvic infection and chronic pelvic pain. Obstet Gynecol Clin North Am 20:699–708, 1993.
5. Mareta LD, Swanson DW, McHardy MJ: Three years follow-up of patients with chronic pelvic pain who were treated in a multidisciplinary pain management center. Pain 41:47–51, 1990.
6. Milburn A, Reiter RC, Rhomberg AT: Multidisciplinary approach to chronic pelvic pain. Obstet Gynecol Clin North Am 20:643–661, 1993.
7. Peters AA, Trimbos-Kemper GC, Admiraal C, et al: A randomized clinical trial on the benefit of adhesiolysis in patients with intraperitoneal adhesions and chronic pelvic pain. Br J Obstet Gynecol 99:59–62, 1992.
8. Reiter RC: A profile of women with chronic pelvic pain. Clin Obstet Gynecol 33:130–136, 1990.
9. Reiter RC, Gambone JC: Nongynecologic somatic pathology in women with chronic pelvic pain and negative laparoscopy. J Reprod Med 36:253–259, 1991.
10. Stewart DE: Chronic gynecologic pain. Gen Hosp Psychiatry 18:230–237, 1996.
11. Walling MK, Reiter RC, O'Hara MW, et al: Abuse history and chronic pain in women: I. Prevalences of sexual abuse and physical abuse. Obstet Gynecol 84:193–199, 1994.

61. Pelvic Mass

Gary R. Newkirk, M.D.

I. The Issues

The majority of pelvic masses are found by the clinician during physical examination. The mass may be found during evaluation of specific complaints or symptoms, such as abdominal pain or in asymptomatic women presenting for routine Papanicolaou smear and pelvic examination. In either instance, the pelvic mass demands evaluation because of the potential for malignancy at all ages. Even the clinical presentation of a likely benign process eventually warrants diagnostic clarification if the mass persists or enlarges. Certain clinical settings, such as postmenopausal patients or patients with a family history of ovarian malignancy, imply an ominous etiology and demand expeditious diagnosis. Primary care providers can play an irreplaceable role in evaluation of the pelvic mass by affording ample time to elicit a detailed history, to perform a thorough pelvic examination, and to coordinate the work-up, which, in many cases, will entail referral to various subspecialists.

II. The Theory

A. A pelvic mass can arise from any pelvic organ
  1. Ovary, adnexal structures, uterus, cervix
  2. Bladder, ureter
  3. Gastrointestinal (GI) structures
     a. Bowel, appendix, omentum
     b. Bowel variants (diverticula, Meckel's diverticulum)
  4. Vasculature
  5. Lymphatic node systems
  6. Congenital variants (pelvic kidneys, adrenal tumors, pelvic testes)
  7. Retroperitoneum
     a. Nodes
     b. Sarcomas

B. **Conditions resulting in pelvic masses**
  1. Infection (abscesses)
  2. Pregnancy (intrauterine, ectopic, molar)

3. Cysts (ovarian, omental, peritoneal, fallopian)
4. Endometriosis implants

C. **Symptomatic pelvic masses**
1. Toxic presentation
   a. Fever, abdominal pain
   b. With or without nausea, vomiting, weight loss
2. Possible etiologies
   a. Abscesses
      i. Tubo-ovarian abscess
      ii. Abscesses of GI origin (appendiceal, diverticular)
      iii. Renal abscess, renal obstruction
   b. Pregnancy complications
      i. Septic abortion
      ii. Ectopic pregnancy
      iii. Previously undiagnosed intrauterine pregnancy with complication (abruptio placentae, amnionitis)
   c. Torsion phenomenon (bowel, omentum, ovary, fallopian tubes)
   d. Acute hemorrhage complicating existing mass (malignant mass, various hemorrhagic cysts, lymph nodes)
   e. Other
      i. Bowel infarct
      ii. Ruptured viscus
      iii. Bladder obstruction, retention
      iv. Hematomas, e.g., psoas muscled, abdominal wall (rectus sheath)

D. **Asymptomatic pelvic masses**
1. Found during routine pelvic examination
2. Etiology often age-related
   a. Women younger than 30 years
      i. ovarian cysts
      ii. Congenital anomalies
      iii. Unsuspected pregnancy
      iv. Lymphoid tumors
   b. Women over 30, premenopausal
      i. Same as for women < 30
      ii. Increased likelihood of cancerous sources, especially ovarian, endometrial, and cervical
   c. Postmenopausal women
      i. Same as for premenopausal women
      ii. Primary GI, bladder cancer
      iii. Metastatic cancers increasingly likely, especially breast and GI tract

III. **An Approach**

A. **Careful history**
1. Prior known pelvic diagnoses
2. Prior abdominal surgery
3. Careful history of obstetric/gynecologic, urinary, GI infections
4. Family history
   a. Especially with ovarian cancer

B. **Physical examination**
1. Complete general exam
   a. Thyroid, breast masses, skin tumors, basic neurologic screen, congenital variants, scars, organomegaly, edema
2. **Pelvic examination**
   a. Careful inspection and palpation of vulva, vagina, cervix
   b. Bimanual exam
      i. Uterine size, contour, tenderness, mobility
      ii. Ovarian size, tenderness
      iii. Rectal/vaginal tissue palpation

      iv. Uterine ligament palpation
   c. Rectal exam
      i. Masses
      ii. Occult blood testing
      iii. Palpate cul-de-sac

C. **Laboratory evaluation**
1. Pregnancy test when appropriate, beta–human chorionic gonadotropin
2. Complete blood count, erythrocyte sedimentation rate, chemistry panel
3. Urinalysis
4. Cultures if infectious etiology suspected
   a. Cervix
   b. Blood
5. Consider CA-125 if ovarian or other gynecologic malignancy suspected
6. Carcinoembryonic antigen (CEA) for GI sources

D. **Imaging studies**
1. Ultrasound
   a. Transabdominal and transvaginal
      i. Doppler flow studies for vascular tumors
   b. Especially helpful if pelvic exam difficult because of
      i. Tenderness or obesity
2. Abdominal series radiographs
   a. Helpful for potentially calcifying processes (e.g., dermoid cysts, renal stones, calcified nodes)
   b. Bowel obstruction suspected, basic bowel air pattern, free air
3. Barium enema for suspected bowel source or involvement, consider water soluble contrast if leakage of contrast possible (perforation)
4. Urologic work-up
   a. For suspected urologic sources
   b. Cystoscopy
   c. Intravenous pyelography (IVP), retrograde cystography
5. Computed tomography (CT)
   a. Especially if source not identified by above imaging studies
   b. Spiral CT tomography
6. Magnetic resonance imaging (MRI)
   a. Most helpful if congenital anomaly suspected
   b. May help locate GI source (e.g., hepatic metastatic disease)

E. **Histologic studies**
1. Colposcopy-directed biopsies, endocervical curettage (ECC) if:
   a. Abnormal appearance to vulva, vagina, cervix
   b. Abnormal cytology on Papanicolaou smear
   c. Abnormal palpatory texture to vulvar, vaginal, cervical tissue
2. Endometrial biopsy (nonpregnant women)
   a. Irregular bleeding problems with and without uterine enlargement
   b. To help determine status of ovulatory function
      i. Secretory epithelium is evidence of ovulation
3. Dilatation and curettage (D&C)
   a. Need for thorough sampling of endometrium
      i. Control bleeding
      ii. Endometrial cancer suspected from biopsy histology
      iii. Often preceded by hysteroscopy in this setting
   b. Fractional sample obtained to stage cervical and endometrial cancer
4. Sigmoid/colonoscopic biopsy
   a. Mass suspected
      i. By pelvic examination
      ii. Positive screening for occult GI blood
      iii. GI source suspected by imaging study (barium enema, CT, or MRI)
   b. Prior to laparotomy to evaluate involvement of lower GI tract

     5. Image-guided transcutaneous biopsy
        a. Example: GI malignancy presenting as rectal mass
        b. Mass demonstrated by initial screening imaging (barium enema, CT, or MRI)

F. Other methods
   1. Hysteroscopy
   2. Laparoscopy
   3. Laparotomy

G. Management: According to probable site of origin
   1. **Adnexal origin suspected**
      a. Premenopausal women
         i. Ultrasound (US)
      b. If mass < 5 am with simple cystic architecture, negative pregnancy test
         i. Hormonal management with birth control pills Depo-Provera, oral progestins
         ii. Repeat pelvic examination and US if mass persists
      c. If mass > 5 cm, complex US architecture, or significant symptoms
         i. Laparotomy
      d. If mass persists or enlarges or becomes symptomatic, laparoscopy is indicated regardless of original US size estimation
      e. Postmenopausal women
         i. Most require definitive surgery
         ii. Consider serum CA-125, although normal levels do not preclude need for surgery

   2. **Urologic origin suspected**
      a. Urologic referral for IVP, cystoscopy, surgery

   3. **GI source suspected**
      a. Occult blood testing
      b. Flexible sigmoidoscopy
      c. Barium enema
      d. Colonoscopy
         i. If barium enema and flexible sigmoidoscopy are not diagnostic
         ii. Colonoscopy may performed first and replace flexible sigmoidoscopy if transverse or right colon source suspected, prior history of polyps and/or bowel malignancy
      e. Small bowel studies if above nondiagnostic
         i. Enterocolysis
         ii. Angiography
      f. CT, MRI for evaluation of pancreatic, liver, pelvic extension, or nodal involvement
      g. Consider liver function tests, CEA

   4. **Uterine source suspected**
      a. Routine studies
         i. Pregnancy test if pregnancy possible
         ii. Papanicolaou smear
         iii. Consider colposcopy with biopsy, ECC
         iv. Endometrial biopsy
      b. Benign fibroids suspected
         i. Serial pelvic US evaluation every 2–3 months
         ii. If mass enlarges or symptoms increase, consider surgery
      c. Malignant process suspected—surgery indicated
      d. Unclear uterine source
         i. Consider hysteroscopy; D&C often follows
         ii. Hysterosalpingography

   5. **Source of mass unclear**
      a. Extensive imaging to clarify source (CT, MRI, barium enema)
      b. Exploratory surgery often performed for concerns about malignant process, enlarging masses, increasing symptoms

   6. **Role of laparotomy**
      a. Diagnosis
         i. Anatomic inspection, culture, biopsy

  b. Diagnosis/treatment
      i. Torsion reduction
      ii. Excision (e.g., appendix)
      iii. Abscess, adhesion reduction
      iv. Laser, electroablation (endometriosis)
  c. For suspected operative cancer
      i. Diagnosis, staging, treatment, palliation
7. Nonoperative management, malignancy not initially suspected
  a. Therapeutic trial of antibiotics
      i. For example, if pelvic inflammatory disease, abscesses suspected
      ii. Diverticular disease
  b. Careful serial examination follow-up

SUGGESTED READING

1. Russell DJ: The female pelvic mass: Diagnosis and management. Med Clin North Am 79:1481–1493, 1995.
2. Roman LD, Muderspach LI, Stein SM, et al: Pelvic examination, tumor marker level, and gray-scale and Doppler sonography in the prediction of pelvic cancer. Obstet Gynecol 89:493–500, 1997.
3. Siegel MJ: Pelvic tumors in childhood. Radiol Clin North Am 35:1455–1475, 1997.
4. Sladkevicius P, Valentin L, Marsal K: Transvaginal Doppler examination for the differential diagnosis of solid pelvic tumors. J Ultrasound Med 14:377–380, 1995.
5. Weinreb JC, Barkoff ND, Megibow A, Demopoulos R: The value of MR imaging in distinguishing leiomyomas from other solid pelvic masses when sonography is indeterminate. Am J Roentgenol 154:295–299, 1990.

62. Endometriosis

Gary R. Newkirk, M.D.

I. The Issues

Endometriosis remains one of the most common gynecologic diseases in women during their reproductive years, and its incidence is increasing. Approximately 10% of premenopausal women are affected. About 60–70% of women with endometriosis are nulliparous, and a majority have a positive family history. Endometriosis is found in 30–60% of women who present for infertility evaluation. Endometriosis substantially affects the individual secondary to pain and loss of work time as well as the health care system with well over a million hospital days for management. Endometriosis is rarely life-threatening but frequently becomes "life-altering."

II. The Theory

  A. **Definition**
      1. Endometriosis: presence of tissue that is biologically and morphologically similar to normal endometrium in locations beyond endometrial cavity
      2. "Typical" patient in late 20s or early 30s, Caucasian, and frequently nulliparous
      3. In reality, endometriosis occurs in all races from early adolescence to peri-menopausal ages

  B. **Pathophysiology**
      1. Incompletely characterized
      2. Most widely accepted explanation focuses on concept of retrograde flow of menstrual fluid through fallopian tubes with implantation of viable endometrial tissue in free pelvis
      3. Coelomic metaplasia theory argues that undifferentiated coelomic epithelial cells remain dormant on peritoneal surface until ovaries produce enough hormones to stimulate ectopic tissue

III. **An Approach**
   A. **Clinical presentation**
      1. Wide range of clinical symptoms
      2. Poor correlation between symptoms and extent of endometrial implants within pelvis
      3. Most common complaints
         a. Dysmenorrhea (50%)
         b. Infertility (25–50%)
         c. Pelvic pain and/or dyspareunia (20%)
         d. Menstrual irregularities (12–14%)
         e. Pain may be diffuse or localized to involved organ
      4. Less common complaints
         a. Low back pain, dysuria, hematuria, diarrhea
         b. Classically occur before or during menses
      5. Patient may present with some, none, or all of above symptoms, which may or may not correlate with menstrual cycle
   B. **Infertility and endometriosis**
      1. Endometriosis should be considered in women initially presenting for evaluation of infertility
      2. Exact relationship not known; more than one mechanism probably involved
         a. Altered anatomy, ovulatory dysfunction, hormonal abnormalities, autoimmunity, toxic pelvic factors, altered sexual functioning, increased spontaneous abortions
      3. Although number of pelvic implants does not correlate well with severity of dysmenorrhea and dyspareunia, probability of successful conception appears to be inversely related to severity of disease
   C. **Diagnosis**
      1. Neither history nor physical exam confirms diagnosis of endometriosis
      2. Pelvic pain, dyspareunia, dysmenorrhea, abnormal bleeding, or infertility should raise suspicion
      3. Physical findings include uterosacral nodularity, retroversion of uterus, limited pelvic mobility, adnexal masses, and diffuse or focal tenderness
      4. Diagnosis requires direct visual and histologic confirmation by laparoscopy or laparotomy
         a. During laparoscopy or laparotomy, endometriosis may appear as classic brown lesions, either focal (e.g., ovarian) or diffuse (e.g., peritoneal)
         b. Reddish-blue nodules on peritoneum, uterine ligaments, or pelvic viscera also common
         c. Focal scarring or retraction of peritoneum, diffuse adhesions, and distortion of uterine, ovarian, and tubal anatomy also may be seen
         d. Ovarian implants may result in formation of endometrioma ("chocolate cysts")
            i. May explain tender adnexal mass on pelvic exam
            ii. Presence of endometrioma, confirmed during laparotomy, may constitute initial finding for endometriosis
      5. Extrapelvic (e.g., vulva, vagina) or pelvic endometriosis should be considered if mass or lesion becomes painful in cyclic fashion with menses
      6. Uniform system of classification based on presence, location, and quality of adhesions, endometriomas, and tubal distortion has been formulated by American Fertility Society (AFS)
         a. Stage I—minimal, stage ii—mild, stage iii—moderate, stage iv—severe
   D. **Imaging tests**
      1. CT and MRI
         a. Provide presumptive evidence of endometriosis but are not diagnostic because of lack of characteristic appearance or location for implants
         b. Rarely justified for initial work-up
      2. Pelvic and transvaginal ultrasound
         a. Not diagnostic but may be helpful in detecting and characterizing pelvic pathology if pelvic exam is limited by tenderness or obesity

      b. Common availability, lower cost, safety in pregnancy, and nonradiographic nature prompt many clinicians to include pelvic ultrasonography in work-up

E. **Blood test**
1. CA-125 is a cell surface antigen found on derivatives of coelomic epithelium, including endometrial tissue
2. Despite correlation of CA-125 levels with both degree of endometriosis and response to therapy, sensitivity of assay too low to be used as screening test
3. May be useful for evaluating ovarian cysts

F. **Management**
1. **General comments**
   a. No universally effective cure, but treatment relieves symptoms
   b. Wide variety of treatments betrays poorly defined etiology and pathophysiology
   c. Factors to consider before treatment
      i. Patient's age
      ii. Desire for fertility
      iii. Severity of symptoms
      iv. Extent, location, and severity of disease
   d. Treatment should be preceded by careful confirmation and staging with laparoscopy or laparotomy
   e. Treatment options
      i. Expectant management
      ii. Conservative surgical therapy
      iii. Medical therapy
      iv. Extensive surgery with castration
      v. Superovulation therapies for infertility (e.g., *in vitro* fertilization or gamete intrafallopian tube transfer [GIFT])
   f. Endometriotic implants behave like normal endometrial tissue and are supported by ovarian hormones
      i. Hormonal management takes advantage of biologic response of endometriotic tissue to alterations of hormonal environment
      ii. In either hypoestrogenic or hyperandrogenic environment, endometriotic implants become atrophic
   g. More advanced endometriosis involves greater likelihood that surgical intervention will be required
   h. Surgical removal of both ovaries invariably induces remission but should be reserved for women with advanced endometriosis who are over 35 years of age and have completed their family
2. **Expectant management (watchful waiting)**
   a. May be reasonable strategy for younger woman who desires pregnancy and has mild symptoms
   b. Identify and correct other infertility factors as necessary (see Chapter 26)
   c. Pregnancy rates as high as with medical therapy or conservative surgery (50%)
3. **Conservative surgery**
   a. Entails either laparoscopy or laparotomy
   b. Indications
      i. To confirm diagnosis
      ii. If fertility is desired, to determine tubal occlusion or peritubal, pelvic, or ovarian adhesions
      iii. To aspirate chocolate ovarian cysts
      iv. To evaluate pelvic pain unrelieved by medical therapy
   c. Initial treatment at time of diagnostic laparoscopy often accomplished with electrocoagulation and/or laser ablation of implants through laparoscope
   d. Partial ovarian resection for endometrioma and lysis of adhesions as necessary
4. **Definitive surgery**
   a. Includes total hysterectomy and bilateral salpingo-oophorectomy
   b. Indicated in women who do not desire pregnancy and for whom all previous medical and conservative surgical efforts have failed

5. **Medical management**
   a. Includes danazol, progestogens, oral contraceptives, and gonadotropin-releasing hormones (GnRH)
   b. Goals are to control symptoms and/or to improve fertility
   c. Most medical regimens involve treatment for at least 6 months to allow adequate regression of implants
   d. Unfortunately, hormonal therapy does not improve adhesive disease or regress ovarian endometriomas; surgery is required in such circumstances
      i. Danazol (Danocrine) induces hyperandrogenic state, whereas GnRH agonists produce hypoestrogenic state
         (a) Both induce regression of endometriotic implants
      ii. Progesterone therapy
         (a) Medroxyprogesterone acetate (Amen, Cycrin, Provera)
         (b) Induces decidual or atrophic changes in endometriotic implants
      iii. Combined estrogen-progestogen contraceptives (pseudopregnancy regimen)
         (a) Produce acyclic hormone environment similar to pregnancy
         (b) Cause endometriotic implants to atrophy

6. **Other management issues**
   a. Severe endometriosis and infertility require organized treatment approach that combines both surgery and prolonged medical treatment
   b. Arranging for consultation, monitoring of medical treatment, and long-term emotional support are required of primary care provider

G. **Prevention**
   1. At present no known effective interventions to prevent endometriosis
   2. Positive family history and deferring childbearing lead to higher likelihood for development of symptomatic endometriosis
   3. Hormonal contraceptives appear to delay symptoms in some individuals

H. **Long-term results**
   1. Endometriosis usually recurs despite medical or conservative surgical treatment
   2. Long-term hormonal therapy without surgery helps to prevent progression in some patients with severe symptoms
   3. Definitive surgery (e.g., abdominal hysterectomy with bilateral salpingo-oophorectomy) combined with resection of all endometrial implants yields highest likelihood for resolution of symptoms
   4. Laparoscopic finding of minimal endometrial disease in women not desiring pregnancy frequently managed with cyclic birth control pills to lessen further seeding
   5. More advanced disease usually requires 6 months of danazol or medroxyprogesterone acetate followed by cyclic birth control pills

I. **Family and community issues**
   1. Effective management challenges family physician to remain informed patient advocate because comprehensive care frequently involves referral and familiarity with long-term treatment modalities not routinely used by family physicians
   2. Education ideally should begin in early adolescence as part of comprehensive health education
   3. Women should be encouraged to seek medical help for symptoms of endometriosis
   4. For many women, endometriosis becomes chronic affliction requiring ongoing education, treatment, and compassion
   5. If patient requests, physician should meet with other members of family to offer information and address questions or concerns
   6. Patients and families may benefit from contracting the Endometriosis Association to obtain educational materials and information about support groups
   7. Women with documented endometriosis who desire pregnancy should be counseled about relationship to infertility; desires and timing of childbearing should be discussed

SUGGESTED READING

1. Farquhar C, Sutton C: The evidence for the management of endometriosis. Curr Opin Obstet Gynecol 10:321–332, 1998.

2. Hurd WW: Criteria that indicate endometriosis is the cause of chronic pelvic pain. Obstet Gynecol 92:1029–1032, 1998.
3. Ingamells S, Thomas EJ: Endometriosis: A continuing enigma? Hosp Med 59:437–441, 1998.
4. Ledger WL: Endometriosis and infertility: An integrated approach. Int J Gynaecol Obstet 64(Suppl 1):S33–S40, 1999.
5. Moghissi KS: Office management of endometriosis. In Stenchever MA (ed): Office Gynecology. St. Louis, Mosby, 1992, pp 413–429.
6. Pittaway DE: CA-125 in women with endometriosis. Obstet Gynecol Clin North Am 16:237–252, 1989.
7. Reddy S, Rock JA: Treatment of endometriosis. Clin Obstet Gynecol 41:387–392, 1998.
8. Saltiel E, Garabedian-Ruffalo SM: Pharmacologic management of endometriosis. Clin Pharmacol Ther 10:518–530, 1991.

PART VII

BREAST ISSUES AND DISORDERS

63. Breastfeeding

Cynda Ann Johnson, M.D., M.B.A.

I. The Issues

How can an act as natural as breastfeeding be so difficult? The answer is that breastfeeding was lost from American society as "old-fashioned" or even "unhygienic." Reintroducing it has not been easy. Breastfeeding is a skill that now must be actively taught to achieve the best results. The mid 1970s and early 1980s saw a significant increase in the number of women in the U.S. who initiated and continued breastfeeding, reaching a peak in 1982 when 61.9% of women initiated breastfeeding and 27% continued for 5–6 months. Numbers declined and hit a nadir in 1991, when 51% initiated breastfeeding and only 18.5% continued for 5–6 months. Currently the incidence of breastfeeding has begun to rise again (initiation rate 59.4%, continuance rate 21.6% at 6 months), but only slowly and with little hope of reaching the level targeted in the government's "Healthy People 2000" report, a goal in which 75% of women would breastfeed early in the postpartum period and 50% would continue for 5–6 months. The barriers to successful breastfeeding are many, but unfortunately physicians have been a significant obstacle. When physicians are unfamiliar with the process of breastfeeding and unable to assist patients with solving breastfeeding problems, the tendency is to recommend bottle feeding or to brush off the problem; undoubtedly, this indicates to the patient that continuation of breastfeeding is of little importance. Primary care physicians need to have enough knowledge about breastfeeding to assist patients with problem-solving initially and to obtain consultation for more difficult problems, while conveying their support at all times.

II. The Theory

- A. **Breast structure: nipple vs. areola**
    1. Areola surrounds nipple
        a. Enlarges and becomes darker in pregnancy
        b. Montgomery's tubercles, which become enlarged and look like small pimples during pregnancy and lactation, contain ductular openings of sebaceous and lactiferous glands
            i. Secrete substance that lubricates and protects nipples and areola
            ii. Also secrete small amount of milk
        c. Sweat glands and free sebaceous glands are also present
        d. For successful breastfeeding, infant must pull adequate amount of areola as well as nipple into mouth
    2. Nipple
        a. Ductal system of breast terminates at nipple (Fig. 1)
            i. Highly vascularized secretory cells (alveolar cells) extract water, lactose, amino acids, fats, vitamins and minerals from maternal blood, converting these components into breast milk
            ii. Milk droplets migrate through the cell membrane into alveolar ducts for storage
            iii. Myoepithelial cells are muscle-containing cells that surround groups of alveoli (acini) and are positioned along the entire ductal system; when many of these cells contract together, milk is forced upstream
            iv. Alveolar ducts empty into system of progressively larger lactiferous ducts
            v. Milk ducts within nipple dilate at nipple base into cone-shaped ampullae (lactiferous sinuses) for temporary milk storage
            vi. Milk ducts may merge again before exiting at 15–20 pores at nipple surface

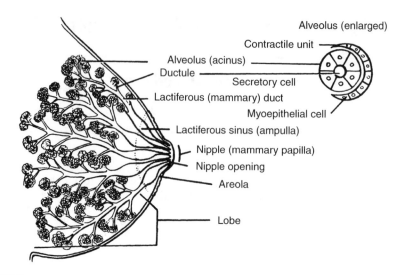

FIGURE 1. Anatomy of the breast. (Adapted from Riordan J, Auerbach KG (eds): Breastfeeding and Human Lactation. Sudbery, MA, Jones & Bartlett Publishers, 1999, p 95.)

B. **Stages of lactogenesis** (initiation of milk secretion)
   1. Stage 1
      a. Begins about 12 weeks before parturition
      b. Increase in substrates needed for milk production
      c. Continues until postpartum day 3 or 4, but thereafter will not continue without suckling
      d. Colostrum is type of milk produced during stage I
   2. Stage II
      a. Begins 2–3 days postpartum when secretion of milk is copious and alpha-lactalbumin levels peak
         i. Corresponds to clinical observation that "milk has come in;" milk comes in sooner in women who have breastfed previously and women who nurse frequently from delivery
         ii. Composition of milk changes over next 10 days; this is known as transition milk
   3. Stage III
      a. Mature milk produced
      b. Lactation maintained by continued production of oxytocin and prolactin, stimulated by suckling
C. **Composition of breast milk**
   1. Compared with cow's milk, all forms are uniquely suited to human infant
   2. **Colostrum**
      a. Appears clear, yellow, or orange; curds may be suspended in fluid
      b. Low volume
         i. 1 dl per feeding
         ii. Total daily volume increased with increased number of feedings, previous breastfeeding, previous deliveries
      c. Higher concentrations of sodium, potassium, and chloride than mature milk
      d. Protein, fat-soluble vitamins, and minerals present in greater percentages
      e. Antioxidants in colostrum include beta-carotene and vitamin E
      f. Rich in immunoglobulins, especially IgA
      g. Facilitates establishment of *Lactobacillus bifidus* in digestive tract; bifidus flora inhibit pathogenic flora
   3. **Transition milk**
      a. Concentration of immunoglobulins and total protein decreases
      b. Concentration of lactose, fat, and total caloric content increases

4. **Mature milk**
   a. White to bluish in color—87.5% water
   b. Energy content: about 70 kcal/100 ml
   c. **Macronutrients** (composition not greatly influenced by maternal diet)
      i. Lactose—42% of calories
      ii. Lipids—about 50% of calories
         (a) Breast milk contains essential fatty acids; infant formula contains mostly precursors
         (b) Breast milk contains many long-chain polyunsaturated fatty acids, high levels of docosahexaenoic acid which is involved in development of human vision
         (c) Higher proportion of acetic acid in the short chain fatty acid spectra compared to formula-fed infants (acetic acid may contain anti-infective agents)
      iii. Proteins—8% of calories include casein proteins (hard curds) and noncasein proteins or whey proteins (soft curds)
         (a) Casein
             (i) High ratio of cystine to methionine, overcoming infant's limited capacity to produce cystine
             (ii) High levels of taurine, important for growth
             (iii) Low levels of potentially toxic phenylalanine and tyrosine
         (b) Whey proteins (alpha-lactalbumin, lactoferrin, albumin, immunoglobulins, lysozyme)
             (i) Easily digested
             (ii) 60% of protein in human milk compared with 20% in cow's milk
             (iii) Alpha-lactalbumin assists the synthesis of lactose
             (iv) Lactoferrin inhibits pathogenic bacteria in gut
             (v) Lysozyme, polyamines, nonprotein nitrogen, nucleotides, and carnitine help growth and development of infant
      iv. Premature infants—mother's milk reflects differing needs of premature infant, with less carbohydrate and greater fat and protein content
   d. **Other nutrients**
      i. Low sodium-to-potassium ratio
         (a) May help to protect infant from sodium-responsive hypertension
         (b) In general, low renal solute load presented to kidney, resulting in lower serum urea levels and lower plasma osmolarity
      ii. Calcium-to-phosphorus ratio is 2:1 in contrast to cow's milk (1.2:1)
         (a) Total amount of calcium is lower, but bioavailability is greater
         (b) Rickets not observed in totally breastfed infants if mother's diet is adequate
      iii. Iron
         (a) Concentration in breast milk is low, but absorption is high, nearly 50%, compared with 10% of cow's milk iron and 4% of iron in iron-fortified formula
         (b) Need for supplementation equivocal
      iv. Zinc
         (a) Low-molecular-weight zinc ligand in breast milk is well absorbed
         (b) Breast milk therapeutic in zinc deficiency syndromes
      v. Fluorine
         (a) Reports of fluorine levels in breast milk are conflicting; level is apparently low
         (b) Exclusively breastfed infants have low levels of dental caries
         (c) Supplementation may not be necessary
      vi. Other trace minerals well represented in breast milk, including copper, selenium, chromium, manganese, molybdenum and nickel
   e. **Vitamins**
      i. Vitamin A—adequate supply in breast milk
      ii. Vitamin D

      (a) Water-soluble fraction is high in breastfed infants, but biologic activity is unclear

      (b) Some increase in infant serum levels when breastfeeding mother receives supplement

      (c) Vitamin D deficiency more likely if infant receives little sunshine

      (d) Recommendations for supplement are equivocal

    iii. Vitamin K

      (a) Low levels in first week of life

      (b) All infants should receive vitamin K at birth to prevent hemorrhagic disease of newborn

    iv. Vitamin E—adequate levels supplied in breast milk

    v. Vitamins C and B complex

      (a) Levels in breast milk vary according to maternal intake

      (b) Breastfeeding mothers should maintain adequate intake of these vitamins

D. Hormone release in breastfeeding

  1. Important hormones released from hypothalamus

    a. Prolactin-inhibiting factor (PIF) inhibits prolactin release

    b. Thyroid-releasing hormone (TRH) stimulates prolactin release

  2. Prolactin released from anterior pituitary gland (Fig. 2)

    a. Necessary for milk production

    b. Elevated levels inhibit menstrual cycle and cause decreased vaginal secretion, which may lead to vaginal dryness

  3. Oxytocin released by posterior pituitary gland

    a. Stimulates milk release from breast

    b. Causes uterine contractions and aids in involution of postpartum uterus

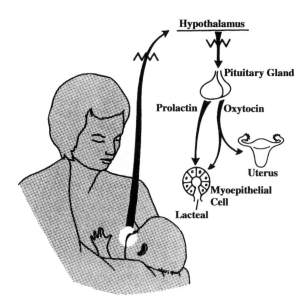

FIGURE 2.   Diagram of ejection reflex arc. When the infant suckles the breast, mechanoreceptors in nipple and areola are stimulated and a stimulus is sent along nerve pathways to the hypothalamus, which stimulates the posterior pituitary to release oxytocin. Oxytocin is carried via the blood stream to breast and uterus. Oxytocin stimulates myoepithelial cells in the breast to contract and eject milk from the alveolus. Prolactin is responsible for milk production in the alveolus. Prolactin is secreted by the anterior pituitary gland in response to suckling. Stresses such as pain and anxiety can inhibit the letdown reflex. The sigh or cry of an infant can stimulate the release of oxytocin, but not of prolactin. (From Lawrence RA: Breastfeeding: A Guide for the Medical Profession, 4th ed. St. Louis, Mosby-Year Book, 1994, with permission.)

E. **Physiology of lactation**
1. Foremilk
   a. Constantly secreted into lactiferous ducts between nursings
   b. Low in fat content and protein
   c. Constitutes one-third of milk available to infant at feeding
2. Hindmilk
   a. Higher fat and protein content
   b. Secreted after nursing begins
   c. Requires "let-down reflex"
3. Let-down reflex
   a. Neurohumoral response in which nipple stimulation by suckling infant causes hypothalamus to stimulate anterior pituitary to secrete increased prolactin and posterior pituitary to secrete oxytocin
   b. Prolactin acts on alveoli cells to increase milk production
   c. Oxytocin responsible for contraction of myoepithelial cells, which rupture alveoli cells and release hindmilk
   d. Reflex may be inhibited by severe cold, emotional conflict, pain, fatigue
   e. Reflex may be stimulated by seeing, touching, hearing, smelling, or thinking about infant; only oxytocin is released in these circumstances
   f. Evidence of let-down reflex
      i. Possible tingling sensation in breast may decrease over time with continued nursing or may not present in other breastfeeding women
      ii. Nursing mother will notice spontaneous release of milk from opposite breast
      iii. Infant may suddenly begin to swallow loudly and rapidly or even pull away from breast as large volume of milk is released

III. **An Approach**
   A. **Benefits of breastfeeding**
   1. Psychological effects
      a. Aids in bonding to newborn
      b. Peaceful feelings in mother while nursing
      c. Enjoyable for mother and baby
   2. Convenience
      a. Breast always available when mother present; no other equipment needed
      b. Easier to take infant out
      c. Less disruption when initiating nighttime feeding
   3. Economical compared with formula feeding
   4. Breast milk is optimal food source for infant
      a. Appropriate composition of nutrients for age
      b. Tastes good
      c. Contains immunologic factors
      d. Results in less overfeeding and obesity
   5. Breastfeeding exercises baby's oral musculature
      a. Less distortion of facial musculature
      b. Tooth decay and malocclusion less common
   6. Decreased incidence of allergies in breastfed children
   7. Decreased incidence of both diarrhea and constipation
   8. Decreased incidence of respiratory illnesses, ear infections, and bacterial meningitis
   9. Possible protection against sudden infant death syndrome and insulin-dependent diabetes
   10. Breast milk stools less malodorous
   11. Most breastfeeding women have fewer menstrual periods and decreased fertility (usually perceived as benefit)
   12. Women who continue to breastfeed for several months have less difficulty losing weight
   13. Decreased incidence of premenopausal breast cancer and ovarian cancer, especially with increased duration of breastfeeding

B. **Contraindications to breastfeeding**
1. Hepatitis
    a. Infants of hepatitis B–positive mothers who have received hepatitis B immunoglobulin may be breastfed
    b. Breastfeeding has not been recommended when mother has hepatitis C
        i. Hepatitis C virus would be expected to be transmitted in breast milk though infectivity seems low (high vertical transmission of hepatitis C probably during childbirth, not breastfeeding)
2. Infection with human immunodeficiency virus (HIV)
    a. Centers for Disease Control and Prevention (CDC) and Public Health Service recommend against breastfeeding
    b. Breastfeeding still method of choice in countries where risk of death from diarrhea and other diseases is 50% or more
3. Group B–streptococcal disease
    a. Bilateral mastitis in breastfeeding mother often caused by group B streptococci
    b. Infants may become ill and should not breastfeed
    c. Etiologic agent should be confirmed
    d. Both mother and baby may require treatment
4. Breastfeeding contraindicated in intravenous drug abusers
5. Cytomegalovirus—not contraindication
    a. Breast milk also contains antibodies against CMV, conferring passive immunity to suckling infant
    b. Premature infants, however, are at risk for serious illness if they acquire CMV and should only receive seronegative milk if fed from banked human milk

C. **Other considerations**
1. Breast cancer in mother is not contraindication to breastfeeding
2. Few women with significant other who strongly opposes breastfeeding do so successfully
    a. Talk with patient about this issue
    b. Support patient if she decides to try to breastfeed anyway
    c. Physician may need to help patient deal with guilt if this barrier results in bottle feeding

D. **Preparation for breastfeeding**
1. Discuss breastfeeding with each patient at first prenatal visit
    a. Women who have breastfed previously and successfully
        i. Continue to encourage and support them
    b. Women who are not interested in breastfeeding
        i. Assess reasons for reluctance
        ii. If they are willing to listen, review reasons to breastfeed and give them written and/or audiovisual materials
        iii. Readdress issue throughout pregnancy
        iv. Send women to breastfeeding classes if interested
        v. If they try to breastfeed, they need help and encouragement from entire health care team
    c. Women who assessed previous breastfeeding experience as unsuccessful
        i. Review reasons for failure—often due to lack of proper support and encouragement
        ii. Handle as above if they are willing to attempt nursing once again
    d. All women who breastfeed should be encouraged to identify other women who have breastfed successfully to support their efforts
2. Prenatal preparation of breast
    a. Women in U.S. often have little experience with touching breast
        i. Although newer studies indicate no increase in breastfeeding success with prenatal preparation, breast manipulation probably leads to greater comfort with handling the breast, supporting the eventual focus on the breast during feeding
    b. Breast massage (also useful postnatally)

         i. Most easily done in shower

        ii. Lift breasts from lower outer quadrant and press together

      iii. Cup each breast with both hands to gently rotate and massage

      iv. May help to increase circulation in breast and increase milk supply

       v. Helps to avoid clogged milk ducts, which occasionally occur prenatally

  c. Nipple preparation

         i. Avoid if premature contractions occurs

        ii. Roll and stretch nipples carefully

      iii. Nipples can be used in foreplay

      iv. To provide continuous, mild friction to toughen nipple, nipple-covering portion of bra may be cut out or small-breasted women may go braless

  d. Soap should not be used on nipples; leads to dryness and predisposes to cracking

  e. Women with flat or inverted nipples can place breast shells over breast inside bra to help nipples evert

  3. Nursing bra

    a. Buy nursing bra, which offers good breast support while breasts are enlarging

    b. Choose bra in which cup can be loosened for nursing with one hand

    c. Bra cups secured by Velcro are noisy when released and may pop loose unexpectedly

    d. After breastfeeding is established, fit nursing bra when breasts are full rather than empty

    e. Beware of underwire, which may press on milk ducts if cup is not large enough

E. Initiating breastfeeding (breastfeeding protocol)

  1. Breastfeeding should be initiated as soon as possible after delivery, within several hours or by next day, infant enters sleepy period and is harder to arouse

  2. Hold infant as comfortably as possible

  3. Roll infant in close (tummy to tummy)

  4. Take advantage of rooting reflex

    a. Touch nipple next to infant's mouth

    b. Infant will extend neck, tilt chin up, turn mouth toward nipple, and open mouth

  5. Infant must be encouraged to open mouth widely and grasp large portion of areola as well as nipple

  6. Mother should lift breast from below near chest wall, so that nipple and areola sag down, allowing infant easier grasp

  7. Infant's hands may be tucked out of way

  8. Infant's trunk should be supported and raised slightly above horizontal—tendency is to let it sag, which pulls infant down and away from nipple

  9. Infants are able to breathe even with faces pressed to breast

    a. Depressing breast near nose must be done carefully

    b. Tends to break suction on breast

 10. Latching on

    a. Requires proper position and suction on breast

    b. Mother feels strong pull, which may be assessed as painful, as infant sucks

    c. Infant is swallowing

    d. Latching on is assured when uterine cramping results (from release of oxytocin)

 11. Alternate positions

    a. Mothers should become familiar with all three principle nursing positions

    b. Milk ducts emptied best for each position are in line with infant's nose and chin

        i. Cross-cuddle (Fig. 3)

          (a) Most natural position for most mothers

          (b) Offers good control of nursing position

        ii. Lying down/side lying (Fig. 4)

          (a) Excellent position for nursing at night

          (b) For mother who finds sitting up painful

      iii. Football hold (Fig. 5)

          (a) After cesarean section when patient wants to avoid pressure on abdomen

          (b) For large-breasted women

          (c) For added visibility in getting infant latched on

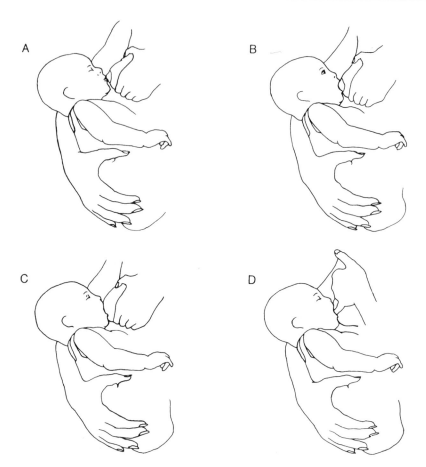

FIGURE 3. Cross-cuddle hold. *A*, Hold infant with head in cubital foci. Support breast well back of the areola, and touch the infant's lips or cheek with the nipple. *B*, When the infant opens wide, place the nipple far into the mouth to contact the upper back palate. *C*, Hold the infant close throughout the nursing and continue to support the breast as needed. *D*, Break suction prior to removing the infant from the breast by inserting a clean finger between the bums. (From Tsang RC, Nichols BI: Nutrition during Infancy. Philadelphia, Hanley & Belfus, 1988.)

        (d) When infant tends to slide down areola onto nipple
        (e) When nursing twins
  12. End of feeding
     a. Suction on breast is great and pulling infant away would be traumatic
     b. To release suction, pull down on infant's chin or insert finger into corner of mouth
     c. Small amount of colostrum spread over nipples and air drying protect them from soreness and cracking
     d. Infant should be burped after feeding on each breast
       i. Pat infant firmly to induce burp
      ii. Some newborns will not burp well until they ingest greater volume of milk
  13. Length and frequency of feeding
     a. "Demand feeding" preferable
       i. Infant may demand to be fed by rooting, mouthing or sucking or by signs of increased alertness or activity; crying is often a late sign of hunger
      ii. Mother may "demand" to feed when breasts become full

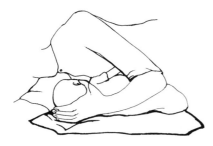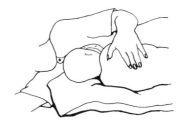

FIGURE 4. Side-lying position. (From Tsang RC, Nichols BL: Nutrition during Infancy. Philadelphia, Hanley & Belfus, 1988.)

    b. With initiation of breastfeeding, newborn should be brought to breast at least every 2–3 hours during day and every 4 hours at night

    c. In first few days of life infant may not take breast at every offering; mother and/or staff should not be discouraged

    d. Infants should continue to be wakened at night to breastfeed until they have regained birth weight

    e. Newborns should nurse 10–15 minutes per breast per feeding during first few days of life

    f. After breastfeeding is established and milk has "come in," infant who is sucking vigorously will empty 75% of milk in breast in 5 minutes and 90% in 10 minutes

    g. Lengthy nursing is not contraindicated for comfort or pleasure, but in newly breastfeeding mother usually leads to sore nipples and more difficulty continuing to breastfeed

    h. Both breasts should be used at each feeding if possible, alternating breast to be used initially

        i. Pin placed on bra strap will remind mother which breast to use first

    i. Early hospital discharge requires early and frequent home or office visits to assess breastfeeding success

        i. Nursing couple should be seen on day 3 or 4 after milk has come in

        ii. Continue to follow frequently until infant gains weight at average of $^1/_2$–$^2/_3$ oz per day

F. **Continuing process of breastfeeding**—a trained observer should evaluate breastfeeding performance 24–48 hours after delivery and again within the first week

   1. Principle of supply and demand

    a. Quantity of milk responds to needs of infant

    b. For nursing couple with established pattern of breastfeeding, quantity of milk made will replace quantity removed from breast

    c. If one feeding is missed, mother's breasts will be overfull, but if feedings are missed repeatedly and/or infant is given bottle, quantity of milk will decrease correspondingly

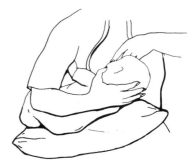

FIGURE 5. Football hold. In this hold, alternative hand should still be under breast lifting from below. (From Tsang RC, Nichols BL: Nutrition during Infancy. Philadelphia, Hanley & Belfus, 1988.)

    d. Growth spurts
       i. Periodically infant enters rapid growth phase and requires increased quantity of milk
       ii. Infant will demand to nurse more frequently (as often as every $1\frac{1}{2}$ hours) for several days to week
       iii. Quantity of milk made will increase accordingly and feeding pattern can return to normal with more milk available per feeding

2. Dietary considerations and supplementation
    a. Mother
       i. Caloric intake should be increased by 500–1000 calories/day over time for fully breastfed infant
       ii. Breastfeeding mothers should respond to thirst and drink water freely; those with inadequate water consumption should drink glass of water each time they breastfeed
       iii. Continue prenatal vitamins
    b. Infant
       i. Before 6 months of age in fully breastfed infant, no dietary supplementation clearly necessary
       ii. Controversy continues about possible supplementation of iron, fluoride, and vitamin D
       iii. Water supplementation not necessary and should be avoided until breastfeeding is well established

3. Clothing
    a. Breastfeeding is easier and more comfortable if proper clothing is selected
    b. Loose-fitting blouses or shirts are easy to pull up and accommodate changing breast size
    c. Dresses and nightgowns made for nursing have slits within folds of material that allow mother to expose her breast

G. **Breastfeeding problems and solutions**
  1. **Problems of infant**
    a. **Slow learner**—infant who has not "latched on" by 24 hours after birth
       i. Position of tongue is often source of problem
         (a) Thrusting or protruding tongue
         (b) Infant sucking on own tongue
       ii. Seek help from hospital personnel experienced in breastfeeding difficulties
       iii. Offer breast frequently but keep sessions short
       iv. Assist infant with pressing tongue down, mouth open wide
       v. Support chin
       vi. Avoid nipple shields
       vii. Discontinue pacifier or any device that may cause nipple confusion
       viii. Begin supplementation by 48 hours
         (a) Lact-Aid Nursing Trainer System dispenses formula (or stored breast milk) through small tube lying against breast
         (b) Allows learning process to continue while infant is reinforced by receiving nutrition at breast
         (c) Withholding supplementation results in less rigorous infant who, in turn, is less likely to learn to nurse properly
         (d) Mother should pump breasts for continued adequate breast stimulation, using electric pump if available
       ix. Infants unable to latch on may be normal, but maintain high index of suspicion for possible neurologic problems
    b. **Sleepy infant**
       i. Before nursing, stimulate infant by unwrapping or changing diapers
       ii. During nursing, continue to stimulate infant who falls asleep while nursing by wiggling feet or patting bottom
    c. **Inadequate weight gain**
       i. Healthy infants born with 5–8% excess water weight, which allows for inadequate intake during first few days of life

    ii. Breastfed infants lose average of 200 gm after birth (compared to 100 gm for bottle-fed infants)

    iii. Intake should be adequate if 6–8 diapers are wet per day after milk has come in (water supplementation makes this guideline useless)

    iv. Breastfed infants may not regain birth weight until as late as 2 weeks after birth but must be followed closely

    v. Observe nursing couple for technique

    vi. Weigh infant before and after nursing to determine adequacy of available milk

    vii. Supplementation between feedings is preferable to finishing feeding with bottle
- (a) Infants who continue to lose weight may become lethargic and are less likely to ultimately nurse successfully

    viii. Reassess mother's caloric intake

    ix. Patient will need much support and encouragement

d. Fussy infant while nursing

    i. If mother is tense or in hurry, infant may respond by fussing

    ii. Infant may have stuffy nose

    iii. During growth spurt, infant may fuss when quantity of milk available at feeding has not yet increased to new level of demand

    iv. Infant may need to be burped before nursing, especially if she or he has been crying

    v. Taste of milk may be unpleasant
- (a) Review foods eaten by mother during several hours before feeding and determine whether baby is repeatedly fussy after mother eats particular foods

e. Jaundice

    i. Early jaundice (2–5 days of age)
- (a) Breastfeeding associated with increased incidence of jaundice, even when controlling for other factors
- (b) When infant is fed early and frequently, incidence of jaundice is less
- (c) Bilirubin levels peak later in breastfeeding infants—at 4–5 days compared with 3 days in bottle-feeding infants
- (d) Bilirubin level does not need to be checked routinely
- (e) Unclear whether high bilirubin levels associated with breastfeeding in an otherwise healthy newborn result in pathology
- (f) Pathologic causes of jaundice should be ruled out, especially Rh or ABO incompatibility in otherwise healthy appearing newborn
- (g) Standard of care in most communities is still to treat bilirubin levels > 20 mg/dl
- (h) In most cases, breastfeeding can be continued while infant undergoes phototherapy (with formula supplementation if intake is inadequate)

    ii. Late-onset jaundice (true breast milk jaundice)
- (a) Occurs at 5–10 days of age
- (b) Caused by substance in milk of some mothers that inhibits hepatic enzyme, glucuronyl transferase
- (c) Other causes of hyperbilirubinemia must be ruled out
- (d) Diagnosis of breast milk jaundice is established if infant with bilirubin level > 16 mg/dl is taken off breast milk for 12 hours and bilirubin level falls at least by 2 mg/dl
    - (i) If bilirubin drops more slowly, infant is kept off breast for up to 24 hours, checking level every 6 hours
    - (ii) If bilirubin rises, another diagnosis must be sought
    - (iii) Phototherapy should be instituted if level of bilirubin reaches 20 mg/dl
- (e) Infant is supplemented with formula until level of bilirubin is < 15 mg/dl; level of bilirubin usually rises only slightly when breast milk is reintroduced
- (f) Bilirubin level should be rechecked at 10 and 14 days of life

f. Diarrhea

    i. Stools of breastfeeding infants are normally frequent and loose; it is not uncommon for infant to have a stool after each feeding

      ii. Stools may be green or yellow/gold (liquid gold), sometimes with curds
      iii. Infants with gastroenteritis should continue to breastfeed
         (a) Diaper usually shows evidence of water ring if infant has true diarrhea
         (b) Appearance of stool and pattern of stooling will change

g. **Constipation**
      i. Breastfeeding infants rarely experience constipation
      ii. Occasionally breastfeeding infants stool as infrequently as once weekly; this pattern is not constipation if stool is soft

h. **Infant wants to nurse continuously**
      i. Assess adequacy of milk production
      ii. Infants like to suck; pacifier is not contraindicated in infant who is otherwise nursing adequately

i. **Nursing blister**
      i. Normal finding in middle of upper lip of nursing infant

j. **Spitting up**
      i. Assess adequacy of burping
      ii. Infants appear to spit up more when intake of milk is greater
      iii. Spitting up blood
         (a) Examine mother's nipples
         (b) Usual source is blood in breast milk from cracked nipples

k. **Biting**
      i. May occur anytime after eruption of first tooth
      ii. Mother should startle infant by saying "ouch!" (she does not usually have to be told to do so)
      iii. After few instances of startling, infant will learn to nurse without biting

l. **Sleeping through night**
      i. Sleeping through night is convenient for parents but cannot be expected for first few months of life
      ii. Some infants will not do so even after several months
      iii. To encourage longer night's sleep
         (a) Do not stimulate infant excessively when nursing
         (b) Nurse frequently during evening
         (c) Put infant to bed 15 minutes earlier each night
         (d) Do not get up immediately when infant wakes; he or she may go back to sleep

2. **Problems of mother**

a. **No let-down reflex**
      i. Successful breastfeeding requires let-down reflex because only foremilk is available without it
      ii. Assess infant factor
      iii. Anxiety often inhibits let-down reflex
      iv. Nurse in quiet, private place
      v. Oxytocin nasal spray is available for women who cannot achieve let-down reflex

b. **Engorgement**
      i. Common when milk first comes in
      ii. Breasts may become full and warm and be accompanied by low-grade fever
      iii. Encourage infant to nurse often
      iv. If breasts become so full that nipple no longer protrudes, express small amount of milk before putting infant to breast

c. **Sore and cracked nipples**
      i. Nearly all women who are breastfeeding for first time experience sore nipples
      ii. Over time nipples become tougher and rarely are sore
      iii. Increase frequency but decrease time of each feeding
      iv. Air dry nipples or use hair dryer on "low"
      v. Apply colostrum or nipple cream to nipples (anhydrous lanolin is hypoallergenic and safe if ingested by infant)

     vi. Do not use soap on nipples

    vii. Do not let breasts become overfull

   viii. Continue to nurse rather than pump breasts

d. **Large breasts**

     i. Choose well-fitting support bra

    ii. Wear bra at night if breasts are uncomfortable

   iii. Experiment with different nursing positions to nurse more comfortably

e. **Apparent inadequate milk supply**

     i. About 2 weeks postpartum, edema and engorgement of breasts decrease; may give false sense of decreased milk supply

    ii. Infant may be experiencing growth spurt

   iii. Review adequacy of mother's intake, especially if she is losing weight

   iv. Mother may need more rest

    v. Try switchback nursing for increasing milk supply, that is, nurse on each breast, then nurse again on first breast

f. **Too much milk**

     i. May result from frequent pumping between feedings

    ii. May result from very frequent nursing

   iii. Increase interval between feedings or pumping slightly

   iv. Nurse on only one breast during a feeding

    v. Offer breast on which infant most recently fed if infant desires to nurse again within an hour

g. **Leaking breast milk**

     i. Common during first 6 weeks

    ii. Place paper or cloth breast pads inside bra

     (a) Replace pads frequently as moist pads lead to maceration of nipple tissue

     (b) Do not select breast pads with plastic shield that holds in moisture

   iii. If leaking or let-down occurs at inopportune moment, pressing palm of hand firmly over breast will stop flow of milk

h. **Change in sex drive**

     i. May be increased or decreased; either pattern moderates with time

    ii. Decreased sex drive may be related to fatigue

   iii. Time alone with partner is important

   iv. Increased prolactin may result in vaginal dryness, which may be improved by use of lubricant

    v. Some women get feelings of sexual arousal while nursing; this is not abnormal

   vi. Breast milk may leak during times of intimacy, especially with orgasm

     (a) Some women prefer to keep bras on if this is uncomfortable

i. **Breast infections**

     i. Whenever milk flow through milk ducts is inadequate, milk may become inspissated in duct

    ii. Clogged or plugged milk duct is first stage in infectious process

     (a) Skin over duct becomes tender, warm, and red; cord may be palpated

     (b) Massage region while in hot shower or use local warm, moist packs

     (c) Change nursing position to empty involved ducts

     (d) Nurse more frequently but perhaps for a shorter time

   iii. Plugged duct that does not resolve is prone to infection; result is mastitis

     (a) Symptoms are same with addition of fever and more systemic, flu-like symptoms

     (b) Begin treatment as above

     (c) Antibiotics required

     (d) *Staphylococcus aureus* and *Escherichia coli* are typical organisms; occasionally *Streptococcus* is isolated

     (e) Amoxicillin and first-generation cephalosporins are reasonable antibiotic choices

     (f) Mother should continue to breastfeed, starting feeding on unaffected breast

      (g) Analgesics usually necessary

      (h) Bed rest and fluids should be prescribed

    iv. Abscess may form in inadequately treated case of mastitis or when treatment is delayed

      (a) Basic treatment guidelines are same

      (b) Surgical drainage usually required; sample should be sent for culture and sensitivity

      (c) Increasing number of oxacillin-resistant strains of *S. aureus* isolated

        (i) Patients require hospitalization and intravenous antibiotics, usually vancomycin

      (d) Nursing can continue if mother can tolerate it and location of drainage site does not interfere

      (e) If nursing is discontinued, breasts should be pumped every few hours

      (f) Sufficient healing usually takes place within 4 days to resume breastfeeding if it was temporarily discontinued

      (g) Occasionally milk leaks from drainage site, but this will seal over with time and breastfeeding can continue

      (h) Complete healing expected within 3–4 weeks

 j. **Colds and flu**

    i. Mothers should be encouraged to continue nursing regularly

    ii. Supplement only if milk supply drops

 k. **Medications**

    i. Many more medications can be taken safely by mother while nursing than during pregnancy

    ii. American Academy of Pediatrics has official statements about compatibility of nursing and many drugs

    iii. *Drugs in Pregnancy and Lactation* is most complete source of information

    iv. *Physicians' Desk Reference* has statement for most entries on use of drug in breastfeeding mother

 l. **Ingestion of other substances**

    i. Caffeine and other methylxanthines not contraindicated in breastfeeding

    ii. Alcohol

      (a) Data are mixed

      (b) Women should not be discouraged from breastfeeding if they have occasional drink

    iii. Cigarette smoking

      (a) Should be discouraged

      (b) Mother should never smoke while nursing infant

      (c) Nicotine is found in breast milk of mothers who smoke

      (d) Committee on Drugs of the American Academy of Pediatrics does not place nicotine cigarettes on list of absolute contraindications to breastfeeding

m. **Exercise and breastfeeding**

    i. Mothers who exercise heavily may experience build-up of lactic acid, which is present in breast milk for 90 minutes

    ii. Mothers should breastfeed infants before heavy exercise

 n. **Oligomenorrhea or amenorrhea**

    i. Decreased menses and decreased fertility are common in breastfeeding women

    ii. Breastfeeding does not offer complete protection from pregnancy

    iii. Progestin-only contraception and barrier methods are good choices while breastfeeding

    iv. Combined oral contraceptives used while breastfeeding often result in decreased milk supply and termination of breastfeeding

 o. **Infant's total dependency on breastfeeding mother**

    i. Two weeks after breastfeeding is established, occasional bottle should be offered

(a) Bottle feeding allows mother to go out without infant periodically

(b) After nursing is established, nipple confusion is no problem

(c) Different artificial nipples should be tried if bottle is refused

(d) Person other than mother may need to introduce bottle

(e) If bottle is not introduced until several months of age, infant may refuse it altogether

(f) Mother should learn to pump breasts

(g) Occasional bottle feeding allows significant other to be more involved

    ii. Significant other can help with other activities of child care to give mother a break and to enhance bonding

H. **Breastfeeding and working mothers**

  1. Several options allow mother to continue breastfeeding while returning to work

  2. Some offices have on-site day care facility that allows mother to continue full-time nursing.

  3. Mother may pump entire supply of milk that infant consumes while she is away

    a. Usually she needs to pump 3 times during full shift

    b. Additional milk can be collected in morning before infant awakens

    c. Pumping in evening (for mother who works days) is less successful because infant will want to nurse frequently during evening

  4. **Part-time nursing**

    a. Mother may nurse infant while not at work and allow formula feeding while she is away

    b. Mother choosing this option may have less stress than those trying to pump entire day's supply of milk

    c. Part-time nursing can be continued indefinitely

    d. Even part-time nursing is more successful if mother is able to pump breasts once or twice daily to maintain adequate milk supply

    e. Mother may wish to nurse throughout day on her days off

      i. Formula supplement may still be necessary

      ii. Mother may be somewhat engorged when she returns to work

  5. Child care provider should always have formula on hand to feed infant in emergency

    a. Powdered formulas are most cost-effective

    b. Only required amount needs to be mixed at any one time

I. **Expressing breast milk**

  1. All nursing mothers should have some skill in breast milk expression

  2. To express milk successfully, let-down reflex must be induced

    a. Let-down is enhanced in quiet room where mother can think about infant as she rolls nipple between fingers

    b. Let-down induced most easily with electric breast pump

    c. Oxytocin nasal spray can be used by mothers who cannot otherwise achieve let-down

  3. Hand expression

    a. Most difficult to learn, but requires no equipment other than clean container

    b. Cup breast with hands, with fingers just behind areola

    c. Squeeze thumbs and fingers together rhythmically while pushing back toward chest wall

    d. Rotate hands periodically

  4. Hand pumps generally of little use

  5. Cylindrical pumps

    a. Two all-plastic cylindrical tubes that fit inside one another to create a vacuum

    b. Flange to accommodate nipple and areola at top of inner tube has gasket at other end so that suction can be created between two tubes

    c. Outer tube collects milk and can be used as feeding unit when nipple is screwed on

    d. As outer tube is pulled out, suction is created and milk flows

    e. Several variations exist; all are inexpensive

  6. "Squeeze-handle" pumps

a. Variation of cylindrical pump with single glass flange attached to collecting jar
b. Trigger handle mechanism creates strong suction that is released by valve
c. Allows free hand to express breast manually while suction is held steady; fingers must be kept close to chest wall or breast will be dislodged from flange and break suction
d. Excellent alternative to electric pump; less expensive and portable
e. Disadvantage: discomfort of longer periods of hard suction

7. Mechanical pumps
   a. Battery-operated models provide inadequate suction in most cases
   b. Electric models
      i. Small electric models
         (a) Portable
         (b) May be powerful enough for fully lactating woman
         (c) Small hole in flange base may be alternately plugged and opened to control pressure and simulate sucking action
      ii. Large electric models are most efficient
         (a) Pump that cycles pressure instead of maintaining constant negative pressure is less likely to cause petechiae or internal trauma to breast
         (b) Hospitals should have these available and large offices should be encouraged to purchase them

J. **Milk storage**
   1. Plastic bottles or bags preferable to glass for milk storage because leukocytes in breast milk stick to glass
   2. Breast milk stays fresh in refrigerator for 48 hours, top freezer for 2 weeks, and deep freezer for up to 1 year
   3. Freezing destroys many of immune properties of breast milk
   4. Milk should be thawed under hot running water
   5. Extreme caution should be used if milk is thawed in microwave
      a. Heating is not even and some portions may be extremely hot when others are cool
      b. Anti-infective factors are destroyed by microwaves

K. **Weaning**
   1. Mothers must not be made to feel guilty whenever they choose to wean children; breastfeeding for any length of time offers benefits to newborn; 12 months or more optimal for the infant
   2. Introduce solid food by 6 months of age whether or not breastfeeding continues
   3. At some time between 6 and 12 months most infants give signs of wanting to be weaned
      a. Weaning is probably easier if mother attends to such clues
      b. Breastfeeding certainly may be carried on beyond that time, but child may be resistant to weaning when mother desires it
      c. Apparent desire to wean on part of infant may be "nursing strike," which may occur from:
         i. Onset of menses
         ii. Dietary indiscretion by mother
         iii. Change in maternal soap, perfume, or deodorant
         iv. Stress in mother
         v. Ear infection or nasal congestion in child
         vi. Teething and startle from mother's response
      d. Slow weaning
         i. Discontinuing 1 feeding/week
         ii. Drop least favorite feeding first (as determined by mother or infant)
         iii. Replace nursing with another interactive activity between mother and infant
      e. Rapid weaning
         i. Appropriate for mother who has breastfed for only several weeks and wants to wean infant before she returns to work
         ii. One feeding should be discontinued each day
         iii. Breasts usually become quite full and should be emptied enough to relieve discomfort but not emptied completely
         iv. Breasts should be inspected for signs of clogged milk ducts

f. Emergency weaning
    i. Should be avoided if at all possible
    ii. Careful attention should be paid to signs of infection in maternal breasts
    iii. Bromocriptine may be used in such cases

SUGGESTED READING

1. Briggs GG, Freeman RG, Yaffe SJ: Drugs in Pregnancy and Lactation, 5th ed. Baltimore, Williams & Wilkins, 1998.
2. Calvo EB, Aspres NB: Iron status in exclusively breast-fed infants. Pediatrics 90:357–379, 1992.
3. Diaz S, Zepeda A: Fertility regulation in nursing women. Contraception 56:223–232, 1997.
4. Duncan B, Ey J: Exclusive breast-feeding for at least months protects against otitis media. Pediatrics 91:867–872, 1993.
5. Huggins K: The Nursing Mother's Companion, Boston, Harvard Common Press, 1990.
6. Greer FR, Marshall S: Vitamin K status of lactating mothers, human milk, and breast-feeding infants. Pediatrics 88:751–756, 1991.
7. Johnson CA, Hassanein R: Factors predictive of heightened third day bilirubin levels. Fam Med 21:283–287, 1989.
8. Lawrence RA: Breastfeeding: A Guide for the Medical Profession, 4th ed. Chicago, Mosby, 1994.
9. Lteif AN, Schwenk WF: Breast milk: Revisited. Mayo Clin Proc 73:760–763, 1998.
10. Martinez JC, Maisels MJ: Hyperbilirubinemia in the breast-fed newborn: A controlled trial of four interventions. Pediatrics 91:470–473, 1993.
11. Mennella JA, Beauchamp GK: The transfer of alcohol to human milk: Effects on flavor and the infant's behavior. N Engl J Med 325:981–985, 1991.
12. Popkin BM, Adair L: Breast-feeding and diarrheal morbidity. Pediatrics 86:874–882, 1990.
13. Powers NG, Slusser W: Breastfeeding update 2: Clinical lactation management. Pediatr Rev 18:147–161, 1997.
14. Riordan J, Auerbach KG: Breastfeeding and Human Lactation, 2nd ed. Boston, Jones & Bartlett, 1999.
15. Whitworth NS: Lactation in humans. Psychoneuroendocrinology 13:171–188, 1988.
16. Yamauchi Y, Uamanouchi I: Breast-feeding frequency during the first 24 hours after birth in full-term neonates. Pediatrics 86:171–175, 1990.

INTERNET SOURCES:

International Lactation Consultants Association: http://www.ilca.org
La Leche League International: http://www.lalecheleague.org
American Academy of Pediatrics: http://www.aap.org
Jan Riordan: http://www.feist.com/~jriordan/jriordan.html
Ameda/Egnell-Hollister, Inc.: http://www.hollister.com
Medela, Inc.: http://www.medela.com
LACTNET—a listserv for professionals in the lactation field. You will receive 3–5 digests per day with an average of 8 posts per digest—e-mail to LISTSERV@LIBRARY.UMMED.EDU; in the body write SUBSCRIBE LACTNET (insert *your* name).

64. Mastalgia

Belinda A. Vail, M.D., and Moya Peterson, R.N., M.A., C.F.N.P.

I. The Issues

Mastalgia, or breast pain, is a common complaint affecting up to 70% of women at sometime during their lifetime. With breast cancer now affecting one in nine women in this country, any abnormality in a breast usually causes alarm. Mastalgia, fibrocystic breast disease and premenstrual syndrome may overlap, but should be evaluated as separate issues and should not be immediately grouped into one diagnosis.

II. The Theory

A. Epidemiology

1. Most mastalgia is not severe; 45% of women report only mild pain
2. 21% report pain severe enough to interfere with their activities of daily living

3. Only 50% of the women with severe symptoms consult a provider
4. Mastalgia is almost always a premenopausal condition, so new, localized pain in the breast of a postmenopausal woman should be carefully evaluated

B. **Classification and etiology**
1. **Cyclical**
   a. This is the most common form occurring in two-thirds of women with mastalgia; onset is usually in their 20s or 30s.
   b. Pain usually lasts about 5 days, beginning in the premenstrual period and resolving with menstruation. It is frequently self-limiting or stops with pregnancy or menopause.
   c. Pain is usually bilateral and diffuse, often in the upper, outer breast quadrants and radiating into the arms
   d. Etiology is unclear, but presumed to be hormonal, based on the pattern of appearance. Many women have decreased plasma levels of gamma-linolenic acid while others have an increased prolactin response to thyrotropin-releasing hormone.
   e. Women who suffer from significant breast pain may also have an increase in other premenstrual symptoms.
   f. The overall response rate to treatment is 92%.
2. **Noncyclic**
   a. This type of mastalgia is less common and usually occurs in women in their 30s.
   b. There is less pattern; pain may be in one or both breasts; and pain may be intermittent or continuous.
   c. Pain is usually described as burning or throbbing and in the lower, inner aspects of the breasts; it may be well localized into "trigger spot pain."
   d. This pain may be associated with fibrocystic disease caused by enlarging or leaking cysts and/or tension on surrounding structures. Although pain is rare in breast cancer its presence does not eliminate the possibility of finding cancer; 1.5–2% of subclinical breast cancer presents with only breast pain.
   e. Caffeine has been implicated in exacerbating the pain from fibrocystic breast disease, but studies are inconclusive.
   f. Overall response rate to treatment is 64%.
3. **Chest wall pain**
   a. Pain from the chest wall may be perceived as breast pain, but the most frequent cause is costochondritis or Tietze's syndrome. Pectoralis muscle strain or spasm or cervical radiculopathy may masquerade as breast pain as well.
   b. This pain is usually localized, unilateral and reproducible on palpation.
   c. Examination of the patient in the lateral decubitus position may facilitate diagnosis by allowing breast tissue to fall away from the chest wall.
4. **Other causes of mastalgia**
   a. Benign breast conditions: ductal ectasia, mastitis, breast abscess, cysts
   b. Referred pain from intercostal neuralgia associated with a respiratory infection, obesity or changes in spinal curvature
   c. Referred pain from surrounding organs: cardiac ischemia, cholelithiasis, peptic ulcer
   d. Hormonal changes: pregnancy, estrogen-secreting ovarian tumors

III. **An Approach**
A. **Evaluation**
1. History
   a. Description of the pain, including location, character, timing with menstrual cycle, and duration
   b. Impact of symptoms on lifestyle
   c. Breast self-examination and mammogram history
   d. Medication use; especially oral contraceptives, hormone replacement therapy, pain medication, and any alternative medications
   e. Personal and family history of benign or malignant breast disease
2. Physical examination
   a. Careful breast examination and instruction on self-breast examination
   b. Examination of chest, heart, lungs, and abdomen.

3. Other evaluation
   a. Mammogram for women over 35, those with a family history of breast cancer, or any abnormal physical findings
   b. Breast pain chart over a 2-month period can be very helpful in establishing diagnosis.

B. **Management**
   1. After a careful evaluation, reassurance that the condition is benign will satisfy about 85% of patients
   2. Conservative lifestyle modifications include: supportive brassiere, reduction in caffeine intake (colas, coffee, tea, chocolate), reduction in foods with salt and saturated fats, and analgesia. The role of caffeine and salt is not proven but may be beneficial in some patients and represents a healthy lifestyle modification.
   3. Medications
      a. Oral contraceptives with low estrogen content are usually helpful, but occasionally higher progesterone levels will exacerbate the symptoms
      b. Evening primrose oil (gamma-linolenic acid) is the first-line treatment for mild symptoms or in addition to oral contraceptives. There are no significant side effects, and it can be purchased over the counter. Usual dose is 1.5 g/bid. Continue treatment for 4 months before re-evaluation. Treatment is usually continued for 12 months with extended effects reported after discontinuation.
      c. Danazol, a gonadotropin releasing inhibitor, is the only FDA-approved pharmaceutical treatment. Usual dose is 100 mg/bid. When pain is resolved, the dosage can be tapered every two months to 100 mg/every other day or daily during the luteal phase of the menstrual cycle. Many women remain pain free after discontinuation, but repeated courses are sometimes necessary. Side effects include menstrual irregularities, weight gain, hirsutism, acne, headaches, and leg cramps. It is contraindicated in patients with a history of thromboembolic disease and can be teratogenic making contraception essential.
      d. Bromocriptine inhibits prolactin release and is most effective with cyclical pain. One third of patients experience side effects, including nausea, headache, and postural hypotension. Side effects are less severe if the medication is introduced gradually. Usual dose is 1.25 mg/at bedtime, increasing by 1.25 mg every 3–7 days until the maximum dose of 2.5 mg bid is reached. Re-evaluate in 6 months.
      e. Tamoxifen, a partial antagonist of estrogen, should only be used in severe, refractory mastalgia. The usual dose is 10–20 mg/day with fewer side effects at the lower dose. Side effects include hot flashes and menstrual irregularities.
      f. Common treatments with no documented benefits: diuretics, narcotics, vitamin E, vitamin B_6, and progesterone.

SUGGESTED READING

1. Clark RV, Tindall GT: Hyperprolactinemia and galactorrhea. In Hurst JW (ed): Medicine for the Practicing Physician, 3rd ed. Boston, Butterworth-Heinemann, 1992, pp 513–515.
2. Cleckner-Smith C, Doughty A, Grossman J: Premenstrual symptoms. J Adolesc Health 22:403–408, 1998.
3. Deckers PJ, Ricci A: Pain and lumps in the female breast. Hosp Pract 67–94, 1992.
4. Gateley CA, Miers M, Mansel RE, Hughes LE: Drug treatment for mastalgia: 17 years experience in the Cardiff mastalgia clinic. J R Soc Med 85:12–15, 1992.
5. Goodwin P, Miller A, Del Giudice M, Ritchie K: Breast health and associated premenstrual symptoms in women with severe cyclic mastopathy. Am J Obstet Gynecol 176:998–1005, 1997.
6. Leis H: Gross breast cysts: Significance and management. Contemp Surg 39:13–20, 1991.
7. Mansel R: Benign breast disease. Practitioner 236:830–837, 1992.
8. Moore MP, Mass: Lump/cyst. In Harris J (ed): Breast Diseases. Philadelphia, J.B. Lippincott, 1991, pp 63–73.
9. Morrow M: Breast pain. In Harris J (ed): Breast Diseases. Philadelphia, J.B. Lippincott, 1991, pp 77–79.
10. Perna W: Pearls for practice. Mastalgia diagnosis and treatment. J Am Acad Nurse Pract 8:579–584, 1996.
11. Preece PE, Mansel RE, Bottom PM, et al: Clinical syndromes of mastalgia. Lancet 2:670–673, 1976.
12. Steinbrumm BS, Zera RT, Rodriguez JL: Mastalgia tailoring treatment to type of breast pain. Postgrad Med 102:183–198, 1997.

65. Nipple Discharge

Belinda A. Vail, M.D., and Diane Ebbert, R.N., M.S.N., C.F.N.P.

I. **The Issues**

Nipple discharge is one of the most common presenting breast problems in women who seek medical care. While presenting a diagnostic challenge to the clinician, it also causes significant anxiety in the patient. Since the majority of nipple discharge is benign, understanding the pathophysiology of the condition can help to alleviate anxiety and eliminate the added financial and emotional burden of unnecessary diagnostic testing. However, because a small percentage of women with nipple discharge will have a malignancy, all women presenting with this complaint must receive a thorough history, careful physical exam and appropriate diagnostic evaluation in order to determine appropriate management strategies. Using a thoughtful, prudent approach to nipple discharge will save lives as well as health care dollars.

II. **The Theory**

   A. **Epidemiology:** Nipple discharge can be divided into 3 categories: physiologic, pathologic, and galactorrhea.

   1. **Galactorrhea** is defined as nonpuerperal secretion of milk, bilateral, spontaneous or expressed and involving multiple ducts.

      a. Idiopathic galactorrhea is a diagnosis of exclusion with no measurable hyperprolactinemia. The incidence is estimated at 0.63–40% of all women with galactorrhea.

      b. The prevalence of pituitary adenomas in women with hyperprolactinemia is unclear. Studies found that 20% of women with galactorrhea had radiologically evident pituitary adenomas; however, autopsies showed pituitary adenomas in 25% of the normal population.

      c. The most common pituitary adenoma is the microprolactinoma. These are defined as prolactin secreting adenomas of < 1 cm. Only 4–11% of these adenomas progress with the majority nonprogressive, or regressing.

   2. **Physiologic discharge** is usually not spontaneous.

      a. The manipulation of nipples during breast self-exam, clinical breast exam, sexual or physical activity can elicit fluid from almost all women of all ages.

      b. Approximately 19% of women will produce nipple secretions with breast massage. With a nipple aspirator, nipple secretions were obtained in over 50% of women.

      c. Underlying cause is thought to be hormonal

   3. **Pathologic discharge** is usually spontaneous, unilateral, originating from a single duct, intermittent and persistent.

      a. The color can vary and may be bloody, watery, cloudy, serous, serosanguinous or green-gray.

      b. Intraductal papilloma and papillomatosis account for about 44% of the cases of pathologic nipple discharge.

      c. Mammary duct ectasia is found in 23% of the cases and 16% are due to fibrocystic disease.

      d. Only 1–5% of all breast cancers present with nipple discharge and only 3–11% of all pathologic nipple discharge is secondary to cancer. However, the likelihood that a bloody discharge will be associated with cancer increases with increasing age, and is 4 to 5 times more likely in women > 60.

   B. **Pathophysiology**

   1. Galactorrhea causes can include:

      a. Pregnancy: milk can be expressed in many women after the first trimester

      b. Conditions affecting the follicle and corpus luteum of the ovary resulting in direct stimulation of mammary glandular tissue and breast lobules include Stein-Leventhal syndrome, Chiari-Frommel syndrome, Forbes-Albright syndrome, and Ahumada-del Castillo syndrome. Oral contraceptives and estrogens induce galactorrhea by this same mechanism. Prolactin levels are not increased.

   c. Breast tissue reacts to cyclic menstrual hormone variations causing an exfoliation of the epithelial lining of the lactiferous ducts into the ducts, and a resulting nipple discharge. This usually occurs at a regular time in the menstrual cycle and is multicolored, bilateral and from multiple ducts.

   d. **Hyperprolactinemia**

      i. Prolactin is a polypeptide synthesized and secreted by pituitary lactotropes, which comprise up to 40% of the cells in the anterior pituitary. It is secreted in a diurnal rhythm, peaking between midnight and 8:00 a.m., and is responsible for the release of milk from the hormonally primed breast tissue.

      ii. The inhibitory feedback mechanism of prolactin is complex, but the main mechanism is inhibition by dopamine. The mechanism is also influenced by histamine, gonadotropin-associated peptides and possibly calcium.

      iii. Suckling is the most potent stimulus for prolactin release; other causes of hyperprolactinemia are listed in Table 1. Neuroleptic agents are the single most common cause, but any medication affecting dopamine synthesis, storage, release, metabolism, reuptake or turnover is suspect. In addition, lesions which affect the hypothalamic production of dopamine can cause hyperprolactinemia.

      iv. Pituitary adenomas directly increase prolactin levels, and as they occupy more space may have accompanying symptoms of headache, infertility, and bilateral temporal visual field defects.

TABLE 1. Causes of Hyperprolactinemia

Physiologic Causes	Drugs Associated with Galactorrhea
Nipple stimulation	Dopaminergic medications
Pregnancy	Tricyclic antidepressants
Intercourse	Psychotropic drugs
Menstrual cycle	Amphetamines
(late follicular/luteal phase)	Benzodiazepines
Stress (emotional or physical)	Cimetidine (possibly all H2 blockers)
Exercise	Ranitidine
High protein food	Monoamine oxidase inhibitors (MAOIs)
Noon-time meal	Metaclopramide
Hypoglycemia	Verapamil (possibly all Ca^{2+}-channel blockers)
Dehydration	Haloperidol
Sleep (stages I, II, REM)	Phenothiazines
Multiple sclerosis	Isoniazid
Tumors compressing the hypothalamus	Methyldopa
Chest wall irritation	Reserpine
Thoracotomy	Anesthetics
Thoracic herpes zoster	Cannabis
Reduction mammaplasty	Dronabinol (Marinol)
Breast implants	Opiates
Ill-fitting brassiere	Estrogen-altering medications
Infections	Oral contraceptives
Schistosomiasis	Exogenous estrogen
Other medical conditions	Conjugated estrogens
Polycystic ovary disease	
Cushing's syndrome	
Hand-Schüller-Christian disease	
Primary hypothyroidism	
Chronic renal failure	
Multiple endocrine adenomas type I	
Estrogen- or prolactin-secreting neoplasms	
Renal adenocarcinoma	
Bronchogenic carcinoma	
Ovarian cyst or teratoma	
Feminizing adrenal carcinoma	

2. **Physiologic discharge** is a serous fluid routinely secreted by breasts of nonpregnant, nonlactating women which is usually absorbed into the blood and lymphatic systems. With manipulation and probably a hormonal influence, this benign fluid can be expressed.

3. **Pathologic discharge** is most frequently caused by benign conditions

    a. Intraductal papillomas are the most common cause of pathologic nipple discharge. They are small (< 0.5 cm) solitary, nonmalignant tumors of the lactiferous duct. Usually found within a centimeter of the areola, they are frequently associated with bloody discharge. They occur in premenopausal women at mid-life. Discharge is unilateral and spontaneous.

    b. Ductal ectasia causes a spontaneous, bilateral, multicolored, sticky discharge. Color ranges from greenish to brownish red. It is thought to be related to chronic inflammation and dilation of the lactiferous ducts resulting in increased glandular secretions.

    c. Mastitis may also cause a milky or purulent discharge, usually unilateral. Pain, swelling, and erythema are prominent. This is discussed further in Chapter 65.

    d. There is a wide spectrum of breast abnormalities which represent aberrations of normal development and involution (ANDIs). These include conditions such as fibrocystic breast disease and may be associated with proliferation, atypia, and/or carcinoma. The most worrisome nipple discharge is bloody, but few breast cancers present with a nipple discharge.

III. **An Approach**

  A. **Evaluation**

    1. **History**

      a. Inquire about characteristics of the discharge: frequency, duration, precipitating factors (e.g., sexual stimulation), color, relationship to pregnancy/menstrual cycle, unilateral or bilateral, location on nipple, and prior symptoms.

      b. Associated breast symptoms: mass, pain, change in appearance

      c. Medication use

      d. Other medical problems

      e. Family history of breast disease

      f. Gynecological, endocrinologic, and neurologic review of symptoms

    2. **Physical exam**

      a. Palpate breast for mass and specify any characteristics

      b. Determine the quadrant of the breast causing symptoms

      c. If galactorrhea is suspected the exam should include a pelvic exam, endocrinologic, funduscopic exam and visual fields, and a neurologic exam

    3. **Initial laboratory tests**

      a. Serum prolactin levels (levels > 200 ng/ml are typical of prolactin-secreting tumors). For reliable interpretation, multiple samples should be obtained in the basal state, because levels are sensitive to stressors such as pain, food intake or breast stimulation.

      b. TSH/T$_4$ (thyroid-stimulating hormone/thyroxine)

      c. Growth hormone or serum cortisol will help differentiate mild to moderate prolactin elevations from those seen in acromegaly or Cushing's syndrome.

      d. Occult blood test on discharge

      e. Cytologic examination of nipple discharge is of questionable benefit. Negative results do not rule out carcinoma as less than half of cancers presenting with nipple discharge have abnormal cytology. Discharge suspicious of cancer requires a biopsy.

    4. **Imaging studies (with normal prolactin levels)**

      a. Mammography may help in diagnosing underlying conditions (e.g., carcinoma or mammary duct ectasia) but a negative mammogram does not rule out an occult carcinoma as only half of patients with cancer and nipple discharge have abnormal mammograms. Decision to biopsy should be made clinically.

      b. Galactography has been used to identify intraductal pathology, but its routine use is controversial. The discharging duct is identified and cannulated, then a water soluble dye is injected and a mammogram performed. It is helpful in identifying intraductal masses but does not differentiate between malignant and benign masses.

   c. Fiberoptic ductoscopy is just being developed and may be quite useful in the future.

5. **Imaging studies (with elevated prolactin levels)**

   a. Computed tomography (CT) displays sellar floor erosions below the pituitary and may be more sensitive in identifying discrete focal lesions within a minimally enlarged or normal sized pituitary gland but will not reveal all microprolactinomas.

   b. Magnetic resonance imaging (MRI) is superior in evaluating pituitary masses in the sagittal and axial planes because it displays lateral margins. It will also not identify all microprolactinomas.

6. **Biopsy**

   a. Indications for biopsy include: hemoccult positive discharge, discharge associated with mammographic abnormalities, and any breast mass suggestive of cancer.

   b. Failure of symptoms to resolve, or questionable diagnosis requires close follow-up and possible biopsy.

B. **Management**

1. If discharge is benign (physiologic or galactorrhea with normal prolactin) or biopsy is negative, reassure patient, treat symptomatically, and arrange for close follow-up

2. Galactorrhea with high prolactin levels, including micro- and macroadenomas

   a. If galactorrhea is medication-induced, medication should be discontinued if at all possible.

   b. Prolactin level needs to be normalized if estrogen levels are low (possible long-term bone loss and resulting osteoporosis), if patient is having fertility problems, in nonsurgically treated macroadenoma, or for persistent wet clothing and patient comfort.

   c. **Pharmacologic therapy**

      i. Bromocriptine (Parlodel) is a dopamine agonist that competes with dopamine for binding in the anterior pituitary inhibiting prolactin synthesis and release.

      ii. It may produce as much as a 50% reduction in volume of 80% of microprolactinomas and 60% of macroprolactinomas with normalization of prolactin and a decrease in galactorrhea and resumption of menses and fertility.

      iii. Doses start at 1.25 to 2.5 mg/qhs and can be increased to 2.5 mg/tid.

      iv. Common side effects include nausea and hypertension which can be significantly improved by delivering medication vaginally. It may exacerbate underlying psychiatric disorders. Less common side effects include: alcohol intolerance, gastrointestinal bleeding, digital vasospasm, hallucinations, delusions, dementia, and depression. Does not appear to be teratogenic but should be discontinued in pregnancy.

      v. Typically used for up to 2 years, then stopped to assess efficacy.

      vi. It has been associated with hypertensive crisis and strokes in postpartum women and is no longer recommended postpartum.

      vii. Possible alternatives for bromocriptine include pergolide mesylate (Permax) 0.05–0.1 mg/d or pyridoxine 600 mg/d (risk of neurotoxicity)

   d. **Microadenomas** may be conservatively managed if prolactin levels are not significantly high, estrogen levels are low, or the tumor does not change or regresses. Must be followed with CT or MRI.

   e. Oral contraceptives should be used with caution in women with microadenomas as they can stimulate lactotrope proliferation.

   f. **Macroadenomas** (> 10 mm in diameter) may be managed surgically through a transsphenoidal approach or craniotomy. Prolactinomas with high prolactin levels have considerably lower cure rates. Surgery promises an immediate cure, but may result in recurrence, infection, postoperative cerebrospinal fluid leak, and transient diabetes insipidus. Radiotherapy is reserved for patients who are not surgical candidates and cannot tolerate the medication. There is a slow response and patient may develop panhypopituitarism.

3. Intraductal papilloma requires excision to rule out cancer.
4. Mammary duct ectasia requires excision if there is an accompanying subareolar mass. If excision is not necessary, treatment is symptomatic, emphasizing good nipple and areolar hygiene with limitation of stimulation.
5. Mastitis is managed with antibiotics, heat, and accelerated nursing. Breast abscesses require surgical drainage
6. In general, suspicious nipple discharge is indication for referral to a surgeon even if no mass can be found.

SUGGESTED READING

1. American Fertility Society: The Use of Bromocriptine: Practice Guidelines of the American Fertility Society. Birmingham, AL, American Fertility Society, 1991.
2. Bohler HC, Jones EE, Brines ML: Marginally elevated prolactin levels require magnetic resonance imaging and evaluation for acromegaly. Fertil Steril 61:1168–1170, 1994.
3. Cady B, Steele GD, Morrow M, et al: Evaluation of common breast problems: Guidance for primary care providers. CA Cancer J Clin 48:49–63, 1998.
4. Corenblum B, Donovan L: The safety of physiological estrogen plus progestin replacement therapy and with oral contraceptives therapy in women with pathological hyperprolactinemia. Fertil Steril 59:671–673, 1993.
5. Deckers PJ, Ricci A: Pain and lumps in the female breast. Hosp Pract 67–94, 1992.
6. Dupont WD, Page DL: Risk factors for breast cancer with women with proliferative breast disease. N Engl J Med 312:146–151, 1985.
7. Edge DS, Segatore M: Assessment and management of galactorrhea. Nurse Pract 18:35–49, 1990.
8. Hindle WH: Fibrocystic breast disease—not a diagnosis. Female Patient 18:41–48, 1993.
9. Hughes LE: Non-lactational inflammation and duct ectasia. Br Med Bull 47:272–283, 1991.
10. Hughes LE: Benign breast disorders: The clinician's view. Cancer Detect Prevent 16:1–5, 1992.
11. Jardines L: Management of nipple discharge. Am Surgeon 62:119–122, 1996.
12. Katz E, Adashi EY: Hyperprolactinemic disorders. Clin Obstet Gynecol 33:622–639, 1990.
13. Leis H: Gross breast cysts: Significance and management. Contemp Surg 39:3–20, 1991.
14. McCool WF, Stone-Condry M, Bradford HM: Breast health care: A review. J Nurse Midwifery 43:406–430, 1998.
15. Morrow M: Nipple discharge. In Harris JR (ed): Breast Diseases, 2nd ed. Philadelphia, J.B. Lippincott, 1991, pp 73–77.
16. Shapiro CL, Henderson IC: Diseases of the breast. In Rakel RE (ed): Conn's Current Therapy. Philadelphia, W.B. Saunders, 1993, pp 1041–1047.
17. Smith S: Neuroleptic-associated hyperprolactinemia: Can it be treated with bromocriptine? J Reprod Med 37:737–740, 1992.
18. State D: Nipple discharge in women: Is it cause for concern? Postgrad Med 89:65–68, 1991.
19. Taber S: The clinical challenge of nipple discharge. J Ky Med Assoc 94:387–892, 1996.

66. Breast Lumps

Belinda A. Vail, M.D., and Moya Peterson, R.N., M.A., C.F.N.P.

I. The Issues

Most cases of breast pain, lumps, and nipple discharge are due to benign conditions, but lumps are a frequent finding in all age groups. In a woman's mind lumps are usually indicative of cancer, and she is often seeking reassurance that the lump is benign. Accurate diagnosis is imperative to avoid missing a malignant lesion, but evaluation is the most difficult part of the puzzle.

II. The Theory

A. Epidemiology

1. Breast cancer occurs in one of every nine women
2. 90% of all breast lumps are discovered by women or their partners through a self-breast examination (SBE); average size of cancerous mass at detection is 2.5 cm and half have metastasized

3. Differential diagnosis of breast lumps is extensive, and a small proportion of lumps in young women are malignant (< 2% in women under 30, but > 85% in women over 70)

4. Risk factors for breast cancer include increasing age, early menarche, late menopause, nulliparity, late first pregnancy, no lactation, positive family history of breast or ovarian cancer

5. Two-thirds of women with malignant masses have no risk factors

6. Only 27% of American women practice self breast examination (SBE) on a regular basis

B. Differential diagnosis

1. **Cysts**
   a. Cysts are fluid-filled, smooth, and round, change cyclically with the menstrual cycle, and may cause pain prior to menses
   b. They are rare before the age of 30 or after menopause. Usually discovered on self-breast or clinical breast examination or on mammograms.
   c. Women who have a cyst have a 30% chance of developing another in the next two years.
   d. There is no evidence which links cysts to later development of cancer, but the relationship is unclear. Some cysts with atypical hyperplasia may be associated. Women with cysts should remain vigilant and not assume all masses are cystic.

2. **Fibrocystic disease**
   a. This disease affects at least 50% of women with the highest incidence in the 20–50 age group. It is rare in postmenopausal women not on hormone replacement.
   b. Breasts are lumpy, nodular, rope-like, or rubbery, and a movable, tender area can vary in size from 1 mm to many centimeters; greatest concentration is usually in the upper outer quadrants.
   c. 85–90% of affected women complain at some time of mastalgia.
   d. There is no increased risk of cancer, but breasts are difficult to examine due to the nodularity.

3. **Mastitis**
   a. Puerperal mastitis occurs in the postpartum period. It begins with pain, swelling, erythema and fever, and can progress to an abscess. The usual pathogen is *Staphylococcus aureus*, which enters through a break in the integrity of the breast nipple.
   b. Nonpuerperal mastitis occurs in women in their forties with symptoms of tenderness, induration and erythema without systemic symptoms. The causative organism is variable, and it can occur from a chronic inflammatory process around the terminal subareolar ducts. This can cause destruction of the duct and lead to ductal ectasia presenting as an irregular, rope-like induration.

4. **Fibroadenomas**
   a. Discreet, smooth lesions that are mobile and nontender. Peak incidence is in the 20–25-year age range and again in the 40–50-year range; they are uncommon after menopause. Usually found in the upper, outer quadrants of the breast.
   b. Clinical course is variable; they can enlarge or completely regress. The condition is benign, but must be differentiated from cancer.

5. **Galactocele**—localized duct dilation of the lactating breast. Can progress to mastitis and/or obstruction of the adjacent ducts.

6. **Ductal ectasia**—an obstruction of the terminal collecting ducts of the breast in perimenopausal or menopausal women and can lead to the accumulation of a greenish black material. This can lead to scarring, fibrosis, or abscess formation.

7. **Papillomas**—benign, unilateral, cylindrical tumors occur occasionally in women forty to sixty years of age. May present as a mass or a bloody brownish or greenish discharge from the nipple. Can occur anywhere in the breast and singularly or in multiples.

8. **Cystosarcoma phyllodes**—rapidly growing, large fibroadenoma-like lesions which usually present in women 40–50 years of age. Sixty percent are benign, but commonly recur locally; 15% are malignant, metastasizing directly to the lungs.

9. **Lipoma/fat necrosis**—lipomas are soft, slow-growing fatty benign tumors. They are often ignored because of their soft consistency. Trauma to the breast tissue causes necrosis and release of fatty acids into the surrounding tissue and an inflammatory response results in fibrosis and calcification.

10. **Carcinoma**—presents an ill defined, firm, immobile mass without pain or cyclic changes.

III. **An Approach**
  A. **Evaluation**
    1. **History**
       a. Review risk factors
       b. When lumps were discovered and if any changes have occurred since discovery; history of pain and/or nipple discharge
       c. Menstrual and reproductive history
       d. Mammogram and self breast exam history
       e. Family history
       f. Medication use (prescription and OTC)
       g. General review of systems
    2. **Physical examination**
       a. Clinical breast examination for size, consistency, margins, and mobility of lesion; associated skin changes (dimpling); lactation/galactorrhea or nipple discharge; and tenderness; and comparison to other breast
       b. Presence of any associated enlarged lymph nodes in the axillary, infraclavicular or supraclavicular areas
    3. **Diagnostic tools**
       a. Screening recommendations for breast self-exam, clinical breast exam, and mammography are listed in Table 1
       b. In patients over thirty years old, bilateral mammograms are essential
       c. In patients under thirty years of age, ultrasonography is indicated because mammography lacks sensitivity due to the increased density of the breast tissue. It is particularly helpful in distinguishing solid from cystic masses.
       d. Fine-needle aspiration (FNA) biopsy may complete the work-up. If the fluid obtained is non-bloody it does not require cytology, and the mass may resolve following the aspiration. Bloody fluid requires cytology. If no fluid is obtained, several passes should be made using strong negative pressure. A thin prep slide should then be prepared for examination by a pathologist.
       e. Excisional biopsy is the most accurate means of diagnosis and should be performed for indications listed in Table 2. The patient should be informed there will be a two to three centimeter scar on the breast, and there is also a high risk of hematoma formation at the biopsy site due to the increased vascularity of the breast. They are costly and inconvenient but should be performed more readily in older patients.
       f. Clinical breast exam, mammography, and fine-needle aspirate together miss < 1% of cancers.
  B. **Management**
    1. **Cysts**
       a. When cystic lesions are present, the quickest route to diagnosis is by simple aspiration of the cyst. If the fluid is clear, and the lesion resolves, the diagnosis is made.

TABLE 1.   American Cancer Society Guidelines for Breast Cancer Screening

Breast self-examination
Monthly for women 20 years of age and older
Clinical breast examination
Every 3 years for women 20–40 years of age
Every year for women over 40 years of age
Screening mammography
Every 1–2 years for women 40–49 years of age
Every year for women 50 years of age or older

TABLE 2. Indications for Excisional Breast Biopsy

Any lesion suspicious for cancer	Mass present after cyst aspiration
Suspicious microcalcifications on mammogram	Persistent or enlarging mass
Bloody fluid from cyst aspiration	

    b. Patients over 30 should still have a follow-up mammogram and all patients should have repeat breast exam in 4–6 weeks.

    c. Any dark or bloody fluid should have cytology performed. Abnormal fluid or recurrence of the cyst requires excisional biopsy

2. **Fibrocystic disease**

    a. Treatment for fibrocystic changes is primarily symptomatic. If pain is present, simple nonsteroidal anti-inflammatory medications are usually sufficient.

    b. Women should be instructed on breast self-examination because the nodularity of the breast makes detection of small malignant lesions very difficult.

    c. Routine mammograms should be encouraged.

3. **Mastitis**

    a. Puerperal mastitis is treated with warm compresses, expression of milk (either manually or with increased nursing), anti-inflammatory medication, and antibiotics with gram-positive coverage.

    b. Nonpuerperal mastitis is also treated with warm compresses, antibiotics and incision and drainage. Recurrence rate is high necessitating surgery.

4. **Fibroadenomas** are benign lesions and require no treatment beyond accurate diagnosis to rule out malignancy. Mammogram or sonogram and fine-needle aspirate may be adequate; however, with increasing age (> 40) excisional biopsy becomes the treatment of choice to avoid missing a malignant lesion.

5. **Galactocele**—aspiration of milk is usually curative, but if unable to resolve or recurs should be excised.

6. **Ductal ectasia**—removal of fluid, anti-inflammatory medication, and hot packs may be curative, but excision is often necessary. Mammogram should be performed since these usually occur in older women.

7. **Papilloma**—discharge from these tumors should be examined cytologically, and excision is the treatment of choice.

8. **Cystosarcoma phyllodes**—mass must be excised with a margin of surrounding normal breast tissue. Occasionally size of tumor necessitates removal of entire breast.

9. **Lipoma/fat necrosis**—no treatment is usually needed beyond reassurance of the patient, but if large, fibrotic or calcified may be excised. Mammography can sometimes be helpful in diagnosis.

10. **Carcinoma**

    a. All masses suspicious of cancer should be removed by excisional biopsy. When fine-needle aspirate or excisional biopsy is positive, patients should be referred to the surgeon.

    b. Management options include lumpectomy with radiation, mastectomy, or bilateral mastectomy.

SUGGESTED READING

1. Andolesk KM, Copeland J: The breast. In Taylor R (ed): Family Medicine: Principles and Practice. New York, Springer-Verlag, 1993, pp 835–845.
2. Bodian C: Biological markers in breast tissue: Benign breast diseases, carcinoma in situ, and breast cancer risk. Epidemiol Rev 15:177–187, 1993.
3. Ciatto S, Cariaggi P, Bulgaresi P: The value of routine cytological examination of breast cyst fluids. Acta Cytol 31:301–304, 1987.
4. Deckers PJ, Ricci A: Pain and lumps in the female breast. Hosp Pract 67–94, 1992.
5. Donegan WL: Evaluation of palpable breast mass. N Engl J Med 327:937–942, 1992.
6. Fiorica J, Schorr S, Sickles E: Benign breast disorders: First rule out cancer. Patient Care April:140–151, 1997.

7. Foxcroft L, Evans E, Hirst C: Newly arising fibroadenomas in women aged 35 and over. Aust N Z J Surg 68:419–422, 1997.
8. Hockenberger SJ: Fibrocystic breast disease: Every woman is at risk. Plastic Surg Nursing 13:37–40, 1993.
9. Hughes LE: Non-lactational inflammation and duct ectasia. Br Med Bull 47:272–283, 1991.
10. Hughes LE: Benign breast disorders: The clinician's view. Cancer Detect Prevent 16:1–5, 1992.
11. Kopicki M: Management of the palpable breast mass. Female Patient 23:45–52, 1998.
12. Leis H: Gross breast cysts: Significance and management. Contemp Surg 39:13–20, 1991.
13. Mansel R: Benign breast disease. Practitioner 236:830–837, 1992.
14. Schnitt SJ, Connolly JL: Pathology of benign breast disorders. In Harris J (ed): Breast Diseases. Philadelphia, J.B. Lippincott, 1991, pp 15–30.
15. Schwartz KL: Breast problems. In Sloan PD, Slatt LM, Curtis P (eds): Essentials of Family Medicine. Baltimore, Williams & Wilkins, 1998, pp 331–345.
16. Smith BL: Fibroadenomas. In Harris J (ed): Breast Diseases. Philadelphia, J.B. Lippincott, 1991, pp 34–37.

67. Plastic and Reconstructive Breast Surgery

Richard Bené, M.D., and Belinda A. Vail, M.D.

I. *Breast Augmentation*
   A. **The Issues**
      Breast augmentation is one of the most common plastic surgery procedures. About 2 million women have undergone breast augmentation since development of breast implant in the early 1960s. Controversy in the early 1990s regarding the safety of silicone implants led to the almost exclusive use of saline implants. Healthy patients with clearly defined motives should seek a qualified plastic surgeon with whom they are comfortable.
   B. **The Theory**
      1. Women seeking breast enlargement often do so to improve their appearance. There is a high level of satisfaction if the patient is motivated by a desire for larger breasts, but patients with ulterior motives (e.g., enhancement of career or social life) are often disappointed.
      2. The controversy about safety of silicone gel breast implants led to a ban by the Food and Drug Administration. Although silicone gel was blamed for the development of connective tissue disorders, no evidence was found that proved a causal relationship between breast implants (silicone or saline) and systemic disease.
      3. Saline-filled implants with a silicone shell are the only type of implant available for use outside study protocols.
   C. **An Approach**
      1. **Techniques:** implants may be placed from 3 different surgical approaches. The implant can be placed in the subglandular (under the breast tissue) or in the submuscular position (below the pectoralis muscle). Patients should understand the implications of the different placements and how they are appropriate for each individual patient.
         a. Inframammary approach uses an incision about 1 to $1^{1}/_{2}$ inches long inferiorly and laterally in the natural crease below each breast.
         b. Periareolar approach uses a circumareolar incision and some dissection through the breast tissue is usually necessary.
         c. Transaxillary approach hides the incision in the axilla, it may be more difficult to position the implants appropriately.
         d. Subglandular placement is below the breast tissue but above the pectoralis muscle
         e. Submuscular placement is between the pectoralis muscle and the chest wall; may reduce incidence of capsular contracture and make mammography easier.
      2. **Risks and complications**
         a. **Infection:** postoperative infections can occur, and may be difficult to treat due to the presence of the foreign body.

    b. **Hematoma:** hematomas may occur in the postoperative period and may require additional surgery to evacuate.

    c. **Capsular contracture:** capsular formation around breast implants is a normal reaction to a foreign body and occurs in all patients with implants. Deformity may occur as the capsule contracts and modifies the shape of the implant. This may lead to pain and palpable and visible changes in breast. Treatment options include:

        i. Open capsulotomy, where an incision is made in the capsule to disrupt contractive force, is most often performed.

        ii. Capsulectomy, removal of capsule, may be necessary in severe cases such as pain or calcification.

        iii. Closed capsulotomy, where external pressure is used to break the capsule, is no longer recommended due to risk of implant rupture

    d. **Implant rupture:** disruption of the implant shell with leakage of implant contents.

        i. Saline implants will be identified by loss of breast volume on the ruptured side. Saline is absorbed by the patient's lymphatic and vascular system without ill effects, but the implant will need to be replaced to restore symmetry. Implants are guaranteed by the manufacturers who often assist with cost of replacement.

        ii. Silicone implants may rupture, and the patient may remain asymptomatic. This occurs because silicone gel is maintained within the capsule that formed around the implant. Implant removal is not indicated in these patients. Many nonspecific symptoms have been associated with rupture of silicone gel breast implants. Although no causal link has been established, silicone gel implants are often removed in these patients. Expenses related to removal may be approved by third-party payors.

3. The presence of breast implants may make mammography slightly more difficult, but does not increase the risk of breast cancer. Special techniques have been developed to improve visualization, and mammography should be performed and interpreted by physicians experienced in viewing mammograms of augmented breasts

II. *Reduction Mammaplasty*

A. **The Issues**

Problems related to large breasts may be physical or psychological.

1. Breast hypertrophy may be responsible for mastodynia, neck pain, back pain, headaches, intertrigo, indentation from bra straps, ulnar nerve paresthesias, skeletal deformity, and breathing problems.

2. Large breasts may be source of embarrassment, and create lifestyle problems. Finding clothing that fits can be frustrating, and some women may have difficulty performing in athletic endeavors.

3. Reductions may be covered by insurance; coverage is dependent on the amount of tissue to be removed, height and weight of patient, and the type of symptoms. Prior authorization should be obtained and may require a photograph of the breasts to document need.

4. Many patients requesting reduction mammaplasty are overweight with a greater percentage of the breast composed of fat. Patients should be encouraged to lose weight before the procedure.

B. **An Approach**

1. Procedure is usually performed under general anesthesia; and may require an overnight stay in the hospital.

2. Blood transfusions are uncommon; but some women may choose to donate autologous blood before the procedure.

3. Several techniques are possible, but the most common procedure produces a scar that surrounds the areola, and extends as inverted T from the areola to the inframammary crease, and then along the crease. The inferior pedicle technique preserves the nipple and areola on a segment of the inferior breast. Various other techniques include superior, medial, lateral, and central pedicles. Excision of the nipple and areola may be performed if the pedicle is too long to provide adequate vascularity; it is then replaced as a free graft.

4. Liposuction can be used concurrently
5. Postoperative considerations: Patients usually miss work for about 2 weeks. Bulky support dressings are applied; drains sometimes required for several days.
6. Risks and complications:
   a. Hematomas, infection, and delayed healing
   b. Breast asymmetry may occur. Explaining to the patient that most women have some breast asymmetry, may help to alleviate postoperative concerns.
   c. Sensation of the nipple may be diminished and should be evaluated before surgery because many women with breast hypertrophy have decreased nipple sensation prior to surgery.
   d. Scarring: the possibility of unsightly, wide, or hypertrophic scarring
   e. Lactation and breastfeeding may be possible after reduction but often are difficult because many ducts are transsected during surgery
   f. Mammography complications: because incisions are made in breast parenchyma, scarring in the breast itself results; small areas of fat necrosis may develop micro-calcifications which can be confused with malignancy on mammograms

III. *Mastopexy*
  A. **The Issues**
  Some women do not have concerns about the size of their breasts but rather about their fullness, position, and appearance. Often after having children and aging, women de-velop ptosis and are no longer happy with their appearance.
  B. **The Theory**
   1. Breast ptosis, which occurs as part of the natural aging process, results from excess of breast skin compared with amount of breast tissue. It is defined by the relationship of the height of the nipple area to the inframammary fold.
   2. Loss of skin elasticity and attenuation of Cooper's ligament contribute to problem. Pregnancy and breastfeeding cause skin stretching and may lead to breast sagging.
   3. Mastopexy is considered a cosmetic procedure and is not covered by third-party payors.
  C. **An Approach**
   1. Degree of ptosis is important in determining the type of mastopexy. The size of the skin envelope is reduced relative to the size of the breast parenchyma. The nipple and areola may need to be repositioned. Mild ptosis may be treated with implant aug-mentation or combination of mastopexy and implant.
   2. Incisions are circumareolar and significant ptosis may require lengthy incisions sim-ilar to those used for reduction mammaplasty.
   3. Risks and complications:
      a. Results may not be permanent because the aging process continues and ptosis may again occur.
      b. Hematoma, infection, delayed healing, scarring, and asymmetry are also risks.

IV. *Postmastectomy Reconstruction*
  A. **The Issues**
  As the incidence of breast cancer continues to rise, more and more women must decide how they will face their postmastectomy body. Changes in insurance regulations have made it mandatory that insurance companies cover reconstruction following mastec-tomy, and an increasing number of women are exercising that option.
  B. **The Theory**
   1. Options after mastectomy include no reconstruction, using a custom-fitted prosthe-sis, or surgical reconstruction of the breast.
   2. Decisions regarding reconstruction are usually made at a difficult time. Women must deal with the cancer issue itself, treatment options of lumpectomy and radiation vs. mastectomy, and the timing of reconstruction if that option is chosen.
   3. Helping the patient to make decisions should be a team approach, including the pri-mary care physician, oncologist, radiation oncologist, onocologic and plastic sur-geons. She should be appraised of all options and the risks and benefits of each. Discussions with other women who have had mastectomy with and without recon-struction may be helpful.

4. Immediate reconstruction is done at the time of mastectomy. It may help to ease the psychological trauma of losing a breast. It does not increase the risk of local recurrence or distant metastases and does not delay adjuvant therapy.
5. Delayed reconstruction is may be more appropriate for women having difficulty in deciding about reconstruction. It may also be better if local control of the tumor is not possible at the time of the mastectomy.
6. Federal regulation now mandates that postmastectomy reconstructive procedures be covered by third-party payors. Procedures on the opposite breast in order to provide symmetry are also covered.

C. **An Approach**
1. Type of reconstruction depends on the health of patient, type of breast to be reconstructed, and preference of the patient. Several procedures may ultimately be required, and depending on the type of procedure a hospital stay may be required.
2. Initial procedure is creation of the breast mound. It may be created by an implant or by use of myocutaneous flap of autologous tissue from the abdomen, buttocks, or back.
3. Implants are usually saline similar to those used for augmentation and may be placed below the pectoralis muscle.
   a. Tissue expanders may be placed below the pectoralis muscle and slowly filled to stretch muscle and skin over several weeks to months. To eliminate the problem of loss of skin, tissue expanders may be placed at time of mastectomy, then filled in office with saline and removed and replaced with implants in a second procedure. Some expanders have a removable filling port and are intended to be left in place as the final implant, after the port is removed.
   b. An advantage of implants/tissue expanders is that the procedures can be done on an outpatient basis.
   c. Risks and complications are similar to augmentation implants of hematomas, infection, delayed healing, breast asymmetry, and scarring. There is some increased risk of exposure of implants compared to those used for augmentation.
4. Autologous reconstruction uses myocutaneous flaps of muscle, skin, and subcutaneous tissue create a breast mound.
   a. TRAM (transverse rectus abdominis myocutaneous) flap uses abdominal skin and tissue vascularized through the rectus abdominis muscle.
      i. The pedicle TRAM procedure depends on the superior epigastric blood vessels coursing through rectus muscle to supply transferred tissue. The flap is tunneled beneath the abdominal skin to reach the chest.
      ii. A free TRAM uses microsurgical techniques to provide vascular supply. The inferior epigastric vessels are microsurgically anastomosed to the internal mammary vessels or vessels in the axilla. This technique requires less muscle harvest, has better vascularity, and it is easier to shape the tissue into a breast. It requires more extensive postoperative monitoring and there is greater risk of flap loss.
   b. Latissimus dorsi myocutaneous flap uses skin of the back and latissimus dorsi muscle. Because the tissue is relatively thinner an implant may need to be added to provide bulk. The back scar may be unsightly.
   c. Buttock and thigh flaps are used much less commonly.
   d. Autologous reconstructions may be lengthy operations and are generally associated with short inpatient stays.
   e. Nipple and areolar reconstruction is usually done as a separate procedure after breast mound has healed. Nipple may be constructed from a small local flap from the reconstructed breast. The areola can be reconstructed by using a graft and/or tattooing.

SUGGESTED READING

1. Beasley ME: The pedicled TRAM as preference for immediate autogenous tissue breast reconstruction. Clin Plastic Surg 21:191–206, 1994.
2. Bostwick J III: Plastic and Reconstructive Breast Surgery. St. Louis, Quality Medical Publishers, 1990.

3. Bryant H, Brasher P: Breast implants and breast cancer—reanalysis of a linkage study. N Engl J Med 332:1535–1539, 1995.
4. Gabriel SE, Woods JE, O'Fallon WM, et al: Complications leading to surgery after breast implantation. N Engl J Med 336:677–682, 1997.
5. Grotting JC: Immediate breast reconstruction using the free TRAM flap. Clin Plastic Surg 21:207–222, 1994.
6. Mathes SJ, Nahai F: Reconstructive surgery: principles, anatomy and technique. New York, Churchill-Livingstone, 1997.
7. McCarthy JG (ed): Plastic Surgery, Vol. 6. Philadelphia, W.B. Saunders, 1990.
8. Trabulsy PP, Anthony JP, Maathes SJ: Changing trends in postmastectomy breast reconstruction: A 13-year experience. Plast Reconstr Surg 93:1418–1427, 1994.
9. Vasconez LO, Lejour M, Gamboa-Bobadilla M: Atlas of Breast Reconstruction. Philadelphia, J.B. Lippincott, 1991.

PART VIII
MENOPAUSE ISSUES

68. Menopause Symptoms

Cynda Ann Johnson, M.D., M.B.A.

I. **The Issues**

Menopausal symptoms result from changes in the hormonal milieu in a woman's body. Although some of these changes (e.g., atrophic vaginitis) can be quantified, all are influenced greatly by the woman's perception of the severity of various symptoms and her expectations of menopause. Two decades ago the scientific community underestimated the psychological and physiologic changes that accompanied the climacteric, believing that only irregular menstrual periods, vasomotor symptoms, and possibly sleep disturbances were significantly associated. Urogenital atrophy and "bone pain" were thought to be potential symptoms of patients well past the menopause. Because many life changes as well as normal changes of aging accompany the fifth and sixth decades, it has indeed been difficult to assign cause and effect to the myriad of symptoms. The primary care physician must remain sensitive to the plethora of change in the lives of menopausal women and work with them, carrying out diagnostic tests when indicated, offering treatment when appropriate, and giving reassurance and continual education about the vagaries of the perimenopausal period.

II. **The Theory**

  A. **Climacteric**

    1. Synonyns include "perimenopause" or "menopausal transition"

    2. The climacteric is the entire period during which the ovary progressively reduces estrogen production and ceases ovulatory function

    3. Structural changes occur in the ovary

      a. Reduced number of follicles; rate of loss accelerates when the total number is < 25,000; in most women this occurs at 37–38 years of age

      b. Reduced number of estrogen-producing cells

      c. Decreased levels of inhibin from granulosa cells

        i. Less negative feedback to pituitary, resulting in increased production of follicle stimulating hormone (FSH)

        ii. Maximum FSH level is 25 mIU/ml during the reproductive years, but may rise to menopausal levels of 35 mIU/ml or more at times during the climacteric

        iii. Secretion of luteinizing hormone (LH) is not affected by inhibin; however, the LH surge before ovulation simulates menopausal levels

    4. Ovulatory and anovulatory cycles unpredictable during climacteric

      a. Long ovulatory cycles are characterized by prolonged follicular phase, low to level estradiol, increased FSH and LH and inadequate luteal phase

      b. Short ovulatory cycles, in contrast, have high FSH, rapid maturation of follicle, and normal luteal phase

  B. **Menopause**

    1. Cessation of spontaneous menstrual periods

    2. Failure of ovarian follicular development in presence of adequate gonadotropin stimulation

    3. Determined in retrospect when no menstrual period for 12 months

    4. Normal age range for natural menopause between 35 and 55 years—95% reach menopause between 45 and 55 years

    5. Premature ovarian failure if age < 35–40 years; etiologies include:

    a. Iatrogenic
       i. Surgical—oophorectomy (gonadotropins increase within 96 hr after castration)
      ii. Cytotoxic chemotherapy
     iii. Ionizing radiation
    b. Genetic—Turner's mosaic
    c. Autoimmune endocrinopathy
    d. Idiopathic/familial
  6. Mean age in U.S. is 51.4 years
    a. Not predictable by heredity, race, or nutritional status
    b. On average, cigarette smokers experience menopause 1–2 years earlier than non-smokers
    c. Increased parity associated with later menopause
  7. FSH and LH both continuously elevated
    a. FSH—10–20-fold increase over premenopause levels
    b. LH—3-fold increase (somewhat lower because of shorter half-life)
  8. Estrogen levels decline
    a. Source is adrenal glands and ovarian stroma—directly and by conversion
    b. Estrone (produced mainly by peripheral conversion of androstenedione); average plasma level of 35 pg/ml compared with premenopausal level of 40–200 pg/ml
    c. Estradiol (from peripheral conversion of testosterone); average plasma level of 13 pg/ml compared with premenopausal level of 40–350 pg/ml
    d. Obese patients convert more androstenedione to estrone (up to 200 µg/day) and consequently have fewer symptoms of estrogen deficiency
    e. Further reduction in estrogens 10 years after menopause
  9. Testosterone levels tend to remain stable or fall slightly

C. Menopause symptoms
  1. Symptoms include vasomotor instability, psychological symptoms, and atrophic changes
  2. Symptoms of early menopause
    a. Vasomotor (hot flush, hot flash)
       i. Recall that hot flush may also be sign of systemic disease, psychological disorder, drug effect, allergic reaction to foods, toxins etc.
      ii. Occurs in 85% of menopausal women (and may precede the actual menopause by months to years in 20%)
     iii. Major symptom during first 2 years of menopause
     iv. While 25% continue to have symptoms more than 5 years after menopause, it is rare to have hot flashes after10 years
      v. Physiology—dependent on low estrogen
        (a) Women with vasomotor symptoms have lower estrogen levels and less sex hormone–binding globulin hormone than those without
        (b) More common in women with less body fat
        (c) Coincides with LH surge and measurably increased heat over entire body surface even though core temperature actually falls
      vi. Description
        (a) Hot flash is sudden onset of feeling of warmth, lasting 2–3 minutes
        (b) Hot flush begins 1 minute after hot flash
          (i) Redness of upper body
          (ii) Profuse sweating in same areas
          (iii) Surface temperature increased by 2.5°C up to 30 minutes
          (iv) 50% of women with hot flushes have at least 1 per day; 20% have more
          (v) Often occur at night, resulting in insomnia
    b. Menopausal syndrome
       i. Relationship to estrogen may be causal or casual
      ii. May include fatigue, nervousness, sweating, headache, insomnia, depression, irritability, joint and muscle pain, dizziness, palpitations, formication

3. Symptoms of intermediate stage (5–10 years after menopause) largely atrophic—including vaginal pain, itching, dryness, and bleeding, dyspareunia, dysuria from urethral atrophy
4. Symptoms of later stage (> 10 years after menopause) related to estrogen deficiency manifestations such as osteoporosis, accelerated atherosclerosis

III. **An Approach**
   A. **Diagnosis of natural menopause**
      1. FSH and LH levels
         a. Not necessary to order routinely unless other hormonal circumstances such as oral contraceptives (OCs)
         b. Patients on combined OCs
            i. Age < 50 years
               (a) Yearly FSH on day 5, 6, or 7 of pill-free (or placebo-pill) week
               (b) 5–7 days enough to allow FSH to rise in menopausal patients
               (c) Diagnose menopause when FSH is > 30 mIU/ml
            ii. Mid-50s
               (a) Empirically switch to hormone replacement regimen
         c. Patients on progestin-only contraception
            i. FSH levels not suppressed so may assess level at any time
         d. Occasionally measure FSH in young patients to prove premenopausal status
         e. Some decrease of FSH in menopausal patient on hormone therapy, but does not normalize
      2. Can determine functional estrogen status from maturation index (see Chapter 109)
      3. No menses for 12 months in women in typical age range is usually enough for diagnosis of menopause (Table 1)
   B. **Diagnosis of premature menopause**
      1. Laboratory results
         a. Weekly LH, FSH, estradiol for 4 consecutive weeks
         b. Erythrocyte sedimentation rate, total serum protein and albumin/globulin ratio, rheumatoid factor, antinuclear antibody
         c. Serum calcium and phosphorus
         d. Thyroid-stimulating hormone and thyroid antibodies
         e. Ovarian antibodies

TABLE 1.   Percent Probability of Menopause According to Duration of First Amenorrhea and Age

Amenorrhea Interval (days)	Age (years)	% Women Menopausal
60–89	45–49	6.0
	50–52	21.6
	> 53	35.2
120–149	45–49	25.1
	50–52	42.4
	> 53	56.2
180–209	45–49	45.5
	50–52	65.2
	> 53	71.9
240–269	45–49	63.5
	50–52	81.5
	> 53	85.3
300–329	45–49	83.0
	50–52	90.3
	> 53	89.5
360+	45–49	89.5
	50–52	93.6
	> 53	95.5

Modified from Wallace RB, Sherman BM: Probability of menopause with increasing duration of amenorrhea in middle-aged women. Am J Obstet Gynecol 135:1021–1024, 1979.

   f. Morning cortisol/ACTH
   g. Karyotype
   h. Ovarian biopsy
  2. Consultation with specialist in gynecologic endocrinology
C. **Hormone replacement therapy**
  1. Begin as soon after menopause as possible for maximal benefit
  2. See Chapter 69 for regimens of estrogen/hormone replacement
D. **Symptom/problem-specific therapies**
  1. Vasomotor symptoms
   a. During perimenopause for the women who has vasomotor symptoms, but regular
       menstrual periods
        i. Measure FSH between days 2–4
       ii. Consider estrogen replacement if FSH level is ≥ 20 ImU/ml
      iii. Prescribe conjugated estrogens (or equivalent) 0.3 mg orally from day 5 to
            the end of the menstrual cycle
   b. Androgens
        i. Methyltestosterone 1.25–2.5 mg by mouth daily
       ii. Combination of estrogen and testosterone (e.g., Estratest®)
   c. Bellergal® (phenobarbital, ergotamine, belladonine alkaloids) 1 tablet in morning
       and noon, 2 tablets at night
        i. No statistical difference from placebo after 4 weeks of therapy
   d. Alpha-adrenergic agonists
        i. Clonidine hydrochloride, 0.1 mg by mouth 1–3 times/day or clonidine patch
       ii. Methyldopa, 250–500 mg twice daily
   e. Progestin-only therapy
        i. Medroxyprogesterone acetate, 10–20 mg/day
       ii. Depot medroxyprogesterone acetate, 150 mg intramuscularly every 3 months
      iii. Megestrol, 40–80 mg/day
   f. Antidopaminergic compounds—veralipride; may be associated with hyperpro-
       lactinemia and galactorrhea
   g. Propranolol, wide dosage range
   h. Vitamin E, 400 u/day
   i. Lifestyle changes—layered clothing, exercise
  2. Disturbance of libido
   a. Androgens (options listed above) oftentimes restore premenopausal libido levels
        i. Androgenic side effects frequently limit therapy
       ii. Deleterious effect on lipids
      iii. Discontinue after several months if not of clear benefit
  3. Headaches
   a. Verapamil hydrochloride, starting at 80 mg/day
   b. Propranolol
  4. Urogenital atrophy
   a. Vaginal estrogen cream daily for 2–4 weeks, then decrease frequency; symptoms
       usually controlled on twice weekly application; low-dose therapy maintains at-
       rophic state of endometrium;
   b. Water-soluble lubricants
   c. Regular sexual activity
  5. Osteoporosis prevention—see Chapter 87
  6. Dysfunctional uterine bleeding during the perimenopause (after appropriate evaluation)
   a. Low-dose oral contraceptive pills (20 µg ethinyl estradiol)
        i. OCs also control vasomotor symptoms and increase bone density
       ii. Contraindicated in the woman who smokes

SUGGESTED READING

 1. Abraham D, Carpenter PC: Issues concerning androgen replacement therapy in postmenopausal women.
     Mayo Clin Proc 72:1051–1055, 1997.
 2. Greendale GA, Sowers M: The menopause transition. Endocrinol Metab Clin North Am 26:261–277, 1997.

3. Hendrix SL: Nonestrogen management of menopausal symptoms. Endocrinol Metab Clin North Am 26:379–390, 1997.
4. Kaunitz AM: The role of androgens in menopausal hormonal replacement. Endocrinol Metab Clin North Am 26:391–397, 1997.
5. Kessel B: Alternatives to estrogen for menopausal women. Proc Soc Exp Biol Med 217:38–44, 1998.
6. McKinlay SM, Brambilla DJ: The normal menopause transition. Maturitas 14:103–115, 1992.
7. Mohyi D, Tabassi K: Differential diagnosis of hot flashes. Maturitas 27:203–214, 1997.
8. Perz JM: Development of the menopause symptom list: Menopause-associated symptoms. Women Health 25:53–59, 1997.
9. Slaven L, Lee C: Mood and symptom reporting among middle-aged women: The relationship between menopausal status, hormone replacement therapy, and exercise participation. Health Psychol 16:203–208, 1997.
10. Speroff L (ed): New Concepts in Managing Menopause (symposium). Patient Care, November 1995.

INTERNET SOURCES:

www.menopause.org.altmed.od.nih.gov/oam
www.healthy.net

69. Hormone Replacement Therapy

Cynda Ann Johnson, M.D., M.B.A.

I. The Issues

Over the last three decades controversies surrounding the safety and efficacy of hormone replacement therapy have been endless. For every argument to prescribe HRT, a counter-argument seems to exist. In the first edition of this book, I wrote, "..only in the last few years [has] the majority of both medical and lay literature strongly supported nearly universal use of hormone replacement therapy." Less than 5 years later, controversies rage on: Is the incidence of breast cancer significantly greater in women exposed to HRT? Should women be prescribed natural rather than synthetic estrogens (see Chapter 70)? Is the beneficial effect of estrogen on cardiovascular disease as great as the initial research purported? What other agents can replace estrogen for its effect of vasomotor symptoms, osteoporosis and urogenital symptoms? Women continue to feel betrayed as the medical literature swings back and forth on these issues. Now our patients bring us articles from the lay press and the Internet. How can we best deal with these complexities? The answer is to stay well-informed, to help our patients assess the endless information, and to stress that the entire picture is not clear, but together, the woman and her personal primary care provider can choose the best option to fit her personal health profile, armed with the information as we know it only at one point in time.

II. The Theory

A. Definitions

1. Estrogen replacement therapy (ERT) refers to administration of estrogen in menopause
2. Hormone replacement therapy (HRT) usually refers to administration of both estrogen and progestin, but also may refer to the use of either hormone alone

B. Rationale for use of ERT

1. To prevent or minimize vasomotor symptoms
2. To reduce discomfort or potential complications of urogenital atrophy
3. To retard bone loss and prevent consequences of osteoporosis
4. To reduce risk of coronary heart disease (by 50% in most studies)

C. Other probable beneficial effects of ERT

1. Mental health may be improved in women using ERT, including fewer stress reactions, less depression, improved memory, later onset and decreased incidence of Alzheimer's disease

    2. Cerebrovascular disease—subarachnoid hemorrhage and intracerebral hemorrhage are markedly reduced with the use of HRT; the risk of thrombotic stroke and ischemic stroke is probably unchanged

    3. ERT may protect against cataract formation

    4. According to studies with dynamic posturography, ERT increases static balance

    5. Skin thickness is enhanced with ERT

    6. ERT reduces the risk of colorectal cancer by about 30%

D. **Negative effects of ERT**

    1. Increased incidence of breast cancer—although the magnitude is unclear, it may be in the range of 10%

    2. The risk of venous thromboembolism is increased in women using ERT

    3. Women on HRT have a greater incidence of gallbladder disease and cholecystectomy

E. The **effect of unopposed estrogen** on the uterus is to stimulate endometrial cell biosynthesis

    1. With continued stimulation, a proliferative endometrium may progress to simple, cystic or adenomatous hyperplasia; adenomatous hyperplasia is more likely than cystic hyperplasia (25% vs. 5% over 20 years) to progress to atypical adenomatous hyperplasia (premalignant) and adenocarcinoma

    2. Adenocarcinoma of the endometrium after estrogen use is generally low-stage, low-grade, and associated with fewer cases of myometrial invasion

    3. The increase in uterine cancer is sixfold compared to nonusers of estrogen, with a 15-fold increase in long-term users

    4. Progesterone counteracts this stimulatory effect; hyperplasia results in only 4% of women who use progesterone 7 days each cycle, 2% using progesterone 10 days each month; and approximately 0% reliably using progesterone for 12 days or more

F. **Lipids and HRT**

    1. Oral ERT

        a. ERT results in decreased LDL within one month of usage; the percent decrease is greater in those women whose initial levels are higher

        b. ERT results in increased levels of HDL; the effect can be measured within three months of therapy

        c. ERT causes increased levels of triglycerides

        d. The rise in HDL is blunted and the rise in triglycerides is exaggerated in diabetic women

    2. Long-term use of transdermal estrogen decreases LDL, increases HDL, and minimally changes triglycerides

    3. Progestin effect on lipid profile

        a. Progestin lessens the benefits of estrogen on the lipid profile; the most negative effect is on HDL

        b. Progestins blunt the negative effect of ERT on triglycerides

        c. Results of the Postmenopausal Estrogen/Progestin Interventions (PEPI) Trial showed preservation of some beneficial effect on LDL and HDL with all regimens of progestins studied, but the most beneficial effect was preserved with the use of micronized progestin, which has recently become commercially available

III. **An Approach**

A. **Evaluation before instituting HRT**

    1. History should include menstrual history, menopausal symptoms, risk factors for osteoporosis and coronary heart disease, such as family history, exercise history, and previous experience with hormonal therapy

    2. Physical exam should include a breast examination, pelvic examination and Papanicolaou smear

    3. Other testing

        a. Mammography—mammograms are more difficult to read in women on ERT

        b. Progesterone challenge test (see Chapter 23) may be carried out in any women in whom it is desirable to know if the endometrium demonstrates estrogen effect; to carry out a PCT, administer 10 mg medroxyprogesterone acetate orally, daily for 10 days; a positive test is any withdrawal bleeding, which usually occurs 2–7 days after completing the course of progestin

    c. Transvaginal ultrasound should not be routine before initiating HRT

    d. Endometrial biopsy should be carried out in any woman who is on or has been on unopposed estrogen therapy; if a transvaginal ultrasound demonstrates ≥ 4 mm of endometrial thickness; if a PCT is positive for bleeding; in a perimenopausal woman being considered for HRT, especially if her menstrual periods have increased in frequency, duration and/or amount

    e. Bone densitometry

        i. Bone densitometry need not be carried out routinely, but with newer drugs that demonstrate additive effect on bone density when used in conjunction with HRT, bone densitometry has greater role (see Chapter 87)

        ii. Offer bone densitometry to women not desiring HRT to assess risk of osteoporosis:

          (a) If bone density is at the mean or within one standard deviation for patient's age, repeat in one year

          (b) If bone density is greater than one standard deviation below the mean, strongly encourage her to use HRT

B. **Follow-up exams**

  1. 3–6 months after initiating HRT to determine adequacy of the regimen and to review any side effects

  2. Yearly once a satisfactory regimen has been established:

    a. Review side effects and menstrual bleeding pattern if any

    b. Carry out breast cancer surveillance with a clinical breast exam and mammography

    c. Perform a pelvic exam (with Papanicolaou smear at least in women with a uterus) with attention to the adequacy of estrogen effect on the vulva and vagina; maturation index can be done if vasomotor or urogenital symptoms continue despite apparent adequate replacement regimen

    d. Perform an endometrial biopsy if the bleeding pattern is not appropriate for the regimen

    e. Transvaginal ultrasound is not useful for follow-up screening in women on HRT as nearly half would have a total endometrial thickness > 4 mm, necessitating an endometrial biopsy; may be useful in patients in whom an endometrial biopsy is unsuccessful or declined when indicated

    f. PCT might be considered yearly in patients opting against HRT, especially if high risk for uterine cancer

C. **Contraindications to the use of HRT**

  1. Known or suspected pregnancy

  2. Undiagnosed abnormal genital bleeding

  3. Active thrombophlebitis or thromboembolic disorder; history of these disorders associated with estrogen use

  4. Known or suspected estrogen-dependent neoplasia

  5. Known or suspected cancer of the breast, except in appropriately selected patients being treated for metastatic disease (in consultation with a specialist in the field)

D. **Special considerations for the use of HRT**

  1. Patients with a history of uterine cancer

    a. In stage I, receptor-negative disease, estrogen may be given after first surgery, even at the time of hospital discharge

    b. Estrogens may be given in steroid receptor–positive disease with only superficial myometrial penetration, negative nodes, and negative peritoneal cytology

  2. HRT may be offered to women previously treated for ovarian and cervical cancer

  3. Women with a past history of breast cancer

    a. Treatment for breast cancers often results induces early menopause

    b. Persistent vasomotor symptoms and urogenital atrophy with dyspareunia may result

    c. Young menopausal women are at high risk for osteoporosis and heart disease 10–15 years later

    d. Strongly consider HRT in women who are disease-free for 5 years

E. **Initiation and duration of therapy**
1. Initiate therapy as soon after menopause as possible—this is especially important as a 6-year period of rapid bone loss follows menopause
2. Starting estrogen replacement in premenopausal patients is not indicated for prevention of osteoporosis
3. Initiating therapy in older women, including those who are ≥ 65 may be indicated
   a. Studies show reduced fracture rates and evidence of bone restoration in this age group and older
   b. Evidence suggests a decrease in cardiovascular risk, subclinical disease and mortality in these women
4. Clinical guidelines in Britain suggest that postmenopausal women after an acute MI should be discharged on HRT unless otherwise contraindicated; however, new study shows decreased survival and increased coronary artery disease in women placed on HRT with pre-existing CAD
5. Duration of therapy
   a. 2–3 years to alleviate vasomotor symptoms
   b. At least 7 years to protect bone
   c. HRT should not be discontinued because of age
F. **Estrogen**
1. Choice of estrogen
   a. Standardized routes of administration include oral, transdermal, vaginal
   b. Alternate forms include subcutaneous pellets, vaginal tablets and rings, gel which is rubbed into the skin, injectable
   c. Some women prefer natural over synthetic estrogens
   d. Controversy exists over the use of conjugated estrogens which are obtained from pregnant mare's urine
2. Dose of estrogen
   a. Standardized doses were determined that would prevent osteoporosis; a serum level of 50–60 pg/ml is required
   b. Typical daily doses are: conjugated estrogens 0.625 mg; estrone sulfate 0.625 mg; estradiol 1 mg; 17β-estradiol cream 1.5 mg; transdermal 17β-estradiol 0.05 mg.
   c. Similar doses seem to be effective in prevention and treatment of cardiovascular disease
   d. Higher doses are often required to alleviate vasomotor symptoms in perimenopause and early menopause
   e. Urogenital symptoms may persist despite apparently adequate blood levels, requiring application of additional vaginal estrogen cream
3. Serum blood levels of estrogen are not routinely indicated; a single estradiol level often inaccurately reflects total estrogen effect; levels may be useful in some circumstances.
   a. Women who are not absorbing estrogen may include those with GI disease
   b. Cigarette smokers may have decreased estrogen levels
   c. Women who believe they have decreased estrogen effect despite standard dosing
   d. Women who believe their estrogen levels are adequate without HRT
   e. Pre- or perimenopausal women who believe they have inadequate estrogen effect
   f. Women with symptoms that may or may not be secondary to estrogen deficiency
G. **Progestins**
1. Choice of progestin
   a. Medroxyprogesterone acetate (MDA) is inexpensive, low in androgen side effects; some reduction in LDL cholesterol persists.
   b. Micronized progesterone (Prometrium™) is now available (best retention of lipid profile when added to estrogen in PEPI trial), but absorption may be irregular, metabolism is rapid and active metabolites may cause sedation and other CNS effects
   c. Norethindrone ("mini" birth control pill) may be used as the progestin, especially for those not tolerating MDA
2. Dose of progestin: 10 mg MDA = 1 mg norethindrone = 200 mg micronized progesterone; use one mini-pill (0.35 mg) or 100 mg micronized progesterone (this was the dose studied) to substitute for 2.5 mg MDA

3. Routes of administration
    a. Standardized routes of administration are oral and transdermal
    b. Natural progestins are also given vaginally
    c. Alternate routes include rings and intrauterine devices

H. **Choice of HRT regimen**—tailor to the individual considering:
    1. Depth of patient's concern about cancer
    2. Previously used regimens and side effects
    3. Tolerance of hormonal side effects
    4. Presence of vasomotor symptoms
    5. Relative contraindications to usage
    6. Patient history of adherence
    7. Stage of menopause

I. **Sample HRT regimens**
    1. Continuous, sequential HRT
        a. Conjugated estrogens, 0.625 mg/day, plus MDA, 10 mg for the first 2 weeks each month
        b. No estrogen withdrawal symptoms
        c. No endometrial hyperplasia expected with at least 12 days of progestin, but 2 weeks is easier for the patient to remember
        d. 80–90% have withdrawal bleeding, but the pattern is predictable
        e. Carry out an endometrial biopsy if the bleeding begins during progestin administration or if the pattern of withdrawal bleeding changes; if no pathology is found in the presence of a proliferative endometrium, increase the progestin (dosage or number of days); if the endometrium is atrophic continue the same regimen or change the type of one or both hormones.
        f. Premphase™ combines conjugated estrogens 0.625 mg and MDA 5 mg into a single tablet for the second half of a 4-week cycle; the manufacturer chose the lower dose of MDA to keep the total dose of hormones as low as possible, although there is a slightly higher incidence of endometrial hyperplasia at this dose; Premphase™ offers ease of adherence, but loss of flexibility in dosing.
    2. Cyclic, sequential HRT
        a. Conjugated estrogen, 0.625 mg, on calendar days 1–25 plus MDA 10 mg on days 16–25
        b. This regimen offers a long history of safety and efficacy with a predictable bleeding pattern (usually on the pill-free days)
        c. Some women have estrogen withdrawal symptoms on the pill-free days
        d. Carry out an endometrial biopsy if the patient has vaginal bleeding during the days of hormonal therapy
    3. Continuous, combined HRT
        a. Conjugated estrogens, 0.625 mg/day (or equivalent) and MDA, 2.5 mg/day
        b. Goal is ultimate amenorrhea
        c. As irregular vaginal bleeding is not uncommon initially, endometrial biopsies should be restricted for the first six months of therapy
        d. If bleeding persists beyond that time, an endometrial biopsy should be carried out; if no pathology is found, increase the MDA to 5 mg/day
        e. Prempro™ combines conjugated estrogens 0.6265 mg and MDA 2.5 mg into one tablet
    4. Cyclic, combined HRT—two approaches
        a. Both conjugated estrogen, 0.625 mg and MDA 2.5 mg on calendar days 1–25 with a pill break for the remainder of the month
            i. Most women on this regimen have withdrawal bleeding for 3–6 months, but the bleeding pattern is predictable and usually only 1–2 days in length, but amenorrhea thereafter
            ii. Hormonal side effects are fewer than with continuous, combined HRT or with regimens using a higher dose of progestin
            iii. Estrogen withdrawal side effects may occur during the pill-free days
        b. Both conjugated estrogens 0.625 mg and MDA 2.5 mg daily Monday through Friday only; this regimen is an alternative for women who have side effects of hormone excess on a continuous combined regimen of HRT.

5. Transdermal estrogen
   a. Transdermal estradiol-17β, 0.05 mg every $3^1/_2$ days (or weekly, depending on the transdermal system), plus MDA for the first 2 weeks each month
   b. The new CombiPatch™ contains progestin within the patch, obviating the need for oral progestin. The CombiPatch™ is the smallest-sized patch available, containing transdermal estradiol 0.05 mg and norethindrone acetate 0.14 mg
   c. Special considerations for transdermal administration—women who:
      i. Are cigarette smokers who maintain adequate serum estrogen levels with usual doses of transdermal estrogen, but may require higher doses of oral estrogen
      ii. Have elevated triglyceride levels (particularly > 300 mg/dl)
      iii. Have migraine headaches on oral estrogens
      iv. Have cholelithiasis; transdermal estrogen does not alter the composition of bile as does oral estrogen
      v. Take oral estrogens who experience increasing symptoms of fibrocystic breast disease
      vi. Have a history of thromboembolic disease; well-controlled studies do not demonstrate a changed in clotting factors
J. **Recommended HRT regimens according to stage of menopause**
   1. During perimenopause, a nonsmoking, low-risk woman may use low-dose oral contraceptive pills containing 20 μg ethinyl estradiol
   2. During perimenopause and early menopause, use a cyclic or sequential regimen. Predictable bleeding is more tolerable than irregular bleeding for most women at this stage.
   3. Several years into menopause, switch to a combined continuous or cyclic, combined regimen. Amenorrhea can usually be achieved in these women.
K. **The ideal HRT regimen** would preserve the positive hormonal effects and eliminate the negative effects. The selective estrogen receptor modulators described in Chapter 101 and currently used for osteoporosis prevention are the most likely candidates.

SUGGESTED READING

1. Beral V, for the Collaborative Group on Hormonal Factors in Breast Cancer: Breast cancer and hormone replacement therapy: Collaborative reanalysis of data from 51 epidemiological studies of 52,705 women with breast cancer and 108,411 women without breast cancer. Lancet 350:1047–1059, 1997.
2. Brace M, McCauley E: Oestrogens and physical well-being. Ann Med 29:283–290, 1997.
3. Calle EE, Hankinson SE, Johnson CA, et al: Postmenopausal hormone replacement and breast cancer. Contemp Ob/Gyn 42(Suppl):S4–S26, 1996.
4. Colditz GA, Hankinson SE, Hunter DJ, et al: The use of estrogens and progestins and the risk of breast cancer in postmenopausal women. New Engl J Med 332:1589–1593, 1995.
5. Cumming DC, Cumming CE: Hormone replacement therapy: Part 1. Should your patient do with—or without—it? Consultant, October 1998.
6. Edozien GY, Edozien LC, Klimiuk PS, Mander AM: The use of hormone replacement therapy in women with acute myocardial infarction: An audit of current practice. Br J Obstet Gynaecol 104:1322–1324, 1997.
7. Gadducci A, Fanucchi A, Cosio S, Genazzani AR: Hormone replacement therapy and gynecological cancer. Anticancer Res 17:3793–3798, 1997.
8. Hulley S, Grady D, Bush T, et al: Randomized trial of estrogen plus progestin for secondary prevention of coronary heart disease in postmenopausal women. JAMA 280:605–613, 1998.
9. Miller KL: Hormone replacement therapy in the elderly. Clin Obstet Gynecol 39:912–932, 1996.
10. Mitlak BH, Choen FJ: In search of optimal long-term female hormone replacement: The potential of selective estrogen receptor modulators. Horm Res 48:155–163, 1997.
11. Petitti DB, Sidney S, Quesenberry CP Jr, Bernstein A: Ischemic stroke and use of estrogen and estrogen/progesterone as hormone replacement therapy. Stroke 29:23–28, 1998.
12. Pedersen AT, Lidegaard Ø, Kreiner S, Ottesen B: Hormone replacement therapy and risk of nonfatal stroke. Lancet 350:1277–1283, 1997.
13. The Postmenopausal Estrogen/Progestin Interventions (PEPI) Trial: Effects of estrogen/progestin regimens on heart disease risk factors in postmenopausal women. JAMA 273:199–208, 1995.
14. Robinson JG, Folsom AR, Nabulsi AA, et al: Can postmenopausal hormone replacement improve plasma lipids in women with diabetes. Diabetes Care 19:480–485, 1996.
15. Sellers TA, Mink PJ, Cerhan JR, et al: The role of hormone replacement therapy in the risk for breast cancer and total mortality in women with a family history of breast cancer. Ann Intern Med 127:973–980, 1997.

16. Silverman SL, Greenwald M, Klein RA, Drinkwater BL: Effect of bone density information on decisions about hormone replacement therapy: A randomized trial. Obstet Gynecol 89:321–325, 1997.
17. Varas-Lorenzo C, Garcia-Rodriguez LA, Cattaruzzi C, et al: Hormone replacement therapy and the risk of hospitalization for venous thromboembolism: A population-based study in southern Europe. Am J Epidemiol 147:387–390, 1998.

70. Natural Approaches to Menopause

Jane L. Murray, M.D.

I. The Issues
A. Overview
Women patients increasingly are asking physicians about approaches to health problems that include more "natural" substances and fewer synthetic ones. Hormonal therapies for common women's health issues are no exception. The popular press has made information about "natural" hormones in place of standard hormone replacement therapy (HRT) widely available, and patients are seeking information from their physicians regarding their potential uses.

B. Why do women eschew standard HRT regimens?
1. A high percentage—about 50%—of women for whom HRT is prescribed do not fill their prescriptions, and 40% of those who do fill the prescription discontinue use after less than a year of therapy.
2. A 1996 survey of women physicians who would be eligible for HRT indicated that less than 50% actually took it.
3. Women report fear of breast cancer stimulation as a major reason for not starting or for discontinuing HRT.
4. Many women experience undesirable side effects from standard HRT, such as weight gain, bloating, depression, poor sleep.
5. Some women dislike breakthrough bleeding, uterine and breast discomfort they can experience on HRT.
6. Some women decry the "medicalization" of what they perceive as a natural aging process, and desire to manage any symptoms they may have with nutrition and lifestyle interventions.

C. Terminology
In this chapter, the term "natural hormone" refers to a substance which is isomolecular to the hormone secreted in the human body. It does not necessarily mean the substance is derived from a natural source. Conjugated estrogens from equine urine, for example, come from nature, but are not bioidentical to human estrogens, and are thus not considered "natural" for the purpose of this discussion.

D. Conditions discussed
Because of the complexity of this topic, only the use of "natural" approaches for menopause and perimenopause are being addressed. Natural hormones, herbal therapies, nutritional supplements, and lifestyle interventions are advocated for a variety of other women's health issues, such as premenstrual syndrome, dysmenorrhea, mastalgia, fibrocystic breast disease, and endometriosis. For discussion of these conditions see Chapter 7 on Alternative Therapies in Women's Health Care.

II. The Theory
A. Ovarian hormonal secretion
1. During reproductive years, the human ovary secretes three estrogens: estriol (E3), estradiol (E2) and estrone (E1). Ass shown in Figure 1, there is interconversion of E2 and E1. Based on studies of circulating serum and salivary free hormones and urinary metabolites, it is estimated that the three main estrogen circulate in the body in approximately a ratio of 80:10:10 of E3:E2:E1.

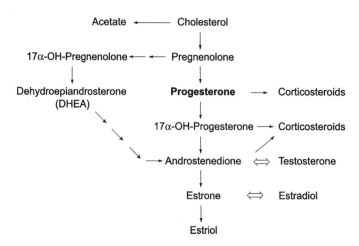

FIGURE 1. Steroid synthesis pathways.

2. During pregnancy, the placenta converts 16-alpha hydroxy-dehydroepiandrosterone to estriol.
3. Estradiol is the most physiologically "potent" human estrogen, while estriol is relatively weak in its estrogenic activity.
4. After menopause, estradiol levels drop but estrone stays near normal, due to conversion of androsterone to estrone. In natural (i.e., nonsurgical) menopause, the ovaries may continue to secrete a small amount of estrogen.
5. About 40% of circulating testosterone in the female comes from ovarian and adrenal sources; 60% is derived from peripheral conversion from adrenal adrostenedione.
B. **Adrenal hormonal secretion**
   1. Adrosterone is made in both the ovaries and adrenals, and is converted to estrone and testosterone.
   2. Dehydroepiandrosterone (DHEA) is secreted in greater quantities by the adrenals than any other adrenal steroid. Adrostenedione declines by 50% after menopause. DHEA declines with age, at approximately 2% per year, until it is only 10–20% of peak levels by age 70.
   3. Estrogens are also manufactured in the adrenal, and with natural menopause, many women will have reasonable circulating amounts of estrogens from adrenal sources.
C. **Potential benefits of natural hormones**
   1. There is evidence that non-isomolecular estrogens may have unintended tissue effects, such as a higher incidence of breast and other cancers, and that all the desirable physiologic effects of natural estrogens, especially estradiol, are not manifested with the use of non-isomolecular hormones.
   2. There is some evidence that estriol may actually be somewhat protective against breast cancer, while higher urinary estrone levels appear to correlate with a higher incidence of breast cancer.
   3. Patient acceptance of "natural substances" is enhanced in some populations, and therefore the known benefits of postmenopausal HRT may be obtained for women with such a philosophy.
   4. In the PEPI trial, the group with the best lipid profile was the group receiving micronized natural progesterone rather than medroxyprogesterone acetate (MPA) as the progestin.
   5. Individualized prescriptions can be written and revised for individual patients with compounded preparations. The prescription fits the patient, rather than vice versa. Serum or saliva levels of hormones can be monitored, and doses adjusted as needed for the individual.
D. **Potential risks of natural hormones**
   1. Various hormonal regimens using triple estrogen with natural progesterone and/or testosterone have not been fully studied; although each component of a typical natural

hormone regimen has a body of supportive literature—mainly from European centers—the combinations have not yet been fully studied in the U.S.

2. No head-to-head comparisons of standard HRT regimens and natural hormone regimens have yet been undertaken to evaluate comparative effects on bone density, lipid profiles, hormone levels, symptom relief, cancer incidence, etc. Clearly, such studies are needed.

3. Many of the natural hormone regimens require individualized compounding by a specialized compounding pharmacy. While accredited pharmacies must meet rigorous quality requirements, there remains the possibility of variations in quality from one prescription to the next, as each is individually manufactured.

E. **Delivery systems for natural hormones**

1. Natural hormones in their native state are rapidly degraded by the digestive process, and therefore are poorly bioavailable in usual oral forms.

2. Micronization of the hormone by surrounding the molecules of hormone in microscopic droplets of oil enhances oral bioavailability.

3. Transmucosal delivery methods bypass the digestive process and liver metabolism entirely. Such systems include rectal and vaginal suppositories, gels and creams, and sublingual or buccal mucosal lozenges or troches.

4. Transdermal creams, gels and patches are an additional mechanism used to bypass the intestinal and liver degradation process.

5. Serum or saliva levels of hormones (as well as patient symptom reports) can be followed to monitor response to therapy. Generally higher doses of hormone are required for oral micronized and transdermal preparations. Most natural hormones need to be dosed twice daily to maintain sufficient serum levels throughout a 24 hour period, as the half-life is shorter than most synthetic HRT regimens.

6. Standard prescription preparations are available (as of the time of publication) for transdermal estradiol patches and oral micronized progesterone capsules. A variety of over-the-counter creams containing various concentrations of progesterone and estrogen, and well as "wild yam" precursors are available. The nonprescription products are more variable in quality, and contain lower amounts of active ingredient so they can be sold as cosmetics and not drugs.

III. **An Approach**

A. **Estrogens**

1. **Phytoestrogens in food** (Table 1)

a. Epidemiology—Japanese women have less breast cancer, endometrial cancer, osteoporosis and consume a diet high in phytoestrogens, especially isoflavones. When they move to a Western diet, the incidence of diseases approximates American women's incidence.

b. Types of phytoestrogens

i. Lignans—present in almost all cereals and vegetables; highest in flax seeds.

ii. Isoflavones—highest in soybeans

c. Properties of phytoestrogens

i. Lignans inhibit breast cancer cell growth *in vitro*

ii. Genistein (a phytoestrogen) equivalent to Premarin in retaining bone mass in oophorectomized rats

iii. Soy-rich diet is associated with lower colon cancer risk

TABLE 1. Isoflavones in Foods

Food	Serving Size	Isoflavones
Tofu, tempeh	100 g	62–112 mg
Miso	120 g	40 mg
Soy milk	250 g	40 mg
Texturized soy protein	100 g	138 mg
Soy beans, roasted	100 g	162 mg
Green soy	100 g	135 mg

    iv. Isoflavones lower LDL and raise HDL

    v. All have antiviral, antibacterial, antifungal, and anticarcinogenic properties

    vi. Flavones have antioxidant, anti-inflammatory, and antimutagenic properties

2. **Herbal products**

    a. Black cohosh (*Cimifuga racemosa*) has estrogenic properties. Sold worldwide as Remifemin, it can thicken the vaginal mucosa and alleviate hypoestrogenic symptoms (hot flashes, irritability, etc.); also used to regulate menses. Lowers LH levels in oophorectomized rats. (NOT related to blue cohosh, which can be toxic due to its mild nicotinic activity). Suggested dose: 40 mg tincture daily.

    b. Dong quai (*Angelica polymorpha*) is advised for numerous gynecologic complaints; little evidence to support its efficacy. Suggested dose: 300–500 mg three times a day.

    c. Evening primrose (*Oenothera* sp.) oil has a high concentration of omega-6-fatty acids, especially gamma-linolenic acid (GLA) which has been shown to lower LDL. It also appears effective in alleviating hot flashes, but has no direct estrogenic effect. Suggested dose: 500-mg capsules 3–6 times daily.

    d. Nettle (*Urtica dioica*): often recommended for menopausal symptoms, has a mild diuretic effect.

    e. Red clover (*Trifolium pratense*): sheep grazing on large amounts have developed sterility. Mild estrogenic effect in humans.

3. **Prescription natural estrogens** (Table 2)

    a. Estradiol: Commonly prescribed alone as oral (Estrace), or transdermal preparation (Alora, Climara, Estraderm, Fempatch, Vivelle); also as vaginal ring (Estring).

    b. Estriol: made by compounding pharmacies as micronized capsule, vaginal cream, transbuccal lozenge or transdermal cream.

    c. Estrone: Found as main constituent of Ogen, Estratab, Orthoest.

    d. "Tri-est" and "Bi-est": Tri-est or triple estrogen usually compounded in ratio of 80–90% estriol, 5–10% estradiol and 3–10% estrone. Bi-est is 90% estriol, 10% estradiol. Made by compounding pharmacies into micronized capsules, transdermal creams, vaginal or rectal suppositories, transmucosal (buccal) lozenges or troches. Nonoral forms bypass liver and intestinal metabolism, so lower doses may be possible with transmucosal forms. Usual dose is 1.25 mg of Tri-est BID (equivalent to 0.625 mg/day of conjugated estrogens, see Table 2). Doses can range from 0.625 mg daily to 2.5 mg BID.

B. **Progesterone**

1. Natural progesterone, unlike synthetic progestins, has been shown to have numerous beneficial physiologic effects: enhanced osteoblastic activity, improved sleep, lowering of LDL, mood stabilization. Often women who experience unwanted side effects from synthetic progestins in standard HRT regimens may improve with natural progesterone supplementation. (Fig. 2).

2. Available in a prescription capsule form as Prometrium, compounded creams, suppositories, or troches, vaginal gel—Crinone, and nonprescription transdermal creams containing a maximum of 450 mg progesterone per ounce of cream.

TABLE 2. Comparative Potency of Estrogens

Conjugated estrogens	0.625 mg
Dienestrol	0.10 mg
Ethinyl estradiol	0.015 mg
Estradiol-17b	1.0 mg
Estrone sulfate	1.25 mg
Estropipate	0.75 mg
Mestranol	0.02 mg
Micronized estradiol	1.0 mg
Tri-est	1.25 mg BID

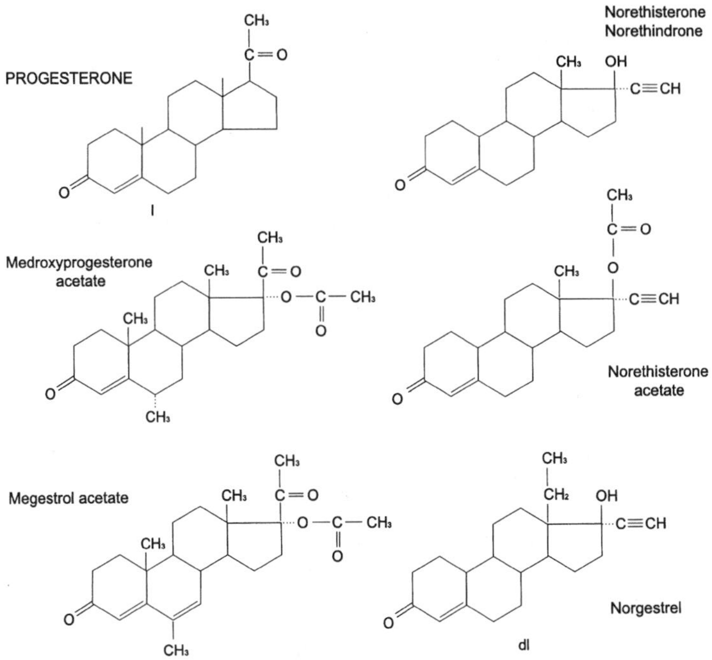

FIGURE 2.   Comparison of natural progesterone and synthetic progestins.

3. Wild yam creams or supplements are often recommended to women as a "natural" substitute for progesterone. Mexican wild yams of the Dioscoreaceae family are used to provide the chemical precursor to progesterone for manufacturing purposes, but there is no evidence that the human can convert this precursor into progesterone *in vivo*.
4. Recommended doses for natural progesterone range from 200–300 mg of transdermal cream per week to 100–200 mg BID of oral micronized progesterone. Compounded troches or suppositories usually contain 50–200 mg once at bedtime to BID.

C. **Testosterone**
  1. Evidence is accumulating that androgen deficiency in the perimenopausal and menopausal periods are largely responsible for declining libido and sexual enjoyment. Replacement with small amounts of testosterone appears to be effective and safe, as long as masculinizing side effects, elevation in blood pressure and other adrogenic effects are monitored. Excess doses of testosterone can result in acne, unwanted hair growth, clitoral hypertrophy, hypertension, and liver disease.
  2. Testosterone has known beneficial effects on osteoporosis and hot flashes, but there is concern that it could induce a poor lipid profile. In the small doses used for women, this concern is unsubstantiated.
  3. Natural testosterone can be added to compounded formulations (creams, micronized capsules, troches, suppositories) in essentially any amount—usually 0.25—5.0 mg BID. A prescription tablet of Estratest is also available in two doses: esterified estrogens 1.25 mg plus methyltestosterone 2.5 mg or esterified estrogens 0.625 plus methyltestosterone 1.25 mg. Estratest does not contain natural hormones, but synthetic ones. A transdermal testosterone patch for women is under development.

D. **Dehydroepiandrosterone** (DHEA)
  1. DHEA is a metabolic precursor to both estrogen and testosterone, so one theory is to provide the body with DHEA and let it decide how to metabolize it. However, not all women are able to make the biomedical conversion from DHEA to testosterone, and in some women the pathway to testosterone is actually more active, so that masculinizing side effects can be pronounced.

2. In many animal and some human studies, higher DHEA levels correlate with increased longevity, decreased heart disease and cancer, enhanced immune function, less obesity and less autoimmune disease in humans. This research, however, remains controversial, and the effects of long-term DHEA supplementation are unknown—especially in supraphysiologic doses.

3. Despite extensive research, the exact mechanism of action of DHEA remains unknown. Excess androgen effects, as described above for testosterone, are also concerns when using DHEA supplementation.

4. DHEA can be administered orally, and is readily available over-the-counter at health food stores. Patients should be advised to take no more than 50 mg of DHEA daily, given concerns about oral administration and liver toxicity.

5. DHEA can also be included in compounded formulations of vaginal creams, transdermal creams, suppositories and transbuccal delivery systems.

SUGGESTED READING

1. Casson PR, Buster JE: DHEA replacement after menopause: HRT 2000 or nostrum of the 90s? Contemp Ob/Gyn 119–133, 1997.
2. Gaby AR: Dehydroepiandrosterone: Biological effects and clinical significance. Alt Med Rev 1:60–69, 1996.
3. Knight DC, Eden JA: Phytoestrogens—a short review. Maturitas 22:167–175, 1995.
4. Lieberman S: Are the difference between estradiol and other estrogens, naturally occurring or synthetic, merely semantical? J Clin Endocrinol Metab 81:850–851, 1996.
5. Murray JL: Natural progesterone: What role in women's health care? Women Health Prim Care 1:671–687, 1998.
6. Northrup C: Menopause. Prim Care 24:921–948, 1997.
7. Sitruk-Ware R, Utian WH (eds): The Menopause and Hormonal Replacement Therapy. New York, Marcel Dekker, Inc., 1991.
8. Taylor M: Alternatives to conventional hormone replacement therapy. Comp Ther 23:514–532, 1997.
9. Warnock JK, Bundren JC, Morris DW: Female hypoactive sexual desire disorder due to adrogen deficiency: Clinical and psychometric issues. Psychopharmacol Bull 33:761–766, 1997.
10. Wright JV, Morganthaler J: Natural hormone replacement. Petaluma, CA, Smart Publications, 1997.
11. Young RL: Androgens in postmenopausal therapy? Menopause Management 21–24, 1993.

RESOURCES:

To locate a compounding pharmacy contact the International Academy of Compounding Pharmacists (IACP), P.O. Box 1365, Sugar Land, TX 77487, (800) 927-4227.

71. Postmenopausal Bleeding

Cynda Ann Johnson, M.D., M.B.A.

I. The Issues

Postmenopausal bleeding is the only significant clinical clue to the presence of endometrial carcinoma, most cases of which occur in postmenopausal women. Until recently the unhesitating response to postmenopausal bleeding was immediate dilatation and curettage (D&C). Numbers as high as 90% were quoted for the prevalence of endometrial cancer in women with postmenopausal bleeding. The incidence of postmenopausal bleeding has risen rapidly with greater numbers of women on hormone replacement therapy. In addition, newer studies suggest that the overall prevalence of endometrial cancer in women with postmenopausal bleeding is certainly no higher than 20% and probably closer to 10%; few women on hormone replacement therapy using both estrogen and progestin have endometrial carcinoma. This recognition has been a major impetus to review the strategy of immediate D&C; moreover, newer studies repeatedly demonstrate the accuracy and cost-effectiveness of in-office endometrial sampling compared with traditional

TABLE 1. Causes of Postmenopausal Bleeding

Ovary	Cervix	Vulva
Cancer	Cervical erosion	Vulvitis
	Cervicitis	Condyloma
Fallopian tube	Cervical polyps	Vulvar intraepithelial neoplasia
Cancer	Condyloma	Cancer of the vulva
	Cervical dysplasia	Vulvar dystrophy
Uterus	Cervical cancer	Eczema/other skin conditions
Atrophic endometrium	Squamous cell	Trauma
Estrogen excess	Adenocarcinoma	
Estrogen replacement	Trauma	Nongenital tract
Endogenous excess		Urinary tract
Leiomyomata uteri	Vagina	Urethral caruncle
Endometrial hyperplasia	Atrophic vaginitis	Urethral cancer
Adenomatous hyperplasia	Infectious vaginitis	Hematuria
Cystic	Condyloma	Gastrointestinal tract
Atypical	Vaginal intraepithelial neoplasia	Hemorrhoids
Endometrial polyps	Vaginal cancer	Other bleeding
Endometrial carcinoma	Trauma	
Endometritis		Idiopathic

D&C. The roles of ultrasound, hysteroscopy and assessment of bleeding patterns (in women on HRT) are also being evaluated.

II. **The Theory**
   A. **Native postmenopausal endometrium**
      1. Endometrial thickness typically 1 mm or less
      2. Cystic atrophy of hormone deprivation not to be confused with cystic variations of endometrial hyperplasia
         a. Most important distinction is overall greater amount of cellular tissue in hyperplastic states
         b. Determination of cellularity
            i. Gross amount of tissue on endometrial sample
            ii. Microscopic evaluation (from pathologic specimen)
   B. **Causes of postmenopausal bleeding** (Table 1)
      1. Menstrual bleeding—women may not be truly menopausal
      2. Atrophic vaginitis: most common cause in patients not on hormone replacement therapy (HRT)
      3. Cause never determined in up to one-third of patients not on hormone replacement
   C. **Patients at greater risk for endometrial cancer**
      1. Nulliparity
      2. Age > 50 years
      3. Age at menopause > 52 years
      4. Unopposed estrogen therapy
      5. Obesity
      6. History of endometrial hyperplasia or adenomatous hyperplasia
      7. Previous pelvic irradiation

III. **An Approach**
   A. **History**
      1. Vaginal bleeding
         a. Bleeding patterns, amount, and frequency
         b. Previous evaluation for postmenopausal bleeding
         c. Abnormal vaginal bleeding before menopause
         d. History of vulvar/vaginal trauma
      2. Other symptoms
         a. Vulvar/vaginal dryness or pruritus; vaginal discharge; vulvar lesions
         b. Abdominal pain or fullness; gastrointestinal symptoms
         c. Urinary symptoms
         d. Other systemic symptoms
      3. Sexual history

   4. Gynecologic history
      a. Gravidity and parity; previous menstrual history
      b. Age at menopause
      c. Previous gynecologic diagnoses/surgery
      d. Radiation exposure
   5. Other history
      a. Systemic diseases (especially diabetes)
      b. Other surgeries
      c. Medications, especially hormonal
   6. Family history of gynecologic cancers
B. **Physical exam**
   1. General
      a. Abdomen
      b. Back and flank
   2. Pelvic exam
      a. External genitalia—lesions, skin condition, hemorrhage
      b. Urethra
      c. Vagina—lesions, atrophy, hemorrhage, discharge
      d. Cervix—friability, lesions, discharge
      e. Uterus—size, mobility, tenderness, surface contour
      f. Ovaries—adnexae, size, tenderness
      g. Rectum, rectovaginal—blood, nodularity, hemorrhoids
C. **Laboratory tests** (as indicated after history and physical examination)
   1. Hematocrit or hemoglobin
   2. Urinalysis
   3. Stool for occult blood
D. **Other diagnostic studies**
   1. Papanicolaou smear in all patients
   2. Maturation index in selected cases of atrophy and hormone replacement
   3. Evaluation of appropriate samples from cervix and vagina
   4. Vulvar, vaginal and/or cervical biopsies of suspicious lesions
E. **When to evaluate uterine bleeding**
   1. Postmenopausal women on HRT—whether to begin evaluation depends on bleeding pattern in relationship to HRT regimen (see Chapter 69)
   2. Postmenopausal women not on ERT—begin evaluation with first episode of bleeding
F. **How to evaluate postmenopausal bleeding**
   1. Endometrial biopsy (see Chapter 117)
      a. First-line evaluation in all patients in whom extrauterine cause of vaginal bleeding not found
      b. Inexpensive office procedure, available to any primary care physician
      c. If biopsy specimen reveals cause of vaginal bleeding, further diagnosis and treatment as indicated
      d. Endometrial hyperplasia
         i. Possibility of spontaneous resolution as high as 70% (> 80% of patients with simple hyperplasia down to 20% with complex atypical hyperplasia)
         ii. There is considerable interobserver variability in the perceived degree of abnormality among pathologists
         iii. First-line treatment for endometrial hyperplasia is prolonged therapy with oral medroxyprogesterone acetate 10–20 mg/day for 1–3 months
         iv. Repeat endometrial biopsy to determine response to therapy
         v. Consider consultation with gynecologist/ oncologist before initiating treatment or after inadequate response
      e. Adequate sample but no pathologic diagnosis—no further work-up at this time (repeat endometrial biopsy if another episode of vaginal bleeding)
      f. Inadequate sample for diagnosis—if sample obtained was appropriately collected, minimal tissue is incompatible with uterine cancer
      g. Unable to obtain sample, usually secondary to stenotic cervical os

   i. If patient is low risk for uterine cancer, repeat sample after local application of vaginal estrogen cream for 2–4 weeks
   ii. Consider pelvic ultrasound, and/or consultation with gynecologist
   h. Recurrent vaginal bleeding of apparent uterine etiology if no pathology found on first specimen—repeat endometrial biopsy
      i. Observation alone is probably most cost-effective with little risk to patient, but medicolegal considerations make most physicians uncomfortable without further efforts at diagnosis and consultation
2. **Dilatation and curettage** (D&C)
   a. Rarely indicated
   b. Possible indication: cervical stenosis; but may dilate cervix in office setting prior to endometrial sampling after injection of local anesthesia
   c. In patients with insufficient tissue for diagnosis on endometrial biopsy, D&C rarely uncovers significant pathology
   d. In some studies, less pathology diagnosed by D&C than by endometrial biopsy
   e. May be therapeutic (at least temporarily) in patients with heavy vaginal bleeding
   f. May be preferred procedure in patients with previous pelvic irradiation
3. **Pelvic ultrasound**
   a. Yield increased by using vaginal probe
   b. Current literature reveals no endometrial cancer or even hyperplasia in patients with < 5 mm total thickness (total of both endometrial walls); negative predictive value is 100% in this group
   c. Usually not cost-effective as first-line evaluation, but some studies recommend vaginal ultrasound as complementary first test along with endometrial biopsy
      i. False-positive rate is high
      ii. 10% of patients on continuous, combined HRT have 5 mm or more of endometrial tissue
      iii. Half of women on cyclic HRT regimens have a total endometrial thickness > 4–8 mm
4. **Sonographic hysterogram**
   a. Inject 10 ml normal saline into uterine cavity—enhances visualization of intrauterine pathology
5. **Hysteroscopy**
   a. Especially useful for diagnosing endometrial polyps in postmenopausal patient
   b. Occasionally diagnose submucous fibroids
   c. May be followed by selective endometrial sampling of abnormal-appearing tissue
   d. More expensive and traumatic than endometrial biopsy alone
   e. Available to some primary care physicians but usually requires consultation
6. **Hysterectomy**
   a. Endometrial sample prior to hysterectomy, even if patient has possible indications for hysterectomy in addition to postmenopausal bleeding

SUGGESTED READING

1. Dubinsky TJ, Parvey HR: The role of transvaginal sonography and endometrial biopsy in the evaluation of peri- and postmenopausal bleeding. Am J Roentgenol 169:145–140, 1997.
2. Feldman S, Berkowitz RS: Cost-effectiveness of strategies to evaluate postmenopausal bleeding. Obstet Gynecol 81:968–975, 1993.
3. Good AE: Diagnostic options for assessment of postmenopausal bleeding. Mayo Clin Proc 72:345–349, 1997.
4. Kendall BS, Ronnett RM: Reproducibility of the diagnosis of endometrial hyperplasia, atypical hyperplasia, and well-differentiated carcinoma. Am J Surg Pathol 22:1012–1019, 1998.
5. O'Connell LP, Fries MH: Triage of abnormal postmenopausal bleeding: A comparison of endometrial biopsy and transvaginal sonohysterography versus fractional curettage with hysteroscopy. Am J Obstet Gynecol 178:956–961, 1998.
6. Weber AM, Belinson JL: Vaginal ultrasonography versus endometrial biopsy in women with postmenopausal bleeding. Am J Obstet Gynecol 177:924–929, 1997.

PART IX

URINARY TRACT DISORDERS

72. Urinary Tract Infections

Belinda A. Vail, M.D.

I. **The Issues**

Urinary tract infections (UTIs) are the most common bacterial infections in women. Most urinary tract infections are uncomplicated and can be treated empirically with short courses of antibiotics. More responsibility for diagnosis and treatment is being given to patients as the cost-effectiveness of this management strategy becomes clear. Complicated or recurrent infections and those in pregnant and elderly women can be difficult to diagnose and treat and require special consideration and evaluation. Physicians are becoming more adept at telephone triage, but must remain vigilant, knowing when a patient must be seen and evaluated.

II. **The Theory**

A. **Epidemiology**

1. Estimates of incidence and prevalence vary widely. About 50% of women report having a UTI sometime in their life.

2. 20% of these women will have recurrent urinary tract infections

3. 90% of urinary tract infections are uncomplicated

4. In the U.S. there are 7 million office visits and 1 million hospitalization each year for urinary tract infections at a cost of more than $1 billion.

B. **Anatomy**

1. Most urinary tract infections are due to ascending infection through the urethra with less than 5% occurring from hematogenous spread.

2. Proximity of the rectum to the vagina allows contamination of the vaginal vault with fecal flora. The urethra is only about 2.5 cm long and allows fairly easy access to the bladder.

3. Vesicoureteral reflux makes access to the kidneys and subsequent pyelonephritis more common, but significant renal involvement may occur even in the absence of anatomic abnormalities or reflux.

4. Physiologic changes during pregnancy increase the risk of infection ascending to the kidneys. The ureters progressively dilate (right > left), and the uterus may even obstruct the ureter. The maternal bladder enlarges, and decreased tone leads to incomplete emptying. Hormonal changes cause ureteral atony allowing for increased access for bacteria.

5. Elderly women are more likely to have neuropathic and obstructive emptying disorders, including a greater incidence of kidney or bladder stones. Decreased mobility and an increase in fecal incontinence give bacteria a logistic advantage.

C. **Pathogens**

1. Cystitis and pyelonephritis are primarily caused by gram-negative enteric bacteria, with *Escherichia coli* responsible for at least 85% of cases. *Staphylococcus saprophyticus* account for about 10% of cases overall and about 20% in young, sexually active women. This limited spectrum of causative organisms and the relative susceptibility of the same also make empiric treatment of UTIs more palatable. *Proteus mirabilis, Klebsiella pneumoniae,* and *Enterococcus* sp. become more common in the elderly. Some bacteria are commonly cultured but rarely cause disease, including *Staphylococcus epidermidis*, diphtheroids, and lactobacilli.

2. Although *E. coli* remains most common, other pathogens increase in incidence during pregnancy, such as group B streptococci, anaerobic bacteria, *Ureaplasma urealyticum*, and *Gardnerella vaginalis*.

3. Urethritis is frequently caused by *Chlamydia trachomatis*, *Neisseria gonorrhoeae*, or herpesviruses.

D. **Pathogenesis**

1. Once bacteria are introduced into the urinary tract, they must adhere to the bladder wall; ordinarily, they are flushed from the bladder with voids so decreased urine volume predisposes the woman to infection. Urine is bactericidal with a low pH and a high osmolarity and urea content. A protective mucin coating inhibits bacterial adherence. Lactobacilli colonize the vagina and inhibit coliform bacteria like *E. coli*.

2. Some women show increased vaginal adhesiveness to pathologic strains of *E. coli*. Certain bacteria show increased affinity for uroepithelial cells by the presence of certain antigens, resistance to host's defenses, or specific metabolic qualities. Bacteria that cause a significant amount of pyelonephritis have certain adhesions (P fimbriae or F adhesin) that bind to receptors on uroepithelial cells. Some women have a genetically determined increase in these receptors and decrease in mucosal secretion of a fucosyltransferase enzyme which blocks bacterial adherence. These women have a predisposition for pyelonephritis.

3. Inflammation usually remains superficial in the bladder, but severe inflammation damages blood vessels, resulting in hemorrhagic cystitis.

4. Women with anatomic abnormalities, particularly vesicoureteral reflux, are much more likely to develop pyelonephritis. Infection in the kidney usually starts at a single focus in the pelvis and medulla and extends in a fan-shaped wedge into the cortex. The medulla contains concentrations of urea and ammonia and has high osmolality, all of which inhibit white blood cell function and complement aggregation. Scarring of the kidney is much less common in adults than in children.

E. **Factors contributing to increased incidence of UTI**

1. Sexual activity—the occurrence of UTIs is highest among sexually active young women. The greater the frequency of sexual intercourse, the greater the incidence of urinary tract infection. It is believed that more bacteria enter the urethra during intercourse, but there is no evidence to support this belief.

2. Contraception—use of spermicides like nonoxynol-9 inhibits lactobacilli in the vagina and allows the pH to rise, leading to growth of coliform bacteria. Use of a diaphragm with spermicide doubles or triples the risk of developing a UTI. Users of cervical caps may also have an increased incidence, but less so than with the diaphragm.

3. Abnormal micturition—inadequate voids or increased time between voids allows more bacterial access to the bladder wall and flushes fewer bacteria from the lower tract. Delayed voiding following sexual intercourse has long been implicated as the cause of postcoital cystitis, but his has not been statistically proven.

4. Diabetes—women with diabetes have twice the incidence of urinary tract infection as healthy women

F. **Factors contributing to pyelonephritis**

1. Anything which impairs or blocks the flow of urine predisposes a woman to developing an upper tract infection. Impaired bladder function, vesicoureteral reflux, ureteral obstruction, renal or bladder calculi, tumor, or a foreign body such as a catheter allow bacteria to ascend the ureters. Pregnant women as noted earlier also fall into this category. Women with congenital abnormalities of the urinary tract are more susceptible, and a history of UTI in childhood is common.

2. Women with chronic illness or immunosuppression are more likely to develop more complicated infections

G. **Clinical features**

1. **Acute cystitis**

a. Cystitis is the most common urinary tract infection, and most cases are uncomplicated. Classic features of cystitis include dysuria, frequency, and urgency. Onset is usually abrupt, and volume of each void decreases markedly. Suprapubic pain is only present in about 15% of women. Although usually present, pyuria is not necessary for the diagnosis. In the presence of symptoms, urine cultures yielding 10^2 colony-forming units (CFUs) per milliliter is adequate for diagnosis.

b. In young women most UTIs are uncomplicated and associated with anatomic abnormalities in fewer than 1%. Aggressive evaluation is unnecessary, and the diagnosis can be made on clinical features alone.

c. Hematuria is sometimes present in cystitis alone, but other pathology should be considered in its presence

d. In elderly women, symptoms may be altered mental status, anorexia, or malaise

2. **Pyelonephritis**

a. When upper tract disease is present, symptoms have usually been noted for several days. Symptoms are similar to those of cystitis, but also include flank pain, fever, chills, nausea, vomiting, and/or abdominal pain. This should always be considered a serious infection and evaluated appropriately. Differentiation of upper and lower tract disease cannot be made on clinical grounds alone.

3. **Asymptomatic bacteriuria**

a. The definition of asymptomatic bacteriuria requires the presence of 10^5 CFU/ml in the absence of symptoms. Only three groups of women with this condition benefit from treatment: (1) pregnant women, (2) renal transplant patients, and (3) patients undergoing genitourinary tract procedures.

b. Asymptomatic bacteriuria is present in 2–11% of pregnant women. Factors that increase the risk of UTI in pregnancy include: increased age, increased sexual activity, increased parity, diabetes, sickle-cell trait, and lower socioeconomic status. All pregnant women with asymptomatic bacteriuria should be treated, as 20–40% of those untreated women progress to pyelonephritis. Complications in pregnancy include low birth weight, prematurity, intrauterine growth retardation, and an increase in perinatal deaths.

4. Urethritis accounts for a significant percentage of culture-negative dysuria. When urethritis appears after sexual intercourse, it usually takes several days to develop. Dysuria is usually the main feature, often perceived as more external, and worse at the beginning of micturition. Frequency, urgency, and small voids may be present, but are usually much less pronounced than in cystitis. Vaginal discharge may be present as well.

5. Recurrent UTI—about 80% of recurrent UTIs are reinfections. The original infection is followed by an asymptomatic period then reintroduction of organisms occurs. Relapse is uncommon and occurs within days after finishing treatment. Relapse implies a hidden focus of organism that was not eradicated with treatment.

III. **An Approach**

A. **Evaluation**

1. **History**—careful evaluation of symptoms and history is usually the key to diagnosis, and therefore, allows some patients to be treated without an office visit.

a. Suspect cystitis with abrupt onset of UTI symptoms, previous similar history, and recent intercourse especially with diaphragm use.

b. Suspect urethritis with gradual onset, recent change in sexual partners, and dysuria worse at start of stream and perceived as external.

c. Suspect pyelonephritis with symptoms present for more than a week, back pain, fever, history of UTI as a child, prior pyelonephritis, pregnancy, diabetes, or immunosuppression.

d. In patients without straightforward symptoms consider other causes such as ectopic pregnancy, pelvic inflammatory disease, or ruptured ovarian cyst.

2. **Physical exam**

a. The abdomen should be examined for generalized or suprapubic tenderness and percussion of the bladder if possible. Kidneys should be palpated and percussed (CVA tenderness).

b. If the history is unclear a pelvic exam should be performed as well, including inspection of the external genitalia, bimanual exam of uterus and adnexa, and vaginal swab and cervical cultures. Presence of rectocele or cystocele may be important in recurrent infections.

3. **Urinalysis**

a. Urine specimen should be a midstream, clean catch. The presence of white cells in the urine (microscopically, by dipstick, or by Gram stain) implies either cystitis or pyelonephritis. It is the only test necessary in young women with straightforward symptoms.

   b. Dipstick for nitrite is usually helpful, but not all organisms convert nitrates to nitrites, including *S. saprophyticus*, *Enterococcus*, and *Acinetobacter*.

   c. Blood and protein in the urine imply cystitis or pyelonephritis but may also be clues to more extensive disease (glomerulonephritis, renal calculi, or tumor). White cell casts are indicative of upper tract disease.

4. **Urine culture**

   a. Culture of the urine is not necessary in young women with previous UTIs, usual symptoms, and reliable history.

   b. Culture should be performed for first UTI, uncertain diagnosis, pregnancy, elderly women, diabetics or immunocompromised, and recurrent infection within six weeks.

   c. Positive urine culture is traditionally 10^5 organisms/ml, but in symptomatic patients, as low as 10^2 organisms/ml of a single organisms may be considered positive.

5. **Imaging studies**

   a. Sonography is noninvasive and helpful in diagnosing renal parenchymal disease. It will also help rule out blockage and incomplete bladder emptying.

   b. Intravenous pyelography (IVP) is useful when there is a suspicion of renal calculi, obstruction, or abnormal urinary tract anatomy.

   c. Renal cortical scintigraphy has > 85% accuracy in distinguishing upper tract disease, but is seldom used secondary to high cost and relative accuracy of clinical diagnosis alone.

6. **Vaginal swab and cultures**

   a. When urethritis is suspected or the diagnosis, the vagina and cervix should be examined and cultures and/or DNA probes performed. There is a correlation between > 5 white blood cells per high power field and chlamydia infection.

   b. *Candida* sp. and *Gardnerella vaginalis* should also be considered.

B. **Management**

1. **Urethritis**—if possible, treatment of urethritis should be culture-based

   a. Gonorrhea can be treated with single-dose ciprofloxacin 250 mg or azithromycin 2 g.

   b. Chlamydia, likewise, may be treated with single-dose azithromycin 1 g or doxycycline 100 mg bid.

   c. If no organism can be found, doxycycline 100 mg bid may be a useful empiric treatment.

2. **Uncomplicated cystitis**

   a. Cystitis is usually easy to cure because infection is superficial and high concentrations of antibiotic are achieved in the urine. Single-dose therapy may be used, but the rate of reinfection is higher, probably due to failure to eradicate organisms from the rectum. Possible antibiotic regimens are listed in Table 1.

   b. Three-day regimens are most often used due to their increased efficacy, probably because they reduce rectal carriage. They also have the same efficacy, reduced side-effects, and lower cost than seven-day regimens.

   c. Fluoroquinolones have a slight increase in efficacy and decrease in side effects, but are not considered first-line therapy due to their significantly higher cost.

3. **Complicated cystitis**

   a. Complicated UTIs occur because of anatomic, pharmacologic, or functional changes that predispose women to persistent or recurrent infections. Recurrent cystitis refers to multiple infections by the same organism, and is treated as a complicated cystitis

   b. Culture and sensitivities are imperative to direct treatment

   c. The same antibiotics may be used, but fluoroquinolones are the drugs of choice. They should be continued for 10–14 days.

4. **Uncomplicated pyelonephritis**

   a. When symptoms are mild to moderate, and women are compliant, oral medication may be considered. They need to be able to tolerate the medication and fluids, and have no other concurrent conditions such as pregnancy.

TABLE 1. Antibiotic Regimens for Treatment of Urinary Tract Infections

Single-dose therapy
Amoxicillin	3 g
Trimethoprim-sulfamethoxazole DS (Bactrim, Cotrim, Septra)[¶][§]	2–3 tablets
Trimethoprim (Proloprim)[§]	400 mg
Ciprofloxacin (Cipro)	100–250 mg|
Fosfomycin tromethamine (Monurol)	3 g
Norfloxacin (Noroxin)	800 mg
Ofloxacin (Floxin)	200 mg

Three-day regimens
Trimethoprim-sulfamethoxazole DS (Bactrim, Cotrim, Septra)[¶][§]	1 tablet bid
Trimethoprim (Proloprim)[§]	100 mg bid
Nitrofurantoin (Macrodantin)	200 mg bid
Amoxicillin (Amoxil)	500 mg tid
Cephalexin (Keflex)	500 mg bid
Norfloxacin (Noroxin)	400 mg bid
Ciprofloxacin (Cipro)	250 mg bid
Ofloxacin (Floxin)	200–400 mg bid
Enoxacin (Penetrex)	200 mg bid
Lomefloxacin (Maxaquin)	400 mg qd
Sparfloxacin (Zagam)	400 mg then 200 mg qd
Levofloxacin (Levaquin)	250 mg qd
Cefpodoxime (Vantin)	100 mg bid
Cefixime (Suprax)	400 mg qd
Amoxicillin-clavulanate (Augmentin)	500 mg bid

Options for prophylaxis
Trimethoprim-sulfamethoxazole DS[¶][§]	½ tablet daily
Nitrofurantoin*	50–100 mg/day
Norfloxacin	200 mg/day
Cephalexin	250 mg/day
Trimethoprim[§]	100 mg/day

Uncomplicated pyelonephritis
Trimethoprim-sulfamethoxazole DS[¶][§]	1 tablet bid
Ciprofloxacin	500 mg bid
Levofloxacin	250 mg qd
Enoxacin	400 mg bid
Sparfloxacin**	400 mg then 200 mg qd
Ofloxacin	400 mg bid
Cefpodoxime	200 mg bid
Cefixime	400 mg qd

Parenteral therapy
Ceftriaxone (Rocephin)	1 g qd
Ciprofloxacin	400 mg bid
Ofloxacin	400 mg bid
Levofloxacin	250 mg qd
Aztreonam (Azactam)	1 mg tid
Gentamicin (Garamycin)	3 mg/kg/day in 3 divided doses q 8h

Complicated and/or severe infections
Ceftazidime (Fortaz)	Imipenem-cilastatin (Primaxin)
Cefoperazone (Cefobid)	Ticarcillin (Ticar)[+]
Cefepime (Maxipime)	Mezlocillin (Mezlin)[+]
Aztreonam (Azactam)	Piperacillin (Pipracil)[+]

¶ Sulfamethoxazole is contraindicated in pregnant women near term and in patients with glucose-6-phosphate dehydrogenase deficiency
§ Contraindicated in patients with folate deficiency
* Exercise caution with nitrofurantoin as long-term use has lead to pulmonary fibrosis; also contraindicated in glucose-6-phosphate dehydrogenase deficiency
** Can cause phototoxicity and prolongation of QT interval
+ Antipseudomonal penicillins should be used in combination with an aminoglycoside

      b. *E. coli* has about a 30% resistance rate to ampicillin, amoxicillin, and first generation cephalosporins, therefore, trimethoprim/sulfamethoxazole or oral fluoroquinolones should be considered.

      c. Therapy should be continued for 10–14 days. If IV medication is used, the patient may usually be switched to oral medication after 72 hours.

5. **Pyelonephritis requiring hospitalization**

      a. Patients should be hospitalized when fever is > 103°F, white count is elevated, patient has protracted nausea and vomiting, and/or the patient appears toxic.

      b. Initial therapy before culture and sensitivity results are known should be with a second- or third-generation cephalosporin or aminoglycoside.

      c. IV antibiotics should be continued until the patient is afebrile and then changed to oral medication for a total of 10–14 days. Follow-up cultures are mandatory.

6. **Recurrent infections**

      a. When a patient has experienced more than three UTIs in 1 year confirmed by culture, further evaluation is necessary

      b. Prophylactic measures include adequate fluid intake, regular urination, voiding after intercourse to flush out the bladder, cotton underwear, rinsing well when showering, avoidance of baths, correct wiping after defecation, finding alternative methods of birth control for diaphragm and spermicidal gel users, and drinking cranberry juice

      c. Treatment options include: (1) acute self-therapy, (2) postcoital $\frac{1}{2}$ tablet of trimethoprim/ sulfamethoxazole, or (3) daily prophylaxis for 6 months. Daily prophylaxis medication options are listed in Table 1. Hormone replacement therapy may be beneficial after menopause.

7. **Hematuria** is a common finding in cystitis or pyelonephritis, but its presence can also be a sign of renal calculi or tumors of the kidneys or bladder. All patients with hematuria should have a follow-up urinalysis to ensure resolution.

8. **Pregnancy**

      a. Asymptomatic bacteriuria should be treated for 3–7 days and acute cystitis for 7–10 days. See Table 1 (previous page) for a list of drug regimens acceptable in pregnancy.

      b. Recurrent infections should be cleared, and the patient should be placed on suppressive therapy, usually until delivery

      c. Pyelonephritis in pregnancy usually requires hospitalization with fluid replacement, blood cultures, and intravenous antibiotics. Selected patients may be managed with outpatient intramuscular ceftriaxone or orally administered cephalexin.

9. **Elderly patients**

      a. Asymptomatic bacteriuria should not be treated in the elderly, as treatment does not alter morbidity or mortality

      b. All patients with symptomatic bacteriuria should be treated, because UTIs are the most common cause of sepsis in the elderly

      c. Treatment duration should be at least 7 days for acute cystitis and at least 14 days for upper tract infection, as urosepsis is one of the leading causes of death in the elderly

      d. Estrogen cream 2 gm vaginally twice a week may help reduce occurrences

SUGGESTED READING

1. Barry HC, Ebell MH, Hickner J: Evaluation of suspected urinary tract infection in ambulatory women: A cost-utility analysis of office-based strategies. J Fam Practice 44:49–60, 1997.
2. Carroll KC, Hale DC, Von Boerum DH, et al: Laboratory evaluation of urinary tract infection in an ambulatory clinic. Am J Clin Pathol 101:100–103, 1994.
3. Fihn SD: UTI in women: The current thinking. Fam Pract Recertif 16:44–53, 1994.
4. Hooton TM, Scholes D, Hughes JP, et al: A prospective study of risk factors for symptomatic urinary tract infection in young women. N Engl J Med 335:468–474, 1996.
5. Kurowski D: The woman with dysuria. Am Fam Physician 57:2155–2164, 1998.
6. Levine MG: The diagnosis of urinary tract infections during pregnancy. Nebr Med J 78:282–285, 1993.
7. Lucas MJ, Cunningham FG: Urinary infection in pregnancy. Clin Obstet Gynecol 36:855–868, 1993.

8. McCarty JM, Richard G, Huck W, et al: A randomized trial of short-course ciprofloxacin, ofloxacin, or trimethoprim/sulfamethoxazole for the treatment of acute urinary tract infection in women. Am J Med 106:290–299, 1999.
9. Nygaard IE, Johnson JM: Urinary tract infections in elderly women. Am Fam Physician 53:175–182, 1996.
10. Schleupner CJ: Urinary tract infections: Separating the gender and the ages. Postgrad Med 101:231–237, 1997.
11. Orenstein R, Wong ES: Urinary tract infections in adults. Am Fam Physician 59:1225–1234, 1999.
12. U.S. Public Health Service: Urinalysis. Am Fam Physician 50:351–353, 1994.

73. Interstitial Cystitis

Belinda A. Vail, M.D.

I. The Issues

Interstitial cystitis (IC) is a chronic inflammatory bladder disease of unknown etiology. Patients often go undiagnosed for years and may search out a variety of physicians in an attempt to find relief from their discomfort and pain. The lack of specific diagnostic criteria and often the absence of specific clinical or histopathologic findings make diagnosis difficult. When a diagnosis is established, there is no clear treatment. All of this uncertainty leaves both patient and physician frustrated, with little satisfactory resolution of the problem; therefore, good communication and understanding are imperative.

II. The Theory

A. Epidemiology

1. An estimated 450,000 people are affected; 90% are female. Median age is 40 years, but 25–30% are < 30 years of age. There is a slightly higher incidence in the Jewish population.
2. The total economic impact is estimated at $1.7 billion/year with direct medical costs average $170 million/year. Patients on average see five different physicians and experience symptoms for 3–4 years before a diagnosis is made. Fifty percent of patients are unable to work full time.
3. Using quality of life questionnaires, patients report lower quality of life than renal dialysis patients. Activities of daily living are adversely affected, and physical activity decreased. Patients tend to have a negative mental outlook and an increase in anxiety and depression. There is a decrease in sexual activity, and 60% stop having sex altogether.
4. Hysterectomies are more than twice as common in IC patients. There is a higher incidence of allergic and autoimmune syndromes, and food sensitivities and intolerance tend to increase with duration of symptoms. Interestingly IC is found less often in diabetics than in the general population.

B. Symptoms and course of disease

1. The most common presenting symptoms are dysuria, urgency, and frequency. Patients may void as much as 60–80 times a day and 10–30 times a night. Pain ranges from mild to excruciating and may involve the lower abdomen, suprapubic area, pelvis, perineum, vagina, low back, and/or thighs. Urination usually relieves the pain temporarily. Dyspareunia is common, and sexual intercourse may exacerbate the symptoms, probably due to mechanical irritation. About 20% of patients experience hematuria. Symptoms may intensify around the time of menses.
2. Onset is usually abrupt with no apparent precipitating factors. Symptoms progress rapidly reaching maximum intensity within about a month. Symptoms then stabilize, but they occur intermittently and may exacerbate or remit. Pregnant women often experience a decrease in symptoms.
3. Symptoms may be intensified by spicy foods, chocolate, bananas, citrus fruits, or alcoholic, caffeinated, or carbonated beverages.

4. Because of the significant psychological and social problems and pain and sleepless-ness, many patients develop depression. This coupled with visits to multiple physicians often leads to a primary psychological rather than physical diagnosis.

C. **Theories concerning etiology**

1. Current theories center on a component of urine obtaining access to bladder wall and inducing inflammatory reaction by toxic, allergic, or immunologic means.

2. Glycosaminoglycan alterans: The mucosal glycosaminoglycan lining of the bladder is broken down (possibly secondary to a prior urinary tract infection). This allows solutes in the urine to irritate the bladder wall and produce an inflammatory response.

3. Chronic bacterial infection: Infection of the bladder by bacteria such as Gardnerella vaginalis may go undetected because bacteria are embedded in the bladder wall.

4. Mast cell–mediated: Mastocytosis occurs in a significant subset of IC patients, and mast cells increase in patients with IC. There are estrogen receptors on mast cells, and symptoms exacerbate with menstruation.

5. Allergic reaction: Many patients have associated food and drug allergies.

6. Vascular or lymphatic obstruction causing dilatation and irritation of vessels.

7. Related to reflex sympathetic dystrophy: Injury to peripheral nerves following infection, surgery, or childbirth may cause an increase in sympathetic receptors and increased transmission of pain stimuli.

8. Autoimmune disorder: Antinuclear antibodies are present more often in patients with IC, and there is an increase in urinary excretion of eosinophilic cationic protein. It is also more common in women.

9. Genetic: IC has been found in siblings and monozygotic twins.

III. **An Approach**

A. **Evaluation**

1. History: A careful history based on the previously listed symptoms is vital. History of urinary tract infections in the past, course of the symptoms, and history of childbirth and surgeries is particularly important. A 24-hour voiding diary can help quantify the actual number of voids a day. The O'Leary-Sant index[12] is a patient-administered questionnaire that is helpful in assessing the history of the disease.

2. Physical exam: A careful examination of the abdomen should include the bladder and kidneys. Pelvic exam is necessary to rule out vaginal or cervical pathology, cystocele, and urethral diverticula. Cultures for chlamydia and tuberculosis and a rectal exam may also be indicated.

3. Urine evaluation: Urinalysis and culture will help rule out infection, and cytology should be performed to exclude transitional cell carcinoma of the bladder.

4. Urologic studies

   a. Cystoscopy under anesthesia is usually the most valuable test. Mucosal ulcerations on the bladder wall surrounded by granulation tissue (Hunner's ulcers) are usually diagnostic and may indicate more severe disease. More common are glomerulations, groups of petechial hemorrhages, evident on bladder distention.

   b. Bladder biopsies can also be taken at this time to rule out carcinoma *in situ*

   c. Passive distention of the bladder to demonstrate reduced bladder capacity may be done in the office or at the time of cystoscopy

   d. If the diagnosis in doubt, a laparoscopy may also be necessary to exclude gynecologic problems causing the symptoms

B. **Management**

1. **Patient education and behavior modification**

   a. Success in treatment requires belief in the disease entity and reassurance of the patient that the disease is not psychosomatic, nor is it cancer. Patients must next understand that there is no cure, and treatment involves management of symptoms. Empathy and tolerance are required.

   b. Patients should be involved in decisions and management. Voiding diaries and quality of life scales can be useful in demonstrating progress to the patient. Developing coping skills, stress reduction, moderate exercise, and dietary modification may all be helpful.

    c. Alternative treatments such as biofeedback, massage, acupuncture, and music or hydrotherapy are all acceptable if they seem to improve symptoms.

    d. Patients may want to become involved with the Interstitial Cystitis Association, P.O. Box 1553, Madison Square Station, New York, NY 10159-1553, telephone 212-080-6057 or 800-HELP-ICA

2. **Oral pharmacologic therapies**

    a. Most medication regimens for IC are off label and have little controlled study support. Improvement in symptoms is usually modest.

    b. Antidepressants amitriptyline (Elavil), doxepin (Sinequan, Zonalon), and imipramine (Tofranil) show a decrease in symptoms in about 35% of patients. They seem to inhibit mast cell secretion. Dose: amitriptyline 25–150 mg/hr; doxepin 10–100 mg/hr; imipramine 75–150 mg/hr

    c. Hydroxyzine (Atarax) is an antihistamine that inhibits neurotransmitters that initiate mast cell degranulation and has anticholinergic properties that decrease frequency. Best given at night. Dose: 25–50 mg/hr

    d. Pentosan polysulfate (Elmiron) is the only oral medication approved for use in IC. It is a heparin-like compound with fewer anticoagulant properties. Its exact mechanism is unknown, but it may augment the glycosaminoglycan mucous lining of the bladder; 12–16 weeks of treatment are needed for symptom relief, but side-effect profile is low. Dose: 300 mg/d

    e. Nifedipine (Procardia) is a calcium channel blocker which relaxes smooth muscle and improves dysuria and pelvic pain. Dose: XL 30–60 mg/d

    f. Nalmefene (Revex) is a long-acting pure opiate antagonist that inhibits mast cell activity and appears to improve suprapubic pain and dysuria.

    g. Cimetidine (Tagamet) 200 mg tid, L-arginine, and azathioprine (Imuran), an immunosuppressive drug, have all shown some success.

    h. Antispasmodics propantheline bromide (Pro-Banthine), oxybutynin chloride (Ditropan), and flavoxate (Urispas) may help with relief of bladder spasm and frequency.

3. **Intravesical therapies**

    a. Hydrodistention: About 25% of patients experience decreased pain and increased bladder capacity following hydrodistention at the time of cystoscopy. If that is the case it may be repeated therapeutically with effects lasting up to several months.

    b. Dimethylsulfoxide (DMSO): This is the only other drug approved for use in IC. It is introduced directly into the bladder, where it appears to have an anti-inflammatory and analgesic effect. Some patients will have a transient worsening of symptoms due to chemical irritation, but 50–70% of patients with classic IC and 50–90% of patients with nonulcer IC have significant relief of pain for up to 2 years. 4 to 8 treatments are given at 1–2 week intervals, and patients can learn to give their own treatments. Nonresponders may have improved response when 100 mg of hydrocortisone or sodium bicarbonate or heparin are added to the DMSO.

    c. Cychlorosene sodium (Clorpactin) can also be used intravesically if DMSO fails, but must be given under regional or general anesthesia due to its painful effects.

    d. Other experimental intravesical medications include bacillus Calmette-Guérin, hyaluronic acid, pentosan polysulfate sodium, and interferon

4. **Other treatments**

    a. Yag laser therapy for patients with Hunner's ulcers

    b. Suprapubic or pelvic floor transcutaneous electrical nerve stimulation (TENS)

    c. Multidisciplinary pain clinic

    d. Surgery is a method of last resort. Transurethral ulcer resection, or a supratrigonal cystectomy with formation of an enterovesical anastomosis to improve bladder capacity are sometimes performed. Total cystectomy with urinary diversion is rarely performed as many patients still have suprapubic and pelvic pain.

SUGGESTED READING

1. Childs SJ: Dimethyl sulfone (DMSO$_2$) in the treatment of interstitial cystitis. Urol Clin North Am 21:85–88, 1994.

2. Fleischmann J: Calcium channel antagonists in the treatment of interstitial cystitis. Urol Clin North Am 21:107–111, 1994.
3. Hanno PM: Diagnosis of interstitial cystitis. Urol Clin North Am 21:63–66, 1994.
4. Irwin PP, Galloway NTM: Surgical management of interstitial cystitis. Urol Clin North Am 21:145–151, 1994.
5. Jepsen JV, Sall M, Rhodes PR, et al: Long-term experience with pentosanpolysulfate in interstitial cystitis. Urology 51:382–387, 1998.
6. Johansson SL, Fall M: Pathology of interstitial cystitis. Urol Clin North Am 21:55–62, 1994.
7. Johansson SL: In consultation interstitial cystitis. Mod Pathol 6:738–742, 1993.
8. Keller ML, McCarthy DO, Neider RS: Measurement of symptoms of interstitial cystitis. Urol Clin North Am 21:67–71, 1994.
9. Koziol J: Epidemiology of interstitial cystitis. Urol Clin North Am 21:7–20, 1994.
10. Kurowski D: The woman with dysuria. Am Fam Physician 57:2144–2164, 1998.
11. Ochs RL, Stein TW, Peebles CL, et al: Autoantibodies in interstitial cystitis. J Urol 151:587–592, 1994.
12. O'Leary MP, Sant GR, Fowler FJ Jr, et al: The interstitial cystitis symptom index and problem index. Urology 49(Suppl 5A):S58–S63, 1997.
13. Ratliff TL, Klutke CG, McDougall EM: The etiology of interstitial cystitis. Urol Clin North Am 21:21–31, 1994.
14. Ratner V, Slade D, Greene G: Interstitial cystitis: A patient's perspective. Urol Clin North Am 21:1–5, 1994.
15. Sant GR: Interstitial cystitis—a urogynecologic perspective. Contemp Ob/Gyn June:119–130, 1998.
16. Sant GR, LaRock DR: Standard intravesical therapies for interstitial cystitis. Urol Clin North Am 21:73–83, 1994.
17. Sant GR, Theoharides TC: The role of the mast cell in interstitial cystitis. Urol Clin North Am 21:41–53, 1994.
18. Stone NN: Nalmefene in the treatment of interstitial cystitis. Urol Clin North Am 21:31–39, 1994.
19. Warren JW: Interstitial cystitis as an infectious disease. Urol Clin North Am 21:31–39, 1994.
20. Wein AJ, Broderick GA: Interstitial cystitis: Current and future approaches to diagnosis and treatment. Urol Clin North Am 21:153–161, 1994.
21. Whitmore KE: Self-care regimens for patients with interstitial cystitis. Urol Clin North Am 21:121–130, 1994.

74. Urinary Incontinence

Belinda A. Vail, M.D.

I. The Issues

Urinary incontinence refers to the involuntary loss of urine in sufficient quantities to be a social or hygienic problem. Although thought by many to be a minor inconvenience, it is a serious and financially significant health problem. It is the leading cause of entry into nursing homes, affecting over 11 million elderly women, as well as up to a third of women over 30 years of age. Unfortunately, fewer than half of the women who suffer from regular urinary incontinence seek medical help, and physicians continue to seriously underestimate the scope of the problem. One quarter of gynecologists, one third of family practitioners and over half of internists believe that less than 10% of elderly women suffer from incontinence. Psychological distress and social dysfunction include embarrassment, anxiety, and depression; limitation of usual or desirable physical activities and travel; and decreased sexual activity. Physical complications include macerated, irritated perineal tissue, rash, pressure sores, skin infections, and an increase in urinary tract infections.

II. The Theory

A. Incidence

1. According to the National Institutes of Health, at least 13 million Americans suffer from urinary incontinence; 75% are women.
2. About one quarter of women under the age of 65 have been or are affected.
3. 25–35% of community dwelling women over 60 are affected, and 50% of those who are institutionalized or homebound.

4. Nearly 75% of hospitalized elderly are reported to have incontinence.
5. Annual cost for diagnosis, treatment, complications, and long-term care is now estimated at over $17 billion.

B. **Anatomy of bladder and urethra**
1. The bladder is composed of a three-layered bundle of smooth muscle called the detrusor muscle. It is controlled as follows:
   a. Contracts in response to parasympathetic stimulation.
   b. Relaxes under sympathetic and beta-adrenergic stimulation.
   c. Activity is initiated by brain stem reflex unless inhibited by cortical control.
2. The bladder neck and proximal urethra contract in response to alpha-adrenergic stimulation
   a. Proximal two-thirds of urethra lies intra-abdominally, supported by the pelvic floor.
   b. Pudendal nerve innervates and causes constriction of the pelvic floor.
   c. Urethral sphincter is made up of elastic tissue, blood vessels, and smooth muscle.
   d. Contraction of the urethral sphincter is aided by increased intra-abdominal pressure, which forces the proximal urethra forward against the pubic symphysis.

C. **Classification of incontinence**
1. **Genuine stress incontinence**
   a. Stress incontinence is the most common type, accounting for about 75% of cases. It results from loss of anatomic support to the vesicle neck and proximal urethra resulting in urethral hypermobility. With an increase of intra-abdominal pressure (e.g., coughing, sneezing, straining) the proximal urethra is no longer pressed against the pubic bone and vesicular pressure overcomes the ability of the relatively weak proximal sphincter mechanism to detain urine.
   b. Although it is the most common type of incontinence in young women, hypoestrogenism and atrophy contribute to the problem accounting for the increase in incidence and severity with advancing age.
   c. Women who are obese, multiparous, postmenopausal, and/or have had pelvic surgery are at greatest risk.
   d. Incontinence is usually only occasional and only with increased intra-abdominal pressure. Postvoid residuals are normal. A cystocele is often present.
2. **Detrusor instability:** Detrusor instability, detrusor hyperactivity, or urge incontinence is more prevalent in the aging population. It occurs when the urge to void is perceived by the patient (whether or not the bladder is full), and she is unable to override the detrusor contraction effectively. These patients complain of frequency and bedwetting. Postvoid residual is usually normal, but neurologic exam is often abnormal. Major causes are:
   a. Idiopathic
   b. Central nervous system or spinal lesions or demyelinating disorders
   c. Urinary tract infection, bladder cancer or stones
3. **Overflow incontinence:** This is the least common type of incontinence. It occurs when the bladder is unable to empty normally and becomes distended, resulting in frequent or constant dribbling of urine. The underlying problem is either inadequate detrusor activity or outflow obstruction. Patients complain of hesitancy and a poor urine stream. Postvoid residual and bladder capacity are increased. Common causes:
   a. Neurologic problems that inhibit detrusor activity, including diabetes mellitus, vitamin B_{12} deficiency, or neurologic insufficiency (i.e., herniated disc).
   b. Obstruction of outflow may result from urethral stricture or urethral sphincter contractions, tumors, or medications (anticholinergics).
4. **Mixed incontinence:** This is usually a combination of stress incontinence and detrusor instability. Many patients have some degree of both disorders, and urodynamic studies can help to differentiate between the two. Treatment is usually aimed at the predominant disorder.
5. **Functional incontinence:** In patients with severe restriction of mobility or cognitive impairment who have intact function of lower urinary tract, but who do not understand the urge to urinate or are unable to reach the facilities. This is common with severe dementia or depression and with significant physical limitation.

III. **An Approach**
A. **Identify problem**
Symptoms of urinary incontinence must be elicited. Women are reluctant to discuss this subject with their physician. Questions about incontinence should be part of a yearly exam in parous women and women over 60. Questions must be specific as follows:
1. Do you ever have trouble with your bladder?
2. Do you ever have trouble holding your urine?
3. Do you ever leak urine when you cough or sneeze or participate in physical activity?
4. Do you ever leak urine when asleep or during sex?
5. Are you ever unable to get to the toilet in time when you feel the urge to urinate?
6. Do you ever wear a pad because you leak urine?

B. **Evaluation**
The first step in evaluation is to rule out transient causes. This can usually be accomplished with a history, physical, and urinalysis. Using the DIAPPERS pneumonic can be helpful:
- D —delirium or confusion
- I —infection
- A —atrophic vaginitis or urethritis
- P —pharmaceuticals (Table 1)
- P —psychological (depression)
- E —excessive urine production from excessive intake or endocrine problems
- R —restricted mobility
- S —stool impaction

1. **History**
a. Obtain a clear description of the problem, including duration of symptoms, frequency, severity or volume of urine loss; activities during urine loss; fluid intake and pattern (including use of caffeine-containing beverages); other lower urinary tract symptoms (nocturia, hematuria, dysuria); previous treatments for urinary incontinence, use of pads or other protective devices, effect on quality of life, and expectations of current treatment. Don't forget to include history of bowel habits and/or incontinence of stool.
b. A number of reversible and contributing causes for urinary incontinence may be elicited in the history. Patients with diabetes, urinary tract disease, and obesity have a higher incidence of incontinence. Respiratory diseases associated with chronic cough will aggravate stress incontinence. Neurologic diseases which affect the bladder or perineal area may cause incontinence.
c. Inquire about underlying neurologic diseases as well as any symptoms of double vision, weakness, numbness, tingling, or tremor.
d. Obstetric and gynecologic history, including operative deliveries and any pelvic surgery is extremely important. See Table 1 for a list of associated conditions. Medications that cause or contribute to incontinence are listed in Table 2.
e. Eliciting this history is usually time consuming. It can be extremely helpful to have available a urogynecologic questionnaire for the patient to fill out in the office or at home. (See starred reference for examples.)

2. **Physical exam**
a. All patients should be examined for signs of systemic diseases, including respiratory and cardiac disease. The abdomen should be examined for masses and suprapubic fullness or tenderness. Particular attention should be paid to the condition of the skin in the perineal area.
b. The vagina and pelvis should be examined for vaginal tone and atrophy, urethral irritation, pelvic prolapse or masses, and the presence of a cystocele, rectocele, or enterocele. Rectal exam for sphincter tone and fecal impaction should be performed.
c. A complete neuologic examination should include strength and sensation in lower extremities, reflexes and Babinski sign, mobility, and cognition.

3. **Urinalysis and postvoid residual**
a. Urinalysis is simple and cost-effective. It can quickly identify reversible causes such as diabetes or urinary tract infection.

TABLE 1. Current or Past Medical or Surgical Conditions that Cause or Contribute to Urinary Incontinence

Metabolic	Obstetric history
Diabetes	Parity
Vitamin B_{12} deficiency	History of prolonged labor
Obesity	Large infants
Renal or urinary tract disease	Operative vaginal deliveries (including forceps
Previous urinary tract infections	and vacuum extraction)
Pyelonephritis	Gynecologic history
Renal calculi	Sexually transmitted diseases (including syphilis)
Pulmonary disease	Age at menopause
Chronic obstructive lung disease	Use of estrogen replacement therapy
Acute respiratory infection	Genital prolapse
Chronic cigarette cough	Sexual activity and dyspareunia
Neurologic disease	Presence of cystocele, rectocele, or enterocele
Multiple sclerosis	Prior pelvic surgery
Stroke	Hysterectomy
Lumbar disc disease	Vaginal repair
Neuropathy	Retropubic surgery

    b. Proteinuria and hematuria (particularly in the elderly) should elicit further work up. If renal dysfunction is suggested blood tests for BUN, creatinine, glucose, and calcium and, in the case of hematuria, an intravenous pyelogram may be warranted.

    c. A postvoid residual is usually determined by catheterization following voiding. If catheterization is difficult or there is evidence of bladder outlet obstruction, sonography may be necessary. Normal postvoid residual is less than 50 ml. Greater than 200 ml is abnormal and indicates urinary retention and overflow incontinence. Values between 100 and 200 ml are equivocal, and repeated positive results are necessary for diagnosis.

  4. **Voiding diary and pad test**

    a. A voiding diary can provide more accurate information than a history or questionnaire. The patient is instructed to keep a diary for at least 24 hours or for several days. It should include time and amount of voids and amount and type of intake. Any episodes of leakage, estimated amount of leakage, position and activity, and presence of urge need to also be recorded.

    b. Having the patient wear a pad at all times and comparing the weight of these pads to the same number of dry pads can help with estimation of volume if this is difficult for the patient to ascertain.

TABLE 2. Medications that Cause or Complicate Urinary Incontinence

Drugs	Causative Mechanism of Urinary Incontinence

Anticholinergics
  Sedative-hypnotics
  Antihistamines
  Tricyclic antidepressants
  Antipsychotics
Nervous system depressants
  Alcohol
  Narcotics
  Calcium channel blockers
	Decrease detrusor contractions leading to retention and overflow incontinence. Sedative-hypnotics also depress central inhibition of micturition.

Alpha-adrenergic agonists Beta-adrenergic blockers	Cause sphincter contractions with outflow obstruction and resulting overflow incontinence
Alpha-adrenergic antagonists	Cause sphincter relaxation and contribute to stress incontinence
Diuretics Caffeine Alcohol	Diuretic-effect drugs that exacerbate urge incontinence

5. **Office stress testing**
    a. Directly observe the urethra while coughing in supine, sitting, and standing positions. In stress incontinence leakage occurs with an increase in intra-abdominal pressure. If the leaking occurs shortly after the cough, it is indicative of mixed incontinence with involuntary bladder contractions. Leakage after obtaining postvoid residual indicates a very low leak point, and these patients typically respond poorly to treatment and require referral.
    b. Urethral hypermobility may be assessed with the "Q-tip test". A sterile, lubricated Q-tip is placed transurethrally to the urethrovesical junction. If the Q-tip moves over 30° from the resting position with the Valsalva maneuver, true stress incontinence can be diagnosed.
    c. Urge incontinence can be evaluated by instilling sterile water or saline through a 12 or 14 French catheter into an empty bladder with the patient in lithotomy position. A 50- or 60-ml syringe without the plunger may be placed on the end of the catheter and held 15 cm above the urethra; 50-ml portions of water are then added to the syringe and allowed to flow into the bladder. The total amount of water added is recorded when the patient feels the urge to void, and when bladder contractions occur as evidenced by a rise in the meniscus of water in the syringe. Severe urgency or bladder contractions at less than 300 ml is indicative of urge incontinence. Normal bladder capacity averages about 500 ml.
    d. Urodynamic testing is indicated when the diagnosis is not clear from above evaluation. It is usually performed by specialists and can be expensive and uncomfortable.
C. **Treatment**
  1. **Behavioral options**
     a. Fluid control is simple and logical, and therefore, often overlooked. Patients should be encouraged to experiment with decreasing coffee, tea, soda, alcohol, and spicy foods which may irritate the bladder. Optimal fluid intake should be no more than 1.5 L/day. Drinking too little fluid, however, should be discouraged as concentrated urine may also irritate the bladder.
     b. Bladder training can be helpful in most cases of urinary incontinence. It is useful in stress incontinence to decrease the amount of bladder distention. It is particularly useful in urge incontinence as the patient can slowly increase the interval between voids to increase bladder compliance. Patient should begin with voids every 30–60 minutes and slowly increase to every 3–4 hours. In functional incontinence it is usually the only viable treatment option. 75% of women will have at least some improvement with this option.
     c. Pelvic muscle exercises are commonly called Kegel exercises and were first described in 1948. They are performed by tightening the vaginal muscles alone and can best be taught by having the patient interrupt flow during urination. Each contraction should be held for10 seconds, repeated 20–25 times, and each set should be performed 3–4 times a day. Best results are seen after about a month, and an adequate trial really takes 3 months. Cure reported in 31–73% and improvement in 43–96% of patients with stress incontinence. These exercises can also be a helpful adjunct therapy in urge incontinence.
     d. Biofeedback can be a valuable aid with Kegel exercises. It is least expensive if finger or perinometer is used. Inserting either of these into the vagina and contracting around it gives the patient evidence that the exercise is being correctly performed. Pelvic floor electrical stimulation has been successfully used in younger patients with stress incontinence. Vaginal weights inserted into the vagina and held for 15 minutes have also been reported effective in 70–80% of patients with stress incontinence.
     e. Intermittent catheterization is often necessary to treat overflow incontinence. Bladder training can be helpful, but the back-up method is self-catheterization on a regular basis.
  2. **Mechanical devices** are designed to catch urine or to block the flow by pressure from the vagina.

a. There are several soft-faced silicone patches, caps and plugs on the market.

b. Pessaries have been used for generations, and there are about 200 different types available. They are helpful but may interfere with intercourse and increase cases of vaginitis.

c. Vaginal diaphragm rings work by pressing the proximal urethra forward.

d. Intraurethral insert is a small disposable, fluid-filled sleeve inserted into the urethra following each void. Efficacy is about 85–90% and adverse effects are minimal, but cost may be an issue as these are not reusable.

3. **Accupuncture** has been used to treat urge incontinence, and does show some promise.

4. **Pharmacologic therapy** may be used alone, especially in urge incontinence, but is usually best if combined with behavioral techniques.

a. Estrogen: Hormone replacement therapy in postmenopausal women strengthens vaginal tissues, increases periurethral blood flow, and increases urethral resistance improving stress or mixed incontinence. The vagina and urethra have similar epithelial linings and react similarly to estrogen, so estrogen should be considered first-line therapy when atrophy is present. It may be effective alone but is usually better when combined with other therapy. The usual dose of oral conjugated estrogen is 0.625 mg/day. Topical preparations can be more effective or may be preferred by the patient. Estradiol cream $^1/_2$ applicator 3–5 times per week can be given initially, then reduced after two months to twice a week. A new form of vaginal estrogen is available as an estrogen-impregnated vaginal ring worn continuously in the vagina for 3 months.

b. Tricyclic antidepressants: Imipramine has both alpha-adrenergic and anticholinergic activity reducing detrusor spasticity and tightening the bladder outlet. It is most useful in urge incontinence but is often helpful for stress incontinence as well, making it an excellent choice for mixed incontinence. Dose from 10–100 mg /day.

c. Alpha-adrenergic agents: Phenylpropanolamine (the sole ingredient in Dexatrim™ or Entex™) increases bladder neck and urethral resistance and improves stress incontinence in over half of patients. Long-acting preparations should be used at 50–75 mg bid. This medication can increase blood pressure and cause tachycardia and should not be used in patients with cardiovascular disease. Pseudoephedrine (15–30 mg tid) is also an option.

d. Anticholinergic agents: These drugs have long been first-line treatment for urge incontinence. They relax the detrusor muscle and decrease bladder spasms. Oxybutynin (Ditropan™) will decrease symptoms of urge incontinence by at least 50% in about half of patients. It has a high incidence of dry mouth, constipation, and gastroesophageal reflux with a relatively high discontinuance rate. A new controlled-release preparation is now available with fewer side effects. Dosage of oxybutynin is 2.5–5 mg bid to tid. The controlled-release version is 5 mg once a day. Propantheline (Pro-Banthine™), dosed at 7.5–30 mg qid, has less antispasmodic properties, must be given fasting. Its difficult dosing schedule and high side effect profile decrease its desirability. Hyoscyamine (Cystospaz™) is a rapid and short-acting medication which can be taken sublingually and is useful if a few hours of protection are desired. Dose is 0.375 mg bid.

e. Competitive muscarinic receptor antagonist: Tolterodine (Detrol™) is similar to oxybutynin with similar efficacy for urge incontinence but a significantly lower discontinuance rate due to side effects. Initial dose is 2 mg twice a day, but may be decreased to 1 mg bid based on efficacy and tolerability.

f. Capsaicin: This extract of chili peppers seems to desensitize hyperactive bladders when injected intravesically. It has been used in interstitial cystitis treatment and may have some benefit in urge incontinence

5. **Surgery**

a. Surgery is the most effective treatment for stress incontinence. It usually follows more conservative trials but may be considered for first-line therapy. The four major surgical procedures are: retropubic suspensions, sling procedures, transvaginal suspensions, and anterior repairs. Retropubic suspension and sling procedures are the most effective. Patients recover most quickly from transvaginal suspensions.

    b. Bladder denervation, selective sacral neurectomy, and augmentation cytoplasty are seldom used surgical procedures for urge or overflow incontinence.

6. **Referral:** Specialists can be extremely helpful in treating this aggravating affliction. Common referrals are to urologists for evaluation, gynecologists or urologists for surgical procedures, and neurologists if a neurologic lesion is suspected. Patients should be referred when:

    a. Diagnosis is uncertain or no treatment plan is reasonable

    b. Failure to respond to treatment plan

    c. Hematuria in the absence of cystitis

    d. Recurrent urinary tract infections

    e. Prior pelvic surgery or failed surgery for incontinence

    f. Evaluation for surgical procedure

    g. Pelvic prolapse beyond the hymen

    h. Abnormal postvoid residual

    i. Abnormal neurologic findings

SUGGESTED READING

1.* Blaivas JG, Sand PK: A straightforward approach to urinary incontinence. Patient Care (Suppl):1–10, 1999.
2. Bourcier AP, Juras JC: Nonsurgical therapy for stress incontinence. Urol Clin North Am 22:613–628, 1995.
3. Brandeis GH, Resnick NM: Pharmacotherapy of urinary incontinence in the elderly. Drug Ther 93–102, 1992.
4. Chancellor MB, Diokno AC, Ouslander JG: Treatment options for urinary incontinence. Patient Care (Suppl):11–16, 1999.
5. Fourcroy JL: Urogynecology update: Incontinence. Hosp Pract 33:63–70, 81, 1998.
6. Fowler GC, Ryan JG, Duiker SS: Evaluating and treating urinary incontinence. Female Patient 18:63–78, 1993.
7. Haygood V, Addison A: Urinary incontinence in women. American Academy of Family Physicians Monograph No. 21, 1983.
8. Luber KM, Bent AE: Clinical management of urge incontinence in women. Female Patient 17:67–81, 1992.
9. McFall S, Yerkes AM, Bernard M, LeRud T: Evaluation and treatment of urinary incontinence. Arch Fam Med 6:114–118,1997.
10. Peggs JF: Urinary incontinence in the elderly: Pharmacologic therapies. Am Fam Physician 46:1763–1769, 1992.
11.* Turzo E, Bavendam TG: Treatment options for urinary incontinence. Women's Health 1:649–657, 1998.
12. Urinary Incontinence Guideline Panel: Urinary Incontinence in Adults: Clinical Practice Guideline. AHCPR Pub. No. 92-0038. Rockville, MD, Agency for Health Care Policy and Research, Public Health Service, U.S. Department of Health and Human Services, 1992.
13. Walters MD, Realina JP: Evaluation and treatment of urinary incontinence in women: A primary care approach. J Am Board Fam Pract 5:289–301, 1992.
14. Wein AJ: Pharmacology of incontinence. Urol Clin North Am 22:557–578, 1995.
15. Weiss BD: Diagnostic evaluation of urinary incontinence in geriatric patients. Am Fam Physician 57:2675–2684, 1998.
16. Weiss BD: Nonpharmacologic treatment of urinary incontinence. Am Fam Physician 44:579–586, 1991.

PART X
SEXUAL ISSUES

75. Sexual Abuse

Elizabeth Alexander, M.D., M.S.

I. The Issues

Sexual assault is a common and ongoing health problem in the U.S. Affected women come to health care facilities as a result of acute assault and with problems related to earlier assault and abuse. Historically, sexual assault has been minimized by health professionals, often because of denial of its prevalence and lack of skills and training to evaluate and intervene in helpful ways. Sexual assault crosses all lines of age, gender, race, and class, although women are predominantly the victims. Because of differences in evaluation and treatment of children who are victims of sexual abuse, this chapter focuses exclusively on the recognition, evaluation, and treatment of sexual assault of adult women.

II. The Theory

A. **Definition:** any sexual contact coerced, manipulated, or forced on one person by another. Legal definitions vary by state, but most involve the use of "threat, duress, physical force, intimidation, or deception; sexual contact; and non-consent of the victim."

B. **Incidence**
  1. **Childhood and adolescent sexual abuse**
     a. 450,000 cases in U.S. per year
     b. 38–45% of adult women report at least one experience of sexual abuse before age of 18 years
        i. Variation in reporting is due to difference in definition and description of sexual abuse
     c. When sexual abuse occurs in childhood, average age of onset is 9.2 years for girls and 7.8–9.7 years for boys
     d. Perpetrators
        i. Intrafamilial: 68%
        ii. Strangers: 20%
        iii. Male perpetrators: 80%
  2. **Adult sexual abuse**
     a. 90% female victims, 10% male
     b. Most frequently committed and underreported violent crime in U.S.
     c. 46% of adult women experience attempted or completed rape at some time during their lives
     d. 12% of married women report forced sexual contact by husbands
     e. Highest incidence in women aged 15–19 years
     f. Perpetrators
        i. Strangers
        ii. Spouse
        iii. Acquaintance
        iv. Gang

C. **Comorbid factors**
  1. Sexual assault has high association with alcohol use, particularly in acquaintance rape of adolescents and young adults.
  2. Many adult victims of sexual assault have been previously victimized, either as children or as adults; survivors of childhood abuse have increased vulnerability to repeated victimization.

D. **Long-term effects**
   1. Symptoms similar to posttraumatic stress syndrome
   2. Depression
   3. Sexual adjustment difficulties
   4. Chronic anxiety
   5. Sleep disturbance
   6. Somatic complaints, such as headache and gastrointestinal distress, although the specific somatic manifestation may be related to the type and location of previous abuse.

III. **An Approach**
   A. **Routine screening** for a history of sexual assault in women yields a significant prevalence of positive histories, evidence of long-term impact on health and is particularly important when women present with sexual dysfunction or chronic depressive symptoms.
   B. **Objectives of evaluation** of acute sexual assault in either the primary care office or emergency department:
      1. To ensure emotional and physical safety of woman
      2. To prevent pregnancy (if desired) and sexually transmitted diseases (STDs) that may result from assault
      3. To collect evidence for prosecution of perpetrator(s)
      4. To arrange for follow-up evaluation and care
      5. To refer to resources for long-term care and recovery
   C. **History in acute sexual assault** is facilitated by presence of an advocate or friend with survivor, and a known and trusted medical examiner (more likely in the primary care setting than in the emergency room).
      1. Format: record in victim's words as much as possible and record on forms provided by law enforcement.
      2. Information recorded to include chronologic details of events; details such as clothing and place that victim recalls; gynecologic history (e.g., last menstrual period, use of reliable contraception); previous pertinent medical problems; and awareness of injury or pain.
   D. **Examination** should be guided by history and include a general physical examination, documentation of all injuries by size, location and color, presence or absence of genital trauma, and a mental status examination.
   E. **Laboratory testing**, guided by history and examination:
      1. Testing for chlamydia, gonorrhea from sites directed by history and examination.
      2. Initial blood tests should include Venereal Disease Research Laboratory (VDRL) test for syphilis; human immunodeficiency virus (HIV); hepatitis B; and human chorionic gonadotropin (hCG) (dependent on history).
      3. Repeat blood tests: HIV at 3 and 6 months, cultures in 1 week if prophylaxis not given, VDRL at 3 months, and pregnancy test if no menses.
   F. **Medical treatment**
      1. Pregnancy prevention: Ovral oral contraceptive pills, 2 pills initially, repeated 12 hours later within 72 hours of assault, 97% effective; or levonorgestrel 0.75 mg in two doses, 99% effective
      2. If not immunized, consider hepatitis B prophylaxis with HB immunoglobulin (0.06 ml/kg), followed by initiation of hepatitis B immunization
      3. Gonorrhea prevention, one of regimens below:
         a. Cefixime, 400 mg orally in a single dose *or*
         b. Ceftriaxone, 125 mg intramuscularly in a single dose *or*
         c. Ciprofloxacin, 500 mg orally in a single dose *or*
         d. Ofloxacin, 400 mg orally in a single dose, plus azithromycin, 1 g orally in a single dose *or*
         e. Doxycycline, 100 mg orally twice a day for 7 days *or*
         f. Spectinomycin, 2 g intramuscularly in a single dose
      4. Chlamydia prevention
         a. Doxycycline, 100 mg twice daily for 7 days *or*
         b. Azithromycin, 1 g orally in a single dose

G. **Charting and documentation** on forms provided by law enforcement
  1. Take photographs of obvious injuries
  2. Follow protocols for collection of specimens and bagging of clothing, with documentation of specimens and recorded, witnessed transfer to law enforcement
  3. Use drawings to document location of injuries
H. **Other therapeutic considerations**
  1. Attend to acute safety needs
  2. Ensure that woman will be with family or friends
  3. Consider whether woman wishes to press charges if assailant identified, although prosecution possible with good documentation without woman filing charges.
  4. Refer for individual therapy
  5. Consider group therapy for validation
  6. Make available community resources known (e.g., sexual assault center)
  7. Consider bibliotherapy (use of books or articles for patients to read)
  8. Recommend therapy and education for family and partners
IV. **Adult Women Survivors of Childhood Sexual Abuse**
  A. **Common responses of adult**
    1. Adaptive at time of abuse—helped child survive
    2. Not adaptive in adult situations
    3. Specific responses include amnesia, repression, denial, and dissociative response
  B. **Common adult health sequelae**
    1. **Somatic manifestations** commonly include insomnia, decreased libido, phobic avoidance of sexual activity, other sexual disorders, increased incidence of abuse of alcohol and other drugs, and increased behaviors that put woman at risk for HIV disease.
    2. **Psychological manifestations** include increased incidence of depression, including suicide attempts and completions; increased incidence of obsessive disorders; increased incidence of victimization as adult; increased incidence of dissociative disorders, including multiple personality; increased anxiety disorders; and lower self-esteem.
  C. **Relationship manifestations** for adult women who have survived childhood sexual abuse are long-term problems with trust and intimacy; a negative impact of lower self-esteem on autonomy and boundaries, the tendency to either avoid relationships or become overly dependent on another; and an increased incidence of marital problems.
  D. **Helpful provider behaviors:**
    1. Obtaining health history in a way that gives permission to discuss previous history of abuse
    2. Attentiveness to clues in doctor–patient relationship that may suggest history of abuse, such as fear of medical situations, overdependence, or overcompliance
    3. Nonjudgmental, empathetic listening to any disclosure
    4. Knowledge of therapists who are skilled in working with posttraumatic stress disorders
    5. Sensitivity to shame and embarrassment that history of sexual abuse engenders in adults
    6. Willingness to talk patient through examinations, procedures that may involve flashbacks or fearful responses
    7. Clarity about and respect of boundaries in therapeutic relationship
    8. Discussion of what is recorded in medical record after disclosure of abuse

SUGGESTED READING

1. Berkowitz CD: Sexual abuse of children and adolescents. Adv Pediatr 34:275–312, 1987.
2. Finkelhor D: The trauma of child sexual abuse: Two models. In: Lasting Effects of Child Sexual Abuse. Newbury Park, CA, Sage, 1988, pp 61–82.
3. Geist R: Sexually related trauma. Emerg Med Clin North Am 6:439–466, 1988.
4. Golding JM: Prevalence of sexual assault history among women with common gynecologic symptoms. Am J Obstet Gynecol 179:1013–1019, 1998.
5. Heinrich L: Care of the female rape victim. Nurs Pract 12:9–27, 1987.
6. Russell DE: Sexual Exploitation: Rape, Child Sexual Assault, and Workplace Harassment. Newbury Park, CA, Sage, 1984.
7. Sexual Assault: An Overview. Washington, DC, U.S. Victims Resource Center, Department of Justice, 1987.
8. Van Look PF, Stewart F: Emergency contraception. In Hatcher RA, Trussell J, Stewart F, et al (eds): Contraceptive Technology. New York, Ardent Media, 1998.

APPENDIX TO CHAPTER 75:

Forms for Evaluation

FSD-97A (10-89)   PART A
MICHIGAN STATE POLICE   Page 2
Forensic Science Division

ASSAULT VICTIM MEDICAL REPORT
RELEASE OF INFORMATION AND EVIDENCE

Please type or print all information clearly.

This report may be completed by any licensed or certified health professional.

---

19. Date of Interview _____   2. Time of Interview _____

3. Patient Name _____   4. Medical File No. _____

5. Patient Birth Date _____   6. Sex _____ Race _____   7. Phone _____

8. Patient Address _____   ZIP _____

---

27. Patients description of assault (pertinent medical details, record in patient's own words, include all spontaneous utterances).

28. Date of assault _____   29. Time of assault _____

30. Significant past medical history.

31. Note identification of pain in patient's own words.*

32. Check pain and symptoms mentioned:

   ☐ skeletal muscular pain   ☐ head ache   ☐ tenesmus

   ☐ abdominal pain   ☐ bleeding   ☐ dysuria

   ☐ pelvic pain   ☐ discharge   ☐ other

33. Has there been recent treatment of any disorder?

   ☐ No   ☐ Yes   Describe _____

I understand that the law considers the examining licensed or certified health professional as an eye witness in the body of events surrounding a potential crime. What a patient/victim says to medical staff may be admissable as an exception to the heresay rule, and these statements may be important in determining the truth before a judge or fury. I agree to preserve these statements as part of the patient's history.

36. Interviewer's Signature _____

37. Interviewer name _____   38. Title _____

39. (If known) Terminiation date of this employment _____

40. Interviewer fluent in English   ☐ Yes   ☐ No

White - Medical Record   Yellow - Place in Kit

FSD-97B (10/88)
Michigan Department of State Police
FORENSIC SCIENCE DIVISION

ASSAULT VICTIM MEDICAL REPORT
PATIENT EXAMINATION FORM

PART B

Please type or print all information clearly.
This examination and report may be completed by any licensed or certified health professional.

41. Date of Examination _____

42. Time of Examination _____

43. Patient Name _____

44. Medical File No. _____

45. Appearance of patient's clothing: (Check if yes)

☐ Missing   ☐ Soiled or muddy   ☐ Leaves, grass embedded
☐ Torn   ☐ Damp or wet   ☐ Other as described
☐ Soiled   ☐ Blood stains   _____

46. Patient changed clothing between assault and arrival at examination?

☐ Yes   ☐ No

47. Itemize clothing placed in containers separately and tagged for evidence:

48. Describe presence of trauma to skin of entire body. Indicate location using chart. Describe exact appearance and size. Indicate possible source such as teeth, cigarette.

49. Itemize photos or X-rays of patient:

AUTHORITY: Act 59, P.A. of 1935
COMPLETION: Voluntary, but information needed
                  for medicolegal purposes.

FSD-97B (10/88)   PART B
Michigan Department of State Police   Page 2
FORENSIC SCIENCE DIVISION

50. Describe external perineal or genito pelvic trauma:

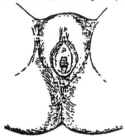

51. Describe internal trauma (Speculum and bimanual examination):
     _____ Lacerations present, Describe:

52. Is there discharge?
     ☐ No   ☐ Yes   Describe:

SPECIMENS COLLECTED (check all that apply)

53. ☐ Air-dried cotton swabs - 2 sets from affected area (list body sources)

54. ☐ Dry unstained slides (list body sources)

55. ☐ Fibers from patient's body

56. ☐ Combing from patient's head

57. ☐ Combing from pubic area

58. ☐ 12 strands pubic hair (pulled)
                                                              ⎫
59. ☐ 12 strands patient's head hair pulled from different regions of head ⎬ Optional
                                                              ⎭

60. ☐ Saliva Sample: paper disc in patient's mouth and air-dried

61. ☐ Tube of whole blood (no preservatives)

I understand that the law considers the examining licensed or certified health professional as an eye witness in the body of events surrounding a potential crime, and that I may be called to testify and be cross-examined about my findings in this examination.

62. Examining health professional signature _____

63. Examining health professional printed name _____

                          Title _____

64. Supervising physician name, if any _____

65. (If known) Termination date of this employment_____

White – Medical Records   Yellow – Police

FSD-97C (10/88)
Michigan Department of State Police
FORENSIC SCIENCE DIVISION

ASSAULT VICTIM MEDICAL REPORT
PATIENT TREATMENT RECORD

PART C

Please type or print all information clearly.

67. Date of treatment _____ 68. Time of treatment _____

69. Patient Name _____ 70. Medical File No. _____

71. Statement of Patient's Rights.

    1. You have the right to considerate and respectful care by doctors and nurses.
    2. You have the right to privacy and confidentiality for yourself and your medical records.
    3. You have the right to full information about treatment.
    4. You have the right to refuse or choose treatment offered, and to leave the location of medical service when you wish.
    5. You have the right to continued care and timely treatment of your future health problems related to this incident.

Tests given to patient:

72. GC culture   ☐ Yes   ☐ No   73. VDRL   ☐ Yes   ☐ No

74. Pap smear   ☐ Yes   ☐ No   75. Pregnancy test   ☐ Yes   ☐ No

76. Chlamydia   ☐ Yes   ☐ No   (pre-existing pregnancy only)

77. Other Information:

Treatment given to patient:

78. VD prophylaxis   ☐ No   ☐ Yes   Describe:

79. Medication given:

80. Medication prescribed:

81. Other Treatment given:

Future treatment planned

82. Transfer to another medical facility   Name _____

83. Appointment in 6 weeks for repeat GC culture, VDRL, and pregnancy test

       Date_____ Time_____ Place_____

84. Referred for couneling, or introduced for follow-up (Refer to counseling center form).

76. Sexual Dysfunction and Counseling

Elizabeth Alexander, M.D., M.S.

I. **The Issues**

The definition of sexual dysfunction is variable across patients and in the same patient across time and within different relationships. Thus the definition of sexual dysfunction is not fixed and defined by an external source; it depends primarily on whether a patient is satisfied with her own sexuality and her level of sexual functioning, regardless of whether she is in an intimate relationship. As we broaden our definition of the many factors that help to make us sexual human beings, coitus becomes only one aspect of sexual functioning. This broader definition adds understanding to the etiology of sexual dysfunction but also makes diagnostic efforts more complex. One can also add the components of intimate relationships in broadening the understanding of a woman's concerns about sexual functioning (Figs. 1 and 2).

II. **The Theory**

A. **Physiology of normal sexual functioning—triphasic model (Table 1)**
1. Introduced by Kaplan, provides a framework for thinking about sexual response cycle in a systemic manner
2. Aids in both diagnosis and treatment

B. **Common sexual complaints of women**
1. **Decreased libido**
   a. Affects 50–70% of women at some point in lifetime
   b. Possible causes: relationship difficulties (most common cause), posttraumatic stress disorder, depression and anxiety, fatigue, and rarely, physical causes in women with chronic disease
   c. Treatment: referral to a therapist skilled in both relationship therapy and sex therapy
2. **Difficulty with arousal**
   a. Possible causes: effect of decreased libido, medications (Table 2), and inadequate information about needed stimulation
   b. Treatment options are sex therapy, bibliotherapy (Table 3), and sensate focus exercise to learn conditions and types of stimulation necessary for arousal (Fig. 3)
3. **Dissatisfaction with frequency of orgasm or type of stimulation required** to reach orgasm
   a. Complaint of over half of women at some point in lives
   b. Possible causes: inadequate information about body, self-observation during sexual arousal, or poor technique or communication about stimulation needs with partner
   c. Treatment options
      i. Group therapy, if available
      ii. Bibliotherapy (Table 3)
      iii. Couple therapy
4. **Painful or uncomfortable sexual activity**
   a. Relatively common, when all ages considered
   b. Ask as part of routine gynecological history
   c. Possible causes
      i. Introital dyspareunia
         (a) Focal vulvitis (most often candidal)
         (b) Infections (Bartholin's or Skene's gland infections, cystitis)
         (c) Scarring (phimosis of clitoris, scarring from episiotomy, vaginal surgery, or irradiation)
         (d) Intact hymen or thick hymeneal tags
         (e) Lack of vaginal lubrication (either hormonal insufficiency or inadequate stimulation)
         (f) Vaginismus
         (g) Clitoral hypersensitivity

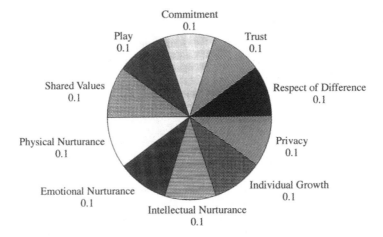

FIGURE 1. Components of being sexual. *1. The use of sexuality as a means of gaining another end; coercive sexual behaviors, use of sex to sell products, etc. *2. What one was taught in childhood about what sexual expression should and should not be. *3. One's conception of self as male or female.

    ii. Deep dyspareunia
        (a) Pelvic inflammatory disease
        (b) Endometritis
        (c) Endometriosis
        (d) Ovarian cysts
    iii. Other
        (a) Pain from movement with arthritis or muscular disease
        (b) Psychogenic pain from previous trauma
  d. Treatment
    i. Teach location of pubococcygeal (PC) muscle and have woman experience difference in tightening and relaxing PC muscle
    ii. Have her practice tightening and relaxing of PC muscle
    iii. Have her insert fingers into vagina, starting with one finger and working up to three

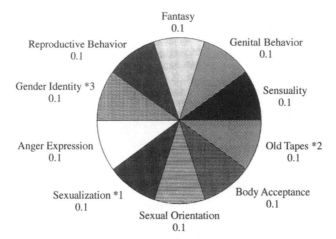

FIGURE 2. Components of an intimate relationship.

TABLE 1.   Triphasic Model of Sexual Function

Phase	Primary Organ System Involved	Innervation	Clinical Presentation
Desire	Brain (subjective desire to experience sexual stimuli)	Dopaminergic/cholinergic in brain	Ask about decreased desire for sex
Arousal	Vascular system (filling of blood vessels in genital organs, breast, skin flush)	Parasympathetic nervous system	Ask about lack of lubrication, lack of arousal
Orgasm	Skeletal muscles in pelvic floor (contraction of pubococcygeal muscle at intervals of 3–7.08 sec)	Sympathetic nervous system	Ask about difficulty in reaching orgasm

     iv. Instruct her to have her partner insert fingers, going from one to three
     v. After foreplay woman should attempt vaginal containment only of penis
     vi. Then woman should initiate thrusting in female superior position
     vii. To help maintain relaxation of PC muscle, woman should bear down slightly while attempting insertion of either finger or penis; it is difficult to contract PC muscle while bearing down
     viii. Success rate: 99%

C. **Less common sexual complaints of women**, all requiring referral to a skilled therapist, are phobic avoidance of sexual contact, fetishism, posttraumatic difficulties with sexual interaction, and sexual identity confusion

TABLE 2.   Effects of Common Medications on Sexual Functioning

Category	Example(s)	Phase(s) Affected	Alternatives
Antihypertensive drugs			
Diuretics	Thiazides	Arousal	Consider calcium channel blocker; more pleasuring in arousal phase
Centrally acting	Clonidine Methyldopa	Arousal	
Beta blockers	Propranolol	Desire, arousal	
ACE inhibitors	Captopril	Arousal	
Antipsychotic drugs	Thorazine Thiothixene Haloperidol	Desire, arousal Priapism, retrograde ejaculation	
Antianxiety drugs	Diazepam	Desire, orgasm	Consider buspirone; decrease medication slowly
Anticholinergic drugs	Atropine Hydroxyzine	Arousal, desire	More emphasis on pleasuring
Estrogen	Premarin	Arousal (improves lubrication, decreases pain)	Topical estrogen for those who cannot take oral estrogens
Progestins	Provera	Desire (may decrease libido)	Use cyclic instead of daily dosing if side effect occurs
H-2 receptor antagonists	Cimetidine	Desire, arousal	Consider alternative drugs
Narcotics	Codeine Barbiturates	Desire, arousal, orgasm	Recognize and treat addictions
Tricyclic antidepressants	Imipramine Amitriptyline	Desire, arousal Delayed muscular phase	Consider fluoxetine, sertraline
Other antidepressants	Trazodone MAO inhibitors	Priapism Arousal, orgasm	Consider fluoxetine, sertraline
Other	Digitalis	Desire, arousal	Treat performance anxiety; reassure fears of cardiac arrest during sex

ACE = angiotensin-converting enzyme; MAO = monoamine oxidase.

TABLE 3. Bibliographic Resources for Patients and Clinicians

Resource	Patient	Clinician	Use
Barbach L: For Yourself. New York, Doubleday, 1975	+	+	Particularly helpful for women with concerns about orgasmic frequency or conditions; also has good sensate focus exercises.
Zilbergeld B: The New Male Sexuality. New York, Bantam Books, 1992	+	+	Has excellent section on separation of emotional, physical, and sexual intimacy needs; excellent sensate focus exercises that are slowly graded.
Annon J: The Behavioral Treatment of Sexual Problems: Brief and Intensive Therapy, vols I and II. Honolulu, Enabling Systems, 1975	–	+	Quick, good references to behavioral treatment for some of the sexual disorders treated best in primary care setting. Specific therapy plans and suggestions outlined.
Kaplan HS: The New Sex Therapy. New York, Bantam Books, 1974	–	+	Good, still current overview of sexual disorders and their causes and treatment.
Kaplan HS: Disorders of Desire. New York, Brunner/Mazel, 1985	–	+	Good clinical reference with more focus on decreased libido in both men and women.
Kaplan HS: The Illustrated Manual of Sex Therapy. New York, Brunner/Mazel, 1987	+	+	Stepwise, basic approach, with illustrations, to therapy for the common sexual dysfunctions.
Lopiccolo J, Lopiccolo L: Handbook of Sex Therapy. New York, Plenum, 1978	+	–	Still current, useful handbook on diagnosis and treatment plans for common sexual concerns.
Barbach L: Pleasures: Women Write Erotica. Garden City, NJ, Doubleday, 1984	+	–	Useful book for women who are having difficulty allowing themselves to have and use sexual fantasies

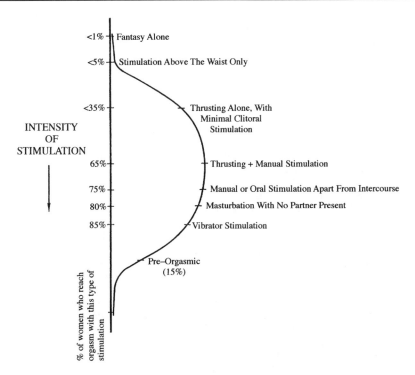

FIGURE 3. Conditions for orgasm in women. (Note: Generally, when a woman can reach orgasm with low-intensity methods of stimulation, she can also reach orgasm with higher-intensity stimulation [farther down the curve].)

TABLE 4.   Issues to Consider in Taking a Sexual History

1. What is the patient's view of the problem?
   The best way to get this information is to ask the woman to describe what usually happens during sexual encounters. This approach avoids the acceptance of diagnostic labels that often have differing meanings for the patient and the caregiver.

2. What is the chronological history of the problem?
   Problems of recent origin are more often readily amenable to treatment, whereas longstanding problems often require long-term therapy. In addition, problems with desire phase disorders that are longstanding suggest repressive developmental teachings about sexuality, longstanding relationship difficulties, or perhaps a history of childhood sexual abuse.

3. If the woman has had other sexual relationships, has this concern been present before?
   An affirmative answer suggests that it is not primarily a relationship problem but a problem that is amenable to education and sexual therapy; a negative answer suggests a relationship component to the problem.

4. Are the woman and her partner able to communicate openly and comfortably about sexual issues, such as preferences for stimulation?

5. Does the woman have any questions or concerns that suggest the need to explore sexual orientation as a part of the diagnostic and therapeutic intervention?

6. How does the woman meet her needs for emotional and physical nurturance, apart from sexual contact?

7. Are the woman and her partner able to resolve conflicts in the relationship openly and nondestructively?

8. Are there any medications or diseases that may explain the phase of the sexual response cycle that is involved?

9. Are there longstanding or acute psychiatric illnesses that may explain the patient's sexual concerns?

10. Is this primarily a relationship problem with a secondary sexual dysfunction, or is the sexual dysfunction primary?

11. Is alcohol or drug abuse a problem for either the patient or her partner?

12. What are the patient's preferences and resources for solution?

13. What is the woman's view of "normal" sexual expression?

14. What are the woman's goals for treatment? Are these goals different from those of her partner, if she is in a relationship?

III. **An Approach**
   A. **Historical information** needed (Table 4)
      1. Timing of onset of symptoms (gradual or sudden)
      2. Masturbatory history
      3. Phase of response cycle most affected (desire, arousal, or orgasm)
      4. Marital or relationship history
      5. Previous sexual functioning
      6. Ability to meet one's needs for emotional intimacy
      7. Desired outcome (what the individual or couple would consider an improvement)
      8. Medications (Table 2)
   B. **Physical examination** should assure the absence of organic brain changes, the integrity of the spinal cord (including bulbocavernosus reflex, perianal sensation, and tone of external sphincter), general muscle tone, status of the cardiovascular system, and amount of estrogen support in genital tissues. Evidence of clitoral size and the presence of adhesions over the clitoral hood should be noted.
   C. **Laboratory tests**, if history and physical information suggest an organic cause, should include HgbA1c; luteinizing hormone (LH); follicle-stimulating hormone (FSH); thyroid-stimulating hormone (TSH); liver enzymes; prolactin; and serum testosterone (bioavailable and total testosterone).
   D. **General treatment options**
      1. Referral for individual or couple therapy
      2. Treatment within primary care setting
      3. Group treatment of anorgasmia
      4. Bibliographic resources for patients and clinicians (Table 3)

    5. Bibliographic resources for clinicians (Table 3)
    6. Reevaluation of current medications (Table 2)
E. **Considerations in treatment options**
    1. Individual or couple therapy
    2. Treatment in primary care setting or referral to outside therapist
    3. Gender of therapist
    4. Education and reading level of patient
    5. Need for relationship therapy prior to work on sexual therapy
    6. Time and skills of primary care provider
    7. Financial resources of patient
    8. Skilled therapists available in community
    9. Sexual orientation, cultural, and ethnic differences between patients and therapists
F. **Treatment principles**
    1. Establishment of realistic and specific goals
    2. Education about body
    3. Self-learning of level and type of stimulation necessary to reach orgasm through masturbation
    4. Permission to use fantasy as focusing aid
    5. Transfer of learned skills to partner, with attention first to development of sexual communication skills
    6. Reinforce permission to be selfish in sexual relationships (sequential focus on each partner)
    7. Separation of emotional from sexual needs
    8. Consideration of sex as being more than intercourse

SUGGESTED READING

  1. Barbach L: For Yourself. New York Doubleday, 1975.
  2. Davis SR: Clinical review 82: Androgens and the postmenopausal woman. J Clin Endocrinol Metab 81:2759–2763, 1996.
  3. Davis SR: The clinical use of androgens in female sexual disorders. J Sex Marital Ther 24:153–163, 1998.
  4. Drugs that cause sexual dysfunction: An update. Med Lett Drugs Ther 34:73–78, 1992.
  5. Halvorsen JG, Metz ME: Sexual dysfunction. Part 1: Classification, etiology, and pathogenesis. J Am Board Fam Physicians 5:51–61, 1992.
  6. Kaiser FE: Sexuality in the elderly. Urol Clin North Am 23: 99–109, 1996.
  7. Kaplan HS: Disorders of Desire. New York, Brunner/Mazel, 1985.
  8. Kaplan HS: The Evaluation of Sexual Disorders. New York, Brunner/Mazel, 1983.
  9. Kaplan HS: The New Sex Therapy. Active Treatment of Sexual Dysfunction. New York, Brunner/Mazel, 1974.
10. Zilbergeld B: The New Male Sexuality. New York, Bantam Books, 1992.

77. Gender-based and Sexual Harassment

Elizabeth Alexander, M.D., M.S.

Sexual harassment, and all forms of gender-based abuse, reinforce the internalization of social stereotypes and prejudices that denigrate women, thereby confirming a sense of devaluation, fragmenting the individual's identity and damaging the self.

Charney and Russell

I. The Issues
Sexual harassment is a common problem for women that affects psychological, somatic, and economic health in many ways. It presents both directly and indirectly within the health care setting and requires knowledgeable discussion and exploration as it relates to the health of women.

Sexual harassment is a relatively new term, coming into use in the past 10–15 years, although it is by no means a new problem. A working definition of sexual harassment is found in federal guidelines issued by the Equal Employment Opportunities Commission:

> Unwelcome sexual advances, requests for sexual favors, and other verbal or physical conduct of a sexual nature constitute sexual harassment when (1) submission to such conduct is made either explicitly or implicitly a term or condition of an individual's employment, (2) submission to or rejection of such conduct by an individual is used as a basis for employment decisions affecting such individual, or (3) such conduct has the purpose or effect of unreasonably interfering with an individual's work performance or creating an intimidating, hostile, or offensive working environment.

Because of lack of research, little is known about the quantitative and measurable effects of sexual and gender-based harassment of the individuals affected, the people who are permitted to continue the abuse, and the organizations in which they work. However, the frequency with which it occurs mandates provider attention to this workplace equivalent of domestic violence.

II. **The Theory**
  A. **Incidence of sexual harassment**
    1. Affects 42–90% of all women at some point in their working lives
       a. Variability due primarily to variations in definition of sexual harassment offered to respondents
    2. Reported by 42% of women and 15% of men in U.S. Government Employees Survey within previous 2 years
    3. Incidence does not vary by type of job; similar for white-collar and blue-collar workers
    4. Incidence among medical trainees reported to range from 36–73%, with much higher prevalence among female trainees
  B. **Characteristics of sexual harassment**
    1. Power differential: hallmark of sexual harassment in workplace
    2. Underreporting to people in positions of authority
       a. Well-documented that women who report sexual harassment experience backlash
       b. Common reasons for silence include fear of job loss; threats of blackmail; self-blame; a belief that nothing will be done to correct problem; and fear of disrupted or increasingly problematic working relationships.
    3. Similarities with other types of abuse
       a. Sexual harassment carries common thread with other forms of abuse, particularly rape and incest
          i. Occurs in context of power differential and abuse of power in relationships
          ii. Accompanied by shame on part of victim
          iii. Invisible to larger society or organization until crises make it more visible
          iv. Long-term impact on health of person exposed to violence similar to post-traumatic stress syndrome
       b. Differences from rape and incest
          i. Occurs most often in workplace
          ii. Threat of very real economic consequences with long-term implications
  C. **Characteristics of perpetrators**
    1. Perpetrators may be either superiors or peers/coworkers
       a. Because men in U.S. culture are often perceived to have more power and influence as result of culturally prescribed gender roles, even coworkers may seem to be in positions of power by women who experience harassment
       b. When persons in authority fail to deal directly with complaints of harassment and ignore, excuse, or cover them up, they become collaborators in abuse
       c. U.S. Merit Systems Protection Board found that only 40% of perpetrators were superiors
    2. Perpetrators are more likely to be men (96% in cases of female victims)
  D. **Impact on victims**
    1. More than 90% of harassment victims report significant degree of emotional or physical distress

2. Somatic effects include headaches, eating pattern changes, sleep disturbance, and increased susceptibility to infection
3. Emotional effects: negative effects on self-esteem, overall life satisfaction, mood, sense of safety, and connection with others.
4. Workplace and economic effects
   a. One in 10 women reports leaving job because of sexual harassment
   b. Affects ability to function in current job
   c. Affects academic progress
   d. Affects career advancement

E. **Responses of women**
   1. **Internal responses**
      a. Intrapsychic and emotional reactions
         i. Confusion
         ii. Self-blame, guilt
         iii. Fear and anxiety over continuing abuse
         iv. Depression
         v. Anger
         vi. Disillusionment, chronic erosion of trust in people and organizations
      b. Depend on whether woman stays in situation, whether harassment is ongoing and repeated, and whether woman files complaint
   2. **External responses**—a continuum from passive to active
      a. Range of passive responses
         i. Submission and acceptance of submission
         ii. Avoidance of situation or perpetrator
         iii. Avoidance of job (by quitting or changing jobs)
         iv. Ignoring perpetrator
      b. Range of active responses
         i. Confronting perpetrator
         ii. Discussion with/getting support from coworkers
         iii. Formal grievance within organization
         iv. Legal action
      c. Individual reactions
         i. Depend on previous victimization and a history of adaptive responses to abuse in family or workplace
         ii. Should not be seen as illness or maladaptations but as learned responses and healthiest response at the time in unhealthy environment
         iii. More active responses require
            (a) Movement from immobilizing self-blame and depression to anger
            (b) Validation by others inside or outside organization
            (c) Ability of organization to deal with repeated victimizations, which are often precipitated by active responses

F. **Responses by persons in authority**
   1. In one study 47% of women who took formal action reported improvement; 33% reported worsening harassment because of complaint
   2. Unsupportive responses are frequent
      a. Denial
      b. Minimization ("This isn't such a problem; you are just overreacting")
      c. Blaming complainer for causing organization trouble
      d. Blaming complainer for causing victimization
      e. Excusing behavior, often because of value of perpetrator to organization
      f. Labeling the problem a personality conflict
      g. Telling complainer to handle it herself without organizational support ("Keep it secret")
      h. Mobilizing support for perpetrator

III. **An Approach**
   A. **Avoid revictimization**
      1. Do not assume that upset or depressed woman brought harassment on herself

    2. Anxiety and depression are most common emotional presentations to health care provider in this form of abuse and should be viewed as normal responses

    3. One must assume considerable self-doubt, ongoing anger, and depression by the time patient comes to health care provider with symptoms

B. **Solidify therapeutic relationship**

    1. As in other forms of abuse therapy, create sense of safety and trust

    2. Allowing person to discuss situation is most important first step in healing

C. **Keep accurate, careful notes**

    1. Avoid conjectures or speculation

    2. Base notes on what patient reports and on clinical diagnosis of impact

D. **Key therapeutic tasks in recovery from harassment**

    1. Validation: reclaiming self-respect

    2. Empathy: accepting and allowing concern of others as deserving

    3. Empowerment: reclaiming anger and right to act to prevent further victimization

E. **Facilitate consideration** of group therapy, individual therapy, or both (concurrently or sequentially)

    1. Advantages of group therapy

       a. Facilitates validation of experience

       b. Expands database about magnitude of problem (in group discussions, things that were not recognized as abusive get discussed by others)

       c. Emotional support from more than one person

       d. Forum for developing strategies and solutions that allows multiple ideas, experiences, and input to come into discussion of options

    2. Advantages of individual therapy (12% of victims of sexual harassment seek individual psychological help)

       a. Greater focus on impact on individual self-esteem

       b. Allows better evaluation of depressive side effects

       c. More effective when patient has family or interpersonal history of victimization because it deals with interaction between past and current experiences

       d. Therapeutic alliance may allow greater sense of safety in working through issues

SUGGESTED READING

1. Baldwin DC Jr, Daughterty SR, Eckenfels EJ: Student perceptions of mistreatment and harassment during medical school: A survey of ten United States schools. West J Med 155:140–145, 1991.

2. Charney DA, Russell RC: An overview of sexual harassment. Am J Psychol 151:1, 1994.

3. Crull P: Stress Effects of Sexual Harassment on the Job. New York, Working Women's Institute, 1981.

4. Equal Employment Opportunities Commission: Guidelines on discrimination because of sex. Fed Reg 45:74676–74677, 1980.

5. Gruber JE, Bjorn L: Blue-collar blues: The sexual harassment of women autoworkers. Work Occup 9:271–298, 1982.

6. Gutek BA: Sex and the Workplace: Impact of Sexual Behavior and Harassment on Women, Men, and Organizations. San Francisco, Jossey-Bass, 1985.

7. Gutek BA, Koss MP: Effects of sexual harassment on women and organizations. Occup Med State Art Rev 8:807–819, 1993.

8. Gutek BA, Nakamura CY, Cahart M, et al: Sexuality in the workplace. Basic Appl Soc Psychol 1:255–265, 1980.

9. Hamilton JA, Alagna SW, King LS, Lloyd C: The emotional consequences of gender-based abuse in the workplace: New counseling programs for sexual discrimination. In Braude M (ed): Women, Power, and Therapy. New York, Harrington Park Press, 1987.

10. Lafontaine E, Tredeau L: The frequency, sources, and correlates of sexual harassment among women in traditional male occupations. Sex Roles 15:433–422, 1986.

11. U.S. Merit Systems Protection Board: Sexual Harassment in the Federal Workplace: Is It a Problem? Washington, DC, U.S. Government Printing Office, 1988.

PART XI

PSYCHOLOGICAL DISORDERS AND SUBSTANCE ABUSE

78. Depression

Mark Larson, M.D.

I. The Issues

Depression is a major cause of disability in the United States. The 1991 estimated cost for major depression exceeded $29 billion; this figure includes costs of treatment (the smallest of the economic costs) and lost productivity due to suicide and absenteeism. Because depression is diagnosed so much more frequently in women than in men, one must consider the effect that family and societal roles play in contributing to its prevalence and identification. One must ask whether, on occasion, the predominance of depression in women represents an understandable, and sometimes logical, adaptation to unacceptable social circumstances that many women feel helpless to change. Understanding the issues of power, uses and abuses of power, and powerlessness is critical in the wider understanding of depression and of individual women who struggle with depression. Clinicians who work with women should be aware of and avoid using the clinical labeling or diagnosis of depression in a way that further oppresses them. Blaming depressed women or labeling them as less competent by virtue of their diagnosis adds to the illness in a socially sanctioned manner in which clinicians routinely participate without thinking. It is critical for a caregiver to adopt a nonvictimizing stance when dealing with this common problem. Useful approaches include helping the woman to uncover the reasons for her sense of powerlessness and hopelessness; to understand that some of these reasons are imposed on her by family, culture, and society; and to know that she has competencies that will be uncovered during recovery.

II. The Theory

A. **Causality**
1. Cognitive models of depression (Beck)
   a. Early development of cognitive ways of processing information in negative, self-effacing manner
   b. Such maladaptive ways of thinking continue through life, exacerbated by life stressors
2. Biologic theories of depression
   a. Neurochemical: complex interactions between neurotransmitter systems and neuroreceptor sensitivity, including norepinephrine, serotonin, and acetylcholine
   b. Neuroendocrine: disturbance of normal hypothalamic–pituitary–adrenal axis
3. Biopsychosocial etiology: integrates biologic with psychological and social factors (Engel)
4. Genetic factors: first-degree relatives of patient with affective disorder have 25–30% chance of developing major or bipolar illness; 50% for monozygotic twins

B. **Types of depression**
1. Major depression (Table 1)
   a. Melancholic type
   b. Seasonal type
2. Bipolar disorders
   a. Bipolar disorder—mixed
   b. Bipolar disorder—manic (Table 2)
   c. Bipolar disorder—depressed
3. Dysthymia (Table 3)

TABLE 1.   DSM–IV Criteria for Major Depressive Episode[1]

1. At least 5 of the following symptoms present nearly every day during the same 2-week period, including one of the first two:
   (1) Depressed mood most of the day
   (2) Markedly diminished interest in, or pleasure in all, or almost all, activities most of the day
   (3) Significant weight loss when not dieting, or weight gain, or decrease or increase in appetite
   (4) Insomnia or hypersomnia
   (5) Psychomotor agitation or retardation
   (6) Fatigue or loss of energy nearly every day
   (7) Consistent feelings of worthlessness, excessive or inappropriate guilt
   (8) Diminished ability to think or concentrate
   (9) Recurrent suicidal thoughts, recurrent suicidal ideation without a specific plan, or a suicide attempt or a specific plan for committing suicide

2. The symptoms do not meet criteria for a mixed episode.

3. The symptoms cause clinically significant distress or impairment in social, occupational, or other important areas of functioning.

4. The symptoms are not due to the direct physiologic effects of a substance or a general medical condition.

5. The symptoms are not better accounted for by bereavement.

C. **Incidence and prevalence**
   1. Lifetime prevalence in all adults: 8.3–20%
   2. Most common psychiatric disorder in women
   3. Female-to-male ratio: 2:1
   4. Higher incidence in lower socioeconomic groups
D. **Risk and protective factors**
   1. Risk factors
      a. Marriage
      b. No work outside home
      c. 3 or more children under 11 years
      d. History of abuse
      e. Family history of depression
      f. Alcohol or substance abuse in family
   2. Protective factors
      a. Confidant, either spouse or significant friend(s)
      b. Employment outside home
      c. Established patterns of self-care, including exercise, recreation
      d. Ability to set limits on expectations of others

TABLE 2.   DSM–IV Criteria for Manic Episode[1]

1. A distinct period of abnormally and persistently elevated, expansive, or irritable mood, lasting at least 1 week.

2. During the period of mood disturbance, 3 or more of the following symptoms have persisted:
   (1) Inflated self-esteem or grandiosity
   (2) Decreased need for sleep
   (3) More talkative than usual or pressure to keep talking
   (4) Flight of ideas or subjective experience that thoughts are racing
   (5) Distractibility
   (6) Increase in goal-directed activity or psychomotor agitation
   (7) Excessive involvement in pleasurable activities that have a high potential for painful consequences

3. The symptoms do not meet criteria for a mixed episode.

4. The mood disturbance is sufficiently severe to cause marked impairment in occupational functioning or in usual social activities or relationships with others or to necessitate hospitalization to prevent harm to self or others, or there are psychotic features.

5. The symptoms are not due to the direct physiologic effects of a substance or a general medical condition.

TABLE 3. DSM–IV Criteria for Dysthymia[1]

1. Depressed mood that occurs most of the day for more days than not for at least 2 years, with at least two of the following criteria, with no more than a 2-month break in symptoms:
   (1) Poor appetite or overeating
   (2) Insomnia or hypersomnia
   (3) Low energy or fatigue
   (4) Decreased self-esteem
   (5) Poor concentration or difficulty making decisions
   (6) Feelings of hopelessness

2. No evidence of:
   (1) Major depressive episode during first 2 years of symptoms
   (2) Manic episode or other diagnosable mood disorder
   (3) Other chronic psychotic disorder
   (4) Direct physiologic effects of a substance or general medical condition

3. The symptoms cause clinically significant distress or impairment in social, occupational, or other important areas of functioning.

E. **Diagnosis**
   1. **History**
      a. Family history of depression
      b. Marital satisfaction, if married
      c. Patient's explanation of depression
      d. History of abuse, current or past
      e. Workplace difficulties or abuse
      f. History suggesting substance abuse or dependence
      g. Recent losses, broadly defined
      h. Support system
      i. Sources of pleasure in life
      j. Lifelong patterns of functioning in caregiver role at expense of self
   2. Rule out **medical illnesses that may mimic depression**, including, but not limited to: hypothyroidism, anemia, dementia and Parkinson's disease.
   3. Consider **depression posing as other medical conditions**
      a. Chronic fatigue
      b. Somatization disorder
      c. Chronic back pain
      d. Chronic headaches
      e. Dementia (pseudodementia)
   4. **Other diagnostic information**
      a. Previous trials with drugs, successful or unsuccessful
      b. Other health conditions that preclude certain drugs
      c. Aggravation of symptoms with hormonal variation
      d. Postpartum history
      e. Availability of therapists
      f. Patient's interest in therapy
      g. Support system availability
      h. **Depression inventories**
         i. Beck Depression Inventory (BDI)
         ii. Hammond Depression Scale (HAM-D)
   5. **Possible laboratory work-up** (depending on history)
      a. Complete blood count
      b. Drug screen
      c. Blood chemistry (liver, renal, iron, electrolytes, glucose, calcium)
      d. Thyroid-stimulating hormone, thyroxine
      e. Depending on history
         i. Venereal Disease Research Laboratory (VDRL) test for syphilis
         ii. Vitamin B_{12}
         iii. Arterial blood gases (if hypoxia present)

      iv. Electrocardiogram

      v. Human immunodeficiency virus (HIV) test

      vi. Heavy metal screen

  6. **Common medications that may cause depression**

    a. Antihypertensives (clonidine, guanethidine, methyldopa, beta blockers, reserpine, thiazides, and spironolactone)

    b. Hormonal agents (danazol, progesterone, oral contraceptives, and adrenocorticotropic hormone)

    c. Psychotropic drugs (anxiolytics, hypnotics, and neuroleptics)

III. **An Approach**

  A. **Guidelines for initiating treatment**

    1. Present clear and hopeful description of what depression is and explain plan to join with patient to treat it, including:

      a. Brief description of presumed biologic mechanism

      b. Recognition of role of psychosocial stressors

      c. Probability of improvement of symptoms with treatment

    2. First establish immediate safety of patient by assessing and managing suicidality

      a. Hospitalization and psychiatric referral are indicated if

        i. In opinion of physician, patient is eminently suicidal and sufficient environmental supports cannot be accessed

        ii. Psychotic symptoms, especially mood congruent delusions, direct patient to harm self

        iii. Patient is so regressed that she is unable to care for self or to assist others in caring for self

        iv. Medical, psychiatric, and social problems are so complex and interconnected that patient cannot be properly treated on outpatient basis

    3. Treat medical conditions that may contribute to depressive symptoms

    4. If possible, eliminate drugs that may intensify or exacerbate depressive symptoms

    5. Address and begin treatment for substance abuse problems

    6. Educate patient about depression, with referral to relevant books and articles, support groups, and frank discussions about significant contributing stresses

    7. Referral for interpersonal or cognitive/behavioral therapy should be entertained

    8. Referral for marital or family therapy should be entertained if marital or family relationships significantly affect patient in negative or counterproductive manner

    9. Because women suffering from depression are usually less physically active, less goal-directed, and more socially isolated, the following behavioral expectations are usually helpful; physician should allow for small incremental steps and not become frustrated or punitive toward patient if tasks are not accomplished

      a. Increase physical activity

      b. Structure daily activities

      c. Increase social contacts

  B. **Psychotherapy**

    1. May be helpful primary treatment in milder depressions and useful adjunctive treatment with medical management for more serious depressions

    2. Primary care physician should become acquainted with several well-trained psychotherapists in order to make timely, appropriate referrals

    3. Cognitive and interpersonal psychotherapy have been shown to be roughly equivalent in efficacy to medications in treatment of mild-to-moderate major depression

    4. Combining medications with psychotherapy appears to increase efficacy and improve outcome in moderate-to-severe depression

      a. Tends to improve cognitive, interpersonal, and self-esteem disturbance first

      b. Antidepressant medications tend to improve vegetative component of depression first, such as sleep disturbance, appetite disturbance, fatigue, difficulty in concentration, and low motivation

  C. **Pharmacotherapy**

    1. Choice of medication should be tailored to health profile of patient, particular symptoms to be addressed, and side-effect profile of medication (Table 4)

TABLE 4. Pharmacotherapy Guidelines*

Predominant Symptom	Drug(s) to Be Considered
Sleeplessness	Amitriptyline
Fatigue, lack of energy	Selective serotonin reuptake inhibitors
Obsessions/compulsions	Clomipramine or fluoxetine
Agitation or panic	Imipramine
Elderly/those with cardiovascular disease	Trazodone, sertraline
Overweight patient	Bupropion, fluoxetine, monoamine oxidase inhibitors

* Drugs mentioned only as possibilities and not as exclusive recommendations.

2. **General guidelines**
   a. Family physician should be able to provide thoughtful, consistent, and effective treatment for uncomplicated major depressive disorders; referral to psychiatrist for
      i. Bipolar disorder presenting as depression
      ii. Chronic depression unresponsive to previous treatment
      iii. Depression with psychotic symptoms
   b. Prescribing of antidepressant should always be preceded by brief description of presumed mode of action, target symptoms, and most common side effects
      i. Make very clear that usual onset of action of all antidepressants is 2–4 weeks
      ii. Patient should not have unrealistic expectations
   c. Many people have strong feelings about taking medications for emotional symptoms; patient's attitude and expectations should be explored and misconceptions clarified
   d. Physician should allow adequate time to address questions and concerns and to set structure for follow-up visits
   e. Return appointments should be scheduled weekly or every other week until symptoms begin to improve
   f. Medications should be ordered in amounts less than lethal dose initially for all patients and always for patients with suicidal ideation
3. **Tricyclic antidepressants** (TCAs)
   a. Mainstay in office treatment of depression for over 30 years
   b. Side effects represent serious obstacle to therapeutic response
   c. Family physician should become thoroughly familiar with dosing regimen, side effects, and therapeutic characteristics of at least one tertiary and one secondary amine TCA
   d. Often require persistence and strong working relationship with patient
   e. To limit side effects, frequently starting dose is 10–25% of ultimate dose needed for therapeutic effect
   f. Caution advised when contemplating use of TCAs in elderly or people with pre-existing cardiac disease
   g. Most effective when side effects can be used to therapeutic advantage
   h. Common **side effects** of all TCAs relate to effect on various receptors
      i. Inhibition of cholinergic receptor is responsible for dry mouth, constipation, blurred vision, urinary retention, sinus tachycardia, sweating, and cognitive deficits (especially in elderly)
      ii. Inhibition of histamine receptor accounts for sedation, weight gain, and hypotension
      iii. Inhibition of adrenergic receptor is responsible for orthostatic hypotension and reflex tachycardia
      iv. Quinidine-like effect on heart can cause prolonged PR and QRS interval and chronic sinus tachycardia
   i. Serious events associated with TCAs include seizures, urinary blockade, paralytic ileus, and delirium or mania; they are more common with tertiary amine tricyclics.

      j. Quite lethal at doses 10 times usual therapeutic dose

          i. Mean lethal dose for adults: about 1500 mg of either imipramine or amitriptyline

          ii. In potentially suicidal patient, care must be taken in prescribing large amounts of medication

      k. **Tertiary amine** TCAs (amitriptyline, imipramine, doxepin, trimipramine)

          i. More anticholinergic, antihistaminic, and antiadrenergic than secondary amine TCAs and thus cause more of above side effects

          ii. May be particularly effective in treatment of depression characterized by intense agitation, insomnia, and loss of appetite

          iii. Imipramine and amitriptyline have been shown to be effective in treatment of panic disorder and some chronic pain syndromes, both of which may be seen as comorbid states in many depressive syndromes

          iv. Total dose usually given at bedtime to take advantage of sedative side effects

          v. Usual starting dose of 25–50 mg at bedtime increased by 25–50 mg every 3–10 days until tolerance or therapeutic effect (usually 100–300 mg/day)

          vi. Reasonably helpful blood levels can be obtained on amitriptyline and imipramine after steady state and should be done at doses of 150 mg/day if no response is noted after 2 weeks; blood levels help to direct future dose changes

      l. **Secondary amine** TCAs (nortriptyline, desipramine, protriptyline)

          i. In general have fewer anticholinergic and antihistaminic side effects but are more likely to cause stimulation and impaired sleep

          ii. For many clinicians, nortriptyline is preferred TCA, due to

            (a) Equal efficacy with more tolerable side-effect profile

            (b) Easy dosing regimen

              (i) Start at 25–50 mg/day

              (ii) Increase by 25 mg every week until tolerance or 100 mg is reached

              (iii) Blood level after steady state helps to direct dosage changes

              (iv) Usual therapeutic dose: 75–150 mg/day

            (c) Accurate blood levels and therapeutic window of effectiveness

              (i) Blood should be drawn 12 hr after last dose of nortriptyline

          iii. Desipramine

            (a) Least sedating of commonly used TCAs

            (b) May be most effective in treatment of depression with prominent symptoms of lethargy, fatigue, and hypersomnia

            (c) Usual effective dose: 100–300 mg/day

            (d) Accurate blood levels help in adjusting dose

    m. **Benefits**

          i. Treatment cost with imipramine and amitriptyline is significantly less than with any other medication (roughly 1/10 the cost)

          ii. Accurate blood levels can be helpful in determining causes for unresponsiveness to antidepressant treatment

4. **Selective serotonin reuptake inhibitors (SSRIs)**

    a. Preferred agents for initial office treatment of depressive orders

    b. **Benefits**

          i. Selectively affect serotonin system and therefore cause fewer side effects related to adrenergic, cholinergic, or histaminergic system; side effects tend to be milder and less frequent

          ii. Lack of serious side effects, including cardiotoxicity, make them preferable agents for elderly

          iii. Lack of serious toxicity in overdoses makes them preferable agents for potentially suicidal patient

          iv. Ease of dosing makes them easier for patient to take and easier for physician to prescribe adequate doses; this limits subtherapeutic dosing, a common problem with TCAs

c. **Common side effects**
   i. Often occur early and slowly improve with continued use
   ii. Gastrointestinal side effects: nausea, stomach cramps, loose stools, diarrhea, anorexia
   iii. Headaches, especially in people already prone to migraine or tension-vascular headaches
   iv. Changes in level of arousal or psychomotor activity
     (a) Anxiety, nervousness, tremor, insomnia
     (b) Somnolence, weakness, fatigue
   v. Sexual dysfunction, particularly decreased libido or anorgasmia,
     (a) Inquire about sexual side effects of all antidepressant medication
     (b) Frequent but often unreported
d. **Comparison of SSRIs**
   i. Fluoxetine
     (a) Dose range: 10–60 mg/day
     (b) Usual dose: 20 mg/day
     (c) Has longest half-life (1–3 days) and active metabolite with longer half-life (4–16 days)
     (d) Potent inhibitor of hepatic isoenzyme P450—may lead to increased plasma levels of certain drugs, such as TCAs and neuroleptics
   ii. Sertraline
     (a) Dose range: 25–200 mg/day
     (b) Usual adult dose: 50–100 mg/day
     (c) Has half-life of 62–104 hr
     (d) Also inhibits hepatic isoenzyme P450
     (e) Most stimulating of SSRIs and may be more likely to cause nervousness and insomnia
   iii. Paroxetine
     (a) Dose range: 10–50 mg/day
     (b) Usual adult dose: 20 mg/day
     (c) Has half-life of 21 hr with no active metabolites
     (d) Most selective for serotonin of all SSRIs
     (e) Also inhibits hepatic isoenzyme P450
     (f) May be more sedating than other SSRIs with fewer GI side effects
   iv. Fluvoxamine
     (a) Dose range: 50–300 mg/day, q d or bid
   v. Citalopram
     (a) Dose range 20–60 mg/day
     (b) Usual adult dose 20 mg/day
     (c) Minimal inhibitor of hepatic isoenzyme P450

5. **Atypical antidepressants**
a. **Bupropion**
   i. Aminoketone and weak dopamine uptake blocker with little effect on serotonin or norepinephrine reuptake
   ii. Mechanism of action yet to be determined
   iii. Efficacy in major depression comparable to TCAs
   iv. Dose range: 225–450 mg/day
   v. Short half-life requires dosing 2–3 times/day
   vi. Side effects
     (a) Increased incidence of seizures at higher doses
       (i) Should not exceed 150 mg at one time and 450 mg total daily dose
       (ii) Should be used with caution in patients with preexisting seizure disorder
       (iii) Not lethal if taken in overdose
     (b) May cause GI disturbances, weight loss, nervousness, restlessness, and insomnia

      (c) Better side-effect profile than TCAs
         (i) Little sedation
        (ii) Few cognitive impairments
       (iii) Few anticholinergic side effects
       (iv) Few cardiovascular effects
        (v) No orthostatic hypotension
      (vi) Probably least likely to cause sexual side effects of presently available antidepressants
    vii. Good alternative to SSRIs as first- or second-line treatment of major depression when sedation not desired

  b. **Trazodone**
     i. First antidepressant not lethal in overdose
    ii. Appears to work primarily through serotonergic system
   iii. Rapid metabolism and half-life of 3–9 hr usually require divided doses
   iv. Dose range: from 200–500 mg/day
    v. Usual therapeutic dose: around 300 mg/day
   vi. If taken with food, drug absorption may improve and limit nausea, dizziness, and acute drop in blood pressure
  vii. Sedation and cognitive slowing may be significant side effects and limit clinical use
      (a) Also may be used to clinical advantage
      (b) Frequently used in lower doses (25–100 mg) with SSRIs when insomnia is significant symptom or side effect of SSRI
  viii. Significantly fewer anticholinergic side effects than TCAs
   ix. May cause significant orthostatic hypotension
    x. May cause priapism in small percentage of men
   xi. Other side effects include headaches and nausea; seldom severe and often improve with continued use

  c. **Nefazodone**
     i. Related to trazodone, but probably more potent 5-HT receptor antagonist at postsynaptic receptor and weaker serotonin reuptake inhibitor
    ii. Short half-life (2–5 hr) requires twice daily dosing
   iii. Relatively high doses necessary for efficacy (400–600 mg/day)
   iv. Appears to have more favorable side effect profile, with virtually no cardiotoxic, anticholinergic, or histaminergic activity
    v. Emergent side effects include sedation, dizziness, asthenia, dry mouth, nausea, constipation, headache, amblyopia

  d. **Venlafaxine**
     i. Newly approved antidepressant chemically unrelated to TCAs or SSRIs
    ii. Probably works by blocking both serotonin and norepinephrine
   iii. Short half-life (3–5 hr) requires twice daily dosage
   iv. Starting dose of 75 mg/day in divided doses can be increased up to 375 mg/day for severe depression
    v. Considered primarily second-line agent by many because of problematic side-effect profile
      (a) Substantial nausea and sexual side effects
      (b) Cardiovascular effects include sustained elevations in blood pressure, heart rate, and cholesterol levels
        (i) Elevations in blood pressure appear to be dose-dependent and range from 3% at doses < 100 mg/day to 13% at doses > 300 mg/day
       (ii) Blood pressure needs to be monitored regularly
      (c) Quite activating and may cause nervousness, insomnia, and anorexia
      (d) Other side effects include headaches, somnolence, and dizziness
   vi. Appears to be particularly effective in treatment of depression unresponsive to multiple medical treatments

D. **Special treatment considerations**
  1. **Depression in women of child-bearing age**

    a. TCAs are only antidepressants that have been around long enough to allow physician to feel confident that significant teratogenicity would be known

    b. Prudent clinical practice still dictates minimal use of any medication during pregnancy

    c. However, serious depression can also have profound impact on pregnancy and mother–child relationship

    d. Cost/benefit ratio can be difficult to determine because physician needs to take into account needs and risks of mother and fetus or nursing child

    e. Following guidelines may be helpful

       i. Significant teratogenic consequences from antidepressants have yet to be shown, but objective information is seriously lacking

      ii. Assume all antidepressants are present in fetal circulation as well as breast milk and that medication side effects or side effects experienced by mother could be experienced by fetus or nursing infant

     iii. Women in child-bearing mode taking antidepressants should be strongly advised to use birth control while taking medication and to stop antidepressants before trying to conceive

     iv. When possible, pharmacotherapy should be reserved till after first trimester; active psychotherapy can be helpful during this time

      v. When potential risks are outweighed by therapeutic need, a secondary amine TCA or SSRI should be used

2. **Psychotic depression**

    a. Depression presenting concomitantly with psychotic symptoms such as auditory or visual hallucinations, delusions, bizarre behavior, or disorganized thinking usually needs to be treated with combination of antidepressant and antipsychotic medication or electroconvulsive therapy

    b. Because psychotic depressions are more unpredictable and more potentially lethal, referral to psychiatrist is strongly recommended

3. **Postpartum depression**

    a. Should be diagnosed early and treated aggressively because it may seriously interfere with mother–infant bonding

    b. Often women prone to recurrent episodes of major depression experience first episode after birth of child; proper education allows early recognition and treatment of future bouts

SUGGESTED READING

1. American Psychiatric Association: Diagnostic and Statistical Manual of Mental Disorders, 4th ed (DSM–IV). Washington, DC, American Psychiatric Association, 1994.
2. Beckham EE, Leber WR, Youll LK: The diagnostic classification of depression. In Beckham EE, Leber WR (eds): Handbook of Depression, 2nd ed. New York, Guilford, 1995, pp 36–60.
3. Cadieux RJ: Practical management of treatment resistant depression. Am Fam Physician 58:2059–2062, 1998.
4. Goetz RP, Fields SA, Toffler WL: Depression. In Taylor R (ed): Family Medicine: Principles and Practice. New York, Springer-Verlag, 1993, pp 234–240.
5. Holder DPO, Anderson CM: Women, work, and the family. In McGoldrick M, Anderson CM, Walsh F (eds): Women in Families: A Framework for Family Therapy. New York, W.W. Norton, 1989, pp 357–381.
6. Majeroni B, Hess A: The pharmacologic treatment of depression. J Am Board Fam Prac 11:98–110, 1998.
7. Pajer K: New strategies in the treatment of depression in women. J Clin Psychiatry 56(Suppl 2):30–37, 1995.
8. Regier DA, Boyd JH, Burke JD, et al: One month prevalence of mental disorders in the U.S. based on five Epidemiological Catchment Area sites. Arch Gen Psychiatry 45:977–986, 1988.
9. Saeed SA, Bruce TJ: Seasonal affective disorders. Am Fam Physician 57:1340–1346, 1998.
10. Torgersen S: Genetic factors in moderately severe and mild affective disorders. Arch Gen Psychiatry 43:222–226, 1986.
11. Williams JW Jr, Rost K, Dietrich AJ, et al: Primary care physician's approach to depressive disorders. Arch Fam Med 8:58–67, 1999.

79. Anxiety

Mark Larson, M.D.

I. The Issues

Anxiety is a normal emotion that becomes problematic when it is excessive, chronic, or inappropriately triggered. Whether anxiety states are pathologic systems or natural consequences of the perceptions and interpretations of life events as shaped by individual history is still an open question. Patients successfully treated with psychotherapy and no medication consistently show the same physiologic changes as patients treated successfully with medication. All categories of anxiety disorders are more common in women than men (Table 1). The DSM–IV differentiates a large number of categories of anxiety disorders, although no evidence suggests a single underlying mechanism that collectively defines them. Anxiety is often mixed with depression and in many cases cannot be reliably differentiated from depression. Anxiety disorders are often concomitant with substance abuse and may be causally interrelated, either preceding or consequent to substance abuse.

II. The Theory

   A. **Basic classification of anxiety disorders in DSM–IV**
   1. **Panic disorders**
      a. Prevalence: twice as high for women as for men
      b. Characterized by severe and intense periods of discomfort and/or fear that come on unexpectedly and rapidly develop to peak intensity, subsiding usually within 10 minutes or less
      c. Dominant symptoms include;
         i. Sudden onset of palpitations
         ii. Chest pain
         iii. Choking sensations
         iv. Dizziness
         v. Feeling of unreality
      d. Nearly all patients with panic disorder have sense of extreme danger and intense need to escape or flee from it
      e. Although unexpected to patient, first identifiable panic attacks almost always occur during periods of high stress
   2. **Agoraphobia**
      a. Usually associated with panic disorder; diagnosis of either without the other is extremely rare
      b. Characterized by extreme anxiety and desire to avoid situations in which escape might be difficult or help unavailable if panic attack were to occur
   3. **Specific phobias**
      a. Characterized by fears and avoidance of specific objects and situations with realization that fear is excessive or unreasonable
      b. Phobias of objects that are avoidable rarely require treatment
      c. Changes in life circumstances such as marriage or employment may bring previously benign fears to crisis proportions, requiring intervention
      d. Begin most often either in late adolescence or in early 30s but onset may be at any age
   4. **Social phobias**
      a. Characterized by persistent marked fear and avoidance of social and/or performance situations
      b. Only anxiety-related disorder with nearly equal prevalence among men and women
      c. Epidemiologic studies show women slightly outnumbering men, but men make up the majority of most clinical samples
   5. **Obsessive compulsive disorder** (OCD)
      a. Characterized by recurrent obsessions and/or compulsions that are time-consuming and disruptive of everyday activities

TABLE 1. Lifetime Prevalence of Various Anxiety Disorders*

Disorder	Women (%)	Men (%)
Panic disorder	2.10	0.99
Agoraphobia	7.86	3.18
Specific phobia	14.45	7.75
Social phobia	2.91	2.53
Generalized anxiety disorder	6.86	4.51
Obsessive compulsive disorder	3.04	2.03

* Data from the Epidemiologic Catchment Area Study.[6]

      b. Realization by patient (at least at some point in history) that they are excessive or unreasonable
      c. May be basis of eating disorder in some cases
  6. **Posttraumatic stress disorder**
      a. Often sequel to violent personal assault
      b. Characterized by recurrent intrusive memories and images regarding trauma
      c. Phobic avoidance of stimuli associated with trauma
      d. Insomnia
      e. Bursts of irritability and anger
      f. Nightmares
      g. Exaggerated startle response
  7. **Acute stress disorder**
      a. Anxiety reaction immediately following traumatic stressor
         i. Some stressors are universal
        ii. Life history may determine or mediate extent to which event is considered stressful
      b. Symptoms include dissociation, de realization, and depersonalization as well as anxiety symptoms
      c. Practitioners with long-standing relationships with victims may be instrumental in identifying disorder
  8. **Generalized anxiety disorder and overanxious disorder of childhood**
      a. Characterized by excessive anxiety and worry over various concerns
      b. Sufferer feels little control
      c. Overlaps substantially with depression and may not exist independently
      d. Unrelenting symptoms for at least 6 months
  9. **Anxiety disorder due to general medical condition**
      a. Anxiety directly attributable to general medical condition (e.g., thyrotoxicosis, pheochromocytoma)
      b. Does not apply to anxiety concomitant with physical changes such as menstruation or climacteric (diagnosed in DSM–IV as adjustment disorder with anxiety)
  10. **Substance-induced anxiety disorder**
      a. Anxiety directly attributable to effects of ingested substance (e.g., cocaine-induced panic)
B. **Causes**
  1. **Neuroanatomic bases:** most areas of brain have been implicated in anxiety, especially frontal cortex, septohippocampal system, amygdala, raphe nuclei, and locus coeruleus
  2. **Neurotransmitter systems**
      a. Gamma-aminobutyric acid (GABA) system
         i. Inhibitory system believed to be deficient in anxiety
        ii. GABAergic systems perhaps exert tonic control over serotonergic systems from median raphe
       iii. Controversy: whether anxiolytic effects of benzodiazepines occur through mechanism of GABA-dependent receptors

b. 5-Hydroxytryptamine (serotonin)
    i. Less substantiated by research
    ii. Implicated by anxiolytic effects of serotonergic drugs, such as buspirone, which are 5-HT receptor subtype-specific ligands

3. **Cognitive perceptual systems**
    a. Anxiety symptoms viewed catastrophically by panic victims
        i. Lead to alarm reactions and increasing cycle of alarm reaction
        ii. Most anxiety disorders can be characterized as intense effort to avoid feeling anxiety symptoms
    b. Avoidance of anxiety-related stimuli reinforces beliefs that sufferer is unable to cope with her responses to such stimuli

4. Conditioning: stimuli associated with traumatic events trigger conditioned responses that may become anxiety symptoms

III. **An Approach**
    A. **Assessment**
        1. Full history and physical exam are necessary to rule out anxiety due to general medical condition or substance abuse
        2. Determine what elicits anxiety
            a. Anxiety log filled out as soon after anxiety occurs as possible
            b. Determine what events precede or predict distress
            c. Determine what kind of thoughts are present before and during anxiety episodes
            d. Collaborative effort that encourages patient to discover her own anxiety triggers fosters general problem-solving perspective that may prevent relapse
        3. Determine what is avoided
            a. Find out what patient feels she cannot do or experience
            b. Encourage patient to contemplate what she believes will happen if she is exposed to avoided stimulus
            c. Explore whether expectations are realistic

    B. **Nonpharmacologic treatment**
        1. **Empathic listening:** general physician can offer openness and understanding
            a. Open and understanding ear can do wonders
            b. Social support predicts recovery from stress better than any other variable
        2. **Education**
            a. Patients benefit greatly from understanding physiologic basis of their feelings and logical rationale for their experience
            b. Suggest self-help books that include programmatic behavioral approaches to overcoming anxiety
        3. **Relaxation and stress management**
            a. Either progressive muscle relaxation training or image-based relaxation can be conducted in office and practiced at home
            b. Teach diaphragmatic breathing
            c. Patients should be encouraged to reduce caffeine use
        4. **Cognitive and cognitive-behavioral therapies**
            a. Acute treatment improvement rates 80–90%
            b. Helping anxious patient to change beliefs about ability to endure symptoms of anxiety
            c. Important step toward eventual exposure and relaxation of vigilance against anxiety symptoms
        5. **Exposure and response prevention**
            a. Gradual exposure to feared situations without fleeing is single most active component in all behavioral treatments for anxiety and has been implicated as most active component even of medication treatment
            b. Physician's desire to monitor and reinforce progress in patient-directed program can make difference between whether plans are merely entertained or actually executed
            c. Feedback should be provided every 1–2 weeks until substantial progress has been made
            d. Prepare patients to expect increase in anxiety during initial stages before improvement occurs

C. **Pharmacotherapy**
1. Possible agents
   a. **Serotonergic drugs**—selective serotonin reuptake inhibitors (sertraline, paroxetine, fluvoxamine, fluoxetine, and citalopram)
      i. Appropriate first-line therapy
      ii. Effective in treating OCD
      iii. Some studies demonstrated efficacy with panic disorder
   b. **Buspirone**—efficacy in panic disorder unresolved
   c. **Tricyclic antidepressants** (imipramine, clomipramine, nortriptyline, and desipramine)
      i. Significant adverse drug effects
      ii. Start low dose, gradually increasing to desired therapeutic effect
   d. **Benzodiazepines**
      i. Early adjunctive treatment for symptom control
      ii. Second- or third-line treatment option
      iii. Demonstrated effective in treatment of generalized anxiety disorder and (in high doses) panic disorder
      iv. Problems with tolerance, dependence, interactions with other substances such as alcohol, and sedative impairment should be considered before prescribing
   e. **Monoamine oxidase inhibitors** (MAOIs)
      i. Shown to be effective in treatment of panic disorder and social phobia
      ii. Severe side effects caution against use
   f. **Beta blockers**
      i. Adjunctive treatment
      ii. Mixed clinical results
      iii. Possibly indirect effect through amelioration of peripheral symptoms
2. **Anxiety or depression?**
   a. Symptoms of anxiety disorders and depression coexist, often posing dilemma to clinician as to which to treat as primary
   b. Many anxiolytic medications are effective antidepressants, and many antidepressants are effective in reducing anxiety
3. **Age considerations:** special precautions necessary when considering pharmacotherapy with children and adolescents and elderly
4. **Medications and pregnancy**
   a. No anxiolytic drug has been shown to be safe during pregnancy
   b. Most clinical trials have excluded women of child-bearing age
5. In most cases final selection of pharmacotherapeutic agent depends on balancing of risk against benefit, considering age, medical status, patient expectations, dependency risks, and potential side effects

SUGGESTED READING

1. American Psychiatric Association: Diagnostic and Statistical Manual of Mental Disorders, 4th ed (DSM–IV). Washington, DC, American Psychiatric Association, 1994.
2. Ballenger JC: Panic disorder in the medical setting. J Clin Psychiatry 58(Suppl 10):11–18, 1997.
3. Barlow DH: Cognitive-behavioral therapy for panic disorder: Current status. J Clin Psychiatry 58(Suppl 2):32–36, 1997.
4. Davidson JR: Use of benzodiazepines in panic disorder. J Clin Psychiatry 58(Suppl 2):26–8, 1997.
5. Hollifield M, Katon W, Skipper B, et al: Panic disorder and quality of life: Variables predictive of functional impairment. Am J Psychiatry 154:766–772, 1997.
6. Robins LN, Regier DA (eds): Psychiatric Disorders in America: The Epidemiologic Catchment Area Study. New York, Macmillan, 1991.
7. Rosenbaum JF (ed): Treatment of Panic Disorder: The State of the Art. J Clin Psychiatry, Vol. 58, Suppl. 2, 1997.
8. Saeed SA, Bruce TJ: Panic disorder: Effective treatment options. Am Fam Physician 57:2405–2412, 1998.
9. Shear MK, Weiner K: Psychotherapy for panic disorder. J Clin Psychiatry 58(Suppl 2):38–43, 1997.
10. Sheehan DV, Harnett-Sheehan K: The role of SSRIs in panic disorder. J Clin Psychiatry 57(Suppl 10):51–58, 1996.

11. van Balcom AJ, Bakker A, Spinhoven P, et al: A meta-analysis of the treatment of panic disorder with or without agoraphobia: A comparison of psychopharmacological, cognitive-behavioral, and combination therapies. J Nerv Ment Dis 185:510–516, 1997.

80. Somatization

Mark Larson, M.D.

I. **The Issues**

It has been estimated that somatization accounts for 50% of American health care costs. Somatization disorder is defined in the DSM–IV as "a pattern of recurring, multiple, somatic complaints . . . [that] cannot be fully explained by any known general medical condition or the direct effects of a substance." Although somatization disorder, when diagnosed according to the DSM–IV, is relatively low in prevalence among the general population, 1% of the American population according to the 1997 Epidemiologic Catchment Area Survey, it is more highly prevalent in practice because of the high rate of help-seeking among somatizers. Somatization disorder is an almost exclusively female disorder.

II. **The Theory**

  A. **DSM–IV diagnostic criteria** include the following:

    1. Multiple, recurring complaints

      a. Begin before 30 years of age

      b. Symptoms occur over "several" years

      c. Frequent treatment-seeking or impairment in social, occupational, or other important areas of functioning

    2. Four pain symptoms: a history of pain related to at least four different sites or functions (e.g.; head abdomen, back, joints, extremities, chest, rectum, during menstruation, during sexual intercourse, or during urination)

    3. Two gastrointestinal symptoms: a history of at least two gastrointestinal symptoms other than pain (e.g.; nausea, bloating, vomiting other than during pregnancy, diarrhea, or intolerance of several different foods)

    4. One sexual symptom: a history of at least one sexual or reproductive symptom other than pain (e.g., sexual indifference, erectile or ejaculatory dysfunction, irregular menses, excessive menstrual bleeding, vomiting throughout pregnancy)

    5. One pseudoneurologic symptom: history of at least one symptom or deficit suggesting a neurologic condition not limited to pain (conversion symptoms such as impaired coordination or balance, paralysis or localized weakness, difficulty swallowing or lump in throat, aphonia, urinary retention, hallucinations, loss of touch or pain sensation, double vision, blindness, deafness, seizures, dissociative symptoms such as amnesia; or loss of consciousness other than fainting)

    6. Either a or b below

      a. After full investigation, none of above symptoms can be explained by physical condition

      b. When physical condition is present, complaints or associated impairment is excessive in relation to condition

  B. **Somatization syndrome:** more than 4 but fewer than the 8 symptoms required to meet diagnosis for somatization disorder

  C. **Comorbidity:** consider the possibility of:

    1. Major depressive disorder

    2. Anxiety disorders

    3. Adjustment disorder

  D. **Factitious disorder or malingering**

    1. Symptoms intentionally produced to achieve desired consequence (malingering)

    2. Symptoms have no apparent gain (factitious disorder)

E. **Cause:** likely multifactorial
  1. **Amplification:** pain sensations that would otherwise go unnoticed are amplified because of either hypersensitivity or hyper vigilance
  2. **Catastrophization:** pain sensations are misinterpreted as signs of serious medical problems
  3. **Stigmatization:** relief from psychiatric problems is sought through more acceptable somatic symptoms
  4. **Communication dysfunction:** inability to articulate nature of acutely felt emotional distress which may lead to descriptions in bodily terms
  5. **Reinforcement:** previous acceptance of somatic symptoms at face value by physicians and family members reinforces somatization
  6. **Family dynamics:** especially in children, somatic symptoms are often concomitant with psychological problems in another family member; family systems sometimes foster one member taking the "sick" role
  7. **Social isolation:** people with low social support have higher levels of health care use
  8. **Economic motivation:** third-party payers may not provide coverage for psychiatric treatment
  9. **Other possible gains:** employer's compensation, pending litigation, avoidance of criminal prosecution, obtaining drugs
F. Some believe that diagnosis of somatization simply reflects inability to identify true physical basis of patient's complaints

III. **An Approach**
  A. **Office management**
    1. Schedule brief appointments and physical exams every 4–6 weeks
    2. Only at set times and not on demand
    3. Avoid laboratory tests, surgery and hospitalization unless absolutely necessary
    4. Avoid suggesting to the patient that the problem is all in her or his mind.
    5. Avoid addictive medications
  B. **Set achievable goals**
    1. Decreased use
    2. Keeping patient to one practice
    3. Improved work or school functioning
  C. **Develop good therapeutic relationship**
    1. Collaborative relationships are best
    2. Stress patient's responsibility for care
    3. Explicitly set out expectations and limits
    4. Consider written agreement or contract
    5. Prescribe treatment and medication on time-contingent basis
  D. **Avoid psychiatric terms and language that implies disability**
    1. Use somatic descriptions and benign somatic diagnoses (e.g., muscle strain)
    2. Be unambiguous in providing information about findings
    3. Educate patient about relationship between stress, anxiety, and somatic symptoms
  E. **Prepare patient for psychological treatment**
    1. Determine that all investigations are complete
    2. Make treatment conditional on no further tests
    3. Develop goals that stress "coping" over "curing"
  F. **Involve family members and other social support**
  G. **Be flexible**
    1. Negotiation always necessary
    2. Expect change to be gradual
    3. Be suspicious of immediate cures

SUGGESTED READING

1. American Psychiatric Association: Diagnostic and Statistical Manual of Mental Disorders, 4th ed (DSM–IV). Washington, DC, American Psychiatric Association, 1994.
2. Barbee JG, Todorov AA, Kuczmierczyk AR, et al: Explained and unexplained medical symptoms in generalized anxiety and panic disorder: Relationship to somatoform disorders. Ann Clin Psychiatry 9:149–155, 1997.

3. Battaglia M, Bernardeschi L, Politi E, et al: Comorbidity of panic and somatization disorder: A genetic-epidemiologic approach. Compr Psychiatry 36:411–420, 1995.
4. Furer P, Walker JR, Chartier MJ, Stein MB: Hypochondriacal concerns and somatization in panic disorder. Depress Anxiety 6:78–85, 1997.
5. Goldberg RJ, Novack DH, Gask MB: The recognition and management of somatization. Psychosomatics 33:55–61, 1992.
6. Gureje O, Simon GE, Ustun TB, Golberg DP: Somatization in cross-cultural perspective: A World Health Organization study in primary care. Am J Psychiatry 154:989–995, 1997.
7. Kroenke K, Spitzer RL, deGruy FV 3rd, Swindle R: A symptom checklist to screen for somatoform disorders in primary care. Psychosomatics 39:263–272, 1998.
8. Liu G, Clark MR, Eaton WW: Structural factor analyses for medically unexplained somatic symptoms of somatization disorder in the Epidemiologic Catchment Area study. Psychol Med 27:617–626, 1997.
9. Portegijs PJ, van der Horst FG, Proot IM, et al: Somatization in frequent attenders of general practice. Soc Psychiatry Psychiatr Epidemiol 31:29–37, 1996.
10. Rief W, Heuser J, Mayrhuber E, et al: The classification of multiple somatoform symptoms. J Nerv Ment Dis 184:680–687, 1996.

81. Eating Disorders

Jane L. Murray, M.D.

I. The Issues

Eating disorders appear to be increasing problem in U.S. with females aged 16–35 being the most vulnerable. In this age group, approximately 0.5–1% of women have anorexia nervosa. The prevalence is as high as 7% among modeling and dance students). Bulimia nervosa affects about 1–3% of women aged 16–35, and other eating disorders, not otherwise specified: about 3% prevalence. The female:male ratio approximates 15–20:1 (i.e., about 0.3% total prevalence in males). Eating disorders are more prevalent in Western cultures and in higher socioeconomic groups, and result in significant morbidity and mortality (as high as 18%)

II. The Theory

A. **Types of disordered eating:** over- and undereating; complex psychophysiologic illnesses
  1. Anorexia nervosa
  2. Bulimia nervosa
  3. Partial syndromes, or eating disorders not otherwise specified
  4. Obesity—not defined as a psychiatric condition

B. **DSM–IV diagnostic criteria**
  1. **Anorexia nervosa**
    a. Refusal to maintain body weight over minimally normal weight for age and height; body weight < 85% of expected weight
    b. Intense fear of gaining weight or becoming fat, even though underweight
    c. Disturbance in way body weight or shape is experienced, undue influence of body weight or shape on self-evaluation, or denial of seriousness of current body weight
    d. In postmenarcheal women, absence of at least 3 consecutive menstrual cycles
    e. Two specific subtypes
      i. Restricting type—during current episode person has not regularly engaged in binge eating or purging behavior
      ii. Binge-eating/purging type—during current episode person has regularly engaged in binge-eating or purging behavior
  2. **Bulimia nervosa**
    a. Recurrent episodes of binge eating
      i. Eating in discrete period (e.g., within 2 hr) amount of food that is definitely larger than most people would eat during similar period and under similar circumstances

      ii. Sense of lack of control over eating during episode (e.g., feeling that one cannot stop eating or control what or how much one eats)

   b. Recurrent inappropriate compensatory behavior to prevent weight gain, such as self-induced vomiting; misuse of laxatives, diuretics, enemas, or other medications; fasting; or excessive exercise

   c. Binge eating and inappropriate compensatory behaviors occur, on average, at least twice per week for 3 months

   d. Self-evaluation unduly influenced by body shape and weight

   e. Disturbance does not occur exclusively during episodes of anorexia nervosa

   f. Two subtypes

      i. Purging type—during current episode person has regularly engaged in self-induced vomiting or misuse of laxatives, diuretics, or enemas

      ii. Nonpurging type—during current episode person has used other inappropriate compensatory behaviors, such as fasting or excessive exercise, but has not regularly engaged in self-induced vomiting or misuse of laxatives, diuretics, or enemas

3. **Eating disorder not otherwise specified**

   a. Spectrum of eating disorders exists; no explicit criteria for diagnosis

   b. Partial syndrome may be precursor to frank eating disorder

4. **Obesity** (see Chapter 99)

   a. Medical definition: 15% over ideal body weight for age and height, or body mass index (BMI) greater than 25

   b. Not strictly considered an eating disorder

C. **Social etiology**

1. Overwhelming preponderance of women

2. Strong cultural and social value on thinness in Western cultures (and increasingly elsewhere); negative stereotyping of obesity

   a. Dieting common

   b. Images of beauty in popular press and television are thin women

D. **Biologic etiology**

1. Studies show 56% concordance for anorexia nervosa among monozygotic twins, 7% concordance for dizygotic twins

2. First-degree relatives of people with eating disorder have 4–5 times greater risk than general public of developing eating disorder

3. Once hypothalamic function (e.g., satiety center) is disturbed, disturbance may contribute to perpetuating disorder

E. **Psychological etiology**

1. Despite social and biologic factors, psychological factors seem to predominate in etiology of eating disorders

2. **Individual personality characteristics**

   a. Anorectics tend to display emotional overcontrol, conceptual rigidity, perfectionism, lack of development of the self

      i. Sense of personal ineffectiveness

      ii. Anorexia may be way to gain feeling of control

   b. Bulimics tend to exhibit greater impulsivity and affective instability

3. **Family dynamics**

   a. Above personality factors may be response to deficits in patient–family relationships

      i. Self-starvation may be attempt to break away from internalized controlling mother and strive for separate identity

      ii. Bulimics may have experienced more overt family dysfunction (such as physical, sexual, or emotional abuse)

   b. Common characteristics in anorectics' families: enmeshment, overprotection, rigidity lack of conflict resolution

4. **Developmental factors**

   a. Onset of eating disorders around early adulthood points to possible developmental issues about maturation

TABLE 1.   Signs of Eating Disorders

Cardiovascular	*Metabolic (cont.)*
Bradycardia (under 40 bpm)	Hypophosphatemia
Hypotension	Decreased bone mineral density
EKG changes and arrhythmias	Hypoglycemia
Peripheral edema	Hypoproteinemia
Cardiomyopathy	Muscle weakness/cramps
Mitral valve prolapse	*Gastrointestinal*
Pericardial effusion	Impaired taste perception
Endocrine	Loss of gag reflex
Menstrual irregularities	Esophagitis, bleeding, perforation
Elevated reverse triiodothyronine (rT_3) with	Gastroparesis, bloating, dilatation, bleeding
normal thyroxine (T_4) and thyroid-stimulating	Malabsorption, steatorrhea
hormone (TSH)	Constipation or rectal bleeding
Hypercortisolism	Pancreatitis (especially during refeeding)
Dental	Fatty degeneration of liver
Erosion of enamel	*Pulmonary*
Loss of vertical height of teeth	Aspiration of vomitus
Pulpitis and pulp necrosis	Hypopnea secondary to metabolic alkalosis
Dermatologic	Pneumothorax or pneumomediastinum
Dry skin	due to vomiting
Yellow hue (carotenemia)	*Hematologic*
Metabolic	Anemia—usually normochromic, normocytic
Dehydration	Leukopenia
Hypokalemia	Thrombocytopenia
Hyponatremia	*Neurologic*
Hypochloremia	Lowered seizure threshold
Metabolic acidosis or alkalosis	Ventricular dilatation (pseudoatrophy)
Hypomagnesemia	

     b. Anorexia nervosa may represent phobic avoidance of sexual maturation, thus protecting individual from turmoils of adolescence

     c. Low self-esteem and poor body image are common at this stage of development

  F. **Signs and symptoms** (see Table 1)

III. **An Approach**

  A. **Assessment of underweight patient**

    1. **Weight history:** current, highest ever, lowest ever, premorbid, perceived ideal, menstrual threshold

    2. **Body image**

      a. Attitudes and feelings—overall size and specific body parts

      b. Cosmetic procedures

    3. **Means of weight control**

      a. Caloric intake

        i. Number of calories

        ii. Number of meals

        iii. Binge episodes: frequency, time of day or night, amount and type of food consumed, subjective experience, associated behaviors—stealing, rumination, pica

        iv. Idiosyncratic nutritional beliefs and practices

      b. Purging behaviors

        i. Vomiting (ipecac use)

        ii. Laxatives

        iii. Drugs to control weight—diet pills, diuretics, caffeine, thyroid

      c. Exercise: type and amount

    4. **Physical exam**

      a. General (height and weight relative to age; hair loss, lanugo, jaundice, edema)

      b. Cardiovascular (blood pressure, arrhythmias, bradycardia, murmurs, clicks)

      c. Gastrointestinal (blood in stool, gastroparesis, diarrhea, abdominal tenderness)

    d. Endocrinologic (goiter, parotid enlargement, hypothermia)

    e. Gynecologic (sexual maturation, amenorrhea)

    f. Dermatologic (signs of malnutrition, perioral irritation from gastric contents on skin, periorbital petechiae from vomiting)

    g. Oral and dental (enamel erosion, loss of vertical height of teeth, pulp necrosis, enlarged salivary glands, lacerations of mouth or throat)

    h. Extremities (abrasions, lacerations or calluses on dorsum of hand, fingers, knuckles [Russell's sign]; acrocyanosis)

  5. **Laboratory studies:** complete blood count, electrolytes, blood urea nitrogen, creatinine, EKG (weight loss, ipecac, hypokalemia), liver function tests (weight loss, alcohol abuse), creatine phosphokinase (ipecac), amylase (GI symptoms)—salivary amylase often high in self-induced vomiters, calcium and phosphorus (amenorrhea or fractures), thyroid profile

B. **Initial feedback to patient**

  1. Cessation of dieting behavior

  2. Regular intake of adequate calories (begin at 1,500 and increase to 2,000–3,000 calories/day)

  3. Proscription of laxatives, diet pills, diuretics

  4. Cessation of exercise if underweight

C. **Indications for immediate hospitalization**

  1. Severe fluid or electrolyte disorder

  2. Cardiac complications

    a. Arrhythmia or conduction disturbance

    b. Cardiomyopathy (ipecac)

  3. Acute rapid weight loss

  4. Acute pancreatitis or gastric dilatation

  5. Convulsions

D. **Ongoing medical management**

  1. Close monitoring of weight, fluid and electrolytes, and cardiac status

  2. Psychiatric consultation

  3. Dental consultation

  4. Nutrition consultation

  5. Periodic hospitalization

    a. Psychiatric crises

    b. Specialized unit for eating disorders

E. **Ongoing psychological management and interventions**

  1. Cognitive-behavioral and interpersonal psychotherapies often effective

  2. Comorbidities common, especially depression—may require pharmacologic treatment

  3. Some eating disorders are first manifestation of multiple personality disorder (MPD); only treatment for MPD will improve eating disorder

  4. Family assessment is crucial; family therapy may be useful, especially in younger patients

  5. Family and parent support groups helpful

F. **Presentations that may obscure eating disorder**

  1. Abdominal pain with elevated amylase

  2. Intermittent diarrhea and/or constipation, undisclosed laxative abuse

  3. Hypoglycemia

  4. Hypothyroidism

  5. Premenstrual syndrome

  6. Systemic candidiasis, chronic fatigue, food allergies

G. **Referral resources**

  1. Academy for Eating Disorders, Montefiore Medical School—Adolescent Medicine: (718) 920-6782

  2. American Anorexia Bulimia Association: (212) 575-6200

  3. Anorexia Nervosa and Related Eating Disorders, Inc.: (541) 344-1144

  4. National Eating Disorders Organization: (918) 481-4044

5. National Association of Anorexia Nervosa and Associated Disorders: (847) 831-3438

SUGGESTED READING

1. Herzog DB, Keller MB, Sacks NB, et al: Psychiatry comorbidity in treatment-seeking anorectics and bulimics. J Am Acad Child Adolesc Psychiatry 31:810–818, 1992.
2. Kaplan AS, Garfinkel PE: Medical Issues and the Eating Disorders. New York, Brunner/Mazel, 1993.
3. Kinoy BP: Eating Disorders: New Directions in Treatment and Recovery. New York, Columbia University Press, 1994.
4. McGilley BM, Pryor TL: Assessment and treatment of bulimia nervosa. Am Fam Physician 57:2743–2750, 1998.
5. Siegel M, Brisman J, Weinshel M: Surviving an Eating Disorder: Strategies for Family and Friends. New York, Harper & Row, 1988.
6. Troop NA, Holbrey A, Trowler R, et al: Ways of coping in women with eating disorders. J Nerv Ment Dis 182:535–540, 1994.

82. Nicotine Dependence and Smoking Cessation

Bruce S. Liese, Ph.D.

I. The Issues

Cigarette smoking is deadly. Nonetheless, millions of men, women, and children in the United States smoke cigarettes. At one time there was a substantial difference in prevalence rates between men and women; that is, many more men smoked than women. Presently, however, women are catching up to men in rates of smoking. This fact is reflected in increased smoking-related morbidity and mortality rates for women. The primary care physician has an important role in helping women to quit smoking.

II. The Theory

A. Epidemiology

1. Prevalence
   a. In 1995, 22.6% of women were cigarette smokers compared with 27% of men
   b. Rate of decline in smoking is higher in men than women (i.e., men are quitting faster than women)—in 1965, 51.9% of men were smokers versus 33.9% of women
      i. Estimated that more women than men will smoke by year 2000
      ii. Converging rates of smoking in men and women can be accounted for by gender differences in initiation rather than cessation
      iii. Smoking begins in adolescence, with prevalence higher in girls than boys
2. Correlates of cigarette smoking
   a. Demographics
      i. Cigarette smoking more likely among minorities and people of low socioeconomic status
      ii. Education accounts for most of variance in smoking prevalence rates, with least educated most likely to smoke
   b. Tobacco and alcohol
      i. Cigarette smoking more likely among heavy drinkers than occasional drinkers
      ii. Similarly, heaving drinking more likely in smokers than nonsmokers
   c. Cigarette smoking and stress
      i. Cigarette smokers report higher levels of stress and psychological concerns (e.g., depression) than nonsmokers

B. **Health effects of smoking**
  1. Health consequences of smoking are well documented and include:
     a. Heart disease
     b. Stroke
     c. Chronic obstructive pulmonary disease
     d. Cancers of lung, breast, mouth, esophagus, larynx, pancreas, bladder, kidney, and more
     e. Osteoporosis
     f. Early menopause
     g. Increased risk of stroke when simultaneously smoking and using oral contraceptives
  2. Cigarette smoking is single most preventable cause of death in U.S.
  3. Estimated that approximately half a million people die in U.S. per year because of cigarette smoking
C. **Cigarette smoking and pregnancy**
  1. Maternal smoking has been studied extensively
  2. Since mid-1960s, cigarette smoking has declined substantially among pregnant women (from approximately 36% in 1967 to approximately 18% presently); nonetheless, relapse rate after pregnancy is extremely high.
     a. Approximately 70% of women who quit smoking during pregnancy relapse within 1 year of delivery
     b. Resembles rates of relapse after smoking cessation clinics
  3. Health consequences related to maternal cigarette smoking during pregnancy: spontaneous abortion, perinatal mortality, stillbirth, abruptio placentae, bleeding during pregnancy, premature rupture of membranes, preterm delivery, low birth weight, intrauterine growth retardation
D. **Passive smoke exposure**
  1. Defined as exposure to environmental cigarette smoke
  2. Effects recently more closely scrutinized
  3. Passive smoke exposure to infants associated with increased rates of upper respiratory infections, pneumonia, otitis media, hospitalizations (3 times higher than for infants of nonsmokers), and sudden infant death syndrome (SIDS)
E. **Cigarette smoking is physically and psychologically addictive**
  1. Active ingredient in tobacco products is nicotine
  2. Withdrawal symptoms may include
     a. Mood changes (e.g., irritability, depression, anxiety)
     b. Physiologic symptoms (e.g., fatigue, restlessness, decreased concentration, craving, headaches, lightheadedness)
     c. Physiologic signs (e.g., EEG changes, decreased heart rate, sweating, constipation)
  3. Smokers have thoughts and beliefs that facilitate continued smoking
     a. "I like to smoke"
     b. "Smoking relaxes me"
     c. "It's my body, and I have a right to smoke"
     d. "I'll quit smoking eventually, before I have any medical problems"
     e. "I can't quit"
  4. In contrast, nonsmokers have such thoughts and beliefs as
     a. "I don't like smoking"
     b. "Smoking would cause me to have medical problems"
     c. "I'm glad I don't smoke"
     d. "Smoking is okay for other people, but it's not okay for me"
  5. Smoking is extremely complex, habitual, ritualized behavior that includes buying, handling, puffing, and so forth
     a. Typical smokers take over 200 puffs/day
  6. Smoking, like other addictions, provides powerful means of mood regulation
     a. People smoke to relieve boredom, depression, anxiety, anger, and other uncomfortable feelings
  7. Women who smoke cigarettes are more likely to report emotional distress than women who do not smoke

    8. Some women smoke cigarettes to self-medicate depression
      a. Many depressed women continue because they lack self-confidence to quit
    9. Smoking cessation associated with weight gain
      a. Many women smoke cigarettes to curb appetites (i.e., for weight reduction)
  F. **Stages of change**—important because they dictate appropriate physician interventions
    1. Precontemplation (denial of problem or some ambivalence)
      Belief: "My smoking is not a problem"
      Behavior: continuation of smoking
    2. Contemplation (some consideration of problem; ambivalence grows stronger)
      Belief: "Perhaps my smoking is a problem"
      Behavior: attempts to cut down, change brands
    3. Preparation (denial mostly ended; focus on potential methods for change)
      Belief: "I'm getting ready to quit smoking"
      Behavior: communicating with others about plans to quit, visiting physician for assistance, enrollment in smoking cessation program, removal of cigarettes and ashtrays from home
    4. Action (cessation program has begun and is maintained for at least 24 hours)
      Belief: "I've begun to change"
      Behavior: learning to substitute positive behaviors for smoking
    5. Maintenance (smoking cessation maintained for at least 6 months)
      Belief: "I'm proud of myself for my success"
      Behavior: new coping strategies have become routine
  G. **Relapse**
    1. Defined as full return to cigarette smoking after successful period of abstinence
    2. Unfortunately, extremely common
      a. As many as 90% of people who quit smoking eventually return to smoking for some period before they quit permanently
      b. Most people relapse within a week of quitting
      c. Similar relapse rates for various addictive behaviors
    3. Certain situations place people at high risk for relapse
      a. External triggers (e.g., relationship changes, vocational difficulties, death or illness of significant other, anniversaries, celebrations)
      b. Internal triggers (e.g., sad feelings, anger, boredom, physical pain, physical withdrawal from substance)
    4. Relapse should not cause frustration to physician or patient; both may potentially benefit from viewing relapse episode as important learning episode
III. **An Approach**
  A. Although physicians understand deadly nature of smoking, many are reluctant to intervene
  B. Physicians have responsibility to **advise all smokers to quit**; research shows that physicians' simple advice to quit is related to increased cessation rates
    1. The Agency for Health Care Policy Research (AHCPR) recently published a clinical practice guideline for smoking cessation, based on smoking cessation research
    2. The AHCPR Guideline recommends that Primary Care Clinicians:
      a. Ask all patients if they smoke (smoking status as one of the vital signs)
      b. Advise all smokers to quit smoking
      c. Identify those smokers ready to quit smoking
      d. Assist the patient in quitting smoking
      e. Arrange follow-up contact
  C. **At least six steps can be taken** by physician
    1. Screen all patients for smoking status
    2. Evaluate psychology of patient who smokes
    3. Assess motivation to quit smoking
    4. Provide brief interventions (e.g,. advise to quit)
    5. Consult and refer when appropriate (e.g., smoking cessation clinics)
    6. Follow-up (including relapse management)
  D. **Screening**
    1. At each office visit ask all patients "Do you smoke?" or "Are you still smoking?"
    2. Record smoking status in prominent place in medical record

3. Be attentive to physical signs of smoking (e.g., smell of cigarette smoke on breath, yellowing of fingers, cough), especially in patients who do not readily admit to smoking (e.g., adolescents)

E. **Evaluate psychology of patients who smoke**
1. Ask patient reasons for smoking (e.g., stress, boredom, physical addiction)
2. Screen for underlying psychiatric problems (e.g., depression, schizophrenia, chronic anger)
3. Inquire about significant others who smoke (e.g., husband, best friend)

F. **Assess motivation**
1. Learn five stages of readiness to change (described above)
2. Understand that each stage may require different type of intervention
3. Do not assume that all patients are prepared to take action; instead assume that some are precontemplators (i.e., in denial)
4. Ask about patient's plans and motivations for smoking or quitting to evaluate stage of change
5. Teach patients to understand their own stage of change

G. **Interventions**
1. Advise all smokers to quit
2. Customize quit message according to demographic data; provide relevant information about risks of smoking; discuss relevant benefits of quitting
3. Customize quit message according to stage of change
   a. Help precontemplators begin to contemplate quitting
   b. Help contemplators prepare for action
   c. Help those in maintenance feel pride in their success
4. For patients contemplating smoking cessation, collaboratively plan quit date
5. The following agencies provide excellent smoking cessation materials:
   • Agency for Health Care Policy Research (800-358-9295) for Physicians' Clinical Practice
   • Guideline and free patient guide entitled, "You Can Quit Smoking"
   • American Cancer Society (800-ACS-2345)
   • American Heart Association (800-AHA-USA1)
   • American Lung Association (800-LUNG-USA)
   • National Cancer Institute (800-4-CANCER)
   • Office on Smoking and Health (800-CDC-1311)
6. Emphasize necessity of cognitive and behavioral changes for cessation; patient must begin to think and act like nonsmoker
7. Discuss potential for relapse and prepare for high-risk situations that may contribute to relapse
8. Recommend structured smoking cessation program (e.g., group treatment) when appropriate (see below)
9. When patient develops disease secondary to smoking, physician should deliver clear, direct, accurate message about effects of smoking and firmly advise patient to quit (all patients in hospital should be advised by physicians to quit smoking)
10. For some time it has been believed that patients should quit one addiction at a time; in fact, this is myth
    a. Smokers who are addicted to other drugs (e.g., alcohol) should undergo lifestyle change
    b. In other words, they should simultaneously make global healthy lifestyle changes
11. Offer nicotine replacement therapy to patients planning to quit smoking
    a. Nicotine gum, transdermal patch, nicotine inhaler, and nicotine nasal spray are currently available
    b. Nicotine replacement is appropriate for those who describe themselves as addicted or having serious withdrawal symptoms
    c. Most effective when used as part of comprehensive behavior modification program
    d. Nicotine replacement therapy is most appropriate after patient has completely stopped cigarette smoking

12. **Specific recommendations for prescribing nicotine replacement**
    a. Nicotine replacement is most appropriate for heavy smokers
        i. More than 20 cigarettes/day
        ii. First cigarette within 30 minutes of awakening
        iii. Strong craving during first week after previous quit attempts
        iv. Nicotine withdrawal symptoms
    b. Offer transdermal nicotine (patch) unless patient specifically requests another delivery system
    c. Two types of patches, designed to be worn either 16 or 24 hours/day
        i. 24-hour patch
            (a) Potential advantage: continuous nicotine delivery that may ameliorate early morning craving
            (b) Potential disadvantage: may have adverse effect on sleep (e.g., awakening, vivid dreams, tachyphylaxis)
        ii. 16-hour patch
            (a) Potential advantage: improved sleep (compared with 24-hour patch)
            (b) Disadvantage: early morning craving
    d. 24-hour patches come in 21-, 14-, and 7-mg/day doses
        i. Patch applied to clean, nonhairy, dry skin site on upper body and replaced every 24 hours
        ii. Heavy smokers (defined above) over 100 lbs without cardiovascular disease generally start with 21-mg patch
        iii. Others start with 14-mg patch (uncommon to start with 7 mg; patients need to step down)
        iv. Use 21-mg or 14-mg patch 4–8 weeks
        v. Step-down periods approximately 2–4 weeks each
        vi. Eventually discontinue patch
        vii. Be flexible
    e. 16-hour patch comes in 15-mg dose
        i. Duration of treatment: approximately 12 weeks
        ii. Patch is placed on morning awakening, removed before bedtime
        iii. Patch applied to clean, nonhairy, dry skin site on upper body
        iv. Again, be flexible
    f. Nicotine gum may be useful for people who want oral gratification during nicotine delivery; however, they tend to use gum improperly (i.e., chewing rather than parking gum)
    g. Main advantages of transdermal nicotine
        i. Delivers steady state of nicotine
        ii. Less likely to be misused
    h. People on nicotine replacement should not smoke; risk of nicotine overdose
    i. Nicotine nasal spray delivers 0.5 mg of nicotine per actuation, 1 actuation per nostril; quick onset (10 minutes); maximum 1–2 doses per hour, 40 per day; maximum length of treatment 3 months; may cause local or ocular irritation; not recommended for patients with nasal or sinus allergies or asthma
    j. Nicotine inhaler releases 4 mg nicotine per cartridge with 2 mg absorbed; maximum 16 cartridges per day; usual length of treatment 3–12 weeks at 6–8 cartridges per day; onset is approximately 30 minutes; may cause local irritation, coughing, dyspepsia; use with caution in patients with COPD and asthma
13. **Bupropion** (Zyban), an antidepressant, has been found effective as adjunct to smoking cessation
    a. Taken orally: begin with 150 mg/day for 3 days then 150 mg twice per day for 7–12 weeks (with at least 8 hours between doses)
    b. Patients should set a quit date within the second week of treatment
    c. Treatment ends after 7 weeks if no improvement in smoking or when patient ready to stop (prior to 12 weeks); tapering not necessary
    d. Known side effects: headache, insomnia, tremor, rash, seizures

      e. Contraindicated with: seizure disorders, bulimia, anorexia; monitor BP if used with nicotine replacement; caution with patients known to have bipolar illness, psychosis, recent MI, CHF, suicidal ideation; do not use with MAOIs

H. **Consultation and referral**
1. Some smokers need additional help with smoking cessation
2. Indications for consultation or referral
    a. Previous unsuccessful quit attempts resulting in extreme pessimism
    b. Extremely negative emotions associated with smoking cessation
    c. Coexisting psychological problems or disorders
3. Consultation and referral should be with reputable specialists (e.g., certified mental health professionals, hospital-based smoking cessation programs)
4. Questionable smoking cessation strategies include hypnosis and acupuncture
5. Provide treatment for coexisting psychiatric disorder (e.g., depression) while helping patient to quit smoking

I. **Follow-up**
1. Arrange follow-up visit within 1–2 weeks after quit date
2. Within 1 week of visit call or send letter to reinforce quit date or plans
3. During all follow-up visits continue to inquire about smoking status
4. When patient maintains abstinence, provide strong reinforcement (e.g., positive effects on health)

J. **Relapse management**
1. When relapse occurs, physician must maintain warm, relaxed, empathetic, supportive, collaborative, inquisitive attitude
2. Inquire about reasons for relapse, paying particular attention to
    a. High-risk situation leading to relapse
    b. Beliefs about smoking that were activated in high-risk situation (e.g., "I need a cigarette to cope with this")
    c. Strength of urges and cravings before actual use
    d. Permissive beliefs that facilitated relapse (e.g., "It'll be okay; I'll just take a few puffs")
3. After relapse teach patients
    a. To anticipate and avoid high-risk situations in future (whenever possible)
    b. When high-risk situations occur, to generate thoughts and beliefs that are antismoking (e.g., "Smoking will only make the problem bigger because I'll have to quit all over again") rather than prosmoking (e.g., "I need to smoke to cope")
    c. To distract themselves when urges and cravings occur; they will pass
    d. Not to give themselves permission to smoke under any circumstances; instead think, "I won't just take a few puffs if I start. It's likely that one will lead to another and another and another..."
4. When relapse occurs, encourage continued efforts to quit ("After falling off a horse it's important to get right back up and ride")

K. **Creating smoke-free office**
1. Most health care settings do not allow cigarette smoking; however, physicians can take additional steps to create truly smoke-free environment in offices
    a. Encourage all currently smoking office personnel (e.g., nurses, receptionists, clerks, secretaries) to become nonsmokers
    b. Post "No Smoking" signs in all office areas
    c. Remove ashtrays from all office areas
    d. Prominently display smoking cessation materials and information
    e. Eliminate all tobacco advertising from waiting room

SUGGESTED READING

1. Beck AT, Wright FD, Newman CF, Liese BS: Cognitive Therapy of Substance Abuse. New York, Guilford, 1993.
2. Benowitz NL (ed): Nicotine Safety and Toxicity. New York, Oxford University Press, 1998.
3. Berman BA, Gritz ER: Women and smoking: Toward the year 2000. In Lisansky Gomberg ES, Nirenberg TD (eds): Women and Substance Abuse. Norwood, NJ, Ablex Publishing, 1993, pp 258–285.

4. Fiore MC, Jorenby DE, Baker, TB: Smoking cessation: Principles and practice based upon the AHCPR guidelines. Ann Behav Med 19: 213–219, 1996.
5. Fiore MC, Smith SS, Jorenby DE, Baker TB: The effectiveness of the nicotine patch for smoking cessation: A meta-analysis. JAMA 271:1940–1947, 1994.
6. Floyd RL, Rimer BK, Giovino GA, et al: A review of smoking in pregnancy: Effects on pregnancy outcomes and cessation efforts. Annu Rev Public Health 14:379–411, 1993.
7. Glynn TJ, Manley MW: How to Help Your Patients Stop Smoking: A National Cancer Institute Manual for Physicians. NIH Publication No. 92-3063. Bethesda, MD, National Cancer Institute, 1991.
8. Jorenby DE, Leischow SJ, Nides MA, et al: A controlled trial of sustained-release bupropion, a nicotine patch, or both for smoking cessation. New Engl J Med 340:685–691, 1999.
9. Liese BS: The KUFP five-visit quit-smoking program: An office-based smoking cessation program. Kans Med 94:294–298, 1993.
10. Liese BS, Franz RA: Treating substance use disorders with cognitive therapy: Lessons learned and implications for the future. In Salkovskis PM (ed): Frontiers of Cognitive Therapy. New York, Guilford Press, 1996, pp 470–508.
11. Liese BS, Chiauzzi E: Alcohol, Tobacco, and Other Drug Use. Kansas City, American Academy of Family Physicians HSSA Program, 1995.
12. Miller WR, Rollnick S: Motivational Interviewing. New York, Guilford, 1991.
13. Orleans CT, Slade J (eds): Nicotine Addiction: Principles and Management. New York, Oxford University Press, 1993.
14. U.S. Department of Health and Human Services: Smoking Cessation: Clinical Practice Guideline (No. 18). DHHS Publication No. (AHCPR) 96-0892. Washington, DC, U.S. Department of Health and Human Services, Public Health Service, Agency for Health Care Policy and Research, 1996.

83. Women and Prescription Drug Abuse

Timothy P. Daaleman, D.O.

I. The Issues

There has been an increased awareness of substance abuse among women in the last decade. A subset of this disorder, prescription drug abuse, is an often unrecognized or ignored presenting problem for the primary care physician. It has been estimated that over 50% of all emergency room visits for drug related problems are connected to prescription drug misuse or accidental overdose. As the most common source for both medical and non medical uses of prescribed medications, the generalist must: be cognizant of the appropriate uses and misuses of his or her pharmacotherapy; attend to the signs and symptoms of abuse in women; and seek to initiate and coordinate a plan of treatment of the identified patient.

II. The Theory

    A. **Continuum of behaviors:** several terms describe the range of drug usage; it is critical to clarify these terms in order to facilitate communication with the patient and other clinicians, and to promote appropriate therapy.

        1. **Abuse:** use of a medication outside of the normally acceptable or standard in such a way that causes adverse consequences; the usage continues, despite negative consequences, and may be characterized by preoccupation with the drug, escalating use, and a chronic, relapsing course.

        2. **Addiction:** a behavior pattern of drug abuse characterized by an overwhelming involvement with the procurement and use of drug.

        3. **Dependence**

            a. Physical—a state of neuroadaptation produced by repeated administration of a drug, necessitating continued administration to prevent a recurrence of the withdrawal or abstinence syndrome.

            b. Psychological—a state of drug craving and compulsive drug seeking that is not based on the experience of withdrawal; can occur with any substance in which a patient has a significant psychological investment.

4. **Tolerance:** the increased dosing of a drug in order to obtain the same effects observed with its initial usage.
5. **Withdrawal:** the physical and psychological reactions cause by the abrupt cessation of a dependence-producing drug.
6. **Intoxication:** an acute state of impaired judgment, cognition, social and occupational functioning, and altered physical homeostasis due to a psychoactive substance.

B. **Drugs of abuse**
1. Prescription drugs with specific pharmacologic properties, such as rapid onset and brief duration of action, high degree of water solubility, and high potency and volatility, are more highly sought after and more commonly abused
   a. **Benzodiazepines** (flurazepam, temazepam, triazolam, diazepam, chlordiazepoxide, alprazolam, lorazepam, clorazepate, oxazepam, halazepam, triazolam, prazepam)
      i. Accepted uses and indications: insomnia, epilepsy and seizure disorder, alcohol withdrawal, anxiety associated with depression, muscle spasm, anxiety disorder, preoperative medication
   b. **Opioids and narcotic analgesics** (hydrocodone, oxycodone, morphine, meperidine, codeine, propoxyphene, buprenorphine, dezocine, methadone, fentanyl, levorphanol, nalbuphine, pentazocine)
      i. Accepted uses and indications: moderate and severe pain
   c. **Amphetamines** (dextroamphetamine, methylphenidate, fenfluramine, pemoline)
      i. Accepted uses and indications: attention deficit with hyperactivity disorder, narcolepsy
   d. **Barbiturates** (amobarbital, phenobarbital, secobarbital, pentobarbital, butalbital)
      i. Accepted uses and indications: insomnia, sedation, tension or migraine headache (butalbital), seizure disorder
   e. **Other drugs** (carisoprodol)
      i. Accepted uses and indications: painful musculoskeletal conditions

C. **Clinician's influence**
1. The therapeutic alliance between physician and patient is frequently challenged when the issue of prescription drug abuse surfaces; the clinician must constantly seek to balance the tension between roles as a caring provider and responsible user of habituating and potentially lethal medications; the misprescribing physician can often be categorized as the following:
2. Dated—unaware of current acceptable prescribing practices
3. Dishonest—seeks financial gain by selling prescriptions
4. Duped—misled by patients who falsify information to obtain medications
5. Disabled—dysfunctional as a result of illness or their own chemical dependence
6. Physicians can act as "enablers" by assisting patients to function despite a disability related to drug abuse; in the setting of drug abuse, the generalist must approach the issue and patient in a direct and confrontational way.

D. **The impaired patient**
1. **The patient who overdoses**
   a. The patient receives medication for an illness and inadvertently takes an overdose; the elderly are particularly susceptible to unintentional overdoses.
   b. Older women are prescribed drugs at rates 2.5 times higher than are older men; these women receive 17% of psychoactive drugs and 20% of sedative hypnotics prescribed.
   c. Analgesics and sedatives are a particular risk, and the physician should prescribe lower, yet therapeutically efficacious, doses.
   d. In the depressed patient, intentional overdoses with antidepressants (especially tricyclic antidepressants) are a particular danger; these medications, either alone or in combination with analgesics or alcohol, can cause respiratory depression, coma, and death.
   e. Patients with a history of "cross-addiction" (a prior or current history of other substance abuse problems) are at increased risk for the combined effects of several medications; these patients should be screened for alcohol and concurrent drug (prescription and OTC) usage; these substances can potentiate many medications and produce potentially fatal consequences.

2. **The chemically dependent patient**
   a. Patient is at risk of dependence while legitimately taking medications for a specific indication.
   b. Physically dependent patients may go through withdrawal symptoms if medications are suddenly discontinued; symptoms may be mild, moderate, or severe, which is dependent upon the medication type, dosage, and duration of use.
3. **The addicted patient**
   a. Patient is often manipulative and tends to falsify their symptoms, and uses several physicians; their often hostile and demanding behavior characterizes the loss of control over drug usage.
   b. Development of a drug-oriented lifestyle typifies the compulsion to continued drug usage despite problems caused by the drug.

III. **An Approach**
   A. **Prevention:** physician behaviors, attitudes, and practice patterns play a crucial role in the development and perpetuation, or prevention of prescription drug abuse; there are two components to implementing an effective preventive approach to prescription drug abuse: identifying patients at risk and rational and careful prescribing practices.
      1. **Identifying patients at risk**
         a. A thorough history and appropriate physical exam are important prerequisites in establishing an indication and use for any medication with abuse potential; key screening information, which includes a current or prior history of drug or alcohol abuse, and a family history of substance abuse, can alert the physician to the possibility of prescription drug abuse.
         b. Prior medical records (ER visits, consultations, etc.) should be reviewed in patients suspected of abuse
         c. Computerized pharmacy personnel are invaluable sources of information for physicians
         d. Signs of prescription drug abuse include: repeatedly losing prescriptions or pills, after hours call for refills, fabricated or incongruent symptoms, multiple physician prescriptions, early refills, sophisticated knowledge of medications, strong preference or questionable intolerance to specific drugs, frequent emergency department visits, evidence of intoxication.
         e. Geriatric patients have a great potential for medication misuse
            i. The generalist should assess for polypharmacy, erratic compliance, self-medication, cognitive or visual impairment, or use of over-the-counter medications in these patients
            ii. The use or misuse of alcohol, which can complicate prescription drug abuse or be a separate abuse problem, is often underestimated in this population
         f. Drug abuse or misuse is overlooked or misdiagnosed in the elderly since it may present in a variety of signs or symptoms, and be a cause or contributor to many comorbid conditions, such as depression, anxiety, insomnia, dementia, sexual dysfunction, falls and trauma, and incontinence
      2. **Rational and careful prescribing practices**
         a. A number of practices may help to limit the problem of prescription drug abuse; limiting access to prescription pads, which should not be left out in examination rooms or patient-frequented areas; and prescription refills and the amount of medication dispensed should be unambiguously noted; DEA number should not be preprinted on any forms.
         b. There are **six important guidelines** to preventive prescribing practices:
            i. **Diagnosis:** the clinician is obligated to attempt to identify the etiology of the presenting problem, rather than simply treat the presenting symptoms; an undifferentiated problem or acute episode may require a tentative diagnosis, but as acute problems become chronic, the process of history taking-examination-assessment-documentation takes on a greater importance to gain an overall clinical picture.
            ii. **Dosage:** the dosage should be appropriate for the diagnosis and severity of the problem while avoiding side effects; as symptoms increase or decrease in severity, medications should be adjusted accordingly.

      iii. **Duration:** the clinician should develop a treatment plan that specifies an expected length of time for therapy

      iv. **Discontinuation:** a therapeutic end-point should be included with the original treatment plan; decisions concerning discontinuation should be determined by adverse drug reactions, resolution or improvement of the symptomatology, expiration of the end-point, and successful nonpharmacologic interventions.

      v. **Dependence:** the physician has a duty to warn the patient about side effects of the medication (including dependence and addiction); the patient should be monitored for possible drug dependence and toxicity.

      vi. **Documentation:** careful documentation is the best defense from legal problems arising from prescription drug abuse; in patients that have a high risk potential for drug abuse, it is critical to note the following: presenting complaints, tentative and formal diagnoses, details of all prescriptions, refills, requests, and refusals, consultations, recommended and actual courses of treatment.

   c. A variety of **nonpharmacologic treatment options** can be considered in clinical situations where psychotropic medications are used (anxiety, mood disorders): therapy (psychotherapy, cognitive, behavioral), stress reduction, support groups

B. **Intervention and treatment**

  1. **Intervening with the problem patient**

   a. When a patient presents with an intentional or unintentional problem of drug misuse, the primary intervention should focus on education, clarification of therapy, and modification of patient behavior

   b. Confusing or misunderstood drug regimens can be simplified, reconstituted, or reinforced with the patient; in the elderly or in cases where visual or cognitive impairment complicate compliance, family members or care givers should be incorporated into the process.

   c. Patients who intentionally misuse medications should first be provided with clear and directed feedback about their usage; the physician should also facilitate a recognition by the patient of the presenting physical and emotional components to the presenting problem; by validating the patient's distress and addressing the problem in a clinical context, an intervention and therapeutic strategy can be outlined.

  2. **Confronting the abusing patient**

   a. In patients suspected of abusing prescription drugs, the physician should express concern in a direct, empathetic, nonjudgmental way with a focus toward exploring the issue; specific questions about drug usage (duration, type, dosage, route of administration, supplementation), and observed and documented behaviors (calls for early refills, escalating usage) are critical.

   b. Family members or care givers can be a significant source of information or corroboration

   c. In patients who are actively seeking drugs:

      i. The clinician should clearly express his or her impression of the drug abuse problem, while validating the clinical relevance of the presenting complaint

      ii. In declining the desired medication, it is important to state the lack of indication or inappropriateness of the request to the patient

      iii. Other therapeutic options for the patient identified problem should be offered

      iv. The patient should be presented with an opportunity to further assess or treat the drug abuse problem

      v. If the patient is amenable to an intervention, he or she should be assessed for withdrawal risk, and appropriate referral or follow-up should be planned

   d. The process of evaluation and intervention may not be accomplished during a single encounter; some clinicians elect to develop a therapeutic relationship or explore the issue of abuse further, with limited use of the desired medication; a therapeutic contract with the patient, which is clearly stated, documented, and followed, is mandatory in this clinical setting.

C. **Treatment of withdrawal**

   1. Medical and psychological risks should be assessed prior to discontinuing any medication; the treatment of withdrawal should be part of a comprehensive plan with a multidisciplinary approach; specialty colleagues in psychiatry, psychology, or addiction medicine can provide assistance in treatment planning.

      a. **Benzodiazepines:** depending upon the individual case, effective treatment can be provided on an inpatient or outpatient basis; therapy and counseling remain cornerstones of care; patients with a history of abusing short-acting agents are usually given longer acting benzodiazepines (diazepam); the long acting agent is then slowly tapered over a period of 4–8 weeks until discontinuation.

      b. **Opioids and narcotic analgesics:** pharmacologic treatment of opioid withdrawal is not essential, although it is sometimes used to ease symptoms; oral clonidine (0.1–0.3 mg) given three to four times daily is effective in reducing opioid withdrawal symptoms but does not shorten the duration of the withdrawal period; methadone is a long acting oral opioid that can prevent withdrawal; by initially dosing to treat withdrawal effects, methadone can be tapered slowly (10–15% per day) or continued at a maintenance dose of 20–40 mg per day.

      c. **Amphetamines:** withdrawal from amphetamines does not require pharmacotherapy; patients who abuse stimulants should be screened for affective and attention deficit disorders since they are more common in these individuals.

      d. **Barbiturates:** barbiturate withdrawal can be a serious or even life-threatening event that requires skilled management

         i. In patients having acute withdrawal symptoms, IV phenobarbital infused at 0.3 mg/kg/min can be titrated until signs of mild toxicity (drowsiness, ataxia, dysarthria, nystagmus) are noted; the patient must be monitored for signs of respiratory depression while the drug concentration slowly declines.

         ii. In a nonacute setting "phenobarbital loading" has been used; the drug is administered in doses of 120 mg every 1–2 hours until the patient shows signs of mild toxicity; after loading is completed, no further drug is given and the patient is observed.

SUGGESTED READING

1. Dougherty RJ: Prescription drug use and abuse. Psych Times Jan:27–30, 1995.
2. Farnsworth MG: Benzodiazepine abuse and dependence: Misconceptions and facts. J Fam Pract 31:393–400, 1990.
3. Finch J: Prescription drug abuse. Prim Care 20:231–239, 1993.
4. Landry MJ, Smith DE, Steinberg JR: Anxiety, depression, and substance abuse disorders: Diagnosis, treatment, and prescribing practices. J Psychoactive Drugs 23:397–416, 1991.
5. Parran T: Prescription drug abuse. Med Clin North Am 81:967–978, 1997.
6. Quinby PM, Graham AV: Substance abuse among women. Prim Care 20:131–140, 1993.
7. Skinner, MH, Thompson DA: Pharmacologic considerations in the treatment of substance abuse. South Med J 85:1207–1219, 1992.
8. Szwabo PA: Substance abuse in older women. Clin Geriatr Med 9:197–208, 1993.
9. Voth EA, DuPont RL, Voth HM: Responsible prescribing of controlled substances. Am Fam Physician 44:1673–1678, 1991.

84. Alcohol Abuse

Bruce S. Liese, Ph.D.

I. The Issues

Ethyl alcohol (ethanol) is a psychoactive drug. It has various effects, depending on the amount consumed and the drinker's physiology (including gender), expectations, circumstances, and environment. At low doses alcohol may have an excitatory effect and reduce inhibitions, resulting in heightened social interaction, feelings of euphoria, and decreased tension. At higher doses it progressively depresses the nervous system, resulting in impairment of attention, disturbances in gait and coordination, impaired short-term memory, and slurred speech. As a result of heavy alcohol consumption some women incur substantial medical, legal, social, and psychological problems. Primary care physicians are well positioned to help women with alcohol problems. Although many physicians effectively do so, some lack the necessary knowledge, skills, or desire.

II. The Theory

A. Classification and diagnosis

1. *Diagnostic and Statistical Manual of Mental Disorders*, 4th edition (DSM–IV), provides diagnostic system for categorizing pathologic alcohol use
2. Main categories of alcohol use disorders are alcohol abuse and alcohol dependence
3. **Alcohol abuse** is defined as maladaptive pattern of alcohol use resulting in at least one of following four criteria
   a. Inability to fulfill major role obligations at work, school, or home
   b. Recurrent use in situations in which it is physically hazardous
   c. Recurrent alcohol-related legal problems
   d. Continued alcohol use despite persistent or recurrent social or interpersonal problems related to alcohol use
4. **Alcohol dependence** is more severe than abuse, meeting at least three of the following criteria
   a. Tolerance (increased need for alcohol to get same desired effect or markedly diminished effect with continued use of same amount)
   b. Withdrawal symptoms (which develop after cessation of heavy, prolonged alcohol use); diagnosis of alcoholic withdrawal requires two or more of following symptoms
      i. Autonomic hyperactivity (e.g., sweating or pulse rate > 100)
      ii. Increased hand tremor
      iii. Insomnia
      iv. Nausea or vomiting
      v. Transient visual, tactile, or auditory hallucinations or illusions
      vi. Psychomotor agitation
      vii. Anxiety
      viii. Grand mal seizures
   c. Increasing quantities of alcohol consumed, often over longer period of time
   d. Persistent desire to drink or unsuccessful efforts to cut down
   e. Great deal of time expended to drink
   f. Important social, occupational, or recreational activities given up or reduced because of drinking
   g. Drinking continues despite persistent or recurrent physical or psychological problems related to drinking

B. Prevalence

1. According to National Center for Health Statistics (NCHS), adult Americans may be classified according to levels of alcohol consumed as follows
   a. Infrequent drinkers (22%) have less than one drink per 2 weeks
   b. Light drinkers (27%) have 1–7 drinks per 2 weeks

    c. Moderate drinkers (13%) have 8–26 drinks per 2 weeks

    d. Heavy drinkers (5%) have 27 or more drinks per 2 weeks

    e. Abstainers (33%) completely abstain from drinking alcohol

  2. Most Americans (approximately 68% or approximately 138 million) over age of 12 years drink alcohol in any given year

  3. Approximately 1.9 million Americans drink daily or almost daily over course of year

  4. Approximately 11% of adult Americans (16 million) drink half of all alcoholic beverages sold

  5. Fewer women (59%) than men (71%) drink alcoholic beverages

  6. Women drink less frequently than men and consume smaller amounts per occasion

  7. Depending on study, fewer women (6–8%) than men (21–31%) drink heavily (defined as 2 or more drinks daily or at least 5 drinks once per week)

C. **Health effects of alcohol problems and chronic alcoholism**

  1. Nervous system disorders

    a. Wernicke's syndrome—acute condition initially characterized by confusion, delirium, and hyperactivity; related to thiamine deficiency

    b. Korsakoff's psychosis—chronic condition believed to be residual of Wernicke's syndrome

    c. Peripheral neuropathy

    d. Degenerative diseases of brain (e.g., alcoholic dementia)

    e. Hepatic encephalopathy

    f. Alcoholic hypoglycemia

    g. Trauma (head injury)

    h. Alcoholic blackouts

  2. Liver diseases (fatty liver, hepatitis, cirrhosis)

  3. Gastrointestinal system disorders (diarrhea, gastritis, peptic ulcers, pancreatitis)

  4. Blood disorders (anemia, leukopenia, thrombocytopenia)

  5. Cardiovascular system disorders (cardiomyopathy, arrhythmias, atherosclerosis, hypertension)

  6. Skeletal muscles—alcoholic myopathy

  7. Reproductive organs

    a. Impotence

    b. Silvestrini-Corda syndrome (coexisting cirrhosis, testicular atrophy, and breast enlargement in men)

    c. Damage to ovaries

  8. Pregnancy (damage to fetus)

    a. Fetal alcohol syndrome (born small, with facial abnormalities and varying degrees of brain damage)

    b. Spontaneous abortion

D. **Differences between women and men**

  1. Women are more susceptible to physiologic consequences of alcohol abuse

  2. Women reach higher blood alcohol concentrations than men from same weight-adjusted levels of consumption

  3. Women may develop liver disorders after lower levels of regular alcohol consumption and earlier in life

E. **Vulnerability to alcohol problems**

  1. Younger women (21–30 years old) have higher rates of alcohol problems than older women (more problems with binge drinking)

  2. Never-married, divorced, and separated women have higher rates of drinking; widowed women have lowest rates

  3. Women in nontraditional career roles more likely to be drinkers and to have drinking problems than more traditional women

  4. Caucasian American women more likely to be drinkers than minorities

  5. Women with drinking partners (i.e., significant others) more likely to be drinkers

  6. Childhood sexual abuse and relationship violence are associated with problem drinking in women

  7. Sexual problems in women are associated with increased drinking

F. Psychological (i.e., cognitive-behavioral) **theory of problem drinking** may help physicians to understand and manage patients with alcohol problems:
  1. Most people use alcohol and other psychoactive drugs for mood regulation (in this context mood may involve any emotional or physiologic condition)
     a. To reduce (i.e., anesthetize or numb) uncomfortable affect (e.g., anxiety, depression, boredom)
     b. To enhance positive moods (i.e., to "party")
     c. To relieve physical pain or discomfort
     d. To enhance quality of or comfort with sex
     e. To avoid psychologic and physiologic withdrawal symptoms (i.e., craving)
  2. As alcoholics increasingly rely on alcohol to regulate emotions (i.e., as coping strategy), they are less able to regulate moods without alcohol
  3. Cognitive-behavioral theory: beliefs, thoughts, and ideas affect drug and alcohol use
     a. Important difference between problem drinker and nonproblem drinker is way he or she thinks about drinking
     b. To make significant changes in alcohol-related behaviors, people must change thought and beliefs about drinking
  4. People with alcohol abuse and dependence tend to drink in high-risk situations (e.g., when they are hungry, angry, lonely, tired)
  5. Examples of alcohol-related beliefs and thoughts
     a. "Life is no fun without drinking"
     b. "A meal without wine is like a day without sunshine"
     c. "Nothing tastes as good as an ice-cold beer"
  6. Alcohol-related beliefs trigger or increase urges and cravings for alcohol
  7. Many people with alcohol problems give themselves permission to drink despite alcohol-related problems; such permissive beliefs include:
     a. "I've worked hard; I deserve a drink"
     b. "Just one won't kill me"
G. **Stages of change**—important because they effectively guide physician interventions
  1. Precontemplation (denial of drinking problem)
     Belief: "My drinking is not a problem"
     Behavior: continuation of drinking
  2. Contemplation (some consideration that drinking problem may exist; ambivalence)
     Belief: "Perhaps my drinking is a problem"
     Behavior: attempts to cut down, change beverage (e.g., from hard liquor to only beer)
  3. Preparation (denial has mostly ended; focus on potential methods for change)
     Belief: "I'm getting ready to make a big change in my drinking"
     Behavior: communication with significant others about plans for change, visit to physician for assistance, enrollment in some type of counseling
  4. Action (cessation program has begun and is maintained for at least 24 hours)
     Belief: "I've begun to change may drinking habits"
     Behavior: learning to substitute positive coping behaviors for drinking
  5. Maintenance (positive change maintained for at least 6 months)
     Belief: "I'm proud of myself for my success"
     Behavior: new coping strategies have become routine
H. **Relapse**
  1. Defined as full return to problem drinking after successful period of abstinence or controlled drinking
  2. Unfortunately, extremely common
     a. As many as 65% of people who quite drinking experience at least 1 relapse before making permanent changes
     b. Similar relapse rate for various other addictive substances (e.g., heroin, nicotine)
  3. Relapse should not cause anger or hopelessness in physicians or patients; both may benefit from viewing relapses as important learning experiences
III. **An Approach**
  A. Many physicians address problem drinking only when it leads to serious medical problems

B. Primary care physician is in ideal position to recognize and address alcohol problems; research shows that physicians' simple advice may have beneficial effects
C. **At least six steps can be taken by physicians**
 1. Screen patients for drinking problems
 2. Evaluate psychological and psychiatric status of patients with drinking problems
 3. Assess motivation to change drinking behavior
 4. Provide brief interventions (e.g., advise to quit or control drinking)
 5. Consult and refer when appropriate (e.g., to alcohol treatment center)
 6. Follow-up (including relapse management)
D. **Screening**
 1. Look for physical or medical signs of drinking problems
   a. Stomach or abdominal pain
   b. Elevated blood pressure
   c. Chronic tension headaches
   d. Insomnia with associated medication requests
   e. Sexually transmitted diseases
   f. Frequent accidents and trauma
   g. Fatigue
   h. Chronic depression
   i. Chronic diarrhea
   j. Memory loss
 2. Be aware of correlates of drinking problems in family members
   a. Frequent office visits by family members
   b. Unexplained medical symptoms (e.g., headaches, abdominal pain in child)
   c. Trauma in family members inflicted by alcohol-abusing person
   d. School problems in child
   e. Attention deficit hyperactivity disorder in child
   f. Depression or anxiety disorder in family member
 3. When index of suspicion is high:
   a. Ask patients at least two questions: "Have you ever had a drinking problem?" and "When did you have your last drink?"
   b. Positive answer (i.e., "yes") to first question, combined with recent use of alcohol, indicates likely current alcohol abuse or dependence
 4. **Be aware of and use questions from various screening tests**, such as CAGE*
   C Have you felt the need to **C**ut down on your drinking?
   A Have people ever **A**nnoyed you by criticism of your drinking?
   G Have you ever felt **G**uilty about your drinking?
   E Have you ever taken a morning **E**ye-opener to steady your nerves or get rid of a hangover?
   * Affirmative answer to 2 or more of these questions indicates likely alcohol problems
 5. Laboratory findings suggestive of alcohol problems (i.e., biologic markers)
   a. Blood alcohol concentration (BAC)
     i. Above 0.1% in routine examination
     ii. Above 0.15% in patient showing no signs of intoxication
     iii. Above 0.3% at any time
   b. Increased gamma-glutamyl transferase (GGT) levels
   c. Increased mean corpuscular volume (MCV)
E. **Evaluate psychological status of patients with drinking problems**
 1. Ask reasons for drinking
 2. Screen for underlying mood or other psychiatric disorders
 3. Inquire about significant others who use alcohol (e.g., husband, best friend)
F. **Assess motivation**
 1. Learn five stages of change (described above)
 2. Do not assume that all patients are prepared to take action
 3. Ask about patient's plans for changing drinking behaviors to evaluate stage of change
 4. Teach patients to understand their own stage of change

G. **Brief interventions**
   1. Discuss problem drinking with patients who drink heavily
   2. Not all patients with drinking problems need to abstain completely from alcohol; thus, it is important for physician
      a. To customize advice
      b. To provide relevant information about risks of heavy drinking
      c. To discuss relevant benefits of changing behavior
   3. Customize advice according to stage of change (and inform patients about changes that will occur with continued alcohol consumption)
      a. Help precontemplators begin to contemplate change
      b. Help contemplators to prepare for action
      c. Help patients in maintenance to feel pride in their success
   4. Suggest self-help reading (bibliotherapy)
      • *Alcoholics Anonymous* (Alcoholics Anonymous World Services, 1976): "The Big Book," which forms foundation for all 12-step (e.g., AA) programs
      • *Sex, Drugs, Gambling, & Chocolate: A Workbook for Overcoming Addictions* (Horvath, 1998): outstanding, well-written handbook written by one of the founders of SMART Recovery
      • *The Addiction Workbook: A Step-by-Step Guide for Quitting Alcohol and Drugs* (Fanning and O'Neill, 1996): Contains practical exercises based on the cognitive-behavioral model of addictive behaviors (described in this chapter)
      • *Rational Recovery: The New Cure for Substance Addiction* (Trimpey, 1996): handbook for Rational Recovery movement
      • *The Recovery Book* (Mooney, Eisenberg, and Eisenberg, 1992): excellent comprehensive text that covers all bases
      • *Moderate Drinking* (Kishline, 1994): somewhat controversial book because it advocates controlled drinking in those with histories of alcohol problems
      • *Staying Sober* (Gorski and Miller, 1986): good text with many practical ideas for staying sober
      • *Understanding the Twelve Steps* (Gorski, 1989): excellent introduction to Alcoholics Anonymous (AA)
   5. Emphasize necessity of cognitive and behavioral changes for cessation
   6. Discuss potential for relapse and plan for high-risk situations that may contribute to relapse
      a. Example: "Mr. Smith, in order to change your drinking pattern it will be necessary to change how you think about alcohol"
   7. Offer medication when appropriate
   8. The National Institute on Alcohol Abuse and Alcoholism (NIAAA) recommends that physicians engage in four steps, described in a free 12-page guide, The Physicians' Guide to Helping Patients with Alcohol Problems:
      a. Ask about alcohol use
      b. Assess for alcohol-related problems
      c. Advise appropriate action (i.e., set a drinking goal, abstain, or obtain alcohol treatment)
      d. Monitor patient progress
H. **Consider drinking trial vs. abstinence** for patients who are alcohol abusers and heavy drinkers (not alcohol-dependent)
   1. First determine whether patient's problem is alcohol abuse, heavy drinking, or alcohol dependence (defined above)
   2. Patients abusing alcohol and heavy drinkers are prescribed trial of controlled drinking: maximum of 2 standard drinks/day, 4 days/week, for total of 8 eight standard drinks/week (NIAAA recommends that women drink no more than one drink per day)
   3. Standard drink defined as 12 ounces of beer, 5 ounces of wine, 4 ounces of sherry or liqueur, or 1.5 ounces of distilled spirits
   4. Patients successful with controlled drinking should be evaluated every few months to assess continued success

5. If success continues, physician may taper check-ups to annual basis
6. Patients dependent on alcohol should be encouraged to engage in trial of complete abstinence for 90 days
7. If alcohol-dependent patient fails at abstinence, formal treatment should be initiated
8. If alcohol-dependent patient succeeds at abstinence, encourage lifetime abstinence
9. Be alert for alcohol withdrawal symptoms when drinking trials are begun—patients should be encouraged to call physician immediately if withdrawal symptoms occur

I. **Consultation and referral**
1. Some problem drinkers need additional help with recovery
2. Recommend self-help groups (e.g., Alcoholics Anonymous, Rational Recovery)
3. Indications for professional consultation or referral
   a. Previous unsuccessful attempts to quit resulting in extreme pessimism
   b. Extremely negative emotions (e.g., annoyance) associated with changing behavior
   c. Coexisting psychological or psychiatric problems
4. Consultation and referral should be with reputable specialists (e.g., certified mental health professionals, highly recommended alcohol treatment programs)
5. Provide treatment for coexisting psychiatric problem (e.g., depression)

J. **Intoxicated patients**
1. Occasionally patients visit physicians intoxicated
2. Recognize and address signs and symptoms of alcohol intoxication
   a. Odor of alcohol
   b. Emotional lability
   c. Cognitive impairment
   d. Impaired judgment
   e. Perceptual problems
   f. Problems in wakefulness
   g. Difficulties with attention
3. Avoid directly confronting patient with such comments as "You're drunk today"
   a. Tentatively (but precisely) reflect obvious and subtle behavioral indicators of intoxication and "check them out" with patient
   b. Example: physician may say, "You seem particularly tired today" or "You seem to be having trouble concentrating today"
4. Maintain empathy and acceptance
5. Inquire about substance(s) used most recently, including quantity and recency (e.g., ounces of alcohol)
6. With patient's permission, get blood alcohol level
7. Discuss circumstances of current use (may be useful for later relapse prevention)
8. Avoid excessive structure, persuasion, and lecturing; intoxicated patients unlikely to benefit from such efforts
9. Plan future treatment
   a. When appropriate, may provide opportunity to anticipate or suggest more intensive treatment to patients who have previously avoided such treatment
   b. Involve significant others when possible
10. Consider safety issues (for example, individual's ability to drive and potential harm to self or others)
11. When patient is impaired or potentially self-destructive, hospitalization is encouraged
12. Follow-up as soon as possible

K. **Follow-up for alcohol counseling**
1. Arrange follow-up visit within 1–2 weeks after initial visit for alcohol problem
2. Within 1 week of visit, call to reinforce alcohol-related changes and plans
3. During all follow-up visits continue to inquire about drinking status
4. When patient maintains abstinence, provide strong reinforcement (e.g., positive effects on health)

L. **Relapse management**
1. When relapse occurs, physicians should maintain warm, relaxed, empathetic, supportive, collaborative, inquisitive attitudes
2. Inquire about reasons for relapse, paying particular attention to

      a. High-risk situation leading to relapse

      b. Beliefs about drinking activated in high-risk situation (e.g., "I need a drink to relax")

      c. Strength of urges and cravings before actual use

      d. Permissive beliefs that facilitated relapse (e.g., "I'll be okay; I'll just take one drink")

   3. After relapse, teach patients the following:

      a. Anticipate and avoid high-risk situations in future (whenever possible)

      b. When high-risk situations occur, generate thoughts and beliefs that are antidrinking (e.g., "Drinking will only make the problem bigger because I'll have to quit all over again") rather than prodrinking (e.g., "I need a drink to cope")

      c. When urgings and cravings occur, distract yourself; they will pass

      d. Do not give yourself permission to drink if abstinent; instead think, "It's more likely that one drink will lead to many more"

      e. When relapse occurs, encourage continued efforts to quit

M. **Several classes of medications** have been shown to be effective in treatment of alcohol problems

   1. Anticraving medication—naltrexone, an opiate antagonist shown to reduce relapse to heavy alcohol consumption; relatively new in treatment of alcoholism

   2. Aversive medication—disulfiram (Antabuse) is appropriate for motivated patients who plan to abstain completely from alcohol

   3. Medications for alcohol withdrawal—benzodiazepines most commonly used for treating moderate-to-severe alcohol withdrawal

      a. May cause excessive sedation

      b. Have high addiction potential

      c. Medications that decrease norepinephrine activity (e.g., clonidine and propranolol) have also been used but do not block seizures

   4. Psychotropic medications—recommended in patients with comorbid psychiatric and alcohol disorders (e.g., antidepressants), depending on problem

   5. Acamprosate, another anticraving medication, has not been used clinically in the United States; however, it has been found effective for reducing drinking frequency in clinical trials conducted in Europe and it is presently undergoing testing in the United States

N. **Physicians' personal reactions to patients with alcohol problems**

   1. Physicians' reactions vary, depending on educational, professional, and personal experiences

   2. Problematic physician reactions include hopelessness, anger, despair, and denial

   3. Beneficial physician reactions include empathy, emotional support, acceptance, and hopefulness

   4. Physicians' responses substantially affect physician–patient relationship, which affects success of treatment

O. **Resources for physicians**

   • National Institute on Alcohol Abuse and Alcoholism (NIAAA; 301-443-7003)

   • American Society of Addiction Medicine (ASAM; 301-656-3920)

   • National Council on Alcoholism and Drug Dependence (NCADD; 212-206-6770)

SUGGESTED READING

1. Alcoholic Anonymous World Services: Alcoholics Anonymous, 3rd ed. New York, Alcoholics Anonymous, 1976.
2. American Psychiatric Association: Practice Guideline for Treatment of Patients with Substance Use Disorders: Alcohol, Cocaine, Opioids. Washington, DC, American Psychiatric Association, 1995.
3. Beck AT, Wright FD, Newman CF, Liese BS: Cognitive Therapy of Substance Abuse. New York, Guilford, 1993.
4. Fanning P, O'Neill JT: The Addiction Workbook: A Step-by-Step Guide to Quitting Alcohol and Drugs. Oakland, CA, New Harbinger Publications, 1996.
5. Garbutt JC, West SL, Carey TS, Lohr KN, Crews FT: Pharmacological treatment of alcohol dependence: A review of the evidence. JAMA 281:1318–1325, 1999.

6. Gorski TT: Understanding the Twelve Steps. New York, Prentice Hall, 1989.
7. Gorski TT, Miller M: Staying Sober: A Guide for Relapse Prevention. Independence, MO, Herald House, 1986.
8. Hill SY: Genetic Vulnerability to Alcoholism in Women. In Lisansky Gomberg ES, Nirenberg TD (eds): Women and Substance Abuse. Norwood, NJ, Ablex Publishing, 1993, pp 42–61.
9. Horvath AT: Sex, Drugs, Gambling, & Chocolate: A Workbook for Overcoming Addictions. San Luis Obispo, Impact Publishers, 1998.
10. Kishline A: Moderate Drinking: A New Option for Problem Drinkers. Tucson, AZ, See Sharp Press, 1994.
11. Lieber CS: Women and alcohol: Gender Differences in Metabolism and Susceptibility. In Lisansky Gomberg ES, Nirenberg TD (eds): Women and Substance Abuse. Norwood, NJ, Ablex Publishing, 1993, pp 1–17.
12. Liese BS, Franz RA: Treating substance use disorders with cognitive therapy: Lessons learned and implications for the future. In Salkovskis PM (ed): Frontiers of Cognitive Therapy. New York, Guilford Press, 1996, pp 470–508.
13. Liese BS, Chiauzzi E: Alcohol, Tobacco, and Other Drug Use. Kansas City, American Academy of Family Physicians HSSA Program, 1995.
14. Lowinson JH, Ruiz P, Millman RB, Langrod JG (eds): Substance Abuse: A Comprehensive Textbook, 3rd ed. Baltimore, Williams & Wilkins, 1997.
15. Miller WR, Rollnick S: Motivational Interviewing. New York, Guilford, 1991.
16. Mooney AJ, Eisenberg A, Eisenberg H: The Recovery Book. New York, Workman, 1992.
17. National Institute on Alcohol Abuse and Alcoholism: The Primary Care Setting: Recognition and Care of Patients with Alcohol Problems. Alcohol Health Res World 18(2)[special issue], 1994.
18. National Institute on Alcohol Abuse and Alcoholism: Women and Alcohol. Alcohol Health Res World Vol. 18, No. 3 [special issue], 1994.
19. National Institute on Alcohol Abuse and Alcoholism: Advances in Alcohol Treatment. Alcohol Health Res World Vol. 18, No. 4 [special issue], 1994.
20. National Institute on Alcohol Abuse and Alcoholism: The Physicians' Guide to Helping Patients with Alcohol Problems (NIH Publication No. 95-3769). Bethesda, MD, NIAAA, 1995. (Note: this 12-page guide can be ordered from NIAAA at no charge.)
21. Trimpey J: Rational Recovery: The New Cure for Substance Addiction. New York, Pocket Books, 1996.
22. Wilsnack SC, Wilsnack RW: Epidemiological Research on Women's Drinking: Recent Progress and Directions for the 1990s. In Lisansky Gomberg ES, Nirenberg TD (eds): Women and Substance Abuse. Norwood, NJ, Ablex Publishing, 1993, pp 62–99.

85. Illicit Drug Use

Bruce S. Liese, Ph.D.

I. The Issues

A. Illicit drugs include marijuana, cocaine, opiates, phencyclidine, inhalants, and hallucinogens
   1. About 66 million Americans have tried marijuana
   2. About 1% of Americans (1.9 million) have tried heroin; about one-half of these are current users
   3. Approximately 3 million people in U.S. use cocaine; approximately 500,000 of these use crack cocaine
B. Fewer women than men use illicit drugs; nonetheless:
   1. More than 10% of women between 18 and 34 years old have used some illicit drug in past month
   2. Approximately 10% of women in same age group admit to marijuana use in past month
   3. Approximately 1% of women admit to cocaine use
   4. Approximately 3% of women in same age group use marijuana at least once per week
   5. Approximately 1% of these women use cocaine weekly

C. About 30% of alcohol-dependent people are also dependent on other psychoactive drugs, especially marijuana

D. Alcoholism is common in people dependent on cocaine (84%), opiates (67%), hallucinogens (64%), and marijuana (36%)

E. Multiple drug dependence rises to 50–90% in inpatient addiction settings

F. Mental disorders increase by 3.8 times with marijuana use, 11.3 times with cocaine use, 6.7 times with opiate use, and 8 times with hallucinogen use

G. Cocaine addicts have higher prevalence of depression, bipolar disorder, and attention deficit disorder than general public

H. Opiate addicts have lifetime risk of psychiatric disorders of 86.9% with depression most common (53.9%)

II. **The Theory**

A. Psychoactive drug use may result in

1. **Intoxication**—the "high"; development of reversible, substance-specific syndrome related to recent ingestion

2. **Withdrawal**—substance-specific syndrome that develops as result of cessation of use

3. **Abuse**—maladaptive or problematic pattern of use leading to significant impairment

4. **Dependence**—more severe than abuse, often involving tolerance, withdrawal, use of increasing dosages, and persistent desire for substance

B. Illicit drugs vary in potential for dependence

1. **Physically**—drugs typically associated with dependence: cocaine (especially crack), opiates, and marijuana

2. **Cognitively**—drug users have thoughts and beliefs that facilitate drug use; for example:

a. "Drug use is fun"

b. "All my friends do it"

c. "I can't possibly stop as long as my husband uses drugs"

d. "Drugs relax me"

e. "I'll quit before I develop medical problems"

f. "People who don't use drugs are boring"

g. In contrast, those who abstain from drug use might think

i. "Drug use is deadly"

ii. "I don't understand why people use drugs"

iii. "Drugs cause problems"

iv. "I would never use drugs"

3. **Behaviorally**—drug use can become extremely complex, habitual, ritualized behavior

4. **Emotionally**—addictions provide powerful means of modifying moods; many women use drugs to self-medicate depression

5. **Socially**—many women use illicit drugs because their friends and significant others (e.g., husbands) use drugs

C. **Cocaine** ("coke," "snow," or "crack")

1. Effects: stimulation, anesthesia, increased energy, improved self-image, increased mental acuity, decreased need for sleep, increased sensory awareness, euphoria

2. Enhanced physical and mental skills may lead to hypervigilance and paranoia, reaching psychotic proportions

3. May increase sexual appetite and arousal, leading to high-risk behaviors (e.g., unprotected sex, multiple partners, compulsive sex)

4. Effects on hypothalamus may contribute to significant weight reduction in compulsive users

5. Some people combine cocaine and sedatives to titrate excitatory effects; some alcoholics use cocaine to drink longer

6. Effects vary significantly with routes of administration

a. Routes associated with abuse and dependence—intranasal ("snorting"), intravenous, and smoking ("freebasing" and "crack" smoking)

b. Intranasal usage involves inhaling "lines" of cocaine hydrochloride powder through straw or rolled-up currency

        i. Each line approximately 30 mg
        ii. Desired effects typically occur in approximately 2–3 minutes
        iii. Effects last 30–45 minutes
     c. Intravenous usage involves injection of cocaine hydrochloride in solution
        i. Initial onset of action in about 30–45 seconds
        ii. Drug effect lasts about 10–20 minutes
     d. Most addictive route of administration appears to be smoking
        i. Delivery to brain within 8–10 seconds
        ii. Brief duration of "high" (approximately 5–10 minutes)
  7. Withdrawal symptoms
     a. Generally mild immediately after cessation of use
     b. Increase over next 12–96 hours
     c. Resemble depression (i.e., sad mood, lethargy, boredom, tension, anhedonia)
  8. Powerful reinforcing effects of cocaine make relapse highly likely
D. **Cannabis** (popular and prevalent)
  1. Most commonly smoked in cigarettes and pipes
  2. Two forms available in U.S.
     a. Marijuana ("pot," "grass," "weed")—most popular form in U.S.
     b. Hashish ("hash")
  3. Effects: euphoria or dysphoria, distortions in perception, spatial and temporal disorientation, depersonalization, increased sensitivity to sound, heightened suggestibility, false sense of "deeper" thinking
  4. Effects of smoking marijuana last 2–4 hr; effects of oral ingestion can last 5–12 hr
  5. Intoxication varies with user's mood and surroundings
     a. Users with predisposition to anxiety or psychoses may experience severe emotional reactions
     b. Use in calm state may lead to feeling of sedation
     c. Use in unfamiliar, secretive, or nonsupportive environment may increase feelings of anxiety or paranoia
  6. In 1960s and early 1970s marijuana considered safe and socially acceptable; presently thought to result in cognitive deterioration, depression, amotivational syndrome, or progression to other drugs
  7. Characteristics of amotivational syndrome: passivity, aimlessness, apathy, uncommunicativeness, low ambition; often difficult to separate from personality traits that predispose to drug use
  8. Often considered gateway drug (i.e., stepping stone to "harder" drugs)
     a. People who use marijuana are more likely to frequent drug-using environments
     b. Availability of other drugs may facilitate "kindling" effect
E. **Opioids** (especially heroin) have recently become popular again
  1. People may use illegal opiates when unable to procure prescription refills for such medications as codeine, hydrocodone (Vicodin), pentazocine (Talwin), meperidine (Demerol), oxycodone (Percodan), or propoxyphene (Darvon); opposite is also true
  2. Signs and symptoms: drowsiness, analgesia, exaggerated sense of tranquility, decreased apprehension, hypoactivity, decreased concentration, falling asleep, itching, apathy
  3. Intravenous users may evidence "track marks" on arms, legs, hands, feet, and other body parts due to repetitive use of veins for injection
  4. Overdose may result in: shallow breathing, depressed levels of consciousness, convulsions, clammy skin, mitotic pupils, coma, death
  5. Opioid withdrawal
     a. Symptoms vary but most likely resemble severe influenza
        i. Develop within 2–48 hours, peak at 72 hours, and last 7–10 days
        ii. Within 8–12 hours diaphoresis, nausea, anxiety, yawning, lacrimation, and rhinorrhea may become evident
        iii. At 12–48 hours anorexia, gooseflesh, abdominal spasms, chills, flushing, diarrhea, elevated vital signs (temperature, blood pressure, pulse, respirations), dehydration, and depression may occur

        b. Common misconception: results in death
           i. Temporarily debilitating, but not generally life-threatening
          ii. Two exceptions—meperidine and propoxyphene—may result in seizures
         iii. Procedures used for administering opioids (e.g., needles) more dangerous than withdrawal
        c. Addicts may plead, demand, or attempt to manipulate others to procure drug of choice during withdrawal

F. **Phencyclidine** (PCP, "angel dust")
    1. Developed in 1950s as general anesthetic
    2. Use was discontinued when patients evidenced severe side effects (e.g., flat faces, sightless staring, rigid posturing, waxy flexibility, dissociation)
    3. Most commonly smoked with marijuana but also may be consumed orally, intranasally, or by injection
    4. Effects
        a. Depend on dose and route of administration
        b. When it is smoked, effects are felt in < 5 min with peak effects in 5–30 min
        c. Typical effects: agitation, numbness, increased muscle tone, negativism, social withdrawal, cognitive dysfunction, bizarre responses, concrete thinking, catatonic posturing
    5. Animal studies indicate that discontinuation of PCP may cause significant withdrawal response

G. **Hallucinogens**
    1. Examples: lysergic acid diethylamide (LSD), psilocybin, methylenedioxyamphetamine (MDMA), and mescaline
    2. Nicknames include "acid," "candies," "Lucy in the sky with diamonds," "dots," "shrooms," "magic mushrooms"; MDMA, a relatively new chemical analog (i.e., designer drug), has been known as "ecstasy" or "XTC"
    3. Most potent hallucinogen: LSD
        a. 100–200 times more potent than psilocybin
        b. Usual street dose equals 200 µg
    4. Effects
        a. Central sympathomimetic stimulation, including mydriasis, hyperthermia, tachycardia, and slightly elevated blood pressure
        b. Effects on perception and mood range from mild changes (i.e., heightened awareness) to severe hallucinations with panic and psychotic depression (i.e., "bad trips")

H. **Inhalants**
    1. Substances inhaled for psychotropic effects (e.g., glue, rubber cement, paint thinners, cleaning fluids, lighter fluid, nail polish remover, gasoline)
    2. May contain halogenated hydrocarbons, fluorocarbons, ketones, toluene, nitrous oxide, and so forth
    3. Acute psychological effects may resemble alcohol intoxication
        a. Effects range from mild euphoria to severe disorientation and confusion
        b. Physical effects may include slurred speech, dizziness, and decreased reflexes
    4. Aftereffects may include headache, gastrointestinal symptoms, cerebellar dysfunction, and paresthesias
    5. Toxic effects may include damage to multiple organ systems (e.g., brain, heart, liver) as well as bone marrow suppression and immunosuppression

I. **Stages of change**
    1. People who use drugs are in one of five stages of change
        a. Precontemplation (denial of problem or some ambivalence)
        Belief: "My drug use is not a problem"
        Behavior: continuation of drug use
        b. Contemplation (some consideration of problem; ambivalence grows stronger)
        Belief: "Perhaps my drug use is a problem"
        Behavior: attempts to cut down, change-related behaviors
        c. Preparation (denial mostly ended; focus on potential methods for change)

Belief: "I'm getting ready to quit using drugs"

Behavior: communications with significant others about plans to quit, visit to physician for assistance, enrollment in treatment program, 12-step program

    d. Action (cessation program begun and maintained for at least 24 hours)

Belief: "I've begun to change"

Behavior: learning to substitute positive behaviors for drug use

    e. Maintenance (cessation of drug use maintained for at least 6 months)

Belief: "I'm proud of myself for my success!"

Behavior: new coping strategies have become routine

J. **Relapse**
1. Defined as full return to drug use after successful period of abstinence
2. Unfortunately, extremely common
3. Certain situations place people at high risk for relapse; most triggers for women involve interpersonal relationships
   a. External triggers (e.g., relationship changes, vocational difficulties, death or illness of significant other, anniversaries, celebrations)
   b. Internal triggers (e.g., sadness, anger, boredom, physical pain, physical withdrawal from substance)
4. Relapse should not cause frustration; both physician and patient may benefit from viewing relapse episodes as important learning experiences

III. **An Approach**

A. Illicit drug use tends to be sensitive topic; discussions may be difficult for both physician and patient

B. Physicians who wish to help addicted patients should avoid behaviors likely to contribute to defensiveness
1. Forcing patient to accept label of "addict"
2. Presenting limited options
3. Expressing frustration, anger, or hopelessness
4. Using "scare tactics" or dramatic statements
5. Meeting denial with argumentation
6. Presenting unilateral treatment goals
7. Forcing conclusions and interpretations

C. **Six steps can be taken by physicians**
1. **Screen all patients for illicit drug use**
   a. During measurement of vital signs ask all patients: "Do you drink alcohol, smoke cigarettes, or use any recreational drugs?"
   b. Be attentive to physical signs of illicit drug use (especially in adolescents)
   c. When index of suspicion is high, screen urine (with patient's permission)
2. **Evaluate psychology of women who use illicit drugs**
   a. Ask reasons for drug use
   b. Screen for other psychiatric problems
   c. Inquire about significant others who use drugs (e.g., husband, lover, best friend)
   d. Inquire about history of violence (including current and past verbal, physical, and sexual abuse)
3. **Assess motivation to change illicit drug use**
   a. Learn five stages of change (described above)
   b. Do not assume that all patients are prepared to take action; accept even precontemplators
   c. Ask about patient's plans for behavior change or quitting to evaluate stage of change
   d. Teach women to understand their own stages of change
4. **Provide brief interventions**
   a. Customize behavior change message according to each woman's needs and interests
   b. Provide relevant education about risks of drug use (for example, teach about effects during pregnancy, risk of AIDS, transmission of other infectious diseases)
   c. Discuss relevant benefits of behavior change

    d. Customize behavior change message to woman's stage of change
       i. Help precontemplators begin to contemplate quitting
       ii. Help contemplators prepare for action
       iii. Help those in maintenance feel pride in their success
    e. Provide self-help readings (i.e., bibliotherapy), such as:
       • *The Recovery Book* (Mooney, Eisenberg and Eisenberg, 1992)
       • *The Addiction Workbook* (Fanning and O'Neill, 1996)
       • *Sex, Drugs, Gambling, & Chocolate: A Workbook for Overcoming Addictions* (Horvath, 1998)
    f. Emphasize necessity of lifestyle change as well as changes in drug use
    g. Discuss potential for relapse and plan for high-risk situations that might contribute to relapse
    h. Focus on significant others who might use drugs (for example, ask, "Is your husband planning to quit using drugs? What will you do if he pressures you to resume drug use?")
    i. Treat physical and medical problems associated with addiction
    j. Treat psychological problems associated with addiction (e.g., depression, suicidal ideation)
    k. Provide parenting education to women with children
    l. Recognize need for child care services when appropriate
  5. **Consultation and referral**
    a. Most illicit drug users need help with change
    b. Indications for consultation and referral
       i. Previous unsuccessful quit attempts resulting in pessimism
       ii. Extremely negative emotions associated with change
       iii. Coexisting psychological problems
    c. If there is coexisting psychiatric problem (e.g., depression), provide treatment
    d. Make extensive use of "grass roots" programs (e.g., Narcotics Anonymous, Cocaine Anonymous, SMART (Self-Management and Recovery Training), Secular Organization for Sobriety)
    e. Phone numbers
       • 1-800-COCAINE—referrals to inpatient/outpatient drug treatment (primarily cocaine but also other drugs)
       • 1-800-347-8998—Cocaine Anonymous (CA) referrals
       • 1-216-292-0220—SMART Recovery
  6. **Follow-up**
    a. Arrange follow-up visit within 1–2 weeks after each drug-related visit
    b. During all follow-up visits continue to inquire about substance use status
    c. After patient makes initial changes, provide strong reinforcement (e.g., positive effects on health)
D. **Pharmacotherapy**
  1. Primarily for opiate withdrawal; no real withdrawal syndrome for marijuana, hallucinogens, or inhalants
  2. **Opioid withdrawal**
    a. Narcotics may be used temporarily (up to 3 days) until patient enters detox program
    b. Methadone is drug of choice (20 mg after signs, not self-report, of withdrawal)
    c. Narcotics and methadone prescriptions require license
    d. Clonidine relieves signs but not symptoms; does not require license
    e. Specific recommendations
       i. Treat early
       ii. Outpatient treatment generally most appropriate (if withdrawal is not severe and patient is otherwise medically healthy)
       iii. Provide comprehensive medical evaluation
       iv. Provide empathy and support
       v. Pharmacotherapy not always appropriate or necessary
  3. **Methadone maintenance** (MM)
    a. Appropriate treatment for opiate addiction

    b. Methadone hydrochloride reduces craving for opiates
    c. MM programs are controlled and regulated
    d. MM greatly improves pregnancy outcome for mother and child
    e. Three phases of MM
       i. Stabilization (up to 3 months)
       ii. Treatment planning (with substantial social services)
       iii. Maintenance (with reduced social services)
    f. **Criteria for treatment**
       i. Minimum of 1 year of opiate addiction (including current addiction)—1-year requirement is waived for pregnant women (who are likely to benefit greatly from MM)
       ii. Minimal age of 18 years or parental consent
       iii. Medical problems (e.g., AIDS) should not prohibit use of MM
  4. **Alternative pharmacotherapies**
    a. Clonidine, while limited, has been shown to reduce some symptoms (e.g., restlessness, lacrimation, rhinorrhea, sweating)
    b. Opiate antagonists, partial agonists, and mixed agonist/antagonists (e.g., naltrexone) block certain subjective effects of opiates
    c. Levo-alpha acetylmethadol (LAAM) is an analogue of methadone used to reduce opioid withdrawal
       i. LAAM has a longer half-life than methadone and therefore it can be administered less frequently
       ii. A single dose of LAAM can prevent withdrawal and craving for 2 to 4 days
    d. Buprenorphine is a newly developed partial opiate agonist; advantage is that discontinuation of buprenorphine results in less severe withdrawal
E. **Relapse management**
  1. When relapse occurs, physician should maintain warm, nonjudgmental, empathetic, collaborative, inquisitive attitude
  2. Inquire about reasons for relapse, paying particular attention to
    a. High-risk situations leading to relapse
    b. Beliefs about drug use that were activated in high-risk situation
    c. Strength of urges and cravings before actual use
    d. Permissive beliefs that facilitated relapse (e.g., "It'll be okay; I'll just smoke a little")
  3. After relapse, teach following strategies
    a. Anticipate and avoid high-risk situations in future (whenever possible)—especially intimate relationships with men who have drug problems
    b. Discuss importance of developing anti-drug thoughts and beliefs (e.g., "Drugs only make my problems bigger") vs. pro-drug beliefs (e.g., "I need to use drugs to have fun")
    c. Find alternative behaviors when urges and cravings occur; they will pass
    d. Do not give yourself permission to use drugs under any circumstances; instead, think, "I won't just use a little if I start"
    e. Find interpersonal relationships that do not support drug use
  4. When relapse does occur, continue to be supportive and encourage efforts to quit

SUGGESTED READING

1. American Psychiatric Association: Practice Guideline for Treatment of Patients with Substance Use Disorders: Alcohol, Cocaine, Opioids. Washington, DC, American Psychiatric Association, 1995.
2. Beck AT, Wright FD, Newman CF, Liese BS: Cognitive Therapy of Substance Abuse. New York, Guilford, 1993.
3. Blondell RD (ed): Substance Abuse. Primary Care Clin Office Pract Vol. 20, special issue, 1993.
4. Fanning P, O'Neill JT: The Addiction Workbook: A Step-by-Step Guide to Quitting Alcohol and Drugs. Oakland, CA, New Harbinger Publications, 1996.
5. Fleming MF, Barry KL (eds): Addictive Disorders. St. Louis, Mosby, 1992.
6. Frances RJ, Miller SI (eds): Clinical Textbook of Addictive Disorders, 2nd ed. New York, Guilford, 1998.

7. Horvath AT: Sex, Drugs, Gambling, & Chocolate: A Workbook for Overcoming Addictions. San Luis Obispo, Impact Publishers, 1998.

8. Liese BS, Franz RA: Treating substance use disorders with cognitive therapy: Lessons learned and implications for the future. In Salkovskis PM (ed): Frontiers of Cognitive Therapy. New York, Guilford Press, 1996, pp 470–508.

9. Lisansky Gomberg ES, Nirenberg TD (eds): Women and Substance Abuse. Norwood, NJ, Ablex Publishing, 1993.

10. Lowinson JH, Ruiz P, Millman RB, Langrod JG (eds): Substance Abuse: A Comprehensive Textbook, 3rd ed. Baltimore, Williams & Wilkins, 1997.

11. Marlatt GA, VandenBos GR (eds): Addictive Behaviors: Readings on Etiology, Prevention, and Treatment. Washington, DC, American Psychological Association, 1997.

12. Mooney AJ, Eisenberg A, Eisenberg H: The Recovery Book. New York, Workman, 1992.

PART XII

SPECIAL MEDICAL PROBLEMS OF WOMEN

86. Hirsutism

Valerie Gilchrist, M.D., and Bruce E. Johnson, M.D.

I. **The Issues**

Hirsutism is a symptom of dual concern for women. Some hair growth occurs with aging, accelerating at the menopause, and some hair growth causes little alarm, occurring with a family history or ethnic background of increased hair. Excessive, dark hair in an androgenic distribution is a cause of considerable distress to most women, affecting, as it does, ones appearance and perhaps even the self-image of femininity. In addition, hirsutism, especially if it is of relatively recent onset or progression, carries concern for a serious diagnosis. Fortunately, the diagnosis of tumor is infrequent but still emotionally wrenching, especially when the work-up for tumor is coupled with a change in appearance. A major challenge for the generalist is to decide when hair growth is atypical enough to warrant a thorough evaluation, which can be both expensive and even invasive.

II. **The Theory**

A. **Definition of hirsutism**

1. Dark, terminal hair developing in androgen-sensitive skin zones, including upper lip, chin, sideburns, neck, chest, lower abdomen, inner thighs (Fig. 1)
2. Differentiated from normal hair growth variation and hypertrichosis
   a. Familial or ethnic pattern (e.g., Mediterranean ancestry) of some facial hair, periareolar hair and partial male escutcheon
   b. Hypertrichosis consists of fine lanugo or vellus hair distributed evenly over the body—not dark, terminal hair
   i. Hypertrichosis may result from diseases such as anorexia nervosa, hyperthyroidism, and head injuries or medications such as phenytoin, cyclosporine, corticosteroids, and minoxidil
3. Hirsutism may be associated with other signs of virilization such as breast atrophy, increase in muscle mass, temporal hair loss, amenorrhea and infertility, and clitoromegaly
   a. Concern of androgen-secreting tumor but virilization occurs in < 1% of women with hirsutism

B. **Sex hormone–responsive hair cells** have receptors for androgens and the enzyme 5 alpha-reductase
1. Converts testosterone to its biologically active form, dihydrotestosterone (DHT)
2. Most responsive areas in normal women are the axillae and perineal areas; normal women convert vellus hair to terminal hair in these areas at puberty

C. **Hirsute women convert vellus hair to terminal hair in areas of the body more typical of a male distribution**; hirsute women demonstrate following changes:
1. Hair follicles in androgen sensitive areas metabolize circulating androgens more avidly to the biologically active form.
2. Most of the causes of hirsutism cause reduction in steroid-binding globulin (SBG), which results in more biologically active testosterone in the circulation.
3. About 80% of hirsute women have increased androgens
   a. Normally, females produce 250 mg of testosterone over 24 hours; 25% is ovarian in origin, 25% is adrenal in origin, and 50% results from the peripheral conversion of androstenedione to testosterone.

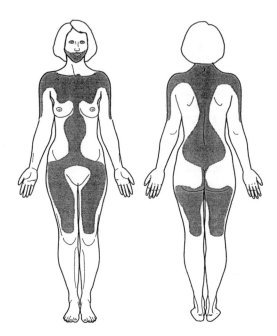

FIGURE 1. The shaded areas indicate regions of the body where hirsutism can occur. (From Excess Facial and Body Hair: A Guide for Patients. Patient Information Series of the American Fertility Society. Birmingham, AL, The American Fertility Society, 1991, p 5.)

  D. **Obesity and insulin resistance** are associated with increased circulating levels of androgens and increased transformation of androgens to testosterone in peripheral sites
    1. Hyperinsulinism stimulates ovarian androgen production
  E. **Polycystic ovary syndrome**, perhaps the most common cause of hirsutism, is syndrome of increased androgen production, decreased SBG production, increased corticosteroids, and obesity—combining virtually all mechanisms of hirsutism
  F. **Other potential causes** of androgen, or androgen-like, stimulation of terminal hair growth includes prolactin, adrenal precursors of androgens, excessive production or ingestion of corticosteroids, exogenous sources of androgens, medications
  G. **Differential diagnosis** (Table 1)
    1. Idiopathic hirsutism and polycystic ovary syndrome account for 90–95% of all cases of hirsutism
III. **An Approach**
  A. **History** (Table 2)
    1. Emphasize:
      a. Use of any medication
      b. Presence of galactorrhea
      c. Signs of virilism
      d. Menstrual history and fertility

TABLE 1. Differential Diagnosis of Hirsutism

Idiopathic hirsutism	Pituitary
Polycystic ovary syndrome	Cushing's syndrome, prolactinoma
Hyperthecosis variant	Medications
Congenital adrenal hyperplasia	Anabolic steroids
Late-onset, including incomplete deficiencies	Testosterone
of 21-hydroxylase, 11-β-hydroxylase,	Oral contraceptives (especially those containing
3-β-hydroxysteroid dehydrogenase	the progestins norgestrel, levonorgestrel,
Ovarian tumors	and norethindrone)
Primary and metastases	Corticosteroids
Adrenal	Danazol
Adenoma, carcinoma, Cushing's syndrome	

TABLE 2.   Key Components of the History and Physical Examination of a Woman with the Complaint of Excessive Hair Growth

History	Physical Examination
Hair growth (onset and speed of progression, distribution, response to treatment)	Height, weight, and blood pressure
Medication use	Amount, distribution, and characteristics of hair growth
Menstrual, contraceptive, and reproductive history	Signs of virilization (breast atrophy, increase in muscle mass, redistribution of body fat with development of male physique, temporal recession of scalp hair, deepening of voice, clitoral enlargement)
Family history of hair growth	
Galactorrhea	Physical features of Cushing's syndrome ("moon" facies, "buffalo" hump, central obesity, striae, acne, proximal muscle weakness)
Symptoms of virilization (voice changes, muscle bulk)	
Abdominal complaints (pain, increased girth)	Galactorrhea
Skin changes (acne, striae, bruising)	Abdominal palpation for masses
Weight gain	Pelvic exam with bimanual evaluation of ovarian size
	Dermatologic abnormalities (acne, acanthosis nigricans, striae)

  e. Family history of hirsutism—may suggest or lead to evaluation for:
   i. Genetic factors affecting hair follicles
   ii. Presence of polycystic ovaries
   iii. Congenital adrenal hyperplasia (late-onset form, inherited as recessive trait)
  f. Temporal course of hirsutism (one of most important factors)
   i. Slow increase over years since puberty
   ii. Acute onset over preceding 1–2 years
 2. Significance
  a. In women with normal menses, positive family history, and slow onset, etiology likely familial/ethnic or idiopathic
   i. With no other clues in history or physical, probably warrants no further diagnostic evaluation and treatment focusing on cosmesis
  b. If hirsute woman has irregular menses and slow onset since puberty, most likely diagnosis is polycystic ovary syndrome (PCOS)
  c. Acute onset, especially with features of virilization, highly suggestive of androgen-secreting tumor
B. **Physical exam** (Table 2)
 1. 50% of hirsute women are > 20% above ideal weight
 2. 30% present with galactorrhea and/or hyperprolactinemia, but women with prolactinoma rarely present with hirsutism
 3. Acanthosis nigricans indicates increased androgens with insulin resistance and hyperinsulinemia
 4. Hirsute women often have mild acne
C. **Laboratory evaluations**
 1. Typical initial blood tests usually normal (e.g., CBC, chemistry panels, UA, thyroid stimulating hormone)
 2. Figure 2 gives proposed algorithm for evaluation—dependent on history and physical exam evidence for virilization and/or menstrual irregularity
 3. All proposed tests for idiopathic hirsutism will be negative (since idiopathic hirsutism is thought to be an abnormal sensitivity of the androgen receptors in the hair follicle)
 4. Since PCO will account for most of the diagnoses, this is the principle target of testing
  a. Enlarged polycystic ovaries often detected on pelvic exam though it is appropriate to proceed to pelvic ultrasound
  b. Measure free testosterone, LH, FSH
   i. PCO characteristically has normal to mildly elevated testosterone, and LH:FSH ratio > 3:1
 5. Other diagnoses will require measurement of prolactin, dihydroepiandrosterone (DHEA), 17-hydroxyprogesterone, cortisone (and its stimulating and suppression

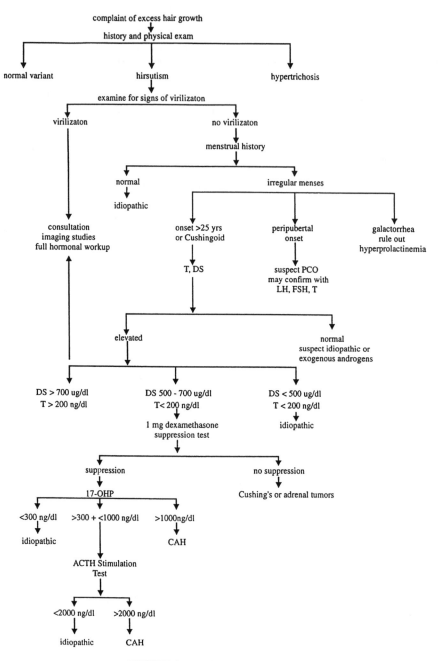

FIGURE 2. Evaluation of hirsutism.

tests) and other investigations beyond the scope of this chapter, although Table 3 gives the basis for interpretation of these tests

6. **Significance**

   a. Serum testosterone > 200 ng/dl or signs of virilization increases concern for ovarian tumor, whereas elevation of both serum testosterone and DHEA suggests adrenal origin of androgens

TABLE 3. Investigations and Management of Hirsutism

Diagnosis	C	T	DS	LH	FSH	P	17-OHP	Management
CAH	↑	N/↑	N/↑	–	–	–	↑	Antiandrogens ± low-dose gluco-corticoids
PCO	–	↑	↑/N	↑	↓/–	↑/–	–	Antiandrogens, oral contraceptives
Idiopathic	–	–	–	–	–	–	–	Antiandrogens
Exogenous	–	–	–	–	–	–	–	Remove offending agent
Tumor	↑/N	↑↑	↑↑	–	–	–	–	Surgery; treat cause

CAH = congenital adrenal hyperplasia; PCO = polycystic ovary; C = cortisol; T = testosterone; DS = dehydroepiandrosterone; LH = luteinizing hormone; FSH = follicle-stimulating hormone; P = prolactin; 17-OHP = 17-hydroxyprogesterone; N = normal.

      b. DHEA level > 500 µg/dl suggests adrenal source of androgens
         i. Cushing's syndrome (25% of female patients have hirsutism)
         ii. Most women with hirsutism and elevated DHEA have congenital adrenal hyperplasia (CAH) with late onset of symptoms
            (a) 95% of CAH due to deficiency of 21-hydroxylase, which results in increase of 17-alpha-hydroxyprogesterone
               (i) Levels > 300 ng/dl after adrenocorticotropic hormone (ACTH) stimulation test confirm diagnosis
      c. If prolactin level is increased, hirsutism is part of amenorrhea/galactorrhea syndrome
      d. If DHEA, LH, and FSH are normal, suspect either iatrogenic or idiopathic hirsutism
         i. Iatrogenic hirsutism associated with drugs that stimulate androgens
         ii. Drugs that cause hyperprolactinemia, such as phenothiazines, may be associated with hirsutism

D. **Treatment**
    1. **For mild hirsutism** local measures may be all that is necessary
      a. Bleaching
      b. Shaving
      c. Plucking or waxing
         i. May stimulate hair growth by increasing blood supply to follicle
         ii. Also may given illusion of increased growth by synchronizing growth cycle
      d. Depilatories
         i. Associated with high incidence of hypersensitivity reactions
      e. Electrolysis
         i. Needs to be done by qualified, licensed operator
         ii. Home units have greater risk of pitting and scarring
         iii. Major side effects: local infection and irritation
    2. **Encourage obese women to lose weight**
    3. **Treatment of polycystic ovary determined by woman's desire for fertility**
      a. If fertility is not desired, low-dose contraceptives are effective
         i. Estrogens increase SBG and antagonize androgen effects at level of hair follicle
         ii. Progesterones increase clearance of testosterone
         iii. Testosterone levels should be decreased when rechecked in approximately 3 months
         iv. Ultrasound of ovaries may show decrease in size after 6 months treatment with OC
      b. If woman desires fertility, stimulation of ovulation with clomiphene citrate may be indicated
    4. **Other therapies dictated by diagnosis**, e.g., tumors are removed and treated, congenital adrenal hyperplasia often responds to low-dose corticosteroid suppression, prolactinomas are either removed or treated with bromocriptine, etc.
    5. In addition to specific therapies, **antiandrogen therapy** is helpful
      a. Treatment of choice for idiopathic hirsutism
      b. Two drugs available in U.S.

   i. **Spironolactone** (most commonly used)
      (a) Potassium-sparing diuretic
      (b) Blocks synthesis of ovarian androgen and binding of DHT to androgen receptors in hair follicles as well as decreasing 5-alpha reductase activities in hair follicles
      (c) Dose ranges from 50–200 mg/day
      (d) Contraindicated in pregnancy and in patients with hyperkalemia or renal disease
   ii. **Flutamide**
      (a) Nonsteroidal antiandrogen approved for treatment of prostate cancer
      (b) Noted to be effective for hirsutism but not FDA-approved for this indication
      (c) May prove superior to spironolactone but side effects can be severe and include possible hepatotoxicity and teratogenicity
      (d) Costly
   c. **Other drugs**
      i. Cyproterone acetate
         (a) Potent antiandrogen derived from hydroxyprogesterone
         (b) Not approved in U.S. but has been used for many years in Europe
      ii. Finasteride
         (a) 5 alpha-reductase inhibitor, FDA-approved only for treatment of prostatic hypertrophy
         (b) Currently under investigation as treatment for hirsutism
6. If treatment is successful, change from coarse to vellus hair is evident in 3–6 months in 60% of hirsute women
   a. Local measures may still be necessary
   b. Response to treatment is highly individual but an attempt is warranted in any woman disturbed enough by her appearance to have sought medical evaluation

SUGGESTED READING

1. American Society of Reproductive Medicine: Excess facial and body hair: A guide for patients. Patient Information Series of the American Society of Reproductive Medicine. Birmingham, AL, American Society of Reproductive Medicine, 1991.
2. Barth J: Hirsute women: Should they be investigated? J Clin Pathol 45:188–192, 1992.
3. Delahunt JW: Hirsutism: Practical therapeutic guidelines. Drugs 45:223–231, 1993.
4. Ehrmann DA, Rosenfield RL: Hirsutism—beyond the steroidogenic block. N Engl J Med 323:909–911, 1990.
5. Givens JR, Kurtz BR: Hirsutism, virilization, and androgen excess. In Hurst JW (ed): The Practicing Physician, 3rd ed. Stoneham, MA, Butterworth-Heinemann, 1992, pp 568–571.
6. Hatasaka HH, Wentz AC: Hirsutism—facts and folklore. Part II: Management options. Female Patient 16:73–81, 1991.
7. Kalve E, Klein JF: Evaluation of women with hirsutism. Am Fam Physician 54:117–124, 1996.
8. McKenna TJ: Screening for sinister causes of hirsutism. N Engl J Med 331:1015–1016, 1994.
9. Rittmaster RS: Evaluation and treatment of hirsutism. Infertil Reprod Med Clin North Am 2:511–530, 1991.
10. Watson RE, Bouknight R, Alguire PC: Hirsutism: Evaluation and management. J Gen Intern Med 10:283–292, 1995.

87. Osteoporosis

Bruce E. Johnson, M.D.

I. The Issues

Osteoporosis is one of the most common medical conditions that afflict women in the U.S.—perhaps 1 in 4 white women over the age of 65 years will have manifestations of the disease. Osteoporosis is inextricably tied with estrogen loss, making this disease one of the quintessential concerns in women's health. The consequences of osteoporosis are a significant source of morbidity and mortality as well as economic loss. The disease, however, should be largely preventable. Prevention requires a concerted educational effort directed at younger women who must be convinced that current efforts will have benefits 40 or more years in the future. Prevention also involves modifications in diet, exercise, and lifestyle, changes that are difficult to implement under the best of circumstances over a much shorter time. In the foreseeable future, efforts will be made to identify and treat women at risk for the consequences of osteoporosis. However, this approach involves screening on a vast scale with technology that currently is not inexpensive and not always readily available. The economics of screening and treatment is troublesome despite the potential savings in cost and reduction in morbidity.

II. **The Theory**
   A. **Prevalence**
      1. Probably 10 times more common in women than men
         a. Related to cessation of sex hormone production
         b. Men with low testosterone also at risk
      2. Affects 1 in 4 white women over 65 in U.S.
         a. Also common in Asians living in industrialized countries
         b. Less common in blacks or Hispanics, probably because of greater bone mass entering menopause
   B. **Normal bone metabolism**
      1. Bone turnover occurs continuously
      2. Basic cells involved are osteoclasts and osteoblasts
         a. Osteoclasts
            i. Involved in bone resorption
            ii. Create microscopic lacunae in bone matrix
         b. Osteoblasts
            i. Move into lacunae and begin process of bone formation
            ii. Secrete hydroxyapatite, an amorphous, calcium-based "cement" material between cells
      3. Approximately 10% of bony skeleton is resculpted each year
         a. During periods of growth and repair (childhood, young adulthood, fractures) slight overproduction by osteoblasts results in new bone formation with lengthening and strengthening
         b. Bone density and strength greatest at sites of stress and tension—muscle attachments, gravity-resisting sites
         c. During adult years, bone metabolism in close balance between osteoclasts and osteoblasts
         d. After menopause, loss of sex hormone results in slight overactivity by osteoclasts which, over many years, results in loss of bone density
      4. Maximal bone density for most women occurs in late 20s
         a. After this age, slight decline in BMA as a consequence of aging alone
            i. Amounts to < 1% per year
         b. Maximal bone density very important at menopause
            i. Higher bone density results in less osteoporosis
      5. Estrogen (and most other therapeutic agents used to treat osteoporosis) has effect of decreasing osteoclastic activity thereby decreasing bone turnover
   C. **Factors in maximal bone density at menopause**
      1. Calcium intake
         a. People (cultures) with high calcium intake have lower prevalence of osteoporosis
            i. Most commonly, milk product intake
            ii. Calcium may be found in drinking water in certain areas
      2. Parity
         a. Greater parity (with proper nutrition) usually gives greater BMA
            i. Pregnancy is a high estrogen state with increased gravity stress on bones promoting bone strength
      3. Breastfeeding
         a. Benefit probably related to persistent estrogen effect
         b. Short-term breastfeeding, even with multiple children, has no adverse effect on eventual bone density if nutrition is adequate

    4. Menstrual regularity
       a. Prolonged amenorrhea poses risk of low BMA
         i. Hypoestrogen state mimicking menopause
    5. Body habitus
       a. Obesity has positive effect on bone density
         i. Effect of gravity pull on bone strength
         ii. Fat tissue converts androgens to mild estrogenic hormones such as estrone; more fat tissue, more estrone
       b. Very thin women do not have adequate bone mass
         i. Often inadequate diet such as women with anorexia nervosa and bulimia
         ii. Less body fat associated with hypoestrogenism, menstrual irregularity/amenorrhea, and decreased bone deposition
    6. Exercise
       a. Moderate exercise has benefit
         i. Salutary effect of muscle tension on bony strength
         ii. Lifestyle requiring hard physical labor, regardless of ethnic influence, has low prevalence of osteoporosis
       b. Excessive exercise may pose risk
         i. Exercise-induced amenorrhea (female triad syndrome; see Chapter 6)
    7. Alcohol—excessive intake, presumably at expense of more balanced diet
    8. Smoking—clearly associated with low density
    9. Medications, treatments associated with osteoporosis
       a. Corticosteroids, phenytoin, heparin, warfarin chemotherapeutics, immunosuppressives, others

D. Menopause: defining event
    1. Cessation of estrogen production associated with inevitable decline in BMA
       a. For most of the first decade after menopause, BMA declines 3–5% per year
       b. 10–15 years after menopause, rapid decline plateaus but bone loss still occurs
    2. Estrogen replacement halts rapid decline
    3. Decline begins at any age estrogen production ceases
       a. Premature menopause for whatever reason
         i. Premature ovarian failure
         ii. Surgical oophorectomy
         iii. Inadequate diet, excessive exercise
    4. Estrogen replacement even many years after premature menopause may halt rapid decline—even adds modest amount of BMA

E. Differential diagnosis of osteopenia (Table 1)
    1. Osteoporosis is actually a "diagnosis of exclusion"—the causes listed in Table 1 should be considered in any woman evaluated for osteopenia

F. Consequences of osteoporosis
    1. Fractures
       a. Hip most serious
         i. In elderly women, often occurs with minimal trauma, such as simple falls or even stumbling or twisting motion
         ii. Morbidity of surgery and rehabilitation
            (a) After hip surgery for fracture, 2 in 3 leave hospital in poorer functional status than prior to fracture, often requiring nursing homes or home health aid
         iii. Mortality
            (a) Up to 5–10% operative mortality
            (b) 15–20% mortality 1 year after fracture
            (c) Mortality almost always associated with underlying medical illnesses or debility and not totally due to consequences of fracture itself
       b. Other long bones
         i. Wrist—Colles-type fracture most common
         ii. Humerus—prolonged disability with sling
         iii. Ankle—cast, crutches make mobility difficult

TABLE 1. Differential Diagnosis of Osteopenia

Primary osteoporosis	**Secondary osteoporosis** *(cont.)*
Menopause-related	Renal disease
Age-related	Renal failure
Lifestyle-related	Hematologic disorders and malignancies
Strong family history of osteoporosis, especially	Sickle cell disease
fracture of hip or development of kyphosis	Mastocytosis
	Multiple myeloma
Secondary osteoporosis	Rheumatic diseases
Endocrine	Inflammatory arthritis (e.g., rheumatoid arthritis)
Thyroid	Scoliosis
Hypothyroidism	Medications
Hyperthyroidism	Corticosteroids
Graves' disease	Phenytoin
Iatrogenic	Heparin
Cushing's syndrome	Chemotherapy
Hyperparathyroidism	Immunosuppressants
Premature ovarian failure	Anorexia nervosa and bulimia nervosa
Hypopituitarism	Osteomalacia
Digestive disorders	
Malabsorption (multiple causes)	
Inflammatory bowel disease	

      c. Vertebrae
         i. Osteoporotic vertebral fracture typically between T6 and L1
           (a) Above T6 or below L1 raises concern of secondary cause, especially malignancy
        ii. Fractures occur with minimal trauma
           (a) Usually asymptomatic and painless except for vague ache
        iii. Anterior compression (wedging)
           (a) Reduces anterior height greater than posterior
           (b) Leads to kyphosis
        iv. Occasionally burst vertebra and central compression
  2. **Kyphosis** (dowager's hump)
      a. Loss of height
      b. Changes balance
         i. Thrusts center of gravity forward, leading to imbalance and may contribute to falls and fractures
      c. Forces rib cage into abdomen
         i. Reduces distance between ribs and iliac crests
         ii. Causes pain if ribs rest on iliac crest
      d. Compresses abdominal contents, resulting in protuberance of abdomen ("pouchy stomach")
         i. May be mistaken for obesity
         ii. Alters bowel function causing early satiety, delayed bowel transit, constipation
      e. Changes neck/back curvature, exaggerating cervical lordosis and putting strain on posterior neck muscles to keep head up, eyes forward
         i. Cause of neck pain and headache
      f. Advanced kyphosis may limit respiratory capacity—rare cause of restrictive lung disease
      g. Alters body carriage
         i. Combination of thoracic hump, foreshortened waist, and protuberant abdomen makes clothes selection difficult
 G. **Screening**
  1. Conceptually, all postmenopausal women at risk
      a. Identifying those women with low BMA identifies those at risk of developing complications of osteoporosis
  2. Consideration of risk factors allows more selective approach

TABLE 2. Factors Associated with Risk for Osteoporosis

White or Asian race	Low calcium intake
First-degree female relatives with osteoporosis, hip fracture	Scoliosis
	Prior or current disease (as listed in Table 1)
Thinness	Medications (especially corticosteroids, phenytoin)
Early menopause without hormone replacement	Smoking
Amenorrhea during reproductive years	Excess alcohol

    a. Women with risk factors may then be counseled regarding tests to identify BMA or followed regularly with BMA measurements

    b. Factors associated with risk for osteoporosis (Table 2)

3. **Technology**

    a. Plain film radiography

        i. Requires 40% bone loss before evident

        ii. May give impetus to accurately measure BMA but of little sensitive value itself.

    b. Ultrasonography of patella or calcaneus

        i. Detects changes in sound wave transmission dependent on bone density

        ii. Reliability and reproducibility still unclear

        iii. Preliminary studies suggest a role to identify women who should have more accurate BMA measurement

        iv. Portable, easy to use, should be inexpensive

    c. Quantitative computed tomography (QCT)

        i. Accurate though difficult reproducibility

        ii. Expensive, time-consuming

        iii. Relatively large radiation exposure

    d. Single-photon absorptiometry (SPA)

        i. Fairly reproducible, portable and inexpensive

        ii. Poor correlation with hip or vertebrae density

        iii. Not accurate enough for screening

    e. Dual photon absorptiometry (DPA)

        i. Accurate and reproducible

        ii. Long exposure time though low radiation

        iii. Nuclear isotope requires special handling

    f. Dual-energy x-ray absorptiometry (DEXA)

        i. Accurate and reproducible (< 0.5% variance)

        ii. Low radiation, easily adapted to office practices

        iii. Rapid (< 30 minutes)

    g. Blood and urine markers of bone turnover (Table 3)

        i. Most commonly marketed are osteocalcin, cross-links, N-telo

        ii. Not likely to be useful in diagnosis—better used if question arises regarding efficacy of therapy chosen for patient

    h. Consensus that DEXA most accurate test for diagnosis and evaluation of therapy even though DEXA is somewhat expensive (typically > $125)

TABLE 3. Biochemical Markers of Bone Turnover

Bone formation	**Bone resorption**
Serum	Serum
Alkaline phosphatase	Tartrate-resistant acid phosphatase ("TRAP")
Osteocalcin	Urine
C- and N-propeptides of type I collagen	Pyridinium cross-links of collagen ("cross-links")
	C- and N-telopeptides of collagen ("N-telo")
	Galactosyl hydroxylysine
	Hydroxyproline

III. **An Approach**
  A. **Prevention and education**
    1. **Diet**
      a. Balanced, especially with calcium sources
        i. Milk (amount of calcium per volume increases as fat content decreases, such that skim milk actually has more calcium per volume than regular milk)
        ii. Milk products (cheese, yogurt, cottage cheese)
        iii. Certain vegetables (cauliflower, brussel sprouts)
      b. Many young women (teens, young adults) stop ingestion of milk products; need to be encouraged to continue
        i. Typical calcium intake for adult American women often not more than 500 mg/day
        ii. Recommended daily allowance for calcium for premenopausal, nonpregnant women—1000 mg/day; for postmenopausal women (not on estrogen replacement)—1000–1500 mg/day
      c. Majority of blacks and many Asians develop lactase deficiency; need sources of calcium other than milk
      d. Other cations—e.g., magnesium—also needed
        i. Found in meats
      e. Vitamin D
        i. While studies demonstrate vitamin D supplementation alone can treat osteoporosis, should be certain calcium intake also adequate
        ii. Evidence that vitamin D deficient in institutionalized, elderly and chronically ill who are not/cannot be in sunlight
      f. Appropriate weight
        i. Obesity actually is preventive of osteoporosis, but other health risks preclude
        ii. Excessive thinness, especially through anorexia nervosa or bulimia poses high risk and should be diagnosed
    2. **Exercise**
      a. Generally recommend weight-bearing (e.g., walking, jogging, gardening)
        i. Other exercises, including even swimming, better than no exercise
      b. Caution against excessive exercise
        i. Exercise-induced amenorrhea poses risk
      c. Ideal to advise for lifelong physical activity
    3. **Medical conditions** (e.g., those listed in Table 1)
      a. Many chronic diseases predispose to osteoporosis
      b. Special caution regarding premature menopause
        i. Early identification and intervention
      c. Scoliosis
        i. May be mild enough not to require intervention while a youth but still poses risk as adult for accelerated osteoporosis
      d. Medications (associated with osteoporosis)
        i. Because of prevalence of use, heightened concern regarding corticosteroids, phenytoin, over-replacement of thyroxine
      e. Whenever these diseases occur or medications are used, the consideration should be given regarding the eventual development of osteoporosis—if evaluation not appropriate at that time, patient should be informed so that she can raise the issue with her physician at a later time (e.g., at menopause)
  B. **Screening**
    1. Virtually by definition, all women are at risk for osteoporosis and screening could be considered. It is unreasonable to screen all women, so thought must go into recommendation to screen.
    2. Three important situations should prompt consideration for osteoporosis screening
      a. Premenopausal medical risk factors
      b. Perimenopausal status
      c. Postmenopausal complications

3. **Premenopausal medical risk factors**
   a. Even premenopausal women can develop osteoporosis; if a condition in Table 1 develops, consideration should be given to testing for osteoporosis.
      i. Greatest concern with chronic, debilitating diseases (e.g., inflammatory bowel disease, rheumatoid arthritis, cancer treatment, amenorrhea, prolonged use of corticosteroids)
4. **Perimenopausal status**
   a. Critical time to consider intervention since estrogen production ceases and BMA falls
   b. In course of discussing menopause with patient, a decision to use estrogen replacement (ERT) for reasons other than osteoporosis obviates need to test for BMA
   c. If patient unsure about ERT, knowledge of BMA might be enough to decide
      i. If BMA adequate, may decide not to use ERT; if BMA low, may be deciding factor to proceed with ERT
   d. If patient has numerous risk factors, knowledge of BMA may compel decision to use some therapy, even if patient chooses not to use ERT
   e. Potential algorithm Figure 1
5. **Postmenopausal complications**
   a. Medicare Bone Mass Measurement Coverage Standardization Act has concluded the indications for BMA include individuals with:
      i. Estrogen deficiency at clinical risk of osteoporosis
      ii. Long-term glucocorticoid therapy
      iii. Vertebral abnormalities
      iv. Primary hyperparathyroidism
   b. Other conditions which might prompt BMA measurement include hip, wrist, femur fracture, loss of height, multiple other medical conditions but Medicare would have to be petitioned for coverage
C. **Evaluation and work-up**
   1. Evaluation should have several aims
      a. Search for secondary illness requiring specific treatment
      b. Assess degree of osteopenia
      c. Guide appropriate treatment
      d. Identify special circumstances (e.g., pain control, significant kyphosis)

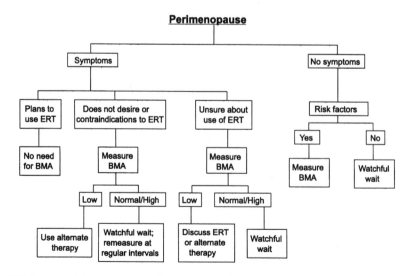

FIGURE 1. Algorithm proposing role of bone density measurement in treatment decisions for perimenopausal women. ERT, estrogen replacement therapy; BMA, bone mineral analysis.

2. **History and physical examination**
   a. Special attention to medical history, high-risk diseases or conditions, degree of kyphosis, identification of other diseases
3. **Laboratory tests**
   a. Complete blood count, chemistry profile, urinalysis, thyroid tests should be standard
   b. Consideration of vitamin D level if circumstances warrant
   c. Follow up other conditions identified by history and physical exam
4. **Radiology**
   a. Not always useful unless patient has kyphosis, known "arthritis" or degenerative joint disease of back, or back pain
   b. Radiographs can identify sclerosis of lumbar region which can give falsely elevated BMA
5. **Bone mineral analysis** (BMA)
   a. Considered diagnostic test of choice (in addition to value in following efficacy of therapy—see below)
   b. Standardized measurements at lumbar spine (with average taken of L2, L3 and L4) and at hip (3 locations)
      i. Sclerosis or other artifacts raise BMA—if result seems unexpectedly normal or high, consider plain radiographs to look for artifact
   c. BMA reported as an absolute density (in mg/cm^3) and as comparison to standard
      i. Standard chosen is "young normal"—typically a group of women at approximately age 30
      ii. Report often also gives comparison to "age matched" which is of little value since, for most older groups, the age matched is already dangerously low bone density and at risk of fracture—should ignore "age-matched" value
   d. Report also given as t-score
      i. t-score is simply the number of standard deviations the observed value differs from a "young normal"
   e. World Health Organization (WHO) has determined the following regarding t-score:
      i. t-score > –1 standard deviation (SD)—within normal limits
      ii. t-score –1 to –2.5 SD—moderate osteopenia
      iii. t-score < –2.5 SD—severe osteopenia
   f. According to WHO, any t-score < –1 SD should prompt careful discussion and probably treatment
6. **Other tests**
   a. Other radiology tests of limited additional usefulness
   b. Blood and urine tests should be saved to monitor therapy
   c. Bone cortex biopsy with histomorphography
      i. Gold standard for certain causes of osteopenia such as osteomalacia, mastocytosis, hyperparathyroidism
      ii. Costly to obtain biopsy, complicated for pathology to read accurately, usually reserved for research/tertiary settings

D. **Treatment**
1. **Calcium intake**
   a. Adequate calcium intake essential to all aspects of therapy
   b. Ideal to increase dietary sources of calcium
      i. Dietary consult may determine sources and quantity of calcium in current diet and suggest means to increase intake
   c. Supplement to recommended daily allowance (RDA)
      i. Premenopausal, nonpregnant female—1000 mg/day
      ii. Postmenopausal female—1000–1500 mg/day
      iii. Unless dietary intake can be increased, may have to supplement 400–600 mg/day since most American women ingest only about 600 mg/day
   d. Choice depends on patient preference
      i. Calcium carbonate (e.g., OsCal, Tums) often least expensive, well tolerated
      ii. Calcium citrate (Citracal), calcium lactate or calcium gluconate occasionally recommended if calcium carbonate poorly tolerated

e. Often suggested that dose be taken at bedtime to counteract modest increase in calcium mobilization with supine position; this suggestion more theoretical than practical

2. **Exercise**
   a. Strongly encourage weight-bearing exercise such as walking, gardening
   b. Instruction in upper-back extension exercises
      i. Kyphosis changes angle of neck, thrusting head forward and down; neck muscles and upper back compensate by contracting to keep eyes forward
      ii. Upper back extension exercises strengthen the entire upper back to lift the neck and head from further back down the neck
      iii. Results in better posture, less neck pain and fatigue, even modest increase in height
      iv. Instructions by physical therapist

3. **Estrogen replacement therapy** (ERT)
   a. Treatment of choice for osteoporosis if appropriate
      i. Especially important in premature menopause
   b. Effective even 10–15 years after menopause
      i. Often induces modest BMA gain; certainly helps prevent further loss
   c. More effective at maintaining BMA than any other therapy
      i. Multiple studies demonstrate that ERT indefinitely maintains the "plateau" phase—but that bone loss occurs shortly after stopping ERT
   d. Most studies confirm that dose equivalent of 0.625 mg conjugated estrogens (Premarin) or 1 mg estradiol (Estrace) adequate to maintain BMA
      i. Lower dose might be satisfactory but evidence still somewhat conflicting
   e. In theory, ERT can be continued indefinitely
   f. Multiple other considerations for ERT (see Chapter 69)

4. **Bisphosphonates**
   a. Pyrophosphate analogs bind to hydroxyapatite and inhibit osteoclast-mediated bone resorption
   b. Etidronate first studied and used in cyclic fashion but alendronate (Fosamax) now largely supplanted etidronate
      i. Multiple other bisphosphonates in trials (e.g., pamidronate, risedronate)
   c. Studies confirm reduction in hip fracture with use—similar to strength of data regarding ERT
      i. Often next therapy chosen if ERT not indicated, not desired or not tolerated
   d. Good data supports dose of alendronate 10 mg/day with increase BMA of 7–8% and continuing after 3 years
      i. Early results suggest dose of 5 mg/day increases BMA by at least 3–4%
   e. Poorly absorbed (< 10%) so cannot be taken with any other medication, food, or calcium supplement
      i. Also persistent reports of esophageal or gastric ulceration if not taken with adequate water
      ii. Instruct patient to take alendronate on empty stomach with full glass of water, not to lie down, and no food, medication or supplement for at least 30 minutes
   f. Must have adequate calcium intake as well
   g. Alendronate studied for at least 5 years, perhaps longer

5. **Calcitonin**
   a. Inhibitor of bone resorption (similar to estrogen)
   b. Good evidence that markers of bone turnover decrease with use of calcitonin and that BMA stabilizes (if not actually increases)
      i. Early studies with nasal calcitonin confirm hip fracture reduction
   c. Only product available in U.S. is salmon calcitonin (though investigating porcine and eel)
      i. Available in injectable and nasal spray formulation; nasal spray better accepted
      ii. Must have adequate calcium intake
   d. Nasal spray calcitonin dose of 200–400 IU daily

e. Injectable calcitonin (and to lesser degree nasal) effective as analgesic—presumably by release of endogenous opiods
   i. Makes calcitonin treatment to consider in painful fractures, especially vertebral

6. **Selective estrogen receptor modulators** (SERMs)
   a. Newest class of drugs to be used for osteoporosis
      i. Prototypical agent is tamoxifen, which has been available for years as treatment for breast cancer
   b. Often called "antiestrogen"—function by binding to estrogen receptors and either blocking or enhancing estrogen effect
      i. Tamoxifen, for example, blocks estrogen action on breast tissue while stimulating uterine tissue
      ii. Because of stimulatory effect on uterine tissue, patients on tamoxifen at increased risk of developing uterus cancer
   c. SERMs being investigated for "ideal" blocking/ enhancing profile—select the best features of estrogen to enhance, and block the less desirable effects
      i. "Ideal" would include estrogen-like effects on bone, lipids and menopausal symptoms while not stimulating breast or uterine tissue
      ii. There is no ideal SERM
   d. Raloxifene (Evista) now available—stimulates bone and lipids while blocks estrogen effect on breast and uterus
      i. Unfortunately, often induces menopausal symptoms such as hot flashes which limits acceptance
   e. Typical dose of raloxifene is 60 mg/day
   f. Not known if time limit to use

7. **Vitamin D supplement**
   a. Frank osteomalacia from vitamin D deficiency not common
      i. Special circumstances in which it may occur include elderly/nursing home residents, malabsorption syndromes, renal disease, vitamin D–resistant syndromes
      ii. Relative deficiency more common
   b. Several studies suggest that supplement, even when measured vitamin D is adequate, may prevent fractures
      i. Always accompanied with adequate calcium intake
   c. If dietary history, lack of sunlight, or measured value suggests insufficiency, supplement with cholecalciferol, 400 IU/day
      i. Except in renal disease, more expensive vitamin D_2 (calcitriol) preparations not necessary
   d. Supplements of cholecalciferol 800 IU/day and calcium 600 mg/day do not result in hypercalcemia/hypercalciuria

8. **Fluoride**
   a. Incorporated into bone matrix, providing increased density
      i. Only therapy that actually induces bone formation
   b. Dosage important—too little has no beneficial effect, too much induces excessively brittle bones
   c. Usual dose: 1 mg/kg or about 50 mg/day for typical thin female
      i. Recent, nonrandomized study with 20 mg/day
   d. Therapy has not been FDA-approved though reports in medical literature date back decades
   e. Some nausea and vomiting may occur
      i. Most unusual side effect is tenosynovitis, often of feet or ankle
      ii. Discontinuation resolves side effect—may even restart fluoride without reinducing pain
   f. Rarely give fluoride > 2 years, but effect may be long-lasting

9. **Thiazide diuretics**
   a. Use in patients with hypercalciuric urine
      i. Defined as > 200–250 mg/day excretion of calcium
   b. Thiazides block calcium excretion, preserving calcium and preventing bone resorption
   c. Typically use hydrochlorothiazide, 12.5–25 mg/day

10. **Androgens**
   a. Occasionally still used in women with estrogen deficiency, contraindication to ERT, and/or failure of other therapy
      i. Low-dose androgen occasionally helpful in women with low libido
   b. Side effects clearly undesirable, but may be limited with low dose
11. **Braces and devices**
   a. Occasionally needed because of significant kyphosis
   b. May help with posture and balance
      i. Use in conjunction with upper back extension exercises
   c. Fitting often a problem, with frequent pain where brace rests on iliac crest, and shoulders
   d. Should be considered, but most women choose not to wear brace even when properly fitted

SUGGESTED READING

1. Consensus Development Conference: Diagnosis, prophylaxis, and treatment of osteoporosis. Am J Med 94:646–650, 1994.
2. Cummings SR, Nevitt MC, Browner WS: Risk factors for hip fracture in white women. N Engl J Med 332:767–773, 1995.
3. Dawson-Hughes B, Harris SS, Krall EA: Effect of calcium and vitamin D supplementation on bone density in men and women 65 years of age or older. N Engl J Med 337:670–676, 1997.
4. Eastell R: Treatment of postmenopausal osteoporosis. N Engl J Med 338:736–746, 1998.
5. Gregg EW, Cauley JA, Seeley DG: Physical activity and osteoporotic fracture risk in older women. Ann Intern Med 129:81–88, 1998.
6. Hosking D, Chilvers CED, Christiansen C: Prevention of bone loss with alendronate in postmenopausal women under 60 years of age. N Engl J Med 338:485–492, 1998.
7. Johnson BE, Lukert BP: New diagnoses in a specialty osteoporosis clinic: Opportunities for consultants. South Med J 85:706–710, 1992.
8. Larcos G: Predicting clinical discordance of bone mineral density. Mayo Clin Proc 73:824–828, 1998.
9. Lindsay R, Tohme JF: Estrogen treatment of patients with established postmenopausal osteoporosis. Obstet Gynecol 76:290–295, 1990.
10. Ott SM: Estrogen therapy for osteoporosis—even in the elderly. Ann Intern Med 117:85–86, 1992.
11. Overgaard K, Hansen MA, Jensen SB: Effect of salcatonin given intranasally on bone mass and fracture rates in established osteoporosis: A dose-response study. BMJ 305:556–561, 1992.
12. Pocock NA, Eisman JA, Yeates MG, et al: Physical fitness is a major determinant of femoral neck and lumbar spine bone mineral density. J Clin Invest 78:618–622, 1986.

88. Fibromyalgia

Bruce E. Johnson, M.D., and Jane L. Murray, M.D.

I. The Issues

Women with chronic pain are not infrequent visitors to the generalist's practice. In many cases, such as cancer or arthritis, the cause of pain is readily apparent. In other cases, such as headache or dysmenorrhea, the cause is frustratingly elusive. Fibromyalgia (FM) is certainly one of the conditions in which the cause of pain is difficult to pinpoint; in many respects, the diagnosis and treatment are as elusive as the cause. The existence of the fibromyalgia syndrome, however, should not be questioned. Probably related to other difficult-to-define syndromes, fibromyalgia causes considerable morbidity. In recent years, a consensus for diagnosis has been developed. The challenge of diagnosis is to consider the condition early and neither to miss other disease nor to overtest. Treatment is probably the most challenging aspect of FM. Because the disease tends to wax and wane, treatment is variably effective. Among the additional challenges of FM is the maintenance of satisfactory rapport in the face of patient frustration and physician self-doubt.

II. **The Theory**
   A. **History**
      1. Symptoms that may be attributed to FM are described by Hippocrates
      2. In late 19th–century Germany extensive literature referred to "nodules" or "muscle callus" or "inflammatory hyperplasia"
      3. Term "fibrositis" coined in 1904 and widely accepted in 1915 after publication of book by that name; however, authors concede that no true inflammatory changes seen in histology of affected muscles
      4. By 1960s and 1970s characterization of muscle pains was made along with observations of associated sleep disorders and psychological dysfunctions
      5. Further defining studies led to name change (fibromyalgia) and more specific description by American College of Rheumatology
   B. **Epidemiology**
      1. True prevalence in community unknown, probably between 2 and 4%
      2. Only data come from rheumatology clinics, representing mostly referred patients
      3. Fibromyalgia accounts for 7–20% of new or continuing patients in many rheumatology practices
      4. Extrapolation has resulted in figure of 3–6 million Americans with syndrome—up to 3% of adult population
      5. Largely in young white women
         a. Some series report up to 90% of cases in young white women
         b. Typical age of onset between 20 and 50; also seen in elderly, in association with other rheumatologic diseases (e.g., rheumatoid arthritis)
         c. Most series find low occurrence in African-Americans, Hispanics, Asians
         d. When present in men, usually in association with other diseases
         e. Diagnosed in teens; rarely in younger children
      6. Economic impact
         a. One study found that 30% of women with FM changed type of employment; 17% stopped working altogether
   C. **Pathophysiology**
      1. Current thinking puts fibromyalgia into a group of disorders characterized largely by derangement of the hypothalamic-pituitary axis (HPA), pain-processing pathways and the autonomic nervous system
         a. There appears to be a heterogeneous type of neuroendocrine dysfunction initiated by a combination of genetic predisposition and insult to the central nervous system (physical trauma, severe emotional stress, infection, etc.) resulting in a spiraling cycle of altered pain sensation, fatigue, depression, poor posture with spinal stress and more pain, deconditioning, altered sympathetic activity and more pain, fatigue and disordered sleep.
         b. Many patients with FM have immune and endocrine function disorders as well
         c. Recent studies indicate that FM patients have low levels of insulin-like growth factor 1 (IGF-1), and may improve with administration of growth hormone.
      2. Biopsy of tender nodules (trigger points) shows no characteristic changes, especially inflammatory
      3. Several observations
         a. Decreased blood flow, lower high-energy phosphate metabolism at general areas of nodules, however these findings overlap with normal tissues and are of uncertain significance.
         b. Dermal-epidermal immune complex deposition in small subset of women with FM, which may offer an autoimmune link to FM
         c. Endocrine dysfunction, including abnormal dexamethasone suppression associated with depression
         d. Decreased serotonin levels, associated with pain, sleep, mood disturbances
         e. Decreased IGF-1 levels occur in about one-third of FM patients; IGF-1 deficiency is associated with fatigue, decreased energy, weight gain, sleep disorders, poor cognition, reduced exercise capacity, cold intolerance, muscle weakness

D. **Clinical features**
1. **Fibromyalgia syndrome**
   a. Characterized by musculoskeletal aching and stiffness, tender and painful trigger points, fatigue, poor sleep and other sleep disorders, and associated clinical syndromes
   b. Symptoms vary from morning to evening and day to day
   c. Variation often attributed by patients to environmental changes (e.g., cold weather, humidity), recent increased physical activity (or, conversely, inactivity), emotional stress, poor sleep
2. **Musculoskeletal complaints**
   a. Described as widespread achiness and stiffness
      i. Somewhat more common in morning but present throughout day
      ii. Gelling (increased stiffness and discomfort following sitting or recumbency) described, although sedentary lifestyle does not improve symptoms
   b. Patient localizes pain to joints: typical presentation is patient self-description of "arthritis" with subjective "swelling" of joints or periarticular regions; however swelling and erythema are not objectively present. Discomfort related, in part, to movement; hence patients make association with joints, calling it "arthritis"
   c. Discomfort is chronic, widespread, tends to fluctuate in intensity, and may involve different sites at different times
   d. Occasional association with changes in weather, alternatively made worse by cold weather as well as by humid conditions
3. **Trigger points and tender points**
   a. Crucial aspect to diagnosis
   b. Presence of discrete, identifiable, reproducible points of pain upon palpation
      i. Vary from muscle insertions to costochondral junctions to fat pads; locations separate from joints, tendons, or bursae
      ii. Described by one author as "only accessible to the finger of faith"
   c. In previous years, thought to be anatomic nodules, but biopsy failed to show typical inflammatory changes
   d. Trigger points are paired, tend to be clustered around neck, shoulder, upper back and knee (Fig. 1)
      i. Trigger points remarkably reproducible among patients with syndrome
      ii. Not all trigger points present in each patient
   e. Patients often surprised by degree of pain elicited by palpation of trigger points
      i. Do not associate symptoms of achiness and stiffness with discrete points of reproducible pain
      ii. Trigger points may be somewhat tender in controls; patients with syndrome describe actual pain
   f. FM patients may have decreased tolerance to pain
      i. Dolorimeter used to apply reproducible pressure to specific sites
      ii. Although some patients indeed "hurt all over," in most cases dolorimeter pressure at nontrigger points elicits no more pain than in controls
      iii. Higher levels of hyaluronic acid are found in serum of FM patients, suggesting biochemical abnormalities in muscle tissue
   g. American College of Rheumatology requires 11 of 18 positive trigger points for diagnosis; patients diagnosed with FM have significantly more trigger points than controls
4. **Fatigue**
   a. Almost all patients describe chronic fatigue with nonrestorative sleep and sleep which is often disrupted (see below)
   b. Fatigue (along with achiness) limits ability to work, play, interact
   c. Overlaps with chronic fatigue syndrome and other similar syndromes (however FM is differentiated from CFS by presence of trigger points and primary complaint of pain rather than primary complaint of fatigue)
5. **Sleep disorders**
   a. Present in 60–90% of women with FM
   b. Nonrestorative sleep in which patients awaken fatigued, tired, and achy

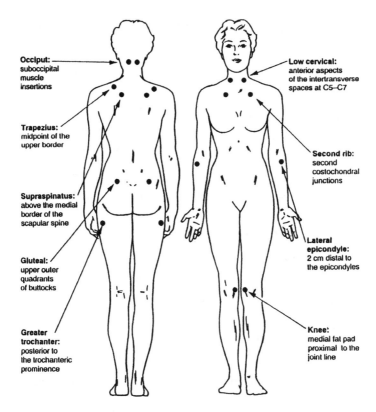

FIGURE 1. Location of trigger points in fibromyalgia. (From Freundlich B, Leventhal L: The fibromyalgia syndrome. In Schumacher HR Jr, Klippel JH, Koopman WJ (eds): Primer on the Rheumatic Diseases, 10th ed. Atlanta, Arthritis Foundation, 1993, with permission.)

    c. Alpha-wave intrusion on delta sleep has been described during sleep electroencephalography (EEG)
      i. Associated with stage IV sleep deprivation
      ii. This pattern not specific to FM; also seen in accident victims and depression without FM
    d. In normal controls, experimentally produced stage IV sleep deprivation results in temporary appearance of musculoskeletal symptoms
  6. **Associated psychiatric and medical conditions**
    a. Women with FM often complain of anxiety, especially regarding concerns about diagnosis of arthritis, free-floating anxiety, and panic syndromes
    b. Depression relatively common
      i. Diagnosed in up to 30% of women with FM
      ii. May predate onset of musculoskeletal complaints
    c. Association with other rheumatologic diseases
      i. FM coexists in 10–15% of patients with rheumatoid arthritis
      ii. Raynaud's phenomenon present in up to 30% of women with FM
      iii. Sicca syndrome described in 10%
      iv. Not believed to have common etiology despite observed associations
    d. HIV disease
      i. One clinic reported that 11% of HIV-positive patients had FM
      ii. In this series, patients more likely to be male and depressed
    e. Increased incidence of other medical complaints in women with FM
      i. Headaches, migraine, or tension

TABLE 1. Synthesis of Proposed Criteria for Diagnosis of Fibromyalgia Syndrome

Defining Criteria	Associated Criteria
Chronic (> 3–6 months), generalized achiness, musculoskeletal pain and/or stiffness	Chronic fatigue
	Disturbed sleep (nonrestorative sleep)
Presence of multiple, often bilaterally symmetric trigger points at characteristic locations (at least 4 sites, up to 11 or more trigger points)	Anxiety, mood disorders, depression
	Subjective swelling
	Paresthesias
Absence of other disease that accounts for symptoms	Headache
	Irritable bowel syndrome

Criteria compiled from Wolfe F, Smythe HA, Yunus MB, et al: The American College of Rheumatology 1990 Criteria for the Classification of Fibromyalgia: Report of the Multicenter Criteria Committee. Arthritis Rheum 33:160–172, 1990; Yunus M, Masi MT, Calabro JJ, et al: Primary fibromyalgia (fibrositis): Clinical study of 50 patients with matched normal controls. Semin Arthritis Rheum 11:151–172, 1981; and Goldenberg DL: Fibromyalgia syndrome: An emerging but controversial condition. JAMA 257:2782–2787, 1987.

      ii. Irritable bowel
     iii. Chronic fatigue syndrome
     iv. Paresthesias
  E. **Laboratory and radiographic findings**
    1. No characteristic abnormalities of blood tests or radiographs
    2. Testing should eliminate other diseases from consideration
    3. Diagnosis of FM is made from clinical findings
III. **An Approach**
  A. **Diagnosis**
    1. Most important step is to consider diagnosis
      a. Many women have had symptoms for a long time
      b. Possibly other diagnoses from other health care workers
      c. Chronicity without progression to more classic rheumatologic disease (e.g., rheumatoid arthritis)
    2. Criteria for diagnosis of FM (Table 1) emphasize chronicity of musculoskeletal complaints, presence of trigger points, and sleep disorder
    3. **Differential diagnosis**
      a. Myofascial pain syndrome
        i. Localized pain with tender points but no associated sleep disturbance, anxiety, fatigue, or multiple, characteristic trigger points
        ii. Believed to be caused by muscle trauma or overuse
      b. Tendinitis, bursitis
      c. Rheumatologic conditions (virtually always show accompanying laboratory, radiographic findings): rheumatoid arthritis, systemic lupus erythematosus, Lyme disease (arthritis), osteoarthritis, polymyalgia rheumatica, polymyositis, ankylosing spondylitis, arthropathy of inflammatory bowel disease
      d. Chronic fatigue syndrome
      e. Hypothyroidism (widespread achiness and fatigue but without other symptoms)
      f. Infections: viral influenza, hepatitis, infectious mononucleosis (Epstein-Barr virus), HIV disease
      g. Sleep disorders: sleep apnea, nocturnal myoclonus
      h. Psychogenic rheumatism—bizarre, musculoskeletal-based complaints
      i. Psychiatric diagnoses (without prominent musculoskeletal complaints): depression, anxiety disorders (including panic attacks), mood disorders
      j. Drugs: alcohol, steroids (steroid pseudorheumatism)
    4. **Laboratory and radiographic tests**
      a. No laboratory or radiographic abnormalities in FM syndrome
      b. Testing done to exclude other diseases, however most of exclusion should be possible by thorough history and physical exam
      c. Reasonable tests to rule out occult disease
        i. Erythrocyte sedimentation rate
          (a) Excludes many rheumatologic disorders

       ii. Liver enzymes

         (a) Chronic or persistent hepatitis

      iii. Thyroid tests

         (a) Exclude hypothyroidism

      iv. Creatine kinase (CK)

         (a) Excludes polymyositis

       v. Other blood tests as clinical situation dictates

         (a) Avoid, if possible, ordering antinuclear antibody or rheumatoid factor tests, as there is a high likelihood of false-positive results, especially in elderly

      vi. Radiographs rarely help without strong suggestion of rheumatologic disease

5. **Diagnosis in elderly**

   a. Sometimes difficult to differentiate symptoms from age-related phenomena

      i. Many elderly have vague aches and pains; not debilitating, as in FM

      ii. Many elderly have altered sleep for other reasons: may require less sleep overall, may nap during day or take frequent nighttime bathroom trips due to nocturia

   b. Applying same criteria as in younger patients simplifies diagnostic process

B. **Treatment approaches**

1. **Education**

   a. Important first step

   b. Assure patient that diagnosis is real and probably chronic but not progressive or fatal

   c. Identify environmental stimuli associated with increase of symptoms

   d. Early in care of patient, frequent office visits are useful to emphasize availability to deal with questions or exacerbations of symptoms

   e. Refer to support groups or national information clearinghouse

2. **Anti-inflammatory medications**

   a. Nonsteroidal anti-inflammatory drugs used in many patients, but infrequently successful as sole therapy—seem to enhance other therapies

   b. Should start with full dosage of chosen drug

   c. FM almost never responds fully to corticosteroids and they should be avoided, as it is difficult to wean patients from drugs and there are considerable side effects with insignificant long-term benefit

   d. Avoid narcotics

3. **Antidepressants and hypnotics**

   a. Studies demonstrate efficacy of tricyclic antidepressants (e.g., amitriptyline) or trazodone

      i. Benefit almost certainly from restoration of appropriate sleep

      ii. Doses often less than used in treating major depression: amitriptyline, 25–50 mg or trazodone 50–100 mg at bedtime

   b. Other hypnotics (e.g., flurazepam) not as useful, perhaps because women with FM have little trouble initiating sleep

   c. Selective serotonin reuptake inhibitors (e.g., fluoxetine) have not been formally investigated but may be useful if tricyclic fails

   d. L-tryptophan shown in some studies to help sleep and pain

4. **Exercise**

   a. Multiple studies confirm importance of exercise in management of FM

   b. Use of muscles and joints around trigger spots seems to decrease tenderness and pain

      i. More flexible body decreases complaint of stiffness

   c. Initiation and maintenance of exercise can be tricky

      i. Exercise may exacerbate symptoms of achiness and muscle pain at first

   d. Goal is to achieve good stretching and mobility before moving into aerobic benefit

   e. Start exercise slowly with gentle movement or walking

      i. Physical therapy consultation if necessary to teach gentle stretching and reaching movements

      ii. Emphasis on upper shoulder girdle, where most symptoms originate

      iii. Need to move muscles and joints around trigger spots

   f. Eventually increase to more vigorous exercise

      i. May have additional benefits of improving sleep, mood

g. Expect setbacks when exercise causes increase in symptoms
  i. Beginning of exercise therapy, particularly in skeptical patient
  ii. Too rapid progression to aerobic level
  iii. When exercise has been halted for some reason and woman attempts return to previous level
5. **Trigger point injection**
  a. Combination of anesthetic and corticosteroid injected directly into trigger points
  b. Should be used judiciously
    i. Aim to inject only a few sites at one visit
    ii. Try to limit injections to occasionally during year
  c. Less invasive therapy: trigger point spray with heat or local anesthetics
6. **Dietary/nutritional approaches**
  a. Large amounts of water intake daily (e.g., 80 oz/day)
  b. Magnesium supplementation
  c. Malic acid supplementation
  d. Avoid foods which exacerbate pain—for some FM patients these include sugars, chocolate, dairy products, citrus fruits, animal fats
  e. Consume foods which contain natural anti-inflammatories: omega-3/6 fatty acids (flaxseed oil, black current oil, salmon, sardines, mackerel), ginger
7. **Other modalities** reported as occasionally effective
  a. Biofeedback
  b. Massage, ultrasound
  c. Hypnosis
  d. Hot baths and whirlpool
  e. Acupuncture
  f. Chiropractic for range of motion and pain improvement
8. **Psychiatric or psychological referral** may be useful if significant disorder suspected or if patient having family or social crises with increase in symptoms

SUGGESTED READING

1. Bennett RM, Clark SC, Walczyk J: A randomized, double-blind, placebo-controlled study of growth hormone in the treatment of fibromyalgia. Am J Med 104:227–231, 1998.
2. Buskila D, Newman L, Vaisberg G, et al: Increased rates of fibromyalgia following cervical spine injury. Arthritis Rheum 40:446–452, 1997.
3. Freundlich B, Leventhal L: The fibromyalgia syndrome. In Schumacher HR Jr, Klippel JH, Koopman WJ (eds): Primer on the Rheumatic Diseases, 10th ed. Atlanta, Arthritis Foundation, pp 247–249, 1993.
4. Powers R: Fibromyalgia: An age-old malady begging for respect. J Gen Intern Med 8:93–104, 1993.
5. Rachlin ES (ed): Myofascial Pain and Fibromyalgia. St. Louis, Mosby, 1994.

89. Arthritis and Collagen Vascular Diseases

Bruce E. Johnson, M.D.

For reasons not fully known, both abnormalities of joints and the collagen vascular diseases are more frequent in women. Because immunologic disorders are implicated in many types of arthritis and collagen vascular diseases, an understanding of immunology is essential. Advances in immunology, even as applied only to arthritis and collagen vascular diseases, are too vast to be covered fully in this chapter. The chapter begins with a discussion of basic components of the immune system and then considers rheumatoid arthritis (RA) as an example of an immune disease afflicting joints and systemic lupus erythematosus (SLE) as an example of a systemic autoimmune disorder.

TABLE 1. Components and Functions of the Immune System
Encounter between antigen and reactive lymphocyte
Recognition in immune system
Activation of lymphocytes
Deployment of immunologic message
Discrimination between self and nonself
Regulation of immune responses

Relevant Aspects of the Immune System
I. **Components and Functions of the Immune System** (Table 1)
   A. **Encounter with antigen**
      1. First step in immune reaction is contact between antigen and scavenger cells, including monocytes, macrophages, histiocytes, dendritic cells
         a. Occurs in all tissues but concentrated in lymphoid tissue
      2. Capture and breakdown of invading organisms or antigens into parts that can be passed to next step of process (recognition)
   B. **Recognition process**
      1. Identifying antigen so that processing results in antibody
         a. System must have enormous flexibility and redundancy
            i. Must respond to each new antigen
            ii. For quicker response at next encounter, must remember antigen through production of relatively specific antibody
         b. Similarities as well as important differences between two arms of immune recognition system
            i. B-cells
               (a) Largely derived from bone marrow
               (b) Manufacture immunoglobulins
            ii. T-cells
               (a) Initially derived from thymus
               (b) Cell-mediated immunity
      2. Key to flexibility of B-cell recognition function is structure of antibody molecule
         a. Multichain molecule constructed of heavy (gamma) chain and light (kappa or lambda) chains
         b. Heavy chains relatively specific to classes of antibody—IgG, IgM, IgD, IgA, IgE
         c. Light chains contain antigen-combining sites and are enormously variable
      3. Precise fit of antibody to antigen is not genetically preset; encounter with antigen "fine tunes" antibody
         a. Because of extensive communication between lymphocytes, antigen gets passed from one to another B-cell lymphocyte
         b. Upon matching with lymphocyte possessing loose fit with antigen, changes in genetic translocation will code for subsequent antibody capable of tight fit—the "one cell, one antibody" rule
      4. Once B-cell lymphocyte develops capability of recognizing antigen, it either is regularly used and multiplies or partially inactivates, becoming a memory cell
         a. If activated, produces clone of cells, all with identical antibody production capability
      5. T-cell memory is similar except T-cell recognizes antigens in conjunction with membrane protein
         a. Processes this larger unit by recognizing and remembering cellular unit
   C. **Activation of lymphocytes**
      1. Activation involves complex cascade of involvement by accessory cells (e.g., CD4 and CD8 cells), production of cellular factors (e.g., interleukin-1), and other soluble messengers, all coordinating cellular responses and eventual manufacture of antibody or attacking cells
      2. System employs not only activating cells but also cells that inactivate or suppress certain functions if they begin to overreact

      a. Suppressor T-cells fulfill this protective role

      b. Failure of suppressor T-cells may lead to unwanted immune response, such as autoimmunity

D. **Deployment of immunologic message**

    1. Soluble messengers

      a. Colony-stimulating factors, interferon, and other factors

    2. Mobility of lymphocytes

      a. Travel from original site of encounter with antigen throughout circulation, allowing rapid response to new invasion by antigen

      b. Other cells reside in lymphocyte centers, such as lymph nodes and become dormant (memory cells), awaiting next encounter with antigen

E. **Discrimination between self and nonself**

    1. "Immunologic tolerance" prevents autoaggression

    2. Early in embryologic differentiation, immune cells (B- and/or T-cells) encounter own tissues ("self")

      a. In most cases, immune cells, having recognized self, are downregulated or suppressed

         i. Supposed to be lifelong suppression

         ii. Release from suppression may be mechanism of some autoimmune diseases

F. **Regulation of immune responses**

    1. Final component of immune system

    2. Helper and suppressor cells modify intensity of response to antigen

      a. Lymphokines activate or suppress responses

    3. Breakdown of any aspect of regulation may lead to disease

      a. Lack of suppressor activity invoked in autoimmune disease

      b. Lack of helper function key abnormality in AIDS

II. **Genetics of Immune Disorders**

A. **Individuality of immune response** determined by genetic variation in two different classes of major histocompatibility complex (MHC or, as alternatively called in humans, HLA molecules)

    1. Antigens reacting with identical portions of MHC may actually stimulate different alleles, resulting in slightly different binding to portion of antigen

      a. Explains variation in immune responses to identical disease stimuli

      b. Explains why identical twins not 100% concordant for autoimmune diseases

    2. Class I and II MHC genes code for HLA system

B. **HLA typing** performed by serologic testing

    1. Human antisera to different HLA alleles

    2. Establishes homology between individuals

      a. Used extensively in tissue typing for transplantation

    3. Experience shows that homology reduces likelihood of, but does not eliminate, serious interaction between self and nonself

      a. Except in immunologically isolated sites (e.g., cornea), any transplant will eventually be rejected due to recognition as nonself

      b. Close HLA typing merely reduces immunosuppressive drugs needed to suppress immune response, permitting maintenance of foreign tissue in body

C. Despite great variability in HLA molecules, **HLA association within ethnic groups is** also potentially strong

    1. For example, HLA-A1-B8-DR3 in northern European Caucasians is associated with SLE

    2. HLA-DR4 is associated with RA among northern European Caucasians but not eastern Mediterranean (Jewish) or Asians

    3. Not so important to disease presentation or management as to epidemiologic study

D. **HLA types also associated with certain diseases**

    1. This association is valuable epidemiologically, occasionally useful clinically

      a. Best known association: between HLA-B27 and ankylosing spondylitis (AS)

         i. Patients with AS 89% positive for HLA-B27 while control population without disease only 9% positive for HLA-B27

        ii. Of course, because general population without AS is so much larger, non-diseased persons with HLA-B27 vastly outnumber AS patients with HLA-B27

    b. Other examples include Reiter's syndrome (85% with HLA-B27), Behçet's syndrome (69% with HLA-B5,W51)

  2. Also find some HLA types associated with more severe disease

    a. Patients with DRB1*0401 are likely to have more severe RA

  3. Finally, association of some diverse diseases may be explained by HLA homology

    a. Graves' disease, myasthenia gravis, and pernicious anemia associated with HLA-B8-DR3

III. Pathology of Immune Responses

  A. **Classic mechanisms characterized by effectors of immune injury**

    1. **Type I, IgE-mediated**

      a. IgE antibodies bind with antigen to basophils or mast cells

      b. Stimulated to release basophilic granules containing vasoactive agents such as histamine, bradykinin, serotonin, slow-reacting substance of anaphylaxis

      c. Most important in clinical allergy, such as asthma, allergic rhinitis

    2. **Type II, antibody-mediated effects on cells**

      a. Cytotoxic or tissue-specific antibody

        i. IgG- and IgM-mediated

      b. Stimulation of complement system and cell killing through phagocytosis or cellular cytotoxicity

      c. Implicated in some types of autoimmune hemolytic anemias, Goodpasture's syndrome

      d. Autoantibodies to cell surface receptors either block (insulin-dependent diabetes) or stimulate (Graves' disease) receptor-mediated function

    3. **Type III, immune complexes**

      a. Soluble antigen and antibodies form complexes, stimulating complement and binding to cellular receptors

      b. IgG-, IgM-, IgA-mediated

      c. Strongly implicated in serum sickness, SLE

    4. **Type IV, delayed hypersensitivity**

      a. T-cells injure tissue containing foreign antigen or bearing autoantigens

      b. Lymphokines released

      c. Often form granuloma

  B. **Variations of these classic mechanisms** implicated in multiple autoimmune or collagen vascular diseases

IV. Autoantibodies and Rheumatic Diseases

  A. Present in most autoimmune diseases

    1. In most instances, function as marker of disease or immune process while not implicated directly in tissue damage

  B. Origin not precisely delineated

    1. Some autoantibodies derive from genes responsible for "natural" autoantibodies

  C. Autoantibodies may reflect site of immunologic damage

    1. For example, anticentromere autoantibodies in systemic sclerosis bind to proteins in centromere where part of abnormality in collagen formation occurs

  D. Stimulation of autoantibody by number of factors

    1. Drugs and infections can stimulate production without characteristic disease

    2. Infectious stimulation of genetically predisposed tissue

      a. Insulin-dependent diabetes associated with viral infection

      b. Reiter's disease associated with Shigella infection

  E. Autoantibody identification often useful in both diagnosis and management

    1. Diagnostically, antinuclear antibody (ANA) sensitive, but not very specific, for SLE

      a. Anti–double-stranded DNA (dsDNA) specific, but not sensitive, for SLE

    2. Anti-dsDNA levels followed for clues to activity of disease

      a. Not always direct concordance, but flare of disease frequently preceded by increase in titer of anti-dsDNA

V. **Autoimmune Disease and Women**
  A. Many autoimmune diseases occur with unexplained greater frequency in women
  B. Tolerance
    1. Ability of immune system to recognize and not attack self is tolerance
    2. At least partly genetically determined
  C. Androgens and estrogens influence tolerance
    1. In mouse model of lupus, castration of male mice results in loss of tolerance while androgen treatment of female mice induces tolerance
    2. Human studies support mice models
    3. In SLE, sex hormones may alter disease
      a. Androgens may limit expression of disease
      b. Estrogens may permit expression of disease, given genetic predisposition and appropriate disease stimulus
  D. Estrogens and antiarthritic, anti-inflammatory effect
    1. For decades, observers note fluxes in disease intensity (e.g., in rheumatoid arthritis)
      a. Most notable during pregnancy when arthritic complaints often diminish
    2. Variance also observed during menstrual cycle
      a. Diary of symptoms demonstrates less morning stiffness and less pain during postovulatory phase coinciding with increased levels of both estrogen and progesterone
    3. Reports of less arthritic pain with use of oral contraceptives and postmenopausal hormone replacement
    4. Estrogen also enhances anti-inflammatory effect of corticosteroids
    5. Estrogen and/or progesterone may be considered adjuncts to treatment when contemplating hormone replacement
    6. Menstrual cycling may also account for variable response to new or different treatment modalities
      a. Therapeutically, it is wise to continue new treatment until several menstrual cycles have passed

Rheumatoid Arthritis
  I. **The Theory**
    A. **Epidemiology**
      1. Afflicts approximately 1–2% of adult population
        a. Age-related, with prevalence reported as high as 10% in persons older than 65 years
      2. Female:male ratio approximately 2.5:1
      3. Incidence increases after menopause
        a. Lends credence to hypothesis that estrogen somewhat protective
      4. Possible decreasing incidence in 30–50-year-old women comparing incidence rates in 1950s with 1970s
        a. Major difference between decades was increasing use of oral contraceptives
      5. Concordance between monozygotic twins only 34%, suggesting genetic penetrance low
    B. **Pathology**
      1. Joints virtually always involved
        a. Rare initial presentation with other manifestations
      2. Injury of synovial endothelial cells
        a. Inflammatory infiltration by both polymorphonuclear cells and monocytes with release of inflammatory mediators
      3. Disease progression to hypertrophic, edematous synovium
        a. Thickened synovium intrudes into joint space
        b. Proliferative fibroblasts and microvascular growth, results in invasive tissue called pannus
        c. Pannus progressively destroys cartilage and, if checked, periarticular bone
      4. Continual inflammatory response and joint destruction lead to pain, deformity, and disability
      5. Disease also has systemic manifestations, including vasculitis

TABLE 2. Diseases Associated with Elevated Serum Rheumatoid Factor

Chronic bacterial infections	Parasitic diseases
Subacute bacterial endocarditis	Leishmaniasis
Tuberculosis	Schistosomiasis
Syphilis	Malaria
Lyme disease	Chronic inflammatory diseases of uncertain etiology
Viral diseases	Sarcoidosis
Rubella	Periodontal disease
Cytomegalovirus	Pulmonary interstitial disease
Epstein-Barr virus (infectious	Chronic liver disease
mononucleosis)	Systemic lupus erythematosus
Influenza	Sjögren's syndrome
Hepatitis B	Mixed cryoglobulinemia
	Hypergammaglobulinemic purpura

C. **Rheumatoid factor** (RF)
   1. Prototypical autoimmune antibody
   2. May be formed of any immunoglobulin class, but IgM most frequently measured
   3. Detected in up to 3% of normal population, increasing in prevalence with advancing age
   4. RF probably not pathologically active but only a marker of RA
   5. Although found in 85% of patients with RA, specificity as test for rheumatoid arthritis is low (Table 2)
D. **Clinical manifestations**
   1. **Articular manifestations** are key to diagnosis
      a. Synovitis, not merely arthralgia, must be present
         i. Joint inflammation and warmth
         ii. Swelling with effusion
         iii. Pain, especially with movement
      b. Classically involves small joints, fingers, and toes, early in disease course
      c. Symmetric involvement, i.e., tends to involve both hands and/or feet equally
      d. Joint symptoms include: morning stiffness of 30–60 minutes, pain, gelling (stiffness of joint with inactivity)
      e. Radiographic evidence of cartilage destruction and bony erosions occurs after months to years of disease activity
   2. **Arthritic manifestations of specific joints**
      a. Hands
         i. Proximal interphalangeal (PIP), metacarpophalangeal (MCP), and wrist joints
         ii. Chronic inflammation causes tendon/ligament stretching and joint laxity resulting in:
            (a) Ulnar deviation (hand locates laterally toward ulnar side)
            (b) Swan-neck deformity (hyperextension of PIP)
            (c) Boutonniere deformity (flexion at DIP)
         iii. Tendon rupture with loss of movement at joint uncommon
         iv. Swelling at wrist may lead to symptoms of carpal tunnel syndrome
      b. Elbows
         i. Proximity to ulnar nerve may cause compressive neuropathy
         ii. Progressive disease may cause inability to fully extend joint
      c. Shoulders
         i. Pain and decreased range of motion without easily detected signs of inflammation
         ii. Restriction of motion occurs subconsciously
         iii. May develop "frozen shoulder" with inability to abduct shoulder fully and prominent symptoms at night
      d. Cervical spine
         i. Neck stiffness and lack of mobility
         ii. Laxity at C1–C2 joint late in disease, resulting in danger of dislocation if neck hyperextended

    e. Feet and ankles
        i. Symmetric involvement early in disease
        ii. Pain with weight-bearing develops early
        iii. Involvement of metatarsophalangeal (MTP) leads to cock-up deformity and subluxation of MTP head at sole
        iv. Involvement of talus and ankle results in altered gait
    f. Knees
        i. Effusion gives symmetric enlargement to joint
        ii. Long-standing effusion may lead to Baker's cyst (evagination of synovial lining and fluid into popliteal space)
        iii. Knee involvement, while often symptomatic, infrequently results in need for knee replacement
    g. Hips
        i. Early manifestations difficult to detect because symptoms not only in groin and thigh but also knee and low back

3. **Extra-articular manifestations**
    a. RA can be multisystem disease with manifestations far from joints
    b. Tendons and ligaments
        i. Ligaments become weakened or severed by erosive activity of synovitis
        ii. Tendons become inflamed (called tenosynovitis) with thickening, nodules, and rupture
        iii. Laxity, instability, and subluxation at joint result in deformity, especially at fingers, wrist and toes
    c. Vasculitis
        i. Not common but may involve skin and nerves sparing kidneys, GI tract
    d. Skin
        i. Rheumatoid nodules found in 25–50% of all RA
            (a) Occur during active phase
            (b) Located on extensor surfaces and pressure points such as olecranon
        ii. Vasculitic lesions, occasionally as leukocytoclastic rash
        iii. Splinter hemorrhages and distal finger pad infarcts from vasculitis
    e. Eyes
        i. Dryness with concomitant Sjögren's syndrome—keratoconjunctivitis sicca
        ii. Episcleritis during exacerbations of RA
    f. Lungs
        i. Interstitial lung disease with fibrosis and/or bronchiolitis obliterans
        ii. Rheumatoid nodules within lung parenchyma
        iii. Pleural disease with effusion
            (a) Characteristically with very low pleural fluid glucose
    g. Heart
        i. Inflammatory pericarditis
        ii. Rarely inflammatory valvular nodules and inflammatory aortitis with aneurysm or aortic insufficiency
    h. Neurologic symptoms
        i. Myelopathies related to cervical spine instability
        ii. Entrapment neuropathies, such as carpal or tarsal tunnel syndromes, from proximate inflammation
        iii. Mononeuritis multiplex from vasculitis

II. **An Approach**
  A. **Clinical presentation**
    1. Two-thirds of patients have insidious onset of inflammatory, symmetric arthritis over weeks to months with morning stiffness, pain, swelling, and warmth over joints
    2. Early systemic symptoms
      a. Fatigue
      b. Anorexia
      c. Weakness
      d. Musculoskeletal complaints (occasionally mistaken for fibromyalgia)

      3. Rare onset with extra-articular or systemic signs
        a. Fever, lymphadenopathy
        b. Vasculitis
        c. Pulmonary disease
      4. Synovitis universal at some point in course of RA
        a. Swelling, tenderness, limitation of motion,
        b. Stretching of synovium with effusion causes pain
          i. Joints often held in partial flexion to minimize stretching
        c. Early involvement of PIP, MCP, and wrist, with other joints in later stages

B. Laboratory tests
    1. No definitive test for RA
    2. Rheumatoid factor (RF) present in 85% of patients with RA
      a. RF not specific for RA; often in other conditions
        i. In addition to list in Table 2, 10–20% of older adults are RF-positive
        ii. Nonetheless, in patients with compatible symptoms, RF has value as confirmatory test
      b. Loose correlation between titer of RF and severity of disease
        i. RF-negative RA tends to be mild and limited
        ii. Very high titers often present in (but do not cause) extra-articular disease
      c. RF titer of little prognostic value in individual patient; once documented, little value in repeated measurements
    3. Erythrocyte sedimentation rate and C-reactive protein typically elevated
      a. Sometimes used to monitor level of inflammation
    4. Anemia
      a. Normocytic, normochromic
      b. Typical for "anemia of chronic disease"
    5. Results of other laboratory tests vary according to degree of inflammation and involvement
      a. For example, patient may have low complement, high platelet and eosinophilia in severe disease with vasculitis and/or nodules

C. Radiography
    1. Early in disease, soft tissue swelling only consistent sign
    2. Progression of disease brings following changes, none of which is specific for RA
      a. Juxta-articular osteopenia
      b. Loss of articular capsule
      c. Bony erosions
      d. Subluxations

D. American Rheumatism Association diagnostic criteria (Table 3)
    1. Developed for epidemiologic and investigative purposes but useful for clinical diagnosis
    2. Persons not fulfilling enough criteria may still have early RA

TABLE 3. American Rheumatism Association Criteria for Diagnosis
of Rheumatoid Arthritis (1987)

Four of seven criteria needed to establish diagnosis

1. Morning stiffness lasting 60 minutes before maximal improvement

2. Arthritis of 3 or more joint areas with simultaneous soft-tissue swelling or fluid in proximal interphalangeal, metacarpophalangeal, wrist, elbow, knee, ankle, and/or metatarsophalangeal joints

3. Arthritis of hand joints: at least 1 joint of wrist, metacarpophalangeal, or proximal interphalangeal joint

4. Symmetric arthritis: simultaneous involvement of same joint area on both sides of body

5. Rheumatoid nodules

6. Serum rheumatoid factor

7. Radiographic changes typical for RA on hand and wrist, including erosions and periarticular osteopenia

Criteria 1–4 must be present at least 6 weeks. Criteria 2–5 must be observed by physician.

E. **Treatment**
1. Evolution in approach
   a. Current emphasis on early rather than late use of disease-modifying drugs
   b. "Toxic" agents are used with evidence of progressive disease
2. **General measures**
   a. Patient education
      i. Interdisciplinary approach to deal with functional and psychosocial interactions
      ii. Identify aggravating activities
      iii. Acknowledge medication toxicities
      iv. Be aware of systemic manifestations
      v. Anticipate interference with work, play, family activities, sex
      vi. Reinforce need for regular follow-up
   b. Rest
      i. RA causes fatigue; regular rest often restorative, allowing better function throughout day
      ii. Full-night sleep (8–10 hours); afternoon nap
   c. Physical therapy
      i. To prevent contractures, limit joint-damaging activities and maintain muscle tone
   d. Occupational therapy
      i. Important in progressive disease
      ii. Assists with adaptation to activities of daily living
      iii. Splints, assistive devices
3. **Nonsteroidal anti-inflammatory drugs** (NSAIDs)
   a. All block cyclooxygenase, which is important in production of prostaglandins, prostacyclin, thromboxanes, all of which are involved in inflammatory response
   b. Multiple choices of NSAIDs
      i. No clearly identified superior agent
      ii. Highly dependent on individual response to NSAID
   c. First-line therapy is full dose of chosen NSAID
      i. Goal is to limit inflammation, improve clinical outlook
      ii. If chosen NSAID does not result in clinical improvement, another should be tried
   d. Most patients are started on and remain on NSAIDs throughout course of RA, most often in combination with other agents
   e. Side effects and complications are common
      i. Most common, and ominous, include GI tract ulcers (esophageal, gastric, intestinal)
      ii. Other important complications include renal insufficiency, bleeding, fatigue/somnolence
4. **Cyclooxygenase 2 inhibitors**
   a. Two isoforms of cyclooxygenase—COX 1 and COX 2; both involved in synthesis of prostaglandins but are found in different concentrations in gastric/intestinal mucosa and synovium.
   b. NSAIDs which selectively block COX 2 might be anti-inflammatory at joints but spare gastrointestinal mucosa—with potentially fewer chances for GI ulcer formation
   c. Diclofenac (Voltaren) and etodolac (Lodine) most COX 2–selective of "traditional" NSAIDs, but still relatively high rate of GI disruption
      i. Attempt to counter ulcer formation by combining relative COX 2 selective diclofenac with GI protective agent misoprostol (Arthrotec)
   d. Celecoxib (Celebrex) recently developed specific COX 2 inhibitor with greatly reduced evidence for GI inflammation/ulcer formation
      i. Celecoxib combines adequate joint anti-inflammatory response with low GI ulceration rate
5. **Corticosteroids**
   a. Have both anti-inflammatory and immunosuppressive effects but whether they modify course of disease controversial

b. Because of high side-effect profile and lack of long-term modifying potential, steroids should be used sparingly

c. Prescribe for serious or life-threatening complications, such as vasculitis or major systemic flare of RA

d. Occasionally used in patients with rapid or explosive initial presentation while awaiting onset of action of slower-acting drugs

e. May use as intra-articular injection when one or two joints flare out of proportion to underlying disease

6. **Estrogens**

a. May be helpful in decreasing inflammation
   i. Response variable and rarely complete

b. Response seen both with oral contraceptives in reproductive-aged women and postmenopausal hormone replacement

c. Estrogen therapy not indicated solely to treat RA, but may be considered if other indications for use exist

7. **Anti-TNF agents**

a. Tumor necrosis factor (TNF) identified in many disease processes, including sepsis, cancer and inflammation (e.g., RA)

b. TNF serves as messenger to attract inflammatory cells along with other factors such as interferon and interleukines

c. Blocking of TNF investigationally used to decrease recruitment of inflammatory cells to joints afflicted by RA

d. Examples of drugs include etanercept (Enbrel) and infliximab (Remicabe)

8. **Disease-modifying antirheumatic drugs** (DMARDs)

a. Patients with any but the most mild forms of RA are considered for therapy with DMARDs

b. DMARDs slow, or halt, the actual progression of RA—a result not possible with NSAIDs or steroids alone

c. DMARDs are often toxic and are prescribed in combinations (similar to cancer chemotherapy regimens)

d. Drugs approved by Food and Drug Administration for use in RA: auranofin and other gold products; azathioprine, methotrexate, leflunomide and other antiproliferative drugs; hydroxychloroquine; penicillamine

e. Drugs approved for other diseases but useful in RA: chlorambucil, cyclophosphamide, cyclosporine, sulfasalazine, minocycline

f. Other experimental procedures and drugs: fish oil, plant oils, total nodal irradiation, apheresis, biologics

g. Combinations of these approaches are common but still investigational and patients should be managed in conjunction with specialists familiar with both efficacy and side effects of therapies

9. **Surgery**

a. Useful for severely affected joints

b. Joint replacement of hip and knee (though this indication not as common as for osteoarthritis)

c. Cosmetic and functional improvement of fingers and hand possible with reconstructive hand surgery

d. Persistent monoarthritis may be helped by synovectomy
   i. Especially indicated for wrist

10. **Complications of RA**

a. Synovial cysts (especially Baker's cyst)
   i. Intra-articular steroids
   ii. Synovectomy may be required

b. Rheumatoid nodules
   i. Difficult management problem
   ii. If interfere with function, may try intralesional steroids or surgical removal but nodules tend to recur

c. Felty's syndrome

      i. Splenomegaly, granulocytopenia, leg ulcers, recurrent infection
      ii. Splenectomy, corticosteroids, gold, methotrexate, penicillamine tried with variable success
    d. Vasculitis
      i. High morbidity, life-threatening
      ii. High-dose corticosteroids
    e. Rheumatoid lung
      i. Very difficult to modify
      ii. High-dose steroids

Systemic Lupus Erythematosus
I. **The Theory**
  A. **Epidemiology**
    1. Disease primarily of young women
      a. Female:male ratio 5:1 or more
      b. Strong female predominance supports role of estrogen in permitting expression of genetic predisposition
    2. Peak incidence between ages 15–40
    3. Secondary peak in older persons (> 60) but female:male ratio of 2:1
    4. Prevalence about 10–15 per 100,000 in general population or about 200,000–300,000 cases in U.S.
      a. Prevalence varies by ethnic and socioeconomic groups with disease more common in African-Americans than whites, Hispanics, or Asians
    5. Concordance in twins only about 25%
  B. **Pathology**
    1. Truly systemic disease with manifestations throughout body
      a. Dominant manifestations through vasculitic effects and immune complex deposition
    2. Most patients with SLE have arthralgia or arthritis
      a. Nondeforming with inflammation of synovium but little cartilage damage and rare bony erosion
    3. Immune complex deposition
      a. Classically involves kidney at glomerulus
        i. Immune complex disease characteristic not only on routine staining but especially with immunofluorescence
        ii. Renal biopsy
          (a) Often used as prognostic indicator in presence of active urinary sediment
      b. In skin associated with rash, vasculitic changes
        i. Under immunofluorescence gives similar band-like appearance as seen in glomerulus
        ii. Occasionally used in making diagnosis
    4. Vasculitic manifestations (severe disease)
      a. Central nervous system with cortical microinfarcts and cerebral vasculopathy
      b. Heart may have nonspecific foci of inflammation at pericardium, epicardium or valves (with "endocarditis" known as Libman-Sacks disease)
      c. Vasculitic changes of skin includes rash, ulcers, infarcts, telangiectasia
  C. **Autoantibodies**
    1. SLE is prototypical autoimmune disease with one of earliest described autoantibody—the antinuclear antibody (ANA)
    2. In contrast to rheumatoid factor, many of antibodies in SLE cause damage
      a. For example, anti-dsDNA complex associated with glomerular damage
      b. Antilymphocyte antibody leads to lymphopenia
    3. Some autoantibodies correlate with disease activity
      a. Titer of anti-dsDNA increases with active kidney disease
      b. Titer of antiplatelet antibody correlates with thrombocytopenia
    4. Most SLE autoantibodies listed in Table 4 are clinically important
  D. **Clinical manifestations**
    1. Waxing and waning of symptoms characteristic, especially in early, mild disease

TABLE 4. Autoantibodies in Systemic Lupus Erythematosus

Autoantibody	Incidence (%)	Clinical Importance
Antinuclear (ANA)	95	Multiple antibodies can be measured; highly sensitive for SLE
Anti-DNA	70	Anti-dsDNA highly specific for SLE; anti-ssDNA not; titer associated with nephritic activity
Anti-Sm	30	Specific for SLE
Anti-RNP	40	High titer in mixed syndromes (e.g., polymyositis, scleroderma, mixed connective tissue disease)
Anti-Ro(SSA)	30	Associated with Sjögren's syndrome, lupus in elderly, neonatal/congenital heart block in infants; causes nephritis
Anti-La(SSB)	10	Always seen with anti-Ro
Antihistone	70	More frequent in drug-induced disease
Anticardiolipin	50	Increased risk for thrombosis, thrombocytopenia, spontaneous abortion, prolonged partial thromboplastin time, positive VDRL test for syphilis
Antierythrocyte	60	Possible hemolysis
Antiplatelet	?	Thrombocytopenia
Antilymphocyte	70	Leukopenia, abnormal T-cell function
Antineuronal	60	In CNS, high titers correlate with CNS lupus

   a. Period of less intense disease activity may be followed by flare
   b. Flares occur with or without obvious precipitating event (e.g., sun exposure)
   c. Flare associated with reemergence of previously quiescent manifestation
        i. For example, previous skin disease may reappear, signifying flare
   d. Flare may initiate new manifestations of SLE for patient
        i. New-onset CNS lupus
2. **Prominent systemic symptoms** include constitutional complaints of fatigue, fever, weight loss: specific organ system manifestations vary from patient to patient and rarely include all manifestations at the same time
3. **Skin**
   a. Most patients with SLE eventually develop skin involvement
   b. Malar, "butterfly" rash, generalized erythema, photosensitivity
        i. Most SLE patients exhibit malar rash
   c. Bullous eruptions
   d. Vasculitic changes such as palpable purpura, digital ulceration, palmar ulcers
   e. Subacute cutaneous SLE seen as nonfixed, nonscarring lesions resembling psoriasis or lichen planus
   f. Discoid lupus typically has erythematous borders with hypopigmented center
   g. Alopecia—diffuse or patchy
4. **Mucous membranes**
   a. Aphthous-like lesions in mouth, nasal septum, and vagina
5. **Joints**
   a. Most (> 80%) patients with SLE have arthralgia or frank arthritis
   b. Any joint, but typically small joints of hands and wrist
   c. Joint involvement may be migratory and evanescent or persistent
   d. Not necessarily symmetric
   e. Unlike RA, not erosive or destructive
        i. Joint deformities (e.g., swan-neck) due to tendon/ligament abnormalities rather than destructive bony changes
6. **Kidneys**
   a. Involvement by immune complexes with autoantibodies
   b. Virtually always involves glomerulus, but occasionally tubules also affected
   c. Early detection by examination of urine

      i. Active urinary sediment (proteinuria, hematuria, casts) strongly suggests kidney damage

   d. Kidney failure from SLE is frequent reason for renal dialysis in young women

  7. **Nervous system**

   a. > 20% of patients with SLE have neurologic involvement

   b. Most significant is CNS lupus with patchy or widespread cerebritis

      i. Symptoms range from focal infarcts to global dysfunction and delirium or even coma

      ii. Confusion, organic brain syndromes, psychosis

      iii. Cerebellar extrapyramidal symptoms

      iv. Subarachnoid hemorrhage, aseptic meningitis, arachnoiditis

   c. Seizure disorder with grand mal, petit mal features

   d. Transverse myelitis with paraplegia

   e. Cranial nerve palsies

   f. Peripheral neuropathy with mononeuritis multiplex or stocking-glove distribution

  8. **Serositis**

   a. Pericarditis may be symptomatic or painless

      i. While found at autopsy in 50–60% of patients dying of SLE, clinically apparent in < 30%

   b. Pleuritis with symptoms of pleurisy—occasionally with effusion

   c. Peritonitis

      i. Abdominal pain

      ii. Peritoneal fluid (ascites) infrequent and rarely becomes chronic with adhesions

  9. **Gastrointestinal findings**

   a. Peritonitis

   b. Mesenteric vasculitis with intestinal angina, malabsorption, even infarct or bowel perforation

   c. Pancreatitis

   d. Hepatomegaly

 10. **Pulmonary findings**

   a. Pneumonitis, hemorrhage, embolism (from cardiolipin-associated thrombosis), pulmonary hypertension

   b. Infiltrates may be patchy, fleeting or persistent with interstitial pattern

   c. Pleural effusion with pleurisy

 11. **Cardiac findings**

   a. Pericarditis

   b. Myocarditis with arrhythmias, tachycardia, conduction defects, cardiomegaly

   c. Endocarditis with bland vegetations (Libman-Sacks disease)

      i. Only rarely requires valve requirement, especially with current practice of early steroid use

 12. **Hematologic findings**

   a. Anemia

      i. Either autoimmune-mediated hemolysis or anemia of chronic disease

   b. Leukopenia

      i. Relatively common

      ii. Not associated with increased rates of infection

   c. Thrombocytopenia

      i. Probably mediated by antiplatelet antibody

   d. Lymphadenopathy common during exacerbations

   e. Splenomegaly

E. **Pregnancy and SLE**

  1. Fertility rate somewhat diminished in women with SLE

  2. Spontaneous abortion rate high (see below)

  3. Presteroid era recognized "rule of thirds"

   a. One-third of women with SLE improved, one-third remained the same, and one-third worsened

    4. Deterioration almost always in patients with renal involvement in whom renal function diminished rapidly
       a. Due in part to increased activity of SLE but also due to inability to handle metabolic demands of pregnancy
    5. Incidence of preeclampsia higher than in general population
    6. In fact, SLE not contraindication to pregnancy in most women with only significant exception being those with moderate/severe renal disease

F. **Antiphospholipid (anticardiolipin) syndrome**
    1. Consists of recurrent vascular thrombosis, thrombocytopenia, and pregnancy wastage associated with positive lupus anticoagulant and/or anticardiolipin test
    2. Thrombosis may be either venous or arterial
       a. Occurs in sites other than leg
          i. Involvement of arms and renal, hepatic, retinal, or even sagittal vein
       b. Arterial thrombosis with stroke, transient ischemic attack, amaurosis fugax, peripheral thrombosis/gangrene, bowel infarction
    3. Other possible manifestations include livedo reticularis, migraine headaches, transverse myelitis, leg ulcers
    4. Prominent sign in women is fetal wastage
       a. Fertility not affected, but spontaneous abortions occur in any trimester
       b. Multiple miscarriages common as antiphospholipid syndrome frequently asymptomatic in young women
    5. Occasionally antiphospholipid syndrome occurs without concomitant SLE
       a. Presentation with thrombosis or fetal wastage
       b. No arthritis, serositis, hematologic or renal changes; ANA-negative

II. **An Approach**
A. **Clinical presentation**
    1. Typical presentation of systemic disease
    2. Constitutional complaints
       a. Malaise, fatigue, fever, weight loss
    3. Skin manifestations
       a. Classic presentation is malar ("butterfly") rash.
       b. Photosensitivity and alopecia also common
       c. Discoid lupus may represent limited manifestation
    4. Musculoskeletal abnormalities
       a. Most patients have myalgias/arthralgias and arthritis
       b. While often symmetric, arthritis usually is not destructive
       c. Hands frequently affected: proximal interphalangeal, metacarpophalangeal, carpal joints
       d. Knees, hips, and feet
       e. Tenosynovitis
          i. May result in swan-neck, ulnar deviations
    5. Mucous membranes: aphthous-type lesions of mouth, nares, vagina
    6. Renal manifestations rarely give symptoms; check for involvement with creatinine, urine studies
    7. Neuropsychiatric symptoms
       a. Headache may be symptom at initial presentation
       b. Later signs more serious: seizures, cerebrovascular accident, cerebritis, transverse myelitis
       c. Depression not uncommon at some time during disease course
       d. Psychosis, organic brain syndrome less likely unless cerebritis is present
    8. Serositis: symptoms of pleuritis, pericarditis, peritonitis
       a. Pleural effusion may be present but rarely massive
       b. Pericarditis may be symptomatic but unlikely to cause tamponade
       c. Abdominal pain may be mistaken for gallbladder, appendix, or pelvic disease
    9. Hematologic manifestations: mostly in laboratory results (see below)
    10. Cardiac, gastrointestinal, pulmonary symptoms uncommon early in course of disease

B. **Laboratory tests**
  1. Hematologic findings
     a. Abnormalities usually reflect presence of autoantibody against involved cell line
     b. Anemia normochromic, normocytic, i.e., anemia of chronic disease
        i. Hemolytic anemia in presence of autoantibody (e.g., Coombs' positive)
     c. Thrombocytopenia—antiplatelet antibodies
     d. Leukopenia—antilymphocyte antibodies
     e. Sedimentation rate elevated and may correlate with severity of disease
     f. Prolonged partial thromboplastin time is suggestive of antiphospholipid syndrome
  2. Chemistry panels
     a. Important to measure creatinine and urea nitrogen levels
     b. Establish presence of renal disease
     c. Other changes in blood chemistries uncommon
  3. Urine—microscopic evaluation essential to establish evidence of renal disease
  4. Misleading tests
     a. False-positive VDRL test for syphilis
     b. RF in 30% of SLE patients
  5. Autoantibodies (ANA and others)
     a. 95% of SLE patients ANA-positive
     b. Other autoantibodies may be helpful in diagnosis
        i. Anti-dsDNA and anti-Sm antibodies highly specific for SLE
     c. Occasional autoantibody useful for documenting flares of disease
        i. Regular screening of anti-dsDNA may detect early evidence of flare of renal disease
C. **Radiography**
  1. No pathognomonic radiographic findings
  2. Arthritis is typically nondeforming
     a. Radiographs show soft tissue swelling only
D. **American Rheumatism Association criteria for diagnosis** (Table 5)
  1. Developed for epidemiologic and investigative purposes
  2. Useful in clinical setting, although treatment of SLE may be started with < 4 criteria in unusual circumstances
     a. For example, initial presentation with neurologic findings, such as CNS lupus or transverse myelitis

TABLE 5. American Rheumatism Association Criteria for the Diagnosis of Systemic Lupus Erythematosus (1982)

For purposes of diagnosis, any 4 of 11 criteria are present, serially or simultaneously, during the interval of observation:

1. Malar rash

2. Discoid rash

3. Photosensitivity: skin rash due to unusual reaction to sunlight

4. Oral or nasopharyngeal ulceration

5. Arthritis: nonerosive, involving 2 or more peripheral joints

6. Serositis: pleurisy (convincing history of pleuritic pain or rub) *or* pericarditis (EKG or rub or evidence of pericardial effusion)

7. Renal disorder: proteinuria > 0.5 gm/day *or* cellular casts (red cell, granular, tubular, mixed)

8. Neurologic disorder: seizures (in absence of other causes) *or* psychosis (in absence of other causes)

9. Hematologic disorder: hemolytic anemia (with erythrocytosis) *or* leukopenia (< 4000/mm^3) *or* lymphopenia (< 1500/mm^3)

10. Immunologic disorder: positive LE cell preparation *or* anti-dsDNA *or* anti-Sm *or* false-positive VDRL test

11. Antinuclear antibody: absence of drugs associated with drug-induced lupus

E. **Treatment**
  1. **Patient education**
     a. Understanding of natural history of disease
        i. Chronic disease with intervals of waxing and waning
     b. Recognition of precipitating events and manifestations of flares
     c. Booklets, support groups
     d. Psychosocial support, physician or nurse or educator availability
  2. **Photosensitivity** may precipitate flare
     a. Avoidance of direct, midday sunlight
     b. Sunscreens, long-sleeved clothing, broad-brimmed hats
     c. May even require physician recommendations against outdoor occupations or office desk near window
  3. **Infections** occur more frequently and tend to be moderately severe in patients with SLE
     a. Early contact with physician when patient feels ill
     b. Early empiric treatment in patients with renal failure, open skin lesions, known cardiac valvular lesions
     c. Immunization for pneumococcus, hemophilus, influenza, hepatitis
  4. **Birth control** (see also below)
     a. Pregnancy is not contraindicated in women with mild, quiescent SLE
     b. Effective birth control important for women with complicated SLE, nephritis, or while taking cytotoxic drugs
  5. **Physical therapy** (PT)
     a. May be useful during active arthritis
     b. Not as important as for patients with RA since SLE arthritis usually not deforming
     c. PT can be valuable for coexistent fibromyalgia
  6. **Medications**
     a. **Nonsteroidal anti-inflammatory drugs** (NSAIDs)
        i. Mainstay of therapy for arthritis, myalgias, serositis
        ii. Salicylates used for arthritis, fever
        iii. Marked variability in response; if one drug unsuccessful, try another
        iv. Use with caution in nephritis
           (a) May worsen renal disease, especially tubular function
        v. Neuropsychiatric side effects, including headache, dizziness, depression
           (a) Reported association in SLE between NSAID use and aseptic meningitis
     b. **Corticosteroids**
        i. Used frequently and extensively for multiple indications
           (a) Topically for skin disease
           (b) Intralesional for discoid lupus
           (c) Low-dose oral administration for moderate arthritis
           (d) High-dose intravenous for severe, life-threatening disease
        ii. In severe disease, use multiple daily dosing
           (a) CNS lupus, worsening arthritis, life-threatening hemolytic anemia or thrombocytopenia, vasculitis
           (b) Some circumstances (e.g., severe nephritis) use "pulse" therapy, i.e., up to 1000 mg methylprednisolone/day for 3–5 days followed by continued, relatively high-dose IV or oral steroid
        iii. Goal is to taper rapidly to discontinue or at least achieve lowest dose
        iv. If high-dose, intravenous steroids needed for 3–4 weeks, consider this a steroid failure and add or substitute cytotoxic agent
     c. **Antimalarial drugs**
        i. Hydroxychloroquine, chloroquine, quinacrine
        ii. Especially useful for cutaneous, arthritic, and musculoskeletal symptoms
        iii. Start at standard doses but frequently can taper to lower dose and maintain efficacy
           (a) Maintenance therapy can be long-term
           (b) Disease often flares if antimalarial drugs discontinued

      iv. Side effects may be typical (GI, dermatologic, constitutional) or specific

        (a) Long-term use associated with myopathy

        (b) Ocular toxicity uncommon at usual low doses; surveillance for retinal changes with periodic (every 6–12 months), slit-lamp, visual field, and fundoscopic exam

   d. **Dapsone**

     i. Useful for cutaneous SLE

     ii. Side effects include dose-related hemolysis

   e. **Cytotoxic agents**

     i. Methotrexate, azathioprine, cyclophosphamide

     ii. Methotrexate frequently indicated in low doses for cutaneous disease

     iii. Used along with steroids or as steroid-sparing agents and in long-term therapy of nephritis

     iv. Although used to spare complications of steroids, these agents have their own problems

       (a) Multiple short-term side effects; liver damage with methotrexate, bladder damage with cyclophosphamide, bone marrow toxicity

       (b) Use may result in ovarian failure, especially in prolonged use of cyclophosphamide

       (c) Contraindicated during pregnancy

       (d) Associated with increased risk of malignancy, especially lymphoma or leukemia

   f. **Danazol**

     i. Attenuated androgen occasionally used as steroid-sparing agent in long-term management of thrombocytopenia

     ii. Side effects include irregular menses, virilization, emotional lability

       (a) Rare appearance of liver tumors

   g. **Investigational therapies**

     i. Cyclosporin A

       (a) Serious effects of hypertension and renal toxicity limit use

     ii. Immunoglobulin

       (a) Some success for treatment of thrombocytopenia

     iii. Plasmapheresis

       (a) Limited experience

     iv. Total lymphoid irradiation

       (a) Slows progression of nephritis

       (b) Multiple complications include increased risk of infection, late-onset leukemia, cardiovascular disease

F. **SLE and pregnancy**

  1. Mild SLE does not limit fertility

  2. Higher fetal wastage (miscarriage, stillbirth) associated with antiphospholipid syndrome

  3. "Rule of thirds" noted above; third whose disease worsens during pregnancy usually had preexisting complications

  4. Flares tend to occur in first trimester and 4–8 weeks postpartum

  5. Stable SLE can be managed during pregnancy, even if steroid therapy required

    a. Placenta metabolizes all steroids except dexamethasone

  6. Immunosuppressive agents avoided despite some experience with azathioprine

  7. Antimalarial therapy avoided due to potential to cause fetal defects

  8. Moderate-to-severe nephritis is serious risk

    a. Pregnancy almost always worsens renal disease, usually irreversibly

  9. Any likelihood of adverse effects requires discussion of abortion, preferably as prenatal discussion or at least early in pregnancy

G. **Antiphospholipid syndrome**

  1. Clinical features noted above

    a. Presentation with thrombosis, pregnancy loss

    b. Cardiac valvular vegetations, livedo reticularis, migraine headaches, thrombocytopenia, anemia, skin lesions

2. Differential diagnosis
  a. Other hypercoagulable states
    i. Deficiencies of protein C, protein S, antithrombin III
    ii. Dysfibrinogenemias
    iii. Thrombotic thrombocytopenic purpura
    iv. Nephrotic syndrome, malignancies, polycythemia vera, Behçet's disease, paroxysmal nocturnal hemoglobinuria
  b. Other causes of pregnancy loss are multiple; antiphospholipid syndrome accounts for only small fraction
3. Laboratory tests
  a. Prolonged PTT
  b. Failure to correct PTT by mixing with normal plasma suggests presence of inhibitor
  c. Normalization of PTT with freeze-thawed platelets or phospholipids
  d. Measurement for lupus anticoagulant or anticardiolipin
4. Treatment
  a. Acute thrombosis treated no differently from any other cause
    i. Heparin, thrombolytics as indicated
  b. Several episodes of thrombosis suggest antiphospholipid syndrome; if detected, woman is at high risk for further recurrence
  c. Prolonged prophylaxis with warfarin (venous and arterial thrombosis) or aspirin (arterial thrombosis)
  d. Use of steroids, immunosuppressives only if vasculopathy or coagulopathy present or if anticoagulants repeatedly fail
  e. Therapy during pregnancy controversial
    i. Warfarin contraindicated during pregnancy
    ii. Heparin successful but associated with high likelihood of osteoporosis
    iii. Aspirin, prednisone, gamma-globulin have been tried
    iv. Increased risk for preeclampsia, intrauterine growth retardation, obstetric complications
H. **Management of asymptomatic, ANA-positive patient**
  1. Usually detected when ANA ordered for symptoms not entirely consistent with diagnosis of SLE
  2. Frequent association of ANA with other diseases as well as with old age
    a. Titer of 1:640 or lower seen with advanced age, hepatitis, Hashimoto's thyroiditis, multiple other rheumatologic disorders (e.g., RA, scleroderma, Sjögren's syndrome, drug-induced disorders)
  3. Careful history and exam for signs, symptoms of SLE, scleroderma, RA, hepatitis, thyroid disease
  4. Laboratory test may include complete blood count, creatinine, urinalysis, liver enzymes
  5. If no abnormal findings, reassurance and follow-up are appropriate
    a. Up to 1–4% of normal population are ANA-positive with no other disease
    b. Possible that SLE or other disease will eventually develop

SUGGESTED READING

1. Boumpas DR, Austin HA, Fessler BJ, et al: Systemic lupus erythematosus: Emerging concepts. Part 1: Renal, neuropsychiatric, cardiovascular, pulmonary, and hematologic disease. Ann Intern Med 122:940–950, 1995.
2. Boumpas DR, Fessler BJ, Austin HA, et al: Systemic lupus erythematosus: Emerging concepts. Part 2: Dermatologic and joint disease, the antiphospholipid antibody syndrome, pregnancy and hormonal therapy, morbidity and mortality, and pathogenesis. Ann Intern Med 123:42–53, 1995.
3. Hahn BH: Antibodies to DNA. N Engl J Med 338:1359–1368, 1998.
4. Hamilton FA (ed): Non-narcotic Analgesics: Renal and Gastrointestinal Considerations. Am J Med 105:1S–60S, 1998.
5. Johnson BE: Adult Rheumatic Disease. Monograph, Edition no. 218, Home Study Self-Assessment Program. Kansas City, MO, American Academy of Family Physicians, 1997.
6. Klippel JH: Rheumatologic diseases. In: Langford CA (moderator): Use of cytotoxic agents and cyclosporine in the treatment of autoimmune diseases. Part 1: Rheumatic and renal diseases. Ann Intern Med 128:1021–1028, 1998.

7. Koopman WJ, Moreland LW: Rheumatoid arthritis: Anticytokine therapies on the horizon. Ann Intern Med 128:231–233, 1998.
8. Latman NS: Relation of menstrual cycle phase to symptoms of rheumatoid arthritis. Am J Med 74:957–960, 1983.
9. Lockshin MD: Antiphospholipid antibody syndrome. JAMA 268:1451–1453, 1992.
10. McCarty GA: Autoantibodies and their relation to rheumatic diseases. Med Clin North Am 70:237–262, 1986.
11. Nossal GJV: The basic components of the immune system. N Engl J Med 316:1320–1325, 1987.
12. O'Dell JR, Haire CE: Treatment of rheumatoid arthritis with methotrexate alone, sulfasalazine and hydroxychloroquine, or a combination of all three medications. N Engl J Med 334:1287–1291, 1996.
13. Rogers MP, Liang MH: Psychological care of adults with rheumatoid arthritis. Ann Intern Med 96:344–348, 1982.
14. Schumacher HR, Klippel JH, Koopman WJ (eds): Primer on the Rheumatic Diseases, 10th ed. Atlanta, Arthritis Foundation, 1993.
15. Sorokin R, Ward SB: Joint pain. Med Clin North Am 79:247–260, 1995.

90. Headache

Bruce E. Johnson, M.D.

I. The Issues

It is estimated that 65–85% of the adult population suffers recurrent headaches; well over half are women. In women, headache onset tends to be at or shortly after the menarche. Headaches frequently are tied to the menstrual cycle and tend to decrease after menopause. Some headaches increase with hormonal manipulation, such as oral contraceptives. Attempts to determine the cause of headache have been frustrated by its multifactorial nature. In contrast to so many other diseases, finding a cause of headache is often less fruitful than working with each woman to identify precipitating events and to manage the consequences of the attack. This approach has led some to embrace a severity model of chronic headache. Newer therapies, especially using serotonin agonists, is bringing hope to this age-old complaint.

II. The Theory

A. Epidemiology

1. Recurrent headache reported by 65–85% of adults
2. Over 60% of all headaches are reported in women
3. Over 50% of all women have disabling headache at some time in life
4. Seventh most common reason for visits to primary care physicians
   a. Women and elderly more likely than men and young to consult doctor
   b. Visit to doctor also more likely with higher socioeconomic status and education level
5. 6–7% of population lose 6 or more days a year from school or work because of headache
6. In 1970s headache estimated to account for half of 30 million pounds of aspirin produced yearly in U.S.

B. Anatomy and pathophysiology

1. **Pain syndromes** may result from stimulation of nerves supplying richly innervated head and neck structures
   a. Skin and subcutaneous tissue
      i. Injuries, trauma, rashes, scars causing facial or scalp pain
   b. Muscles
      i. Implicated in tension headaches (see below)
      ii. Spasm or strain of neck may cause neck or occiput pain
         (a) Irritation of muscles with cervical spondylosis
         (b) Whiplash injuries
      iii. Spasm or strain from temporomandibular joint (TMJ) disorder

        iv. Fibromyalgia with tender nodules (trigger points) near insertion of cervical muscles

  c. Arteries and veins

      i. Implicated in migraine (see below)

      ii. Dull, aching, persistent, diffuse headache from temporal or giant-cell arteritis which is important diagnostic consideration in new-onset headache in the elderly

      iii. Evolving thrombosis (stroke) rarely gives headache

          (a) If present, thrombosis of internal, anterior, or cerebral vessels referred to forehead or temple; of vertebral vessels, to postauricular region; of basilar vessels, to occiput

          (b) Transient ischemic attacks (TIAs) in one series caused headache in 25%

      iv. Thrombus of intracranial veins refers pain to overlying scalp

  d. Periosteum of skull

      i. Trauma, hematoma

  e. Eyes

      i. Pain located in orbit, forehead, or temple; steady, aching quality with overuse of muscles (e.g., hyperopia, impaired accommodation—the familiar "eyestrain")

      ii. Increased intraocular pressure (e.g., acute glaucoma)

      iii. Pain of intracranial aneurysm, cavernous sinus thrombosis, or pituitary tumor referred to eye

  f. Ears

      i. Infection (otitis), trauma (ruptured eardrum)

  g. Nasal and sinus cavities

      i. Pain overlies maxillary and frontal sinuses

      ii. Pain from ethmoid and sphenoid sinuses referred to eyes or vertex

      iii. Sinus pain tends to be throbbing and to recur at same time of day; often the morning because sinuses fill during night—relief comes with emptying sinuses in morning

  h. Parts of dura at base of brain and arteries within dura and pia-arachnoid

      i. Distention of dura and/or arteries from tumor, closed head injury, subdural hematoma refers pain to overlying skin

  i. Cranial nerves V, IX, X and cervical nerves 1–3

      i. Trigeminal pain located at face (e.g., tic douloureux)

      ii. Glossopharyngeal and vagal pain referred to ear or throat

      iii. Cervical nerves 1–3 carry pain impulses from posterior fossa and infradura

2. **Other headaches**

  a. Systemic illnesses give steady or throbbing headache, usually frontal or occipital

      i. Hypothyroidism, obstructive sleep apnea, Cushing's disease, acute anemia, corticosteroid withdrawal, chronic obstructive pulmonary disease with hypercapnia, acute or very severe hypertension, carbon monoxide poisoning

      ii. Accompanied by flushing suggests mastocytosis, carcinoid, pheochromocytoma

  b. Lumbar puncture headache typically occipital-nuchal and resolves when leak covers and pressure of cerebrospinal fluid (CSF) maintained

  c. Cough or exertional headache

      i. Sinusitis

      ii. Rarely arteriovenous malformations, Arnold Chiari malformations, tumor

  d. Coital headache

      i. Women less often than men

      ii. Usually brief, with no underlying pathology

C. **Classification of headache**

  1. Often classified into three or four groups

    a. Migraine

    b. Tension

    c. Combined or mixed

    d. Systemic or secondary

2. Current strategy to move away from precise diagnosis (except for secondary causes where a diagnosis may cure headache)
   a. Clear that in most women headache types overlap ("combined" or "mixed")
   b. As therapy has evolved, it is less useful to reserve one type of treatment for migraine and another for tension headache but choose freely from all treatments
3. Severity model
   a. Developed due to recognition of several factors
      i. Most headache is relatively brief, short-lived, and self-treated
         (a) Persons who come to doctors almost always have recurrent headache, interfering with activities and resistant to self-treatment
      ii. Treatment approaches do not greatly differ, regardless of diagnosis
      iii. More aggressive treatment reflects severity and persistence of headache more than specific diagnosis
         (a) Recognizes differences in quantity rather than quality
   b. In an effort to move away from labels (i.e., "tension") the term "recurrent nonspecific headache" may be used
   c. Uses biopsychosocial approach
      i. Emphasizes patient in her context, equally acknowledging psychological states and social context with anatomic and biochemical contribution as common pathway of headache
   d. Encourages doctor–patient relationship in continuity
      i. Appropriate to primary care setting
      ii. Addresses trust and access
   e. Equal importance to nondrug and drug treatment
D. **Migraine headache**
   1. Throbbing headaches with typical onset in adolescence or early adulthood
      a. Diminish in frequency with advancing age
      b. Small number of women develop migraine, sometimes for first time, with initiation of hormone replacement therapy (HRT)
   2. Frequent positive family history
   3. Afflicts 3 times more women than men
      a. Frequently timed during premenstrual period
      b. Often improves or disappears during pregnancy and after menopause
   4. Pathophysiology both evident and elusive
      a. Symptoms associated with changes in cerebral blood flow
         i. Prodrome with vascular constriction
         ii. Headache coincident with (though not completely associated with) vasodilation of same vessels which had been constricted
   5. Increasing evidence points to role of serotonin depletion in brain, possibly in association with chronic stress, sleep deprivation, depression
      a. Success with serotonin agonists such as triptans
   6. **Four clinical syndromes**
      a. **Classic migraine**
         i. Prodrome such as visual scintillations, photophobia, scotomas, dizziness, tinnitus
         ii. Visual symptoms may even proceed to field blocks or hemianopsia
         iii. Headache occurs after interval of minutes to hours and is usually accompanied by nausea and vomiting
         iv. Relieved by sleep but may persist several days
      b. **Common migraine**
         i. Similar to classic but without prodrome or visual symptoms
      c. **Complicated migraine**
         i. Neurologic symptoms precede or accompany headache
            (a) Not limited to visual disorders but include numbness or tingling of ex tremities, dysphasia, weakness, or paralysis
            (b) Specific manifestation depends on vascular supply involved, e.g., hemiplegia if middle cerebral artery involved

(c) Usually self-limited; stroke a rare occurrence
ii. Basilar migraine
(a) Visual disorders and paresthesias along with confusion or stupor, vertigo, outbursts, dysarthria
(b) Relatively common in children with migraine
iii. Migraine equivalents
(a) Neurologic symptoms without headache but often with pain in thorax, trunk extremities, abdomen, and nausea
(b) Difficult to diagnose without headache, especially at initial presentation
d. **Cluster headache**
i. Four times more common in men who smoke
ii. Constant, unilateral orbital pain, intense, with parasympathetic displays including lacrimation, rhinorrhea, ptosis, flushing
iii. Duration of several hours
iv. Recurrent over days to weeks, then remits and may be absent for months to years
v. Often associated with times of stress, overwork, exertion, emotional overload
vi. Pain so severe and without effective immediate treatment that patients speak frequently of suicide
vii. Etiology and pathophysiology unclear, but features believed to be consistent with migraine variant
7. Triggering features frequent
a. Emotional stress, fatigue, anxiety, sleeplessness
b. Premenstrual status
c. Oral contraceptives, postmenopausal HRT
d. Dietary factors
i. Dairy or wheat products, alcohol (especially red wine), chocolate, coffee, tea, tyramine-containing foods
e. Nitroglycerin medications
f. Sunlight, exercise, other environmental stimuli
E. **Tension headache**
1. Bilateral, bifrontal, or occipital
2. Dull, aching, fullness, tightness ("like a band")
3. Slower, gradual onset
a. Typical onset later in day, after time of stress (e.g., after work)
4. May be persistent for hours or days without remission
a. Able to sleep, but headache present upon awakening
5. Onset any age, but more likely than migraine to have onset in middle or older years
6. Attributed in part to muscle tension in neck and occiput applying tension to galea; pain either occipital (site of muscle strain) or frontal (attachment of galea)
7. Prominent associated symptoms of depression, anxiety, hypochondriasis
a. In selected populations, up to 60% of patients with tension headache are depressed
8. Tension and migraine headaches not infrequently coexist in same patient, making diagnostic separation difficult
III. **An Approach**
A. **Age**
1. Onset of headache most common in adult years, from young adulthood to middle age
2. Child or adolescent
a. Important contribution by eyestrain
b. Anxiety or tension occasionally present
c. Menarcheal onset of migraine
d. Depression
3. Elderly
a. Cranial arteritis or polymyalgia rheumatica
i. Headache onset after age 55–60, occasionally with fever, fatigue, myalgia
ii. More common in women

      b. Tumor, abscess, subdural hematoma
          i. Gradual onset with increasing severity and frequency
      c. Depression

B. **History**
  1. **Recent**
      a. More concerned with systemic, medical disease
          i. Typically other symptoms and signs of systemic illness
             (a) Influenza or viral infection, hypothyroidism, carcinoid, carbon monoxide poisoning
             (b) Hypertension rarely associated with severe headache without recent elevation to severe levels (e.g., diastolic > 120–130 mmHg)
             (c) Increased intracranial pressure may cause headache, e.g., tumor, pseudo-tumor cerebri
      b. Contribution of recent severe stress, personal loss, emotional overload
  2. **Chronic or recurrent**
      a. Signs or symptoms with stereotypic features
          i. Classic migraine or cluster headache
      b. Recent change in pattern suggests systemic disease superimposed on chronic illness
      c. Recurrent patterns should prompt examination of psychosocial context
          i. Psychological stress
          ii. Relationships
          iii. Work or school
          iv. Family life
          v. Economic pressures
          vi. Consider spousal abuse
      d. **Precipitating events**
          i. Environmental factors
             (a) Weather, glare, loud noises, odors
          ii. Activities
             (a) Aggressive dieting, fatigue, inadequate sleep, sexual activity, vigorous exercise, travel
          iii. Foods, beverages
             (a) Tyramine foods (aged cheese, chocolate, yogurt), nitrate or nitrite compounds (in cured foods), monosodium glutamate
             (b) Alcohol, especially red wine
             (c) Caffeinated foods including coffee, tea, chocolate, soft drinks
          iv. Aspartame
          v. Tobacco, marijuana
          vi. Drug withdrawal, including withdrawal from daily use of analgesics as treatment for headache
      e. Menstrual pattern
          i. Often premenstrual
          ii. May improve with pregnancy and menopause
          iii. Aggravated by birth control pills
      f. Some women are concerned about starting postmenopausal HRT for fear of onset of headache, but new or increased headaches not common, even in women who had problems with headache with birth control pill

C. **Physical exam**
  1. Special attention to secondary causes (these are usually of recent onset)
      a. Elevated blood pressure
      b. Evidence for systemic disease
      c. Palpable vessels, especially temporal artery
      d. Vascular bruits
      e. Finding of myofascial nodules (trigger points) or cervical joint abnormalities
      f. Neurologic exam
          i. Papilledema, ophthalmoplegia, visual field cuts, lateralizing weakness

    2. Rarely have specific findings in recurrent headache

        a. Physical exam should be done as part of patient expectation and developing doctor–patient relationship

D. **Laboratory studies and procedures**

    1. No characteristic abnormalities unless suggested by history and physical exam

    2. Complete blood count, chemistry profiles, thyroid tests frequently performed, but diagnostic value slight

    3. Sedimentation rate in new-onset headache over age 50

    4. Skull radiographs and electroencephalogram virtually worthless

    5. Carotid vascular studies of little help

    6. Computed tomography or magnetic resonance imaging often performed in referral headache clinics

        a. Assumption is that referral patients represent more complicated headaches, yet even in this setting, very low yield without neurologic findings

E. **Nonpharmacologic treatments**

    1. **Establish therapeutic doctor–patient relationship**

        a. Assure patient of interest and belief in patient's symptoms

            i. Pain is what the patient says it is

        b. Assert continuity

            i. Availability for consultation and guidance, even if therapy not yet successful

        c. Studies suggest that patients fully satisfied with physician relationship over 3 times more likely to have resolution of headache than patients only partially satisfied

        d. Provide explanation of headache causes, approach to work-up and treatment, and reasons for medication if used

    2. **Treatment of secondary, contributing medical illnesses**

    3. **Identify precipitating causes**

        a. Attempt to modify causes

            i. Avoidance useful for many environmental, food and beverage, or activity-related causes

            ii. Some causes may be temporary or short-lived and supportive therapy adequate while waiting for resolution (e.g., recent death in family, impending divorce proceeding)

    4. **Evaluate for anxiety, depression**

        a. These conditions quite common in recurrent nonspecific headache

        b. Common features (such as weeping, weight loss, anhedonia) may be missing—focus instead on fatigue, poor sleep pattern (non-restorative), conflict avoidance

        c. Anxiety or depression infrequently suspected by patient; not really denial so much as never considered

    5. **Adjustments to menstrual-related headache**

        a. Barrier-type contraception preferred because oral contraceptives may exacerbate headache

        b. Since timing of menstrual-related headache frequently coincides with falling endogenous estrogen, consider applying estrogen patch in premenstrual period

        c. Women already taking estrogen have additional options

            i. Low-dose oral contraceptives may be continuous with infrequent (q 3–4 months) menses

            ii. For women on postmenopausal HRT, anecdotal reports of using danazol, tamoxifen, and bromocriptine

    6. **Regular, aerobic exercise**

        a. Decreases effects of stress and promotes sense of well-being

        b. Releases endorphins (endogenous opiates)

    7. **Physical therapy**

        a. Especially useful in patients with muscular components

        b. Stretching, massage, strengthening

        c. Correction of postural features

    8. **Biofeedback and relaxation training**

        a. Monitor and control physiologic effects of stress

TABLE 1. Classes of Therapy for Acute Treatment of Headache

Over-the-counter preparations	Triptans *(cont.)*
Acetaminophen	Sumatriptan, injection, nasal, oral (Imitrex)
Aspirin	Zolmitriptan (Zomig)
Ibuprofen and other NSAIDs	Antiemetics
Fixed combinations	Chlorpromazine (Thorazine)
Acetaminophen, aspirin, caffeine (Excedrin Migraine)	Hydroxyzine (Phenergan)
Acetaminophen, isometheptene, dichloralphenazone	Metoclopramide (Reglan)
(Midrin)	Prochlorpromazine (Compazine)
Muscle relaxants	Narcotics
Chlorzoxazone (Parafon)	Butorphanol, nasal (Stadol)
Cyclobenzaprine (Flexeril)	Cocaine nasal
Orphenadrine (Norflex)	Codeine
Ergot preparations	Meperidine
Dihydroergotamine injection (DHE 45)	Oxycodone
Dihydroergotamine basal (Migranal)	Propoxyphene
Ergotamine sublingual (Ergomar)	Others
Ergotamine, aspirin (Cafergot)	Corticosteroids
Triptans	Droperidol
Naratriptan (Amerge)	Ketorolac (Toradol)
Rizatriptan (Maxalt)	Lidocaine nasal

    b. Mobilize patient expectation of placebo effect
    c. Involve patient in own therapy
    d. Need not use expensive equipment
      i. Simple relaxation training requires neither equipment nor highly trained personnel
  F. **Drug therapy** (Tables 1 and 2)
    1. Most headache is self-treated with mild analgesics
      a. As headache becomes more severe, features become more vascular-like and patient more likely to seek help
    2. **Mild-to-moderate headache**
      a. Acetaminophen, aspirin, ibuprofen
        i. Recognize early signs of headache and attempt to abort by early and regular use
        ii. Recently the familiar OTC combination of acetaminophen, aspirin and caffeine (previously Excedrin Extra Strength, now Excedrin Migraine) received FDA approval for mild to moderate headache
      b. Premenstrual headaches may be helped with diuretics or nonsteroidal anti-inflammatory agents
      c. Narcotics
        i. Reserved for moderate headache or failure with first-line therapy

TABLE 2. Classes of Medication for Prophylactic Treatment of Headache

NSAIDs	Alpha adrenergic agonists	Anticonvulsants
Ibuprofen (Motrin)	Clonidine (Catapres)	Divalproex* (Depakote)
Naproxen (Naprosyn)	Guanabenz (Wytensin)	Gabapentin (Neurontin)
Others	Antidepressants	Serotonin antagonists
Beta blockers	Tricyclics	Cyproheptadine (Periactin)
Propranolol* (Inderal)	Amitriptyline (Elavil)	Methylsergide* (Sansert)
Timolol* (Blocadren)	Doxepin (Sinequan)	Others
Others	Nortriptyline (Pamelor)	Riboflavin
Calcium channel blockers	Others	
Diltiazem (Cardizem)	Selective serotonin reuptake inhibitors	
Verapamil (Calan)	Fluoxetine (Prozac)	
Others	Sertraline (Zoloft)	
	Others	

* FDA-approval for migraine headache prophylaxis

3. **Moderate-to-severe headache** (Table 1)
   a. Isometheptine, acetaminophen, dichloralphenazone (Midrin), naprosyn sodium (Anaprox), and nasal butorphanol (Stadol) quite different but effective abortive agents with few side effects
   b. Ergotamine tartrate, often formulated with caffeine and/or barbiturates (e.g., Cafergot, Bellergal, Fiorinol), effective abortive agent
      i. Early in headache onset
      ii. Use rectal route if nausea or vomiting prevents oral administration
   c. Oral, nasal, parenteral ergot preparations (e.g., DHE 45 or Migranal) without caffeine or barbiturates useful and nasal preparation has rapid onset but ergots have danger of significant side effects
      i. Important side effects include myalgia, dysphagia, nausea, flushing, gangrene of digits (ergotism), and even myocardial infarct
      ii. Excessive use insidiously promotes dependence; severe headache can result with ergot withdrawal
      iii. If ergots used, cannot use triptans within 24 hours without increased risk of cardiovascular effects
   d. Antiemetics helpful with nausea which frequently accompanies both a migraine headache itself or the treatment
      i. Prochlorperazine and/or hydroxyzine frequently used for this purpose
      ii. Metoclopramide also used for this purpose
   e. Emergency and urgent care settings now often use injectable promethazine (Compazine) or ketorolac (Toradol) for immediate relief
      i. Along with injected narcotics and antiemetics, should allow patient enough relief to fall asleep, arresting headache
   f. The triptans, a class of selective serotonin (5-HT1) agonists, have changed much of the acute treatment of headache
      i. Currently four choices available in oral, nasal and injectable forms
         (a) Sumatriptan and zolmitriptan have rapid onset of action, but frequently more significant side effects; onset of action of naratriptan slower but side effects less pronounced
      ii. Most efficacious at onset of migraine-type headache but useful even after headache well established
      iii. Some concern with overuse—should limit to no more than 3–4 doses per week; if using more than this amount, should be on more effective prophylactic
      iv. Side effects include flushing, tingling, neck tightness; chest pressure or pain simulating angina which may be alarming and limiting in some patients
         (a) Because of coronary artery constriction, contraindicated in patients with ischemic heart disease
         (b) Especially worrisome if accidentally combined with ergot preparations
   g. Prolonged, severe attacks may require chlorpromazine (Thorazine), 50–100 mg over 7–10 days
   h. Prednisone, 40 mg/day, used to abort severe attacks not responsive to other agents
      i. Breaks unrelenting cluster headaches
4. **Prophylactic treatment of headache with vascular features**
   a. If vascular-type headaches frequent (> 1/week) or severe, consider prophylaxis
      i. Used daily for prolonged periods to reduce frequency of headache
      ii. Cannot promise absolute absence of headache
      iii. Treatment for 6–12 months minimum once committed to prophylaxis
   b. Beta blockers
      i. Propranolol used first, in doses up to 320 mg/day
      ii. Less lipid-soluble agents, such as atenolol (Tenormin) and nadolol (Corgard), avoid most central nervous system side effects attributed to propranolol
   c. Calcium channel blockers
      i. All calcium channel blockers seem to have equal efficacy and should choose on basis of potential side effects

    d. Antidepressants
      i. Whether patients fulfill all criteria for diagnosis of depression, these agents frequently helpful in clinical practice
      ii. Since much recent effort is in repletion of serotonin in CNS, these agents make sense
      iii. Tricyclic antidepressants have longest use and often very helpful in patients with disordered sleep
        (a) Amitriptyline, doxepin, nortriptyline
        (b) Start with low dose, e.g., amitriptyline 25 mg/night
      iv. Selective serotonin reuptake inhibitors (SSRIs) in recent years used more since side effects tend to be less than tricyclics
        (a) Fluoxetine, sertraline
        (b) Initial low dose, e.g., fluoxetine 20 mg
      v. Should plan to continue antidepressants for at least 6–12 months before taper or discontinue
    e. Methylsergide (Sansert) used in refractory cases
      i. Doses of 6–8 mg/day eventually effective
      ii. Serious complication of pulmonary and retroperitoneal fibrosis
        (a) Occurrence increases after 6 months' use
    f. Report of use of riboflavin (400 mg/day) as migraine prophylaxis
      i. Precursor to flavoenzymes, a component of brain energy production
5. **Cluster headache**
    a. Quite resistant to treatment, both abortive and prophylactic
    b. Acute attack responds to inhaled oxygen, with or without ergots
    c. Since headaches are usually clustered, additional prophylactic treatment started immediately
      i. Amitriptyline, 100–150 mg/day
      ii. Nifedipine, 30–90 mg/day, or verapamil, 240–480 mg/day
      iii. Methylsergide, 6–8 mg/day
      iv. Prednisone, 40 mg/day, then taper
      v. Lithium carbonate, 750 mg/day, then titrate
      vi. Indomethacin, 50–150 mg/day
    d. Goal is to gain control of headache until cluster discontinues
    e. Since next attack may be months or years hence, little enthusiasm for long-term prophylactic therapy
6. Character of headache may change or features may evolve
    a. Any one treatment may lose effectiveness and require trial of another
    b. May return to previously ineffective treatment after passage of time and trial of other treatments
7. Some of above drugs used only with caution, if at all, during pregnancy
    a. Restrictions regarding ergots, beta blockers, tricyclic antidepressants, SSRIs, NSAIDs, methylsergide, prednisone
    b. Encourage patience; headache tends to become less severe while pregnant

SUGGESTED READING

1. Ferrari MD: Migraine. Lancet 351:1043–1051, 1998,
2. Kumar KL, Cooney TG: Headaches. Med Clin North Am 79:261–286, 1995.
3. Liptin RB, Stewart WF: The burden of migraine. PharmacoEcon 6:215–221, 1994.
4. Smith MJ, Jensen NM: The severity model of chronic headache. J Gen Intern Med 3:396–409, 1988.
5. Welch KMA: Drug therapy of migraine. N Engl J Med 329:1476–1483, 1993.
6. Young WB, Silberstein SD: Migraine treatment. Semin Neurol 17:325–333, 1997.
7. Ziegler DK, Hassenein RS, Couch JR: Characteristics of life headache histories in a non-clinic population. Neurology 27:265–269, 1977.

OTHER RESOURCES

American Council for Headache Education: www.achenet.org
National Headache Foundation: www.headaches.org

91. Fatigue

Bruce E. Johnson, M.D.

I. **The Issues**

Fatigue is an extremely common complaint. Short-term fatigue is expected after conditions ranging from viral infections to surgery. Chronic fatigue is a more complicated complaint. When not associated with a known underlying illness, fatigue is a largely female condition. Many illnesses initially present with fatigue as a symptom; these illnesses must be identified and properly treated. Chronic fatigue syndromes are often frustrating to both doctor and patient. Real progress has been made in identifying underlying abnormalities which, when treated, may result in effective care—in the meantime, a comprehensive management approach is often successful in allowing fatigued women to resume many usual activities.

II. **The Theory**

A. **Definition of chronic fatigue**

1. Tiredness or weariness; lassitude; unrelated to exertion
   a. Usual recovery from exercise or physical work is rapid
2. Fatigue interferes with patient's usual activities
   a. Unable to accomplish usual tasks at home, or work
   b. Limits socializing with family or friends
   c. Decreases sports or recreational physical activities
3. Duration of complaint varies, proposed definitions include:
   a. "Prolonged fatigue"—self-reported, persistent fatigue lasting at least one month
   b. "Chronic fatigue"—self-reported, persistent or relapsing fatigue lasting six or more months
      i. "Idiopathic chronic fatigue"—no medical or psychiatric diagnosis but does not meet CDC criteria for CFS
      ii. "Chronic fatigue syndrome (CFS)"—see definition below
   c. Women who have been "tired all my life" are not usually included in discussions of fatigue since most have a psychiatric basis for this complaint

B. **Historical perspective**

1. For centuries, descriptions of fatigue have been noted
   a. Often in epidemic terms, leading to persistent suspicions that certain fatigue syndromes are infectious
2. Colorful terminology
   a. Terms include febricula, vapors, DaCosta's syndrome
   b. From late 1800s to present frequently referred to as neurasthenia
   c. When occurring in outbreaks, termed myalgic encephalomyelitis or epidemic neuromyasthenia, despite no evidence for a central nervous system inflammatory process
3. In more recent years, unexplained fatigue diagnosed as hypoglycemia, chronic mononucleosis, chronic candidiasis, postviral fatigue syndrome, and yuppie flu

C. **Prevalence**

1. As presenting complaint, fatigue claimed by 25% of adults in primary care settings
   a. Diagnosable medical and psychiatric illnesses account for up to 90% of complaints of fatigue
   b. Chronic fatigue syndrome criteria (see below) met in about one quarter of "undiagnosed" complaints meaning that only 1–2% of all patients with fatigue actually have CFS
      i. This figure highly variable, depending on site of practice and specialty interest of investigators
2. Female predominance: 60% or more of patients with chronic fatigue
3. More common in adults; seen in adolescents, but prevalence unclear

D. **Differential diagnosis** (Table 1)

TABLE 1. Differential Diagnosis of Fatigue*

Infectious disease
    Human immunodeficiency virus (HIV), infectious mononucleosis syndrome (Epstein-Barr virus),
    cytomegalovirus, tuberculosis, osteomyelitis, subacute bacterial endocarditis, Lyme disease, disseminated
    fungal disease

Malignancy
    If undiagnosed, fatigue often due to anemia, hypercalcemia, or fever
    If diagnosed, fatigue often due to treatment (e.g., chemotherapy, radiation therapy)

Endocrine
    Hypothyroidism, Addison's disease, acromegaly, uncontrolled diabetes, estrogen deficiency, pregnancy

Gastrointestinal disorders
    Inflammatory bowel disease, chronic hepatitis

Cardiovascular disease
    Congestive heart failure, chronic ischemic disease, cardiomyopathy

Rheumatologic disorders
    Chronic arthritis (e.g., rheumatoid, lupus, psoriatic), vasculitis, myositis

Renal disease
    Chronic renal failure, glomerulonephritis

Hematologic disorders
    Anemia, polycythemia

Neurologic disorders
    Parkinsonism, dementia, narcolepsy, myasthenia gravis, multiple sclerosis

Medications
    Sedatives, antihistamines, analgesics, nonsteroidal anti-inflammatories, antihypertensives, progestational
    agents

Physiologic disorders
    Increased physical activity; inadequate rest; sedentary lifestyle; recent illness, surgery, or disability; sleep
    alteration (e.g., mother of newborn infant)

Habits
    Caffeinism, alcoholism, other drug abuse

Psychologic disorders
    Depression, grief, anxiety, stress reaction, insomnia, boredom

Controversial possibilities
    Food allergies, tension-fatigue syndrome

Chronic fatigue syndrome

* Partial list only.

    1. Diagnoses reached after thorough history, physical exam, and appropriate laboratory
       studies
       a. Depending on setting, medical diagnosis may account for 70–80% of fatigue
          complaints
       b. Definitive diagnosis may not be evident at first visit supporting repeat visits for
          re-evaluation
    2. Suspicion for psychiatric diagnosis high
       a. After medical conditions accounted, studies suggest 90% of the remainder will
          have psychiatric diagnosis
       b. Likelihood of psychiatric diagnosis increases the longer the patient has had fatigue
  E. **Chronic fatigue syndrome**
    1. Separate, distinct diagnosis accounting for 1–2% of all cases of fatigue
    2. Strict case definition
       a. Newer (1994) case definition differs from earlier (1988) in dropping of require-
          ment for fever, nonexudative pharyngitis, lymphadenopathy (Table 2)
    3. Definition perhaps too confining
       a. May inadvertently exclude persons with milder chronic fatigue syndrome
    4. Cause of disease unknown

TABLE 2. 1994 CDC Diagnostic Criteria for Chronic Fatigue Syndrome

Major criteria (all three must be present)	**Minor criteria** (four or more must be present)
Unexplained, persistent or relapsing fatigue > 6 months	Arthralgias
Fatigue resulting in 50% reduction in previous activity	Muscle pain
Fatigue of new or recent onset (not lifelong)	Sore throat
	Painful nodes
	New headaches
	Unrefreshing sleep
	Post-exertion malaise
	Impaired memory or concentration

      a. NIH investigative approach has identified some viral or immunologic abnormalities
      b. Recent note of mild abnormalities in pituitary-adrenal axis
          i. Slight subnormal urinary free cortisol excretion and decreased response to corticotropin-releasing hormone
      c. Identification of delayed orthostatic hypotension occurring after standing position for > 10 minutes
          i. Variant of neurally mediated hypotension
          ii. Abnormal tilt table test, especially with isoproterenol
   5. Natural history varies
      a. Some patients have prolonged, debilitating fatigue
      b. Fatigue and other symptoms (e.g., fever, lymphadenopathy, pharyngitis) most intense early in course
      c. Evidence that gradual improvement and return of functional state occur without specific intervention in 6–12 months after identification of syndrome, i.e., 12–18+ months after onset of illness
  F. **Special circumstances**
    1. Excessive demands ("super-mom")
      a. Household expectations (e.g., cleaning, cooking, laundry)
      b. Outside-the-home work, especially if shift work, travel from home, or position of responsibility without set hours
      c. Shopping (e.g., food, clothes for self and children, household furnishings)
      d. Spouse
          i. Even if he helps with housework, many other responsibilities remain the wife's, especially child care, "running the household"
      e. Children's activities
          i. Very young children require almost constant care
          ii. When older, transporting to activities such as sports, clubs, lessons
          iii. Self-doubts about being a "good enough mom" if not directly involved in many of these activities
      f. Days characterized by early rising, time pressures at home and work, late evenings, occasional night wakenings
      g. Becomes pathologic when interferes with sleep, sex, weight/appetite, socializing
    2. Biologic interference with sleep
      a. Menstrual periods frequently result in 2–3 days each month of altered or poor sleep—typically first couple days of flow
      b. Pregnancy a time of very poor sleep due to discomfort, fetal movements, frequent urination
      c. Menopause frequently characterized by poor sleep with hot flashes, depression, mood swings
III. **An Approach**
  A. **History and presentation**
    1. Nature of fatigue
      a. Debilitating; interfering; unrelenting
      b. Fatigue in excess of usual physical demands
    2. Duration of fatigue
      a. Present for at least 1 month (CDC criterion—6 months)

        i. Recent onset more likely either medical illness or CFS

        ii. Prolonged duration more likely psychiatric

3. Bed rest not restorative
4. Sleep disorder
   a. Difficulty falling asleep or nighttime awakening
   b. Excessive sleeping but without improvement
5. Reduced activity
   a. Interferes with completing duties at work, housework, children's activities
6. Reduced socialization with friends or family
7. Allergic symptoms (e.g., sneezing, congestion, ear pain, dyspnea)
8. Neurophysiologic symptoms
   a. Headache
   b. Photophobia, visual scotomata
   c. Forgetfulness, irritability, difficulty with concentrating
9. Drug use
   a. Prescription drugs, especially recent onset
   b. Over-the-counter drugs
   c. Alcohol
   d. Recreational/illicit drugs
10. Physical complaints
    a. Weight change, fever, sore throat, lumps (lymphadenopathy), myalgias, transitory or migratory arthralgias, allergic manifestations (rhinitis, conjunctivitis, itching), skin rashes, changes in hair, muscle weakness

B. Physical exam

1. Search for findings that may lead to specific diagnosis (see Table 1 for differential diagnosis)
2. Vital signs
   a. Special attention to fever (even though no longer specific CDC criterion)
   b. Weight loss
   c. Orthostatic changes
      i. Check BP supine and after standing > 10 minutes
3. Head, ears, eyes, nose, and throat
   a. Pharyngitis, thrush, nasal congestion
4. Neck—thyroid enlargement or nodes
5. Nodes
   a. Special attention to anterior/posterior and axillary nodes
   b. Nodes > 2 cm suggest other cause
6. Chest—wheezing, rales (especially posttussive), dullness
7. Heart
   a. Murmurs, especially new, cardiomegaly, S3
8. Abdomen
   a. Hepatomegaly (left lobe), splenomegaly
9. Pelvic
   a. Recurrent vaginitis (especially yeast), pelvic infection
10. Extremities
    a. Vascular deficiencies, muscular atrophy
11. Joints
    a. Effusion, active arthritis
12. Skin, nails, and hair
    a. Hair loss
    b. Jaundice, striae, myxedema
    c. Rashes
       i. Erythema chronicum migrans, intertrigo, unusual pigmentation, vasculitic pattern
    d. Signs of internal disease
13. Neurologic exam
    a. Muscle weakness, lateralizing findings, eye muscle or pupillary changes, posterior column abnormalities

C. **Laboratory tests and procedures**
  1. Complete blood count with differential, sedimentation rate
  2. Electrolytes
  3. Chemistry profile
     a. Include at least glucose, creatinine, calcium, alkaline phosphatase, transaminases (aspartate and alanine), creatine phosphokinase or aldolase
  4. Urinalysis
  5. Thyroid-stimulating hormone
  6. Antinuclear antibody and/or rheumatoid factor (if indicated)
  7. Antibody test for human immunodeficiency virus (if indicated)
  8. Chest radiograph (if signs or symptoms of pulmonary disease)
  9. Purified protein derivative (PPD) if recent exposure
  10. Additional tests to further evaluate or confirm abnormalities guided by findings in history, physical exam, or above studies
  11. Specifically, do not need to perform as part of initial evaluation unless clinical clues support diagnosis:
     a. Epstein-Barr virus antibodies, Lyme disease (*Borrelia*) antibodies, immunoglobulins, cortisol, blood cultures, urine drug screen, urine heavy metal measurement, electrocardiogram, CT or MRI studies, electromyography and nerve conduction studies, myelin basic protein in cerebrospinal fluid
D. **Psychological testing**
  1. May be difficult to get patient's agreement
  2. Assess depression, anxiety, and somatization
     a. Interview or self-completed questionnaires
        i. Beck Depression Score
        ii. NIH Diagnostic Interview Schedule
        iii. Inventory to Diagnose Depression
        iv. Pennebaker Inventory of Limbic Languidness
E. **Treatment of identified medical or psychiatric disease**
  1. Medical disease
     a. Fatigue may precede physical exam abnormality or laboratory/procedure evidence of disease
     b. Multiple visits with repeated questioning and examination coincide with progression to evident disease; specific diagnosis can be made
     c. Fatigue often but not always responds to effective therapy of underlying illness
  2. Treat identified psychiatric disorders
F. **Treatment of CFS**
  1. Counsel both patient and family
     a. Explain that patient has chronic disease
     b. Intermittent symptoms; wax and wane
     c. Avoid situations known to induce stress
  2. Diet should be balanced and nutritional
     a. No special additives or supplements have demonstrated effectiveness
  3. Physical exercise should be monitored
     a. Most patients should be prescribed modest, graduated exercise
     b. Do not initiate abrupt vigorous exercise
        i. Misguided attempt to exercise oneself out of fatigue
  4. Empiric treatments of physical complaints
     a. Symptomatic treatment of myalgia and arthralgia with nonsteroidal, anti-inflammatory drugs
        i. Myalgia may respond to massage therapy
        ii. Anecdotal reports of response to guaifenesin
     b. Control of fever with antipyretics
     c. Antihistamines for allergic symptoms
     d. Analgesics for headache
  5. Empiric treatment of psychological complaints

    a. Many patients respond to therapy for depression with tricyclic antidepressants or
       serotonin uptake inhibitors
        i. Especially helpful if altered sleep cycle
    b. If appropriate, consider anxiolytic therapy
  6. Investigational approaches
    a. Neurally mediated hypotension (abnormal tilt table test)
        i. Use of fludrocortisone, e.g., 0.1 mg qd
        ii. Use of atenolol, e.g., 25 mg qd
        iii. Use of leg support hose
    b. Pituitary-adrenal axis dysfunction
        i. Empiric hydrocortisone "replacement," e.g., 20–25 mg in AM, 5–10 mg in PM
        ii. Symptomatic/functional gain measurable but slight
  7. Unproven treatments (while not usually harmful, these are unproven and may be costly)
    a. Immunologic stimulation
    b. Gamma-globulin infusion
    c. Vitamin/mineral supplements
    d. Herbal "natural" therapies (such as St. John's wort or echinacea)
    e. Antibiotic therapy for EB virus, Lyme disease
  8. Empathetic support by physician
    a. Chronic fatigue is discouraging and depressing illness
    b. Patient needs advocate in physician
    c. Similar support provided to any patient with chronic illness

SUGGESTED READING

1. Bates DW, Schmitt W: Prevalence of fatigue and chronic fatigue syndrome in a primary care practice.
   Arch Intern Med 153:2759–2765, 1993.
2. Cathebras BJ, Robbins JM: Fatigue in primary care. J Gen Intern Med 7:276–286, 1992.
3. Elnicki DM, Shockcor WT: Evaluating the complaint of fatigue in primary care: Diagnoses and outcomes.
   Am J Med 93:303–306, 1993.
4. Fukuda K, Straus SE: The chronic fatigue syndrome: A comprehensive approach to its definition and
   study. Ann Intern Med 121:953–959, 1994.
5. Komaroff AL, Buchwald DS: Chronic fatigue syndrome: An update. Ann Rev Med 49:1–13, 1998.
6. Manu P, Matthews DA: The mental health of patients with a chief complaint of chronic fatigue. Arch
   Intern Med 148:2213–2217, 1988.
7. McKenzie R, O'Fallon A: Low-dose hydrocortisone for treatment of chronic fatigue syndrome: A randomized controlled trial. JAMA 280:1061–1066, 1998.

OTHER SOURCES:

The Chronic Fatigue and Immune Dysfunction Syndrome Association of America (CFIDS)—www.cfids.org
Guidelines to the Management and Treatment of Chronic Fatigue Syndrome—www.cdc.gov/phtn/pg9-
  12.htm

92. Anemia

Bruce E. Johnson, M.D.

I. The Issues

Anemia from all causes is a disease of considerable importance to the health of women. It is estimated that worldwide as many as 40% of all women of child-bearing age are anemic. Most anemias are nutritional, as seen in iron deficiency; in parts of the world, hemoglobinopathies (such
as sickle cell anemia and thalassemia) and parasitic infestations account for an additional burden
of anemia. Iron deficiency in women is usually due to menstruation and pregnancy. Other nutritional deficiencies, such as folic acid and vitamin B_{12} deficiencies, are less common but when

present may cause profound morbidities. Anemia is insidious in development and causes consequences beyond simple fatigue. Because iron deficiency is so prevalent, yet relatively easily diagnosed and treated, much of the following section concerns this specific type of anemia.

II. **The Theory**

   A. **Iron deficiency anemia** (IDA)

      1. **Prevalence**

         a. Worldwide, over 80% of women of child-bearing age have iron deficiency anemia (though not necessarily anemia)

            i. Even in U.S., 5% of women of child-bearing age have IDA

         b. During pregnancy, prevalence rises with as many as 35–50% of women developing IDA if iron supplements not prescribed

         c. After menopause, prevalence decreases so that by age 60 full iron stores is the rule

      2. **Iron metabolism**

         a. On average, iron-replete adult has 3–5 g total body iron (10–20% in hemoglobin and other iron-containing proteins)

         b. Obligatory loss of iron, approximately 1 mg/day, in feces, urine, skin sloughing

         c. Iron loss during normal menstrual period about 20 mg, in addition to obligatory loss

         d. Iron loss during pregnancy ranges from 500–1000 mg

         e. Foodstuffs contain iron in either heme or nonheme form

            i. Meats and liver contain iron in heme form

            ii. Heme iron more easily absorbed and though heme iron accounts for only 10% of oral iron intake it represents 40% of absorbed iron

            iii. Iron in legumes, wheat, and eggs mostly nonheme form and must be solubilized for absorption; little iron in fruits and most vegetables

         f. For absorption iron must be in ferric (Fe^{3+}) state

            i. In acid environment (normal stomach), ferric iron stays soluble and able to be absorbed; achlorhydria of any etiology decreases iron absorption

            ii. Citrate and ascorbate (i.e., vitamin C) forms soluble complex with ferric ion and enhances absorption

            iii. Tannates (such as in tea) and certain plant phosphates tightly bind ferric ion in insoluble complex, decreasing absorption

            iv. Absorption mechanism shared with several heavy metals—e.g., lead, cadmium

         g. Once absorbed, iron transported by transferrin

            i. In iron-replete state, approximately one-third of transferrin saturated with iron (total iron binding capacity—TIBC)

            ii. Transports iron from intestine to iron stores and from stores to cells

         h. Iron storage in reticuloendothelial cells of bone marrow, liver, and spleen and in skeletal muscle cells and hepatocytes

            i. Stored as ferritin or hemosiderin

            ii. Ferritin leaves storage cells in strictly controlled quantities; since plasma ferritin equals about 1/1000 storage ferritin, plasma ferritin is close approximation of storage iron

            iii. Hemosiderin, not as closely regulated, is stainable material in bone marrow examination

      3. **Tests for iron status**

         a. Peripheral blood smear can be suggestive

            i. Early iron deficiency presents only with anisocytosis; more significant IDA leads to microcytosis (mean corpuscular volume [MCV] < 80 fl), hypochromia, poikilocytosis, and cigar-shaped cells

         b. Reticulocyte count low

            i. More accurate test is reticulocyte index, in which double correction is made both for degree of anemia and impact of bone marrow adjustments to anemia

         c. Serum iron inaccurate indicator of iron status

            i. Normal values 50–200 mg/dl, but diurnal variation may be as much as 10–40 mg/dl

      ii. Serum iron reduced in inflammation and malignancy

      iii. Serum iron elevated with supplementation

  d. Transferrin (TIBC) also subject to variation: frequently depressed in inflammation, infection, malignancy

  e. Ratio of iron to transferrin (iron/TIBC) accurate to diagnose IDA in absence of inflammation

      i. Normal ratio above 15%

        (a) If less than 10%, strongly suggestive of iron deficiency

      ii. Ratio above 70–80% suggests iron storage disease such as hemochromatosis

  f. Ferritin accurately reflects iron storage

      i. Levels < 10 mg/dl strongly suggest iron deficiency

      ii. Ferritin is also acute phase reactant; hence difficult to interpret in setting of inflammation, malignancy, liver disease

      iii. Levels > 50 mg/dl unlikely in iron deficiency, even in setting of inflammation

  g. Bone marrow aspirate is definitive test

      i. In addition to morphology of cells, staining of marrow with Prussian blue determines iron stores

      ii. Diagnosis usually made before bone marrow test required though bone marrow aspirate may be necessary when anemia with chronic inflammation is in differential

B. **Other nutritional anemias**

  1. **Folate deficiency**

    a. Prevalence in women probably lower than in men but significance greater during pregnancy

      i. Metabolic demands for folate increase as much as 7-fold during pregnancy

      ii. Without supplement, folate levels fall, especially in latter half of pregnancy

      iii. Folate deficiency associated with neural tube defects, which can be prevented by supplementation

    b. In nonpregnant state, most commonly seen in alcoholism, malabsorption states, urban poor with inadequate diet, hemolytic anemia (e.g., sickle cell anemia), certain drugs

    c. Folate present in many fresh fruits and leafy vegetables

      i. Readily absorbed and transported except in intestinal disorders with malabsorption (e.g., sprue, short bowel) and certain drugs (e.g., anticonvulsants, triamterene, sulfasalazine)

    d. Storage of folate limited; deficiency develops in months without replacement

    e. Deficiency characterized by elevated MCV and macrocytosis

      i. Advanced cases develop diarrhea, cheilosis, glossitis

      ii. Unlike vitamin B_{12} deficiency, no neurologic manifestations

    f. Diagnosis suggested by elevated MCV > 100 fl

    g. Reticulocyte index low

    h. While serum folate is useful, the level can be altered by recent ingestion of folate

      i. Better test is red blood cell folate which reveals tissue status over previous 3 months

  2. **Vitamin B_{12} (cobalamin) deficiency**

    a. Prevalence overall equal between men and women

      i. Association with other autoimmune conditions, such as Graves' or Hashimoto's thyroiditis or Addison's disease

    b. Common causes

      i. Pernicious anemia (lack of intrinsic factor with autoantibody against parietal cells of stomach)

      ii. Gastrectomy

      iii. Absence or disease of terminal ileum (site of absorption of vitamin B_{12}/ intrinsic factor complex)

      iv. Fish tapeworm infestation

      v. Practicing vegans (vegetarians who avoid all animal products, including eggs and milk)

    c. Vitamin B_{12} found naturally in animal meats and dairy products; not synthesized in plants

    d. Storage in liver and elsewhere in body

        i. Stores are adequate for up to 3–6 years

    e. Manifestations

        i. Anemia may be profound, with hematocrit of 15–20 not uncommon

        ii. Deficiency develops gradually and body adapts remarkably to low hematocrit

        iii. Symptoms of weakness, fatigue, lightheadedness

        iv. Skin and eyes may develop icteric coloration

        v. Gastrointestinal changes include glossitis (tender, reddened tongue), anorexia, diarrhea, malabsorption with weight loss

        vi. Neurologic manifestations most ominous

            (a) Demyelination of peripheral nerves, spinal cord (especially lateral and posterior columns), and finally changes in cerebrum

            (b) Early symptoms include numbness of fingers and toes, then progress to ataxia, position sense, and vibratory sense diminution (positive Romberg and Babinski tests), diminished reflexes, and sphincter disorder

            (c) Eventually may develop dementia and/or psychosis

            (d) Neurologic changes frequently not reversible with replacement of vitamin B_{12}

        vii. Neurologic changes may develop before changes noticed in hematocrit or red cell indices

    f. Diagnostic tests

        i. Vitamin B_{12} deficiency should be considered during evaluation of malabsorption, peripheral neuropathy, dementia and, of course, megaloblastic changes

        ii. Increase of MCV > 100 fl should prompt evaluation; MCV > 110 fl is frequently due to vitamin B_{12} or folate deficiency

        iii. Blood smear shows poikilocytosis, macroovalocytes, and characteristic increased segmentation of nuclei in leukocytes

            (a) If deficiency profound, also expect relative leukopenia and thrombocytopenia

            (b) Reticulocyte index low

        iv. Measured serum vitamin B_{12} level often accurate and will be low

            (a) Low serum vitamin B_{12} occasionally seen in pregnancy and oral contraceptives with no other manifestations of disease

            (b) Unfortunately, some aspects of disease, especially neurologic, may precede hematologic changes and be detected only by low serum vitamin B_{12} or other tests

        v. Schilling test next appropriate test

            (a) Several stages of Schilling test help narrow diagnosis among several possibilities with pernicious anemia most common in American women

        vi. Bone marrow may be needed for diagnosis

C. **Hemolytic and other genetic anemias**

    1. Examples include sickle cell anemia, thalassemias, red cell wall abnormalities (spherocytosis, ovalocytosis), and other hemoglobinopathies

    2. Although important to recognize and, occasionally, to characterize, there is no greater likelihood for most of these to occur in women than men

III. **An Approach**

A. **Classification of anemias** (one of several different approaches; useful for quickly evaluating more common anemias in women)

    1. Assuming anemia is present, first useful step is to determine reticulocyte index

      a. Proliferative anemia (e.g., hemolytic) has reticulocyte index > 3%

      b. Nonproliferative anemia (e.g., IDA, deficiency of folate or vitamin B_{12}) has reticulocyte index < 3%

    2. Next test is iron/TIBC ratio

    a. Proliferative anemias have ratio > 20%

    b. IDA and anemia of chronic disease have ratio < 20%

    c. Other nonproliferative anemias have ratio > 20%

3. At this point, categorize proliferative anemia, if present

    a. Hemolytic anemias (many causes)

    b. Hemorrhage and its recovery

    c. Marrow invasion

4. If reticulocyte index < 3%, and ratio < 20%, diagnose either IDA or anemia of chronic disease

    a. Although both diagnoses have low MCV and serum iron, IDA has increased TIBC, low ferritin, and no marrow iron

    b. Anemia of chronic disease has low TIBC, normal or increased ferritin, and marrow iron

5. If reticulocyte index < 3%, and ratio > 20%, diagnostic choices include marrow failure (e.g., aplasia, myelofibrosis, hypothyroid, renal failure) or ineffective erythropoiesis

    a. Ineffective erythropoiesis includes deficiencies of folate or vitamin B_{12}, certain thalassemias, sideroblastic anemia, or refractory anemias

    b. At this point, appropriate testing involves measurement of serum red cell folate, vitamin B_{12}, Schilling tests, hemoglobin electrophoresis, bone marrow examination

6. For most anemias, stepwise approach results in accurate diagnosis

    a. Mistakes in diagnosing common anemias due to mixed causes, e.g., concomitant IDA and folate deficiency

    b. Consultative help may be needed for mixed anemias, hemoglobinopathies, marrow failures, and other less common causes

B. **Iron deficiency anemia**

1. **Classic symptoms**

    a. Fatigue, lassitude, breathlessness, or exertional dyspnea

    b. Tachycardia, palpitations

2. **Other symptoms and signs**

    a. Pallor

    b. Glossitis with red, swollen, smooth, tender tongue

    c. Gastric atrophy with achlorhydria (which, of course, further exacerbates iron absorption)

    d. Koilonychia (spoon nails)

    e. Menorrhagia

        i. Both cause and effect of IDA

        ii. Bleeding becomes more excessive with iron deficiency; unclear whether this constitutes unrecognized clotting factor deficiency

        iii. Excessive bleeding corrects as IDA treated

    f. Some suggestions that certain cognitive functions may be affected by chronic IDA

3. **Pica**

    a. Peculiar symptom rather specific to iron deficiency

        i. Appears more often in women, but this may be either cultural or because IDA much more common in women

        ii. May be present in as many as 50% of all women with IDA

        iii. Etiology unclear but related to iron deficiency, not simply anemia; i.e., pica not present in other anemias

    b. Excessive or compulsive ingestion of material, both foodstuffs or nonnutritive; virtually anything may be ingested (colorful terms frequently applied to compulsion)

        i. In U.S. most common pica is ice (pagophagia)

        ii. Among African-Americans, not infrequent to find geophagia (ingestion of clay or dirt) and amblyophagia (ingestion of starch, often laundry starch)

        iii. Other reports of potatoes (geomelophagia), carrots, peanut butter—almost any foodstuff; even toothpicks, match heads (cautopyreophagia), paper tissues

    c. Some ingestions may lead to serious complications

        i. Bowel obstruction with clay, toothpicks; mercury poisoning reported with ingestion of paper tissues; satiety from starch ingestion with inadequate diet

 d. Some pica may be combination of physiologic and cultural factors
   i. Not infrequently, pica develops during pregnancy, likely time for IDA
   ii. Southern African-Americans frequently recommend clay eating during pregnancy, even suggesting recipes for preparation
 e. Compulsion occasionally embarrassing (women often think they're "crazy") but gentle, persistent questioning useful, explaining that pica is frequent accompaniment of IDA
 f. Compulsion disappears within days of beginning iron replacement, well before anemia corrected
4. **Diagnostic studies**
 a. IDA has low reticulocyte index, low MCV, low serum iron, elevated TIBC (low iron/TIBC ratio), low ferritin, and absent iron stores
   i. Bone marrow aspirate infrequently required
   ii. Some values altered by concomitant disease e.g., inflammation which alters the TIBC and ferritin ratio, or concomitant folate or vitamin B_{12} deficiency—the macrocytosis of folate or B_{12} deficiency mixing with the microcytosis of IDA giving "inappropriately normal" MCV
5. **Differential diagnosis** (Table 1)
 a. Important to perform adequate evaluation in any American woman with IDA—just because she is menstruating is not prima facie evidence for menstrual loss as the etiology
6. **Treatment**
 a. **Oral iron therapy preferred**
   i. Unfortunately, up to 20% have side effects, typically nausea, bloating, abdominal distress, constipation
   ii. Always turns color of stool black/dark green, occasionally alarming patients (stool not hemoccult-positive)
   iii. Standard choice: ferrous sulfate
     (a) Optimal dose: 325 mg (65 mg elemental iron) 3 times/day
     (b) Frequent GI side effects decreased by reducing frequency to 1–2 times/day
   iv. If ferrous sulfate not tolerated, try ferrous gluconate, 325 mg (40 mg elemental iron), or ferrous fumarate, 325 mg (100 mg elemental iron)
   v. Consider stool softener (e.g., docusate) because constipation frequent
   vi. Consider supplementing with ascorbic acid (vitamin C) to improve ingestion
 b. **Parenteral iron therapy** (iron-dextran complex, Imferon) complicated by adverse reactions
   i. Anaphylaxis (< 1% of patients receiving parenteral iron); other complications include arthralgias, fever, hypotension, and abdominal pain
   ii. Injection must be made using Z-track, preferably in buttock since seepage of iron-dextran complex into skin causes permanent discoloration

TABLE 1. Causes of Iron Deficiency

Blood loss	Increased requirements
Uterine	Infants and children
Menstruation/menorrhagia	Pregnancy
Gastrointestinal	Decreased absorption
Peptic ulcer disease	Gastrectomy or achlorhydria
Drugs, esp. NSAIDs	Malabsorption syndromes
Telangiectasia/angiodysplasia	Decreased intake
Pulmonary	Low-meat diets
Hemosiderosis	
Intravascular hemolysis	
Trauma, surgery, hemorrhage	
Phlebotomy	
Blood donor	
Diagnostic/hospitalization	

    c. Transfusion infrequently needed unless patient suffering cardiovascular instability

       i. Transfusion provides 250 mg iron

C. **Folate deficiency**

  1. Recognition involves high index of suspicion in settings other than pregnancy

    a. Routine supplement now advocated before and during pregnancy

    b. Other circumstances not always evident on routine exam

       i. Alcoholism, poor diet frequently denied or not readily appreciated

    c. Should be suspected in work-ups for malabsorption

  2. Earliest suspicion often macrocytosis (MCV > 100 fl)

  3. Combination of macrocytosis (even without anemia) and low red cell folate sufficient to make diagnosis

  4. Treatment

    a. Oral folic acid, 1 mg/day

       i. In some cases of malabsorption, may require up to 5 mg/day

    b. Replacement requires 1–2 months

       i. In circumstances of continued folate requirements (e.g., hemolytic anemias), continuous supplement required

D. **Vitamin B_{12} deficiency**

  1. Onset typically insidious and gradual, usually in older women

    a. Symptoms may be absent or little appreciated, even with hematocrits as low as 15–20

  2. Vigilance needed when following patients with other autoimmune diseases, because pernicious anemia may eventually manifest

  3. Diagnosis involves high index of suspicion, evidence of neurologic disease, anemia, or macrocytosis

    a. Serum vitamin B_{12} fairly accurate

       i. Normal value 200–1200 pg/ml; values below 100 always significant

    b. Schilling test should be performed to document cause of disease

       i. Circulating antibodies to parietal cell highly specific for pernicious anemia (PA), but present only in 60% of patients with PA

    c. In some circumstances, e.g., partial gastrectomy or ileal resection, Schilling test may be falsely positive

  4. **Treatment usually involves parenteral vitamin B_{12}**

    a. In instances of small bowel bacterial overgrowth, terminal ileum disease (e.g., inflammatory bowel disease), or tapeworm, treatment of underlying disease may allow absorption of vitamin B_{12} and obviate need for shots

    b. Shots should be given intramuscularly

    c. Intensity of therapy depends on stage of disease

       i. Advanced disease (profound anemia, neurologic findings) requires daily injection of 100 mg for at least 1 week, followed by 200–300 mg weekly for 6 weeks; maintenance therapy then followed

       ii. Less advanced disease may require only 500–1000 mg/week for 6 weeks

    d. Maintenance injections of vitamin B_{12} required for life for pernicious anemia

       i. May choose 100–500 mg/month or even 1000 mg every 2 months

    e. With replacement, bone marrow begins to correct within hours, reticulocyte count rises, anemia corrects, and GI manifestations, including glossitis, return to normal within days to weeks

       i. Some aspects of neurologic changes may not correct; posterior and lateral column changes in spinal cord along with dementia may be permanent, even with replacement

    f. Rare patient will refuse parenteral treatment; if this occurs, oral replacement of 300–1000 mg/day may be tried, but success is variable and follow-up should be close

  5. Important to avoid inappropriate treatment of vitamin B_{12} deficiency with folic acid

    a. Folate may correct some manifestations of vitamin B_{12} deficiency such as elevated MCV, anemia and glossitis but folate does not prevent progression of neurologic manifestations; hence, inappropriate treatment with folate may actually worsen one of most dreaded consequences of vitamin B_{12} deficiency

E. **Hemolytic anemias**
  1. When following patients with these conditions, need to be aware of potential deficiencies in either iron or folate
     a. Occurs because of high turnover of hematopoietic cells and increased demand
     b. Folate, but not iron, supplement required for sickle cell anemia
     c. Iron may be required for other hemolytic conditions (e.g., microvascular hemolysis)

SUGGESTED READING

1. Beutler E: The common anemias. JAMA 259:2433–2437, 1988.
2. Bini EF, Micale PL: Evaluation of the gastrointestinal tract in premenopausal women with iron deficiency anemia. Am J Med 105:281–286, 1998.
3. Colon-Otero G, Menke D: A practical approach to the differential diagnosis and evaluation of the adult patient with macrocytic anemia. Med Clin North Am 76:581–598, 1992.
4. Crosby WH: Pica. JAMA 235:2765, 1976.
5. Guyatt GH, Oxman AD: Laboratory diagnosis of iron-deficiency anemia: An overview. J Gen Intern Med 7:145–153, 1992.
6. Hallberg L, Hulthen L: Iron balance in menstruating women. Eur J Clin Nutr 49:200–207, 1995.
7. Looker AC, Dallman PR: Prevalence of iron deficiency in the United States. JAMA 277:973–976, 1997.
8. Massey A: Microcytic anemia: Differential diagnosis and management of iron deficiency anemia. Med Clin North Am 76:549–566, 1992.

93. Thyroid Disease

Bruce E. Johnson, M.D.

I. **The Issues**
Diseases of the thyroid gland are common, with greater incidence in women than men and often having different manifestations. Thyroid diseases are insidious in presentation. Several thyroid conditions affect the menstrual cycle; women may undergo extensive evaluations or procedures for menstrual irregularities when the symptom is merely an early sign of thyroid disease. The same may be said for certain presentations of infertility; recognition and correction of thyroid disease may obviate the need for extensive, invasive investigations for the cause of infertility. The presence of estrogen alters the protein binding of thyroxine, making interpretation of thyroid testing different in women. Despite the role thyroid disease may have in infertility, it is not uncommon for young women with thyroid disease to become pregnant, making management of the thyroid condition difficult. Thyroid disease affects other conditions more likely to occur in women; for example, both hyper- and hypothyroidism adversely affect bone mineralization. It is beyond the scope of this chapter to discuss all thyroid disease; rather, the Theory section deals with issues germane to most thyroid conditions, while the Approach section highlights selected thyroid conditions with emphasis on aspects of particular importance in women.

II. **The Theory**
  A. **Protein binding and thyroid-stimulating hormone** (TSH)
     1. Most thyroxine (T_4)—99.97%—carried in blood by thyroid-binding globulin (TBG) and other proteins
        a. Unbound T_4 determines metabolic state
        b. Free T_4 and T_3 not influenced by TBG concentrations
        c. While measurement of free T_4 and free T_3 available, these tests are expensive and frequently do not add much to usual work-up
     2. While variations in concentration of TBG result in increased or decreased measurement of total T_4, hypothalamic-pituitary-thyroid axis maintains free T_4 at appropriate level
     3. TBG may be altered by several circumstances

a. Increased by oral contraceptives, estrogen, tamoxifen, pregnancy, hepatitis, porphyria, or in familial (genetic) cases

b. Decreased by androgens and corticosteroids, chronic cirrhosis, acromegaly, severe systemic illness, nephrosis, or in familial (genetic) cases

4. Laboratory test of thyroxine (T_4) measures total thyroxine, i.e., TBG-bound and unbound T_4

   a. Measurement of total T_4 influenced by quantity of TBG

      i. Explains "high normal" or "high" total T_4 in otherwise euthyroid women on oral contraceptives or estrogen replacement

      ii. Interpretation of total T_4 must include knowledge of medications

5. Laboratories attempt to correct for TBG concentration by performing T_3 resin uptake

   a. Indirect measurement of TBG, allowing correction for measured total T_4

   b. Reported as "free T_4 index," "T_7," or inaccurately as "free T_4"

   c. Less expensive overall than accurate measurement of true free T_4

6. Free T_4 feeds back to hypothalamus and pituitary, regulating release of TSH; measurement of TSH often most useful of thyroid tests

   a. Hypothyroidism (low free T_4) sensed by hypothalamus causing release of thyrotropin-releasing factor (TRF) which results in pituitary stimulation to increase thyroid production of T_4; since the pituitary stimulation is production of TSH, the measured TSH in hypothyroidism is elevated

   b. Hyperthyroidism (high free T_4) generally suppresses the hypothalamus and pituitary; TSH usually depressed

7. In many women in whom TBG may be altered by hormones or medications, measurement of TSH provides necessary decision-making information at less expense than measurement of free T_4, free T_3, or even the resin uptake technology

8. TSH measurement now in third-generation technology—often referred to as "ultra-sensitive"

B. **Menstrual abnormalities, pregnancy, and thyroid disorders**

1. In hypothyroidism, women typically have menorrhagia associated with prolonged menstrual cycles

   a. In hypothyroidism, menstrual changes are, in part, mediated through prolactin

      i. Hypothalamic production of TRF, in addition to stimulating TSH, also cross-reacts to stimulate production and release of prolactin

      ii. Hyperprolactinemia alters leutinizing hormone (LH) and follicle-stimulating hormone (FSH), regulatory hormones for menstrual cycle, resulting in altered menstrual periods and, potentially, infertility

2. In hyperthyroidism, more often oligomenorrhea or amenorrhea with more scanty bleeding

3. Pregnancy results in physiologic changes in thyroid gland

   a. Increased metabolic demands and increased blood flow cause increased size of glands

      i. Small, physiologic goiter present in many pregnant women if gland examined by ultrasound

   b. Due to increased metabolic demands of pregnancy, T_4 production varies during pregnancy

4. Exogenous thyroid replacement varies during pregnancy

   a. Prenatal thyroxine replacement dose does not remain static through pregnancy; need to increase replacement dose early in pregnancy; dose changes toward prenatal level in third trimester

   b. Because of changes in TBG, must measure free T_4 frequently (even TSH often does not respond quickly enough to metabolic changes), every 4–6 weeks in first and second trimester; every 6 weeks in later pregnancy

   c. After delivery, metabolic demands and TBG production fall toward nonpregnant levels within 2–4 months; again, frequent measurement and replacement adjustment until stable

C. **Autoimmune mechanisms of thyroid disease**

1. Several thyroid diseases are autoimmune (e.g., Hashimoto's thyroiditis, Graves' disease)

       a. Autoimmune diseases generally more common in females; possibly explains thyroid disease predominance in women
2. Autoantibodies produced include antithyroglobulin and antimicrosomal
       a. Typically seen in Hashimoto's disease; occasionally seen in Graves' disease
       b. Antibodies may precede clinical disease
          i. Goiter and increased antibodies may occur in early Hashimoto's thyroiditis before changes detected in T_4 or TSH
       c. May be useful in arriving at precise diagnosis; e.g., to differentiate between Hashimoto's thyroiditis and simple goiter
       d. Autoantibody complexes rarely implicated in immune complex deposition conditions
3. Once one autoimmune disease diagnosed, higher risk of developing others
       a. Strong association between thyroiditis and Addison's disease (originally called Schmidt's syndrome); also premature menopause (oophoritis), hypoparathyroidism, diabetes mellitus, and even hypopituitarism
       b. Associations also noted with other autoimmune diseases, such as myasthenia gravis, vitiligo, pernicious anemia, sprue, pure red cell aplasia, and antibody-mediated immunoglobulin A deficiency
       c. Keep such associations in mind when following patients on long-term basis

D. **Head and neck irradiation and thyroid disease**
1. In late 1940s and early 1950s radiation of head and neck in children for various conditions, including "enlarged" thymus, chronic tonsillitis, acne
2. High incidence of thyroid disease, including carcinoma
       a. Nodular thyroid disease develops in up to 20% of persons so exposed but may not become evident until 30+ years after initial exposure
3. Among patients with head and neck irradiation with palpable nodules, one-third have carcinoma at surgery
4. With history of irradiation, current practice favors regular surveillance with physical exam and thyroid scan

E. **Screening for thyroid disease**
1. Until recently, no major organization has advocated routine screening—despite high prevalence (up to 5–10%) of thyroid disorders in women
2. In 1998, American College of Physicians stated that the high prevalence of thyroid disease, especially in postmenopausal women, warranted screening
       a. Recommended screening with sensitive TSH test most women over age 50 (interval undetermined but probably every 2–5 years)
       b. Because of lower prevalence, screening not recommended for asymptomatic premenopausal women (or men of any age)
3. Specific recommendations for treatment once abnormal TSH found not as straightforward as might be expected
       a. Data stronger for asymptomatic suppressed TSH (i.e., hyperthyroidism) than for asymptomatic elevated TSH (hypothyroidism)
       b. Because of controversy regarding treatment, even these recommendations for screening are not widely adopted

III. **An Approach**
A. **Goiter**
1. Simply defined as enlargement of thyroid gland
2. Generally has cause; if none detected, referred to as simple goiter
3. Regardless of cause, symptoms may include
       a. Sensation of fullness or even choking
       b. Hoarseness (due to compression of recurrent laryngeal nerve)
       c. Pain and/or swelling with hemorrhage into nodule
4. Physical findings
       a. Symmetrically enlarged gland with palpable lobes and isthmus
       b. Compression or displacement of trachea or esophagus
       c. Retrosternal thyroid leads to mediastinal enlargement and Pemberton's sign (raising arms above head in retrosternal thyroid gives suffusion of face, lightheadedness, or even syncope)

TABLE 1. Common Symptoms Associated with Hypothyroidism

Lethargy	Hair loss	Late manifestations
Fatigue	Menorrhagia	Myxedema (pretibial edema)
Constipation	Infertility	Puffy eyes
Cold intolerance	Carpal tunnel syndrome	Dull expressionless face
Weight change (usually increase)	Decreased exercise tolerance	Coma
Slowing of intellect	Increased sleep	
Dry skin		

5. Depending on clinical setting, goiter may be due to: iodine deficiency, ingestion of goitrogens, hypothyroidism, hyperthyroidism, thyroid nodules, presence of antibodies, defective iodination in biosynthetic pathways, physiologic enlargement of thyroid in pregnancy

6. Simple goiter followed for possible development of diagnosable abnormality; most common eventual diagnosis is autoimmune hypothyroiditis (Hashimoto's disease)

B. **Hypothyroidism**

1. **Symptoms** familiar and insidious (Table 1)

2. **Physical exam** includes findings noted above as well as enlarged thyroid (except late in disease), cardiomegaly or pericardial effusion, megacolon

3. **Hashimoto's disease** is usual cause in U.S.

   a. Autoimmune disease characterized by antibodies (antithyroglobulin, antimicrosomal) against thyroid tissue

   b. Predilection for females greater than 6:1

   c. Strong association with other autoimmune disease, including diabetes mellitus, adrenal insufficiency, gonadal failure (early menopause), pernicious anemia, systemic lupus erythematosus, rheumatoid arthritis

4. **Other important causes** of hypothyroidism: subacute thyroiditis; endemic iodine deficiency; iodination defects in biosynthetic pathways; postpregnancy thyroiditis (usually transient); drug-induced (goitrogens), including iodides, phenylbutazone, lithium, amiodarone; postsurgical, postradiation thyroiditis; suprathyroid (pituitary, hypothalamus) failure

5. **Laboratory studies**

   a. Most valuable test required for confirmation of clinical suspicion is thyroid-stimulating hormone (TSH)

   b. Serum thyroxine (T_4) should be low; total T_4 is modified by TBG which is often elevated in high estrogen states such as pregnancy, birth control pills, or estrogen replacement; in such states, if T_4 measurement necessary, measure free T_4

   c. Antithyroid antibodies

      i. Antithyroglobulin and antimicrosomal antibodies detectable in Hashimoto's disease but not usually present in other causes of hypothyroidism

      ii. May be discordant, i.e., one might be elevated, the other normal in one patient but vice versa in another patient

   d. Several other blood tests altered by hypothyroidism

      i. Total cholesterol elevated

      ii. Creatine phosphokinase (CPK) often elevated

         (a) Probably represents mild myopathy of hypothyroidism

      iii. Aspartate aminotransferase (ASAT) and lactate dehydrogenase (LDH) also elevated

   e. EKG may show bradycardia, low-amplitude QRS complexes, mild T-wave flattening

   f. Thyroid scan (radioiodine or technetium pertechnetate) not needed in typical cases

      i. More useful in hyperthyroidism, nodular disease, retrosternal or ectopic thyroid

6. **Treatment**

   a. Thyroid replacement with levothyroxine (T_4)

      i. Oral replacement satisfactory except in cases of profound myxedematous coma or initiation of thyroid replacement in patient facing urgent surgery in which case thyroxine may be given intravenously

      ii. Little benefit to substitute levothyroxine with T_3 or combinations of T_4 and T_3 since such combinations make monitoring more complicated

      iii. Dosing given once daily; long half-life of levothyroxine gives flexibility with timing of dosage and, if dose skipped, enough hormone circulates that double dose next day is not necessary

  b. In most patients, initiation at full replacement dose not advised

      i. Start levothyroxine, 0.025–0.05 mg/day, and increase by 0.025– 0.05 mg every 2–3 weeks

      ii. In elderly women, especially with known cardiovascular disease, start at low doses and increase gradually

      iii. Slow increase in dosing allows cardiovascular compensation, may avoid infarct or congestive failure

  c. Replacement dose varies with age and size of patient

      i. Rough rule for estimating replacement levothyroxine dose: 0.0018 mg/kg body weight

      ii. Always individualize, but in general younger women require more replacement than older women; always adjust dose to eventual normalization of TSH

      iii. Dose changes in same patient with aging; dose required in younger woman will usually be decreased as she ages

  d. Manifestations of hypothyroidism correct as replacement dose approached

      i. Size of gland usually normalizes with adequate replacement

  e. Monitoring with serum T_4 and/or TSH

      i. TSH more sensitive and less likely to be modified by protein binding of T_4

      ii. Once final dose determined, lifelong periodic monitoring necessary; typical interval is yearly

      iii. Replacement dose may vary with change in body size, age, metabolic requirements, changes in medication manufacturer

      iv. With periodic monitoring, check for associated autoimmune conditions, if appropriate

C. Hyperthyroidism

1. Symptoms

  a. Nervousness/anxiety, inability to sleep, frequent bowel movements, excessive sweating or heat intolerance, weight loss despite maintained or increased appetite

  b. With advancing disease, proximal muscle weakness (myopathy) develops

  c. In younger women, oligomenorrhea or amenorrhea

  d. In older women, angina, congestive heart failure, or arrhythmias (especially atrial fibrillation) common

      i. Cardiac signs with dulled sensorium in elderly called "apathetic hyperthyroidism"

      ii. Recognized by lack of nervous symptoms, presence of apathy, and cardiac signs

2. Physical findings

  a. Patient appears fidgety, anxious, restless

  b. Goiter usually symmetric and smooth with prominent lobes and isthmus

      i. With multinodular goiter, nodules detected

      ii. May hear bruit over gland from increased blood flow

  c. Skin warm, moist, smooth, almost velvety

      i. In contrast, Graves' dermopathy includes pretibial myxedema which is thickened, infiltrative, pigmented peau d'orange patches or confluence on legs

  d. Hair fine, silky

  e. Arms, hands, and fingers with fine tremor when held out

  f. Graves' ophthalmopathy includes exophthalmos, stare with lid lag, widened palpebral fissures

  g. Cardiac signs include tachycardia or fibrillation, widened pulse pressure, systolic flow murmurs, and, occasionally, heart failure (high-output heart failure)

  h. Neurologic changes include tremor, hyperreflexia, myoclonus and weakness on muscle testing, typically proximal

     i. Psychologically, patients frequently complain of poor sleep, nonproductive activity, anxiousness—but occasionally a curious, aggressive lack of insight into symptoms of disease

3. **Differential diagnosis**
   a. **Graves' disease**
      i. Autoimmune disease characterized by hyperthyroidism and goiter, ophthalmopathy, and dermopathy
      ii. More common in women than men by 7:1
      iii. Immunologic pathogenesis involves antibodies directed at TSH receptor, but resulting in stimulation rather than blockage
      iv. Implicated immunoglobulin referred to as thyroid-stimulating immunoglobulin (TSI)
      v. Stimulation by TSI of TSH receptor results in overproduction of T_4 and hyperthyroidism
      vi. TSI not associated with ophthalmopathy or dermopathy
      vii. Graves' disease subject to exacerbations and remissions
         (a) Even under antithyroid medication, may flare and cause symptoms
         (b) About 40% of cases "burn out" or spontaneously remit within 12–18 months
   b. **Other causes of hyperthyroidism**
      i. Autonomously functioning thyroid nodules and toxic multinodular goiter
      ii. Thyroiditis with immediate or delayed release of T_4
      iii. Extrathyroid production of thyroxine
         (a) Stuma ovarii, follicular carcinoma
      iv. Excessive TSH (rare)
         (a) Pituitary source
         (b) Trophoblastic tumor
      v. Exogenous ingestion (thyrotoxicosis factitia)
   c. **Conjugal Graves' disease** (i.e., Graves' disease occurring more or less simultaneously in a couple), while intriguing from etiologic standpoint, probably represents no more than chance occurrence of relatively common condition in two persons (independent of "infectious" cause)

4. **Laboratory tests**
   a. Increased total T_4
      i. Must interpret in light of possible high estrogen state
      ii. Free T_4 almost always elevated
   b. T_3 elevated
      i. Only rarely (in thyroid previously treated with I-131 for Graves' disease) may find normal T_4 with elevated T_3 (T_3 toxicosis)
   c. TSH depressed, often undetectable
      i. Only exception is rare case of pituitary hyperstimulation or trophoblastic tumor
   d. Autoantibodies present
      i. TSI specific for Graves' disease
      ii. Occasionally see antithyroglobulin and antimicrosomal antibodies, more typical of Hashimoto's disease
   e. Few other blood tests characteristically abnormal
   f. EKG demonstrates tachycardia, even atrial fibrillation
   g. Bone density often decreased in long-standing hyperthyroidism (including inadvertent overdose or thyrotoxicosis factitia)
      i. Most cases of Graves' disease have short premorbid period and are less likely to result in major loss of bone
   h. Thyroid scanning useful, if not essential, in diagnosis
      i. I-131 uptake uniformly increased in Graves' disease
         (a) Also increased in hyperfunctioning nodules of toxic multinodular goiter
         (b) Patchy changes in thyroiditis
         (c) Suppressed in exogenous sources of T_4
      ii. Technetium pertechnetate scanning of lesser value

     i. Sonography detects nodules and differentiates solid from cystic nodules but does not give same functional information as I-131 scanning

5. **Treatment**
   a. **Antithyroid drugs**
      i. Block hormone synthesis
      ii. Effective only as long as drugs are taken
      iii. Propylthiouracil
         (a) In addition to blocking hormone synthesis, inhibits peripheral conversion of T_4 to T_3 giving more rapid control of hyperthyroid symptoms
         (b) Usual starting dose: 100–150 mg every 6–8 hr
         (c) Regular administration important because thyroid escapes effects of drugs after 6–8 hours and production of T_4 ensues
      iv. Methimazole, 10–15 mg every 8 hr, also effective
      v. With both drugs, once control of initial symptoms ensues, dose may be decreased to maintenance level
      vi. Serious complication is leukopenia with propylthiouracil. This is mild and transient in 5–10% of patients but does rarely cause agranulocytosis; regular monitoring of CBC important and any abnormality requires change to another therapy.
      vii. Indications for antithyroid drugs:
         (a) Graves' disease in children, adolescents, young women, and pregnant women, in whom ablative therapy not acceptable
         (b) Frequently given "to cool down" patient before definitive decision on therapy
         (c) Not useful for long-term treatment of autonomous nodules
   b. **Adrenergic antagonists**
      i. Propranolol or other beta blocker
      ii. Do not modify metabolic abnormality but will block sympathetic effects of hyperthyroidism, such as tachycardia, jitteriness, anxiety, tremor, sweating
      iii. Never substitute for more definitive therapy; should be considered only adjunctive
   c. **Iodine**
      i. Temporarily inhibits release of T_4 but not effective on long-term basis
      ii. Reduces symptoms while waiting for antithyroid drugs to become effective
      iii. Reduces gland size and blood flow if surgery
   d. **Radioiodine ablative therapy**
      i. I-131 in large doses—taken up in thyroid follicles, gives off radiation destroying follicles and hence entire gland
      ii. In Graves' disease, ensures no further exacerbations
      iii. Somewhat delayed in onset; need for antithyroid drugs in interim
      iv. Indications vary
         (a) Definitive, nonsurgical treatment eliminating long-term drug use
         (b) Probably treatment of choice for elderly women
         (c) Failure of drug therapy
         (d) Drug toxicity
         (e) Patient noncompliance
      v. Contraindications include pregnant women due to radioisotope crossing to fetus
      vi. Some lay people worry about effect on ovaries in children, adolescents, or women of reproductive age
         (a) All long-term follow-up studies fail to detect increase in birth defects or ovarian neoplasia—reassurance important
      vii. After treatment patients often become hypothyroid and require replacement for life
   e. **Surgery**
      i. Indications vary
         (a) Very large gland with obstructive symptoms
         (b) Nodular disease (especially solitary nodule)

          (c) Noncompliance with antithyroid medication, especially noncompliant pregnant women and young children
- ii. Surgery complicated and liable to complications
  - (a) Most concerning is inadvertent removal of parathyroids, damage to recurrent laryngeal nerve
  - (b) Experienced surgeon should be sought; recent surveys suggest general surgeons have fewer complications than ENT surgeons
- iii. Typically, surgery leaves patient hypothyroid, requiring replacement therapy for rest of life

D. **Thyroiditis**
1. Several different **clinical circumstances** but only three are common
   a. Hashimoto's disease (discussed above)
   b. Subacute thyroiditis
   c. Chronic thyroiditis (including postpartum thyroiditis)
2. **Subacute thyroiditis** (granulomatous, de Quervain's disease)
   a. Believed to be postviral disorder
   b. Usually presents with painful swelling of thyroid after upper respiratory viral illness
      i. Occasionally acute and severe with painful enlargement of gland, referred pain to jaw or ear, fever, and thyrotoxicosis
      ii. More common presentation is insidious with fatigue, malaise, thyroid discomfort, referred pain, and irregular enlargement of gland
   c. Important differentiation from Hashimoto's disease and chronic thyroiditis
   d. Laboratory tests
      i. Almost invariably elevated erythrocyte sedimentation rate (ESR)
      ii. T_4 and T_3 variable; early in disease, may be elevated as damaged follicles release T_4; later, as T_4 depleted, T_4 and T_3 may be low, with resultant elevation of TSH
      iii. Radioiodine scanning
         (a) Patchy and depressed uptake without "hot" nodules
         (b) Technetium pertechnetate scan of less value
   e. Treatment symptomatic
      i. Aspirin, nonsteroidal anti-inflammatory drugs useful for discomfort from swelling
      ii. Rarely, corticosteroids needed in severe, acute painful enlargement of gland
      iii. If needed for thyrotoxic symptoms of tachycardia, jitteriness, anxiety, should use beta blockers
   f. Generally self-limited with eventual return of normal function after weeks to months
      i. Infrequent need for antithyroid medication or radioiodine therapy
3. **Chronic thyroiditis** (painless, with transient thyrotoxicosis)
   a. Female:male ratio approximately 5:1
   b. Etiology unknown
      i. Lymphocytic infiltration but without viral titers or antibodies
   c. Characterized by periods of thyrotoxicosis interspersed with hypothyroid or euthyroid status
      i. Waxing and waning over months or years
      ii. Exacerbation may be associated with pregnancy
         (a) Postpartum thyroiditis, typically hypothyroid, may occur after each pregnancy
   d. Thought to be self-limiting; that is, eventually women resolve thyroid disorder with normally functioning gland
   e. Symptoms usually mild
      i. Gland firm, symmetric, and, at most, mildly enlarged
      ii. If thyrotoxic, symptomatic with tachycardia, jitteriness, anxiety, tremor
      iii. If hypothyroid, symptoms include fatigue, sleepiness, achiness
         (a) When thyroiditis occurs postpartum, symptoms attributed to fatigue from dealing with newborn

      f. Laboratory tests

         i. ESR only mildly elevated, if at all

        ii. T_4, T_3 transiently elevated during toxicosis with concomitant depressed TSH

       iii. Radioiodine scan has depressed uptake

          (a) Differentiates from Graves' disease

    g. Treatment symptomatic

       i. Eventual outcome should be normal gland; hence goal is to treat symptoms while waiting for self-limited resolution

      ii. Beta blockers, mild sedatives for toxicosis

     iii. Transient thyroid replacement if needed

E. **Thyroid nodules**

  1. Since both benign adenoma and malignant carcinoma can exist in nodule, **differentiation between adenoma and carcinoma** is major concern

  2. History important

    a. Many women in 1940s–1950s subjected to low levels of head and neck radiation

       i. Has resulted in relatively high incidence of thyroid nodules, many of which become carcinoma

  3. **Adenoma**

    a. May be solitary or multiple (multinodular goiter)

    b. Often but not always TSH-sensitive

       i. Autonomously functioning adenomas, occasionally producing enough T_4 to cause toxicosis, typically take up radioiodine (referred to as hot nodules)

      ii. If TSH-sensitive, can be reduced in size if TSH suppressed by exogenous thyroxine

    c. Symptoms variable

       i. Often none; nodules are detected on regular physical exam of neck

      ii. Patient may notice enlargement of nodule

     iii. If nodule painful, may signify hemorrhage into (usually) benign nodule

     iv. Hyperfunctioning nodule may produce mild toxicosis symptoms

    d. Difficult diagnostic decisions since adenomas very common with advancing age, especially if sonography done (for other reasons)

    e. Laboratory tests

       i. Few characteristic abnormalities

      ii. T_4, T_3 usually normal except for occasional case with elevated T_4 and resultant suppressed TSH

    f. Radioiodine scan valuable

       i. Autonomously functioning nodule preferentially takes up radioiodine

         (a) Increased uptake called "warm" nodule if surrounding tissue still functional, i.e., TSH not suppressed and "hot" nodule if surrounding tissue suppressed and nodule only site of uptake

         (b) Difference between warm and hot nodules not diagnostically useful—carcinoma more often "cold"

    g. Sonography useful

       i. Cystic nodules, especially if < 2 cm in diameter, not likely to be carcinoma

      ii. Multiple nodules tend not to be carcinoma

     iii. Solid nodules may be adenoma or carcinoma

    h. Fine-needle aspiration

       i. Often first step in evaluation—even before scans

      ii. Straightforward procedure with few risks if done by experienced physician

     iii. Interpretation requires experienced and interested cytopathologist because differences between benign and malignant cells are subtle

     iv. Skilled cytopathologist is very important to decision-making process; if one not available, refer patient to center with experience in both the procedure and interpretation

    i. Decision making difficult and depends on local resources

       i. Adequate cytopathology availability may call for fine-needle aspiration as first step, regardless of whether nodule feels cystic or not

(a) If carcinoma, move immediately to surgery
  ii. If fine-needle aspirate cytology suggests adenoma or is equivocal, perform radioiodine scan
    (a) Both warm and hot scans less likely to be carcinoma and watchful waiting is appropriate
    (b) Cold scan should result in surgical removal, even though only 20% of cold scans are due to carcinoma
  iii. If evaluation starts with sonography, large cystic nodules tend not to be carcinoma and can either be sampled for cytology or watched; solid nodules should result in either radioiodine scan or aspiration
  iv. Decision becomes even more complicated in older women as likelihood of benign nodules increases

4. **Carcinoma**
  a. Except for anaplastic carcinoma, which is inevitably fatal in 6–12 months, most carcinoma treated with subtotal thyroidectomy
  b. Radioiodine scan of prime importance
    i. When performed postoperatively, detects metastatic disease
    ii. Treatment with high-dose I-131 then directed to metastatic disease
    iii. Multiple I-131 treatments possible as long as metastases present
  c. Management of thyroid cancer involves experienced endocrinologist and/or oncologist

F. **Thyrotoxicosis factitia**
  1. Commonly women in health care field with access to thyroxine medication
    a. Increasingly a concern with self-administered "natural" preparations which may contain small quantities of thyroid extract
  2. Initially begin self-administration in attempt to control weight, gain energy, improve wakefulness, "get things done"
  3. May continue for years with few evident symptoms
  4. Long-term complications significant include: osteoporosis, cardiac abnormalities (tachyarrhythmias, even cardiomyopathy), myopathy
  5. Women admit to few symptoms—most frequently comes to doctor's attention with osteoporotic fractures, random screening TSH, or inability by patient to obtain additional medication
  6. Laboratory tests
    a. T_4 usually elevated
      i. Many abusers prefer administration of liothyronine (oral T_3), which is not routinely detected with total T_4 measurement
    b. TSH uniformly depressed—increasing use of TSH as screening test makes suppressed TSH the most common presentation
  7. Radioiodine scan will be depressed (since thyroid gland not stimulated)
  8. Treatment can be tricky
    a. If thyrotoxicosis factitia long-standing, thyroid gland atrophied and not capable of autonomous production; will require physician-ordered thyroid hormone replacement
    b. Goal should be either removal of exogenous thyroid source and recovery of thyroid gland, or carefully monitored levothyroxine administration
    c. Initially expect bitter complaints of fatigue, cold intolerance, weight gain
  9. Special attention should be paid to likelihood of osteoporosis with long-standing hyperthyroidism and at least bone mineral density should be done

SUGGESTED READING

1. Bastenie PA, Bonnyns M: Natural history of primary myxedema. Am J Med 79:91–99, 1985.
2. Burge MR, Zeise T-M: Risks of complication following thyroidectomy. J Gen Intern Med 13:24–31, 1998.
3. Dayan CM, Daniels GH: Chronic autoimmune thyroiditis. N Engl J Med 335:99–107, 1996.
4. Gharib H, Mazzaferri EL: Thyroxine suppressive therapy in patients with nodular thyroid disease. Ann Intern Med 128:386–394, 1998.

5. Helfand M, Redfern CC: Screening for thyroid disease: An update. Ann Intern Med 129:144–158, 1998.
6. Hermus AR, Huysmans DA: Treatment of benign nodular thyroid disease. N Engl J Med 338: 1438–1447, 1998.
7. Mandel SJ, Brent GA: Levothyroxine therapy in patients with thyroid disease. Ann Intern Med 119:492–502, 1993.
8. Ron E, Doody MM: Cancer mortality following treatment for adult hyperthyroidism. JAMA 280:347–355, 1998.
9. Singer PA, Cooper DS: Treatment guidelines for patients with thyroid nodules and well-differentiated thyroid cancer. Arch Intern Med 156:2165–2172, 1996.
10. Surks MI, Ocampo E: Subclinical thyroid disease. Am J Med 100:217–223, 1996.

94. Gallbladder Disease

Bruce E. Johnson, M.D.

I. **The Issues**

"Female, fat, fertile, and forty." For decades this aphorism has characterized the demographics of gallbladder disease. Indeed, although presented in a less than flattering manner, the aphorism is largely true—gallbladder disease afflicts far more women than men. The reasons may lie in the interaction of the female hormonal milieu, the effects of pregnancy and obesity with the saturation of products in the gallbladder. Treatment of symptomatic gallstones is becoming clearer and safer. Although screening is not recommended, management of serendipitously discovered gallstones is still controversial.

II. **The Theory**

  A. **Pathophysiology of gallstone formation**

    1. Bile, as stored in gallbladder, has several constituents:

      a. Cholesterol, in concentrations largely unrelated to serum cholesterol levels

      b. Bile acids (cholic and chenodeoxycholic acids)

        i. Assist in forming micelles in bile to solubilize cholesterol and fatty acids are also important in intestinal absorption of fatty acids

      c. Fatty acids—concentration in part related to serum triglyceride levels

      d. Bilirubin

        i. Concentration depends on liver excretion

      e. Lecithin and phospholipids

      f. Proteins

        i. Immunoglobulin A (IgA) and other proteins metabolized by the liver

      g. Pronucleating and antinucleating factors

      h. Electrolytes, mucus, calcium salts, and others

    2. Formation of gallstones depends on relative concentrations of bile constituents

      a. 80% of gallstones are cholesterol stones

        i. Concentrations of cholesterol vary upward from 70% with mixtures of calcium salts, bile acids, bilirubin pigments, and other factors

      b. 20% of gallstones are largely bilirubin and calcium salts with only small quantity of cholesterol

    3. Cholesterol not soluble in aqueous solution

      a. Must be solubilized with concentrations of bile salts and phospholipids to form soluble aggregates called micelles

    4. Cholesterol remains soluble in usual concentrations

      a. Relatively low concentration of cholesterol (up to 20%), with high concentration of lecithin and bile salts

      b. When soluble, these form micellar liquid or supersaturated liquid—but without crystallizing

TABLE 1. Factors Associated with Gallstone Formation

Cholesterol Stones and Sludge	Pigment Stones
Estrogen states	Chronic hemolysis
Postpubertal females	Sickle cell anemia
Oral contraceptives	Other hemoglobinopathies
Postmenopausal estrogen replacement	Other RBC cell wall abnormalities
Advancing age	Cirrhosis
Pregnancy	Alcoholic
Obesity	Biliary tract infection
Rapid weight loss	Bacteria
Total parenteral nutrition	Parasites
Malabsorption	
Ileal resection	
Drugs	
Clofibrate	
Ceftriaxone	
Ethnic background	
Northern European origin	
Native American	
Others	
Diabetes	
High polyunsaturated fat diet	

    c. If any of these concentrations change (e.g., elevation of cholesterol), possibility of supersaturation with precipitation of cholesterol crystals to form sludge or stones

  5. Also present in bile are ill-defined pro- or antinucleation factors

    a. These factors promote or discourage formation of crystals

      i. Factors are poorly understood but a recent suggestion has aspirin functioning along with antinucleation factors to decrease formation of gallstones

  6. Pigment stones (20% of total stone disease) generally formed by excessive secretion of bilirubin as in hemolytic red cell conditions

  7. Gallbladder stasis

    a. Frequent emptying of gallbladder washes out early crystal formation; stasis allows concentrations to change, microcrystals to form and grow

    b. Probable reason for increased gallstones in spinal cord injuries, total parenteral nutrition

  8. Predisposing factors for gallstone formation (Table 1)

    a. Mechanisms vary from increased cholesterol production (e.g., obesity) to decreased bile salt formation (e.g., estrogen states) or stasis (e.g., total parenteral nutrition)

B. **Epidemiology**

  1. At least 10% of American adults have gallstones

    a. Incidence increases with age; after age 60 as many as 20% of all people have gallstones

  2. Women outnumber men at least 2:1

    a. By seventh decade ratio may increase to 4:1

  3. Each year after age 40, slightly less than 1% of population will form new gallstones

C. **Asymptomatic stones**

  1. Detected serendipitously while investigating another complaint

  2. Most gallstones are asymptomatic

    a. Probably only 10–18% of women ever develop symptoms from gallstones

  3. Risk of complications from asymptomatic stones is low

    a. Surgery required in 7–10% at 5 years, 12–18% at 15 years

  4. In most cases, prophylactic cholecystectomy not recommended

    a. Current recommendation includes gallstones in diabetics, in contrast to strong recommendation to operate just a few decades ago

5. Subgroups in which surgery for asymptomatic stones may be considered:
   a. Children and young adults; likelihood of eventual development of symptoms quite high
   b. Sickle cell disease; prevalence high due to hemolytic state and much higher risks from emergent cholecystectomy
   c. Surgery for morbid obesity; development of gallstones very high in rapid weight loss
   d. Native Americans; greater risk of gallbladder cancer than general population (3–5% of Native Americans with stones develop cancer)
   e. "Porcelain" gallbladder; up to half develop gallbladder cancer

D. **Complications**
   1. **Symptomatic stones without obstruction**
      a. Recurrent episodes of right upper quadrant pain, epigastric pain, back (near right scapula), shoulder pain
      b. Milder symptoms include indigestion, belching
      c. Pain may be constant or intermittent (biliary colic)
         i. Pain often nocturnal, peaking toward midnight
      d. Intolerance to fatty foods common but not specific or pathognomonic
   2. **Acute cholecystitis**
      a. Presumed to occur with obstruction of cystic duct causing dilatation and inflammation of gallbladder—resulting in acute abdomen with abdominal pain, nausea, vomiting, fever
      b. Lab exam shows leukocytosis, elevation of transaminases, alkaline phosphatase
      c. Not always indication for emergent cholecystectomy
         i. With treatment, including antibiotics, frequently inflammation subsides and surgery can be done under elective conditions
      d. Less common complications
         i. Empyema
            (a) Superinfection of bile, often with air-forming organisms invading gallbladder wall; a surgical emergency
         ii. Hydrops
            (a) Chronic cystic duct obstruction with minimal symptoms
            (b) Gallbladder fills with mucus or transudate and grow to large, palpable size
            (c) Removal indicated; high risk for infection
         iii. Perforation
            (a) Localized perforation—walled off by omentum or adhesions
            (b) Free perforation—ruptured viscus with free air in abdomen, peritonitis
         iv. Fistula formation
            (a) Usually localized perforation to intestine
            (b) May be totally asymptomatic but when detected, cholecystectomy indicated because of high risk of infection
         v. Gallstone ileus
            (a) Passage of gallstone to intestine with lodging of gallstone in intestine (frequently ileocecal valve) causing small bowel obstruction
         vi. Porcelain gallbladder
            (a) Rarely, in circumstance of chronically inflamed gallbladder, calcium salt deposition gives halo-type outline on plain film radiograph of abdomen
            (b) Relatively high likelihood of progression to carcinoma
   3. **Choledocholithiasis** (stones in biliary tree)
      a. Symptoms similar to cholecystitis
      b. Occasional totally asymptomatic blockage—one of the few benign causes of painless jaundice)
      c. With infection of bile ducts (cholangitis) patient presents toxic with fever and sepsis, abdominal pain, high white count which is indication for rapid intervention
         i. Always treat with antibiotics but then decide if patient can tolerate interventional endoscopy or requires surgery

4. **Acute pancreatitis**
   a. Obstruction of pancreatic duct proximal to ampulla of Vater
   b. Abdominal pain, boring through to back; nausea, vomiting, ileus with fever, prostration, cardiovascular instability
   c. Leukocytosis, increased amylase and lipase; electrolyte abnormalities, hyperglycemia, hypocalcemia in severe cases
   d. Pancreatitis from gallstones tends to be particularly severe and should be taken seriously by physician
5. **Carcinoma of gallbladder**
   a. Rare cancer, but most cases associated with gallstones
   b. Because of infrequency of cancer of gallbladder (< 6000 cases/year in U.S.) and high likelihood of gallstones (present in over 20 million Americans), mere presence of gallstones is not indication for cholecystectomy to prevent cancer

III. **An Approach**
   A. **Management of asymptomatic gallstones**
      1. Despite prevalence of gallstones (which is much higher than many other conditions for which screening is performed), the complications are low enough that routine screening is not recommended
      2. Usually detected while looking for another condition (if detected as part of an evaluation for abdominal pain, for instance, these would no longer be "asymptomatic")
      3. Low likelihood of progression to symptoms over relatively long time (10 years) and only infrequent (< 5%) presentation with complications
      4. Only circumstances in which removal of asymptomatic gallstones might be considered listed above; in all other situations, watchful waiting is indicated
   B. **Diagnostic studies for symptomatic gallstones**
      1. Plain film abdominal radiographs
         a. Up to 20% of gallstones (mostly pigmented stones) are calcified and can be seen
         b. Useful for porcelain gallbladder, empyema of gallbladder (air in wall), gallstone ileus—but as routine test for diagnosing gallstones, not useful
      2. Oral cholecystogram
         a. Oral ingestion of dye excreted into gallbladder, opacifying bladder and leaving stones apparent
         b. Largely supplanted by ultrasonography
      3. Ultrasonography
         a. Can be performed under most circumstances
         b. Accurately and predictably visualizes gallbladder
            i. If not seen in fasting state, strongly suggests chronic cholecystitis
            ii. Poor quality studies with ascites, excessive bowel gas, massive obesity
         c. Identifies stones down to 2-mm diameter
            i. False-negative rate only about 2%
         d. Can even identify sludge (forms interface with normal bile)
         e. Allows visualization of bile ducts, liver parenchyma, pancreas—helps with diagnosis of biliary tract obstruction, pancreatitis, chronic inflammatory gallbladder
      4. Radioisotope studies
         a. One of several labeled iminodiacetic acids (e.g., PIPIDA)
         b. Rapid clearance from blood and excreted into biliary tree
            i. Effective even with bilirubin values up to 6–10 mg/dl
         c. Failure to visualize gallbladder or cystic duct in presence of intact common duct suggests cystic duct obstruction, chronic cholecystitis, or surgical absence of gallbladder
         d. Greatest use in setting of acute cholecystitis
   C. **Oral dissolution therapy**
      1. Oral dissolution first attempted 25 years ago with chenodeoxycholic acid (chenodiol)
      2. Currently use ursodeoxycholic acid (ursodiol)
         a. More efficacious than chenodiol (approximately 30% dissolution) with less diarrhea and hepatotoxicity
      3. Many problems with oral therapy

      a. Typical therapy must last 1 year or more

      b. High incidence of side effects

      c. Not effective for stones > 20 mm in diameter

      d. Not effective for pigmented, calcified stones

      e. High rate of recurrence of stones once therapy discontinued

         i. First year as many as 20% have recurrence of stones; up to 45% by 5 years

      f. Expensive

         i. Typical therapy costs $1500–2000 for year's treatment plus cost of physician visits and ultrasonography monitoring

    4. Best candidates for oral therapy are women with symptomatic gallstones who refuse or are poor candidates for surgery

      a. Patients should have small noncalcified stones (< 20 mm) and patent cystic duct, and understand risk of recurrence of stones

      b. Another reason for prophylactic oral therapy is to prevent formation of stones in persons undergoing rapid weight loss

D. **Parenteral dissolution therapy**

    1. Investigational instillation of solvents into gallbladder or bile ducts to dissolve stones using methyl-tertiary-butyl ether or n-propyl acetate

    2. Percutaneously placed catheter into gallbladder, infusing solvent directly around stones

    3. Rapid dissolution of most stones

      a. Not limited to cholesterol stones alone

      b. May be successful in as little as 15 hours of therapy

    4. Complications may be frequent, expertise limited and procedure actually little used

E. **Lithotripsy**

    1. Focusing of high-amplitude sound waves on small area to fragment stones to small size, allowing harmless passage via intact gallbladder contraction to bile duct

    2. Often followed with oral dissolution therapy to prevent reformation of stones

    3. Technical complications, high cost, limited expertise have virtually eliminated lithotripsy from America

F. **Open cholecystectomy**

    1. In healthy, low-risk candidates, open procedure has low operative mortality (< 1%), relatively short hospital stay (4–6 days), and good visualization of gallbladder and biliary tree with few complications

    2. Concerns with open procedure:

      a. Complications, often postoperative, and prolonged hospital stay in elderly, chronically ill, or emergent cases

      b. Incision through rectus abdominis muscle associated with considerable pain; recovery period prolonged even in healthy patients

      c. Expense associated with hospital stay and loss of wages from delayed return to work

    3. Open procedure probably still remains gold standard despite rapidly dropping number of procedures performed

G. **Laparoscopic cholecystectomy**

    1. First developed in 1988

      a. Acceptance and spread of procedure truly astounding

         i. Adoption so rapid, no accurate figures on use relative to open procedure

    2. Several advantages

      a. Substitution of the classic large, upper quadrant incision with four small, stab-type incisions for

      b. Pain and disability greatly reduced

      c. Typically requires only overnight hospital stay, saving several days' expense and return to work in as little as 1 week compared with 4–6 weeks for open operation

    3. Limitations

      a. Emergent, seriously ill patient with cholecystitis who is not candidate for open cholecystectomy is also not candidate for laparoscopic procedure

      b. Multiple, upper abdominal operations with resultant scarring

      c. Contraindicated in pregnancy (at least beyond 14–16 weeks)

      d. Contraindicated in known common duct stones

4. Acknowledged higher complication rate
    a. Especially during early learning curve
    b. Most complications involve biliary tree damage with need to convert to open procedure to repair
    c. Complication rate among experienced surgeons should be no greater than for open procedures
5. Approximately 5–7% of laparoscopic procedures need to be turned into open procedures
    a. Typical reason—discovery of common duct stones
    b. Unexpected damage to biliary tree or other structures
    c. Other technical limitations, such as adhesion of gallbladder to liver, intestines, omentum; unsuitable patient habitus
6. Laparoscopic procedure requires more operating room time, partially offsetting hospital stay savings
    a. Surgeon's fee usually higher than for open procedure
7. Laparoscopy is now procedure of choice if no contraindication

H. Management of common duct stones
1. If common duct stones demonstrated and patient does not require emergent surgery, attempts should be made to extract stones
2. Endoscopic retrograde cholangiopancreatography (ERCP)
    a. Combination of sphincterotomy (of ampulla of Vater) and basket removes retained stones in high percentage of cases
    b. Usually accomplished with mortality rate of 1–2%
3. Limitations to ERCP
    a. Cannot remove stones larger than 20 mm
    b. Increased complications if done in patients with cholangitis
    c. Risk of bleeding, perforation, cholangitis, pancreatitis
    d. Unknown whether sphincterotomy prevents subsequent development of gallstones
4. If ERCP cannot extract stones, open procedure generally required
    a. Laparoscopic techniques improving but have not supplanted open procedure for this complication

I. Post-cholecystectomy syndromes
1. Symptoms persisting past postoperative period
2. May occur in 10–25% of patients
    a. Although figures are hard to determine, impression is that most are women
3. The post-cholesystectomy syndrome often represents a missed diagnosis preoperatively (that is, patient may have been investigated for abdominal symptoms but gallstones were not the cause)
    a. Other likely causes include reflux esophagitis, peptic ulcer disease, pancreatitis, irritable bowel syndrome
4. If correct diagnosis missed, no surprise that even "successful" operation does not relieve symptoms
5. Other possible etiologies
    a. Papillary stenosis; spasm of sphincter of Oddi; biliary dyskinesia
        i. Diagnostic criteria vague and response to therapy variable
        ii. If diagnosis suspected or confirmed, attempts at sphincterotomy may be successful
    b. Bile-salt diarrhea and/or gastritis
        i. Diarrhea due to cathartic effect of bile salts
        ii. Reflux of bile salts into stomach with inflammation and gastritis
        iii. Both diarrhea and gastritis may be controlled with cholestyramine, if diagnosis strongly suspected

SUGGESTED READING

1. Bowen JC, Brenner HI: Gallstone disease: Pathophysiology, epidemiology, natural history, and treatment options. Med Clin North Am 76:1143–1157, 1992.
2. Johnston DE, Kaplan MM: Pathogenesis and treatment of gallstones. N Engl J Med 328:412–420, 1993.

3. Kadakia SC: Biliary tract emergencies: Acute cholecystitis, acute cholangitis, acute pancreatitis. Med Clin North Am 77:1015–1036, 1993.
4. Kivioluoto T, Sirén J: Randomised trial of laparoscopic versus open cholecystectomy for acute and gangrenous cholecystitis. Lancet 351:321–325, 1998.
5. Maclure KM, Hayes KC: Weight, diet, and the risk of symptomatic gallstones in middle-aged women. N Engl J Med 321:563–569, 1989.
6. NIH Consensus Development Panel on Gallstones and Laparoscopic Cholecystectomy: Gallstones and laparoscopic cholecystectomy. JAMA 269:1018–1024, 1993.
7. Zubler J, Markowski, G: Natural history of asymptomatic gallstones in family practice office practices. Arch Fam Med 7:230–233, 1998.

95. Irritable Bowel Syndrome

Bruce E. Johnson, M.D.

I. The Issues

Any condition that is claimed by 10–15% of the adult population is going to result in multiple appointments with primary care physicians. Yet the patients who come to the doctor with complaints eventually diagnosed as irritable bowel syndrome (IBS) represent only a fraction of the afflicted group. Most women have mild symptoms and control their symptoms without medical intervention. Those who do present to the doctor certainly are more indisposed but also seem to put an emphasis on symptoms that pass barely recognized by others. One of the important issues in dealing with irritable bowel syndrome is early diagnosis with a reasonable but controlled number of tests. Once a diagnosis has been confidently made, a directed approach to management can be undertaken. However, dealing with this condition means dealing as much with the patient's fears, concerns, and psychosocial milieu as with the symptoms and other manifestations of the disease.

II. The Theory

A. Presentation

1. Condition with alterations of defecation as perceived by patient
   a. Several different presentations
      i. Chronic abdominal pain and constipation
      ii. Intermittent diarrhea, occasionally without pain
      iii. Alternating diarrhea and constipation, sometimes associated with cramping, bloating, and painful defecation
   b. Symptoms may be relieved, at least temporarily, by bowel movement
2. Multiple synonyms include spastic colon, functional bowel syndrome, colitis, and psychogenic mucus colitis

B. Epidemiology

1. Prevalence depends on population studied and definition used
2. Compatible symptoms claimed, at one time or another, by 10–22% of adults
   a. Only 15–40% of persons with symptoms consult physicians for evaluation and treatment
   b. Estimated that up to half of referrals to some gastroenterologists are for IBS
3. Approximately 2:1 female:male ratio, with suggestion that women much more likely to seek medical attention
4. Onset typically in adolescence or young adulthood

C. Pathophysiology

1. Constellation of symptoms, signs, and physiologic observations revolves around **three primary points**
   a. Alterations in colon motility
   b. Alterations in sensation
   c. Associations with other symptoms and psychological complaints

2. **Alterations in colon motility**
   a. Some patients have increased basal colonic motility
      i. Spasms of dysfunctional colonic contractions; not especially useful in moving fecal bolus
   b. Other patients present with decreased resting colonic motility
   c. In addition to resting motility, distal colon in IBS may demonstrate alterations in slow-wave activity
      i. Increase in colonic segmental contractions at 3 cycles/minute, which may interfere with normal peristaltic wave formation
      ii. By interfering with normal peristalsis, such contractions contribute to static, nonpropulsive action by colon (i.e., constipation)
      iii. Slow-wave activity may be stimulated by arrival of bolus at cecum
   d. Alterations in motility in small bowel
      i. Clusters of paroxysmal contractions in duodenum and jejunum
      ii. Either alter propulsive function or simply cause cramping pain
      iii. Paroxysmal contractions disappear during sleep, coinciding with clinical clue of absence of irritable colon symptoms during sleep
   e. Although alterations in motility are observed in patients with IBS, they are not always present during painful attacks
      i. Raises question whether motility causative or simply reactive to other stimuli
3. **Alterations in sensation**
   a. Originally suggested because of frequent patient complaints of excessive abdominal gas (flatus)
      i. Measurements did not confirm excessive gas production
   b. Experimental balloon distention of sigmoid colon and rectum in patients with IBS results in increased pain at volumes that do not cause pain in normal people
      i. Presumably due to altered sensation of pain rather than excessive intestinal contractions or altered compliance of bowel wall
   c. Sensations seem to be greatest at right lower quadrant, location of ileocecal valve
   d. Increased sensation also may feed back to motor activity of bowel
      i. May result in heightened motor activity (contractions and motility)
   e. Patients with IBS have higher incidence of complaints regarding other organ systems, such as indigestion, esophageal dysfunction, bladder irritability
      i. Common pathophysiology to all these disorders may be altered visceral perception of distention
4. **Psychosocial factors**
   a. Most studies find increased prevalence of psychiatric diagnoses
      i. Personality disorders
      ii. Obsessive/compulsive tendencies
      iii. Anxiety disorders
         (a) Panic attacks
      iv. Depression
      v. Somatization disorders
      vi. Phobias
   b. Symptoms of IBS frequently improve with effective treatment of psychosocial problems
   c. Most symptoms of IBS are exacerbated during stress
      i. Normal persons under stress may develop symptoms of irritable bowel, even demonstrating motility and sensory changes seen in IBS
   d. Several studies demonstrate that prior physical and sexual abuse rates are high among patients with IBS
5. **Intestinal irritants**
   a. Agents in intestine that primarily or secondarily contribute to symptoms
   b. Malabsorbed sugars
      i. Lactose, maltose, fructose, and sorbitol
         (a) For example, mild lactase deficiency can give symptoms of IBS or exacerbate pre-existing IBS

        ii. Sorbitol important in U.S. because it is frequently used as nonabsorbed, noncaloric sweetener (chewing gum, some candies)

        iii. If not digested, function in part as osmotic agents, inducing diarrhea

    c. Food "allergens"

        i. Difficult to identify and quantify (and usually is not a real "allergy"

        (a) Consciously or subconsciously, patients often develop own avoidance behaviors

        ii. Avoidance and elimination diets (planned or from patient experience) may improve symptoms

    d. Bile acids

        i. Large intestine irritant not uncommon in some postcholecystectomy patients who develop altered bowel habits

        ii. Mechanism of bowel irritation not known but relief frequent when treated

    e. Short- and medium-chain fatty acids

        i. If, for some reason, these are not absorbed in small intestine, they may act as irritant in large bowel or as osmotic agents

III. **An Approach**

  A. **Clinical presentation**

    1. Typically female and young

      a. Men may describe symptoms on questionnaire studies; women more likely to seek medical advice

      b. Syndrome usually has onset in adolescence or young adulthood

    2. Broad range of symptoms that may be continuous or intermittent

      a. Because everyone may have transient alterations in bowel patterns, symptoms should be present more than 3–6 months before diagnosing IBS

    3. Symptoms almost always involve abdominal pain and altered bowel habits

      a. Additional symptoms more common in IBS than other gastrointestinal diseases include:

        i. Abdominal distention, pain relief with bowel movement, more frequent stools with onset of pain, looser stools with onset of pain, passage of mucus, sensation of incomplete evacuation

      b. Not all additional symptoms present in all patients

    4. Table 1 offers consensus criteria that helps in confirmation of diagnosis

      a. Many patients helped by treatment do not have frequent abdominal pain

    5. Many of these criteria diminish with advancing age

      a. Diagnosis much more likely in younger than older women

      b. Symptoms, even those in Table 1, in older women more likely associated with organic gastrointestinal disorder

    6. Criteria more reliable in women than men at all ages

  B. **Additional historical information**

    1. Noncolonic symptoms associated with IBS: gastroesophageal reflux, dysphagia, globus sensation, noncardiac chest pain, urologic dysfunction, gynecologic disorders, fatigue, psychosocial disorders

TABLE 1.   Symptom Criteria for Irritable Bowel Syndrome

Continuous or recurrent symptoms
    Abdominal pain or discomfort relieved with defecation or associated with a change in frequency or consistency of stools
        and/or
An irregular pattern of defecation (consisting of three or more of the following):
    Altered stool frequency
    Altered stool form (hard or loose and watery)
    Altered stool passage (straining or urgency, feeling of incomplete evacuation)
    Passage of mucus
    Bloating or feeling of abdominal distention

From Drossman DA, Thompson WG, Talley NJ, et al: Identification of sub-groups of functional gastrointestinal disorders. Gastroenterol Int 3:159–172, 1990, with permission.

    2. Important to exclude symptoms suggestive of organic gastrointestinal disease

       a. Weight loss or fever; bloody diarrhea; explosive, large-quantity diarrhea; diarrhea that awakens patient from sleep; abdominal pain that awakens patient from sleep

    3. Identify other sources of disordered gastrointestinal function

       a. Medications

           i. Anticholinergics or sympathomimetics

           ii. Antibiotics (especially taken long-term)

           iii. Hormones, including birth control pills

       b. Travel

       c. Dietary

           i. Especially additives, such as sorbitol, aspartame

           ii. Lactose or other carbohydrate intolerance

    4. Identify sources of recent stress or psychosocial disorder

C. Physical exam

    1. Usually normal unless an underlying disease detected

       a. Pain elicited by abdominal exam is diffuse and usually nonlocalizing, though if pain present more likely over cecum (right lower quadrant)

    2. Any specific or reproducible findings should prompt further work-up

D. Differential diagnosis

    1. Table 2 lists important differential diagnostic considerations

    2. With such an extensive, broad differential diagnosis, a careful, thorough structured history essential

       a. Important emphasis on dietary and psychosocial aspects

E. Evaluation

    1. Because there are no specific diagnostic findings, extensive work-up is usually nonproductive

    2. Frequent pressure from patient for more testing to find "cause"

    3. Many patients are frustrated and doctor shop

       a. Want repeat tests, investigations

TABLE 2.   Differential Diagnoses for Irritable Bowel Syndrome

Neoplasm	Endocrine and metabolic disorders
Adenocarcinoma of colon	Diabetes (with autonomic dysfunction, either
Villous adenoma	diarrhea or constipation)
Other (metastatic), including ovarian	Thyroid (hyperthyroidism with diarrhea; hypo-
Inflammatory bowel disease	thyroidism with constipation)
Chronic diarrhea	Others (with alterations in catecholamines,
Drugs, including alcohol	corticosteroids, cations, electrolytes)
Intestinal infection (e.g., giardiasis)	Dietary and food additives
Celiac disease	Lactose
Other malabsorption syndromes	Sorbitol
Collagenous colitis	Fructose
Chronic constipation	Aspartame
Drugs	Travel-related alterations
Pseudoobstruction	Travelers' diarrhea (toxigenic *Escherichia coli*)
Impaction	Giardiasis
Postoperative changes	Amebiasis
Bacterial overgrowth	Psychosocial disorders
Cholecystectomy with cholerrheic diarrhea	Stress reactions
Previous gynecologic surgery with constipation	Anxiety disorders
Vascular insufficiency	Panic disorders
Ischemic colitis	Previous sexual or emotional abuse
Abdominal angina	Somatization disorders
Gynecologic alterations	Depression
Multiple deliveries with pelvic floor relaxation	
Rectocele, enterocele	
Endometriosis	

4. Initial tests
   a. Complete blood count (CBC)
   b. Erythrocyte sedimentation rate (ESR)
   c. Chemistry panel
   d. Thyroid-stimulating hormone
   e. Stool hemoccult
   f. Flexible sigmoidoscopy
      i. Reasonable in younger patient to exclude inflammatory bowel disease or in older patient to exclude neoplasm
      ii. If high suspicion of IBS, full colonoscopy or barium enema not needed
5. Other tests as conditions warrant
   a. For persistent diarrhea
      i. Stool for ova and parasites, fecal fat and leukocytes, stool volume
      ii. Lactose-hydrogen breath test
      iii. Colonoscopy and barium enema
      iv. Small bowel enema (enteroclysis) for inflammatory bowel disease
      v. Small bowel biopsy for parasites, sprue
   b. For persistent constipation
      i. Small and/or large bowel transit time
      ii. Anorectal manometry
      iii. Pelvic floor function tests

F. **Management**
1. Most patients have symptoms that are
   a. Mild with minimal functional interference
   b. Moderate with occasional dysfunction
   c. Severe and intractable with significant functional disorder
2. Important aspects of long-term management for IBS
   a. Chronic functional disorder
   b. Benign, no progression to organic, life-threatening consequences
   c. Symptoms often intermittent, with exacerbations and remissions
      i. Cannot extrapolate from one patient's pattern to next
      ii. Exacerbations often correspond to periods of psychological stress
   d. Repeated testing has little value
   e. Education is essential and flows both ways—physician to patient and vice versa
      i. Issues include nature of disease, dietary manipulation, medication responses, trial-and-error findings
   f. Reassurance that physician understands reality of symptoms and is available for assistance upon exacerbations
3. **Management of mild symptoms**
   a. Identification of symptom triggers
      i. Mild disease typically is intermittent; symptoms occur after alterations in diet, health, or habits
         (a) Episodic illnesses
         (b) Travel
         (c) Job, home, or relationship stresses
         (d) Menstrual changes or irregularities
      ii. Encourage symptom diary
         (a) Detailed collection of diet and habits
         (b) Include relationship to menstrual periods (even though periods may not be modifiable this information may lead to greater understanding of symptoms
   b. Diet
      i. Trial elimination of certain dietary items
         (a) Lactose, sorbitol, caffeine, fatty foods, legumes
         (b) Many patients have already discovered foodstuffs to eliminate; may reintroduce items to prove or disprove consequences
      ii. Trial ingestion of fiber

        (a) More valuable in constipation than diarrhea

        (b) Adjustment of fiber content leads to patient involvement in disease management

        (c) Significant side effect is gas production and bloating—often same symptoms as IBS

        (d) Dietary sources (e.g., wheat bran) or commercial (e.g., psyllium)

  c. Medication

    i. Not commonly needed

    ii. Patient frequently self-medicates with OTC products

4. **Management of moderate symptoms**

  a. Identification of symptom and diet triggers

  b. Drug therapy is not encouraged but often necessary

    i. IBS is chronic and remitting yet benign; concern with drug dependence and eventual loss of efficacy of therapy

    ii. If used, tailor drugs to symptoms (e.g., do not use same approach for every patient with IBS)

  c. Drug therapy for symptoms of constipation

    i. Fiber or bulk products

    ii. Stool softeners (e.g., docusate)

    iii. Nonabsorbable osmotic products

        (a) Lactulose (Chronulac) is carbohydrate used in hepatic encephalopathy, but its predictable diarrheagenic side effect may be useful

        (b) Sorbitol is less expensive, almost equally effective agent as lactulose, but not as readily available

    iv. Cathartics (stimulant laxatives) should be strongly discouraged

    v. Prokinetic products

        (a) Cisapride (Propulsid) originally developed for gastroparesis; may have efficacy in constipation

            (i) Another prokinetic product, metoclopramide, not as effective

        (b) Investigations suggest that certain calcium channel blockers, serotonin antagonists, and other agents may stimulate intestinal motility

  d. Drug therapy for symptoms of diarrhea

    i. Recommended use for short periods only because of development of dependence

    ii. Loperamide (Imodium) preferred over diphenoxylate (Lomotil), which crosses blood–brain barrier

    iii. Avoid opiates (codeine)

    iv. Trial of cholestyramine

        (a) May be effective in sequestering bile acids and reducing diarrhea

        (b) Causes almost universal constipation in high enough doses

  e. Drug therapy for symptoms of pain

    i. Perhaps most difficult symptom to evaluate and treat

    ii. Pain associated with bloating and gas may respond to dietary intervention

    iii. Pain after meals often from heightened sensation and may respond to anticholinergics

        (a) Dicyclomine (Bentyl) perhaps least likely to cause other side effect

        (b) Propantheline (Pro-Banthine), belladonna, tincture of opium also used

        (c) Peppermint oil promoted in Great Britain

    iv. Any anticholinergic should be used with caution in elderly populations due to risk of glaucoma exacerbation, urinary retention, dry mouth

    v. Use of opiates and narcotics strongly discouraged

    vi. Tricyclic antidepressants may be useful as adjunct similar to use in other chronic pain syndromes

  f. Drug therapy for symptoms related to menstrual cycle

    i. Consider instituting oral contraceptives (OCP); IBS symptoms associated with painful menses may decrease along with dysmenorrhea

    ii. If on OCP, consider altering hormonal mix (i.e., estrogen content relative to progestin)

g. Other therapies
  i. Relaxation therapies, biofeedback
    (a) Early identification of stressors/triggers allows relaxation techniques to abort IBS exacerbation
  ii. Psychotherapy
    (a) May be of considerable assistance in circumstances of anxiety disorders, panic attacks, depression; previous or current physical or sexual abuse
    (b) Anxiolytics should be avoided because of early habituation and problems with rebound after withdrawal

5. **Management of severe symptoms**
   a. Therapies listed under moderate symptoms may be tried
   b. Patients have high likelihood of psychological underpinning of IBS, especially anxiety and somatization disorders
   c. Unrealistic expectation of "diagnosis" and "cure" of organic disease along with frequent doctor-shopping and gastroenterology consultation
   d. Psychosocial and behavioral techniques
     i. Establishment and maintenance of supportive doctor–patient relationship
     ii. Intensive education, especially of benign nature of disease and nonfatal, nonmorbid outcome
     iii. Assurance of doctor's availability on exacerbation of symptoms with frequent, regular visits emphasizing patient control rather than disease symptoms
   e. Drug therapy of symptoms
     i. Antidepressants often useful
     ii. Sedating tricyclics may be tried in patients with anxiety or sleep disorders
     iii. Occasional use of anxiolytics may be unavoidable
   f. Pain clinic referral
     i. Multidisciplinary approach may offer comprehensive approach patients demand

6. Associated conditions (bladder dysfunction, esophageal spasm, possibly also pelvic pain or even anxiety disorders)
   a. Cross-over of characteristics in diseases with few diagnostic specifics
   b. Effective treatment of one may assist management of others
   c. Argues for comprehensive, "holistic" approach perhaps as part of team

SUGGESTED READING

1. Camilleri M, Prather CM: The irritable bowel syndrome: Mechanisms and a practical approach to management. Ann Intern Med 116:1001–1007, 1992.
2. Drossman DA, Leserman J: Sexual and physical abuse in women with functional or organic gastrointestinal disorders. Ann Intern Med 113:828–833, 1990.
3. Drossman DA, Thompson WG: Identification of subgroups of functional gastrointestinal disorders. Gastroenterol Int 3:159–172, 1990.
4. Drossman DA, Thompson WG: The irritable bowel syndrome: Review and a graduated multicomponent treatment approach. Ann Intern Med 116:1009–1016, 1992.
5. Lynn RB, Friedman LS: Irritable bowel syndrome: Managing the patient with abdominal pain and altered bowel habits. Med Clin North Am 79:373–390, 1995.
6. Manning AP, Thompson WG: Towards positive diagnosis of the irritable bowel. BMJ 276:653–654, 1978.

96. Mitral Valve Prolapse

Bruce E. Johnson, M.D.

I. **The Issues**

Mitral valve prolapse, a syndrome occurring largely in women, is frequently misunderstood. Although this condition is usually benign and often asymptomatic, the finding of mitral valve prolapse leads to concern, even panic, in the patient. Unfortunately, this worry may be a direct result of comments made by the physician. Mitral valve prolapse is rather common and frequently noted in young women. Associated symptoms may have led the woman to medical evaluation. However, the click or murmur is often picked up during a routine exam and overstating the consequences of such a finding may do the woman a disservice, labeling her "ill" for the rest of her life. A clear understanding of the circumstances in which appropriate concern should be expressed is important; knowing when to offer simple reassurance is every bit as valuable.

II. **The Theory**

   A. **Background**
   1. Reports attributed to mitral valve prolapse (MVP) found in writing of William Osler (1908) and other before him
   2. Although auscultatory descriptions varied, Reid (1961) and Barlow (1963) fully characterized syndrome
      a. In addition to auscultatory findings, they noted changes on echocardiography
   3. Further characterization and identification of complications proceeded over past two decades
   4. Additional synonyms: Barlow syndrome; floppy valve syndrome; systolic click/murmur syndrome; billowing mitral leaflet syndrome

   B. **Epidemiology**
   1. Broad range of clinical and echocardiographic findings, from minimal to significant, leads to variability in definition of syndrome
      a. Prevalence depends on definition, i.e., whether by physical exam, echocardiography, or both
   2. Accepted values now suggest that MVP occurs in 2–3% of general population
   3. Probably > 70% of cases in women
      a. Ironically, in men, especially older men, prognosis of more concern

   C. **Causes of prolapse**
   1. Displacement of mitral leaflets from normal location during systole
      a. Degree of prolapse from mild without regurgitation to marked billowing with moderate regurgitation
      b. Murmur of MVP occurs after snapping of chordae tendinae, billowing or ballooning of leaflet, and then incompetence with regurgitation
      c. Mitral leaflets relatively larger than ventricular annulus leading to initial closure with redundancy, but, at late systole, prolapse into atrium
   2. Microscopic changes in collagen arrangements tie MVP to other connective tissue abnormalities
      a. Marfan's syndrome
      b. Ehlers-Danlos syndrome types I and III
      c. Less well defined but recognizable conditions collectively thought to be abnormalities of connective tissue
         i. Primary scoliosis (of young women)
         ii. Thoracic skeletal abnormalities, including pectus excavatum
         iii. Arched palate
      d. Sequel to rheumatic heart disease, postmitral valvulotomy, and, in association with ostium secundum, atrial septal defect
   3. Most cases are primary

     a. May have heritable component—autosomal dominant

     b. Inherited syndrome expression modified by age and sex

        i. Early development in young women

        ii. Later development appears in older men

D. **Characteristics**

  1. **Anatomic and pathologic features**

     a. Mitral valve tissue shows myxomatous degeneration and increased mucopolysaccharide

     b. Posterior valve affected more than anterior

     c. Mitral annulus frequently enlarged compared with left ventricle

     d. Elongated chordae tendinae

     e. Posited that chronic tension on chordae tendinae may elongate or irritate papillary muscle

     f. Increases tension on ventricular wall, leading to EKG changes and ventricular irritability

  2. **Physical findings**

     a. Most characteristic finding is midsystolic click and late systolic murmur

     b. Timing of midsystolic click important

        i. Click is late systolic in supine or squatting position or with isometric exercise

        ii. Click moves earlier in systole (mid or even early position) with maneuvers decreasing ventricle size such as sitting, standing Valsalva maneuver, use of amyl nitrate

     c. Murmur is late systolic, located at cardiac base, and follows click

        i. Crescendo/decrescendo murmur occasionally with whooping or honking

        ii. Other causes of mitral regurgitation lack preceeding distinctive click

     d. Physical findings tend to vary from exam to exam, especially in mild cases

        i. Fluctuations in audible click, timing of click, presence of murmur

        ii. Explains discordance in prevalence studies

        iii. Findings also tend to diminish somewhat with advancing age

  3. **Electrocardiography**

     a. Most commonly normal

     b. Abnormalities usually nonspecific, including biphasic or inverted T waves in inferior leads (II, III, aVF); nonspecific ST-T wave abnormalities, especially repolarization changes in inferior leads; prolongation of Q-T interval

     c. Atrial arrhythmias

        i. Premature atrial contractions

        ii. Atrial tachycardias

     d. Ventricular arrhythmias

        i. Premature ventricular contractions

        ii. Ventricular tachyarrhythmias

  4. **Echocardiography**

     a. Criteria for diagnosis continually refined and narrowed

     b. Agreement on following: M-mode recording of posterior systolic motion of leaflet behind valve's closing point

        i. Prolapse of 2 mm in late systole or 3 mm for holosystolic prolapse

        ii. Applying these criteria, incidence is approximately 3–4% of population

     c. Two-dimensional echo can be helpful if billowing seen across annular plane

        i. Subject to overinterpretation, depending on view of annulus taken (long-axis vs. apical)

     d. Pulsed Doppler evaluation useful for determination of regurgitation, especially volume of regurgitation

     e. Measurement of mitral leaflets

        i. Strong association with MVP if leaflet > 5 mm thick

  5. **Angiography**

     a. Less accurate than echocardiogram due to poor reproducibility and poor differentiation from normal variants

     b. Used when regurgitation substantial enough to consider replacement

E. **Associated findings and complications**
  1. **Psychiatric associations**
     a. Several studies suggest greater complaints in women with MVP of nonanginal chest pain; dyspnea; panic attacks; high anxiety trait
     b. Most studies note markedly higher report of anxiety-type symptoms in women than men
     c. Very real question of which came first—MVP with subsequent reaction or true association of anxiety-related disorders with anatomic valvular abnormality
  2. **Variations in cardiovascular and autonomic systems**
     a. Relative hypotension, especially systolic blood pressure or orthostatic hypotension
     b. Palpitations and relative tachycardia
  3. **Illness syndrome**
     a. Otherwise healthy young women, when given diagnosis, adopt ill persona
        i. Miss work, lose income, avoid household activities, avoid sports, avoid sex
        ii. High use of medical services
        iii. Early retirement
     b. Findings independent of echocardiographic or other determinations of severity of MVP
  4. **Bacterial endocarditis**
     a. Most extensively studied complication of MVP
     b. Relative risk increased 3–8 times compared with adults without MVP
        i. Up to 4,000 cases of endocarditis in U.S. each year in patients with MVP
     c. Highest risk in patients with hemodynamically important regurgitation
     d. Distribution of organisms causing endocarditis in MVP no different from other series of endocarditis
  5. **Sudden death**
     a. Relative risk may appear high but only because absolute number of cases so low in typical age group
     b. Most sudden death believed to be due to arrhythmia, probably ventricular
     c. Also associated degree of valve deformity
     d. Patients at risk for sudden death often have baseline EKG abnormalities
  6. **Progressive mitral regurgitation and ruptured chordae**
     a. Not inevitable consequence of MVP but increased MVP over general population
     b. Rapid decompensation and heart failure if chordae rupture
     c. Progressive regurgitation may result in eventual need for mitral valve replacement especially in older women with hemodynamically important regurgitation
  7. **Cerebrovascular embolization**
     a. Assumed to be platelet emboli
     b. Risk higher for MVP than general population, but investigators unable to determine criteria for risk within MVP groups

III. **An Approach**
  A. **Identification and diagnosis**
     1. Most cases detected during one of three presentations
        a. Serendipitous auscultation of click or murmur or both on routine exam
        b. Auscultatory findings while investigating complaints of atypical chest pain or palpitations
        c. Evaluation due to detection of MVP in family member
     2. Physicians often detect auscultatory changes when examining women with thoracic abnormalities, scoliosis, underweight (> 10% under ideal body weight)
     3. Auscultatory findings relatively specific for MVP
        a. MVP click not a widely split S_1 or opening snap of mitral stenosis
        b. Click of MVP shows mobility depending on maneuver (e.g., squat, Valsalva)
        c. Murmur of MVP late, after billowing of leaflet; murmur of mitral regurgitation tends to occur at onset of systole (holosystolic)
  B. **Evaluation**
     1. Auscultation of typical click followed by soft murmur or isolated midsystolic click, both showing mobility with maneuvers, considered definitive diagnosis

2. Electrocardiogram
   a. Findings nonspecific and unlikely to be useful unless atypical features in presentation
3. Echocardiogram
   a. Should be considered in several circumstances
     i. If appropriate criteria applied, confirms diagnosis
     ii. Helps to quantitate degree of regurgitation (valuable prognostic information), especially for older women
     iii. Helps to quantitate thickness of leaflet (also valuable prognostically)
   b. May be useful to expunge earlier, incorrect diagnosis
4. Radiographs, blood and urine tests, stress tests, even angiography not helpful

C. **Risk stratification**
1. Most important data are auscultation and echocardiogram
2. Important risks for which interventions are possible; decision must be based on information about leaflet thickness and amount of regurgitation
   a. Loud, harsh, almost holosystolic murmur suggests hemodynamically significant regurgitation
   b. Echocardiogram suggesting hemodynamically significant regurgitation
   c. Mitral leaflet > 5 mm thick
3. Several conditions for which abnormal findings, as noted above, suggest increased risk
   a. Stroke
   b. Endocarditis
   c. Progression to severe mitral regurgitation
   d. Rupture of chordae tendinae
4. Presence of severe findings leads to need for treatment or prophylaxis

D. **Treatment**
1. Most women are asymptomatic and require no specific therapy
   a. No therapy affects prolapsing mitral valve itself
2. Beta blockers used for symptomatic arrhythmias
   a. Useful for palpitations, atrial and ventricular contractions and tachyarrhythmias
   b. Help with anxieties and panic attacks
   c. If above symptoms prominent and beta blockers do not work, try calcium channel blockers
3. Infrequently, arrhythmias become major symptom, prompting attempts at therapy
   a. Antiarrhythmics (e.g., quinidine, procainamide)
4. Specific therapy for psychiatric disorders may be necessary
   a. Usually ansiety disorders, panic attacks (see Chapter 79)

E. **Prophylaxis**
1. Endocarditis
   a. Prophylaxis recommended for significant regurgitation, thickened leaflets
     i. Same as prophylaxis for other damaged valves
   b. May not be needed for minor abnormalities of valve (e.g., click without murmur, soft intermittent murmur)
   c. Applies to most surgical procedures, dental work, certain procedures (colonoscopy with biopsy, cystoscopy, cryotherapy, or laser treatment of cervix), and other "dirty" procedures
     i. Not necessary for Papanicolaou smear and pelvic exams, removal of skin lesions, routine exams
   d. 1–2 hours before procedure give oral penicillin (e.g., Pen V-K, 1 g) followed by same dose 4 and 8–12 hours after procedure
     i. Alternative choice for penicillin-allergic patients: erythromycin, 500 mg
     ii. For especially damaged valve, consider adding aminoglycoside
2. Stroke and transient ischemic attack
   a. Prophylaxis with significant regurgitant murmur and/or leaflet thickness
     i. Not necessary for mild degree of MVP
   b. Use aspirin 80–325 mg/day
   c. Use ticlopidine or Coumadin if embolus occurs despite aspirin

3. Progression of mitral regurgitation and rupture of chordae
   a. Probably applies only to 2–4% of patients with MVP
   b. Control hypertension if present
      i. Lower blood pressure decreases strain on valve and chordae, lessening chances of progression

SUGGESTED READING

1. Alpert MA, Mukerji V, Sabeti M, et al: Mitral valve prolapse, panic disorder, and chest pain. Med Clin North Am 75:1119–1133, 1991.
2. Clemens JD, Horwitz RI, Jaffe CC, et al: A controlled evaluation of the risk of bacterial endocarditis in persons with mitral-valve prolapse. N Engl J Med 307:776–781, 1982.
3. Devereux RB, Kramer-Fox R, Kligfield P: Mitral valve prolapse: Causes, clinical manifestations, and management. Ann Intern Med 111:305–317, 1989.
4. Enriquez-Sarano M, Orszulak TA: Mitral regurgitation: A new clinical perspective. Mayo Clin Proc 782:1034–1043, 1997.
5. Marks AR, Choong CY, Sanfilippo AJ, et al: Identification of high-risk and low-risk subgroups of patients with mitral-valve prolapse. N Engl J Med 320:1031–1036, 1989.
6. Retchin SM, Fletcher RH, Earp J, et al: Mitral valve prolapse: Disease or illness? Arch Intern Med 146: 1081–1084, 1986.
7. Wynne J: Mitral valve prolapse. N Engl J Med 314:577–578, 1986.
8. Zimetbaum P, Josephson ME: Evaluation of patients with palpitations. N Engl J Med 338:1369–1373, 1998.
9. Zuppiroli A: Natural history of mitral valve prolapse. Am J Cardiol 78:245–250, 1995.

97. Coronary Artery Disease

Bruce E. Johnson, M.D.

I. **The Issues**

More women die of myocardial infarction (MI) than any other disease. Coronary artery disease (CAD) remains the most common precursor to MI, constituting a major public health concern. Arguments that women have been systematically excluded from study of CAD are exaggerated, although it is true that women of child-bearing age have not been included in many intervention trials. The most likely cause of CAD is cholesterol deposition in coronary arteries; hyperlipidemia is addressed in Chapter 100, but the consequences of hyperlipidemia are considered in this chapter. Topics germane to generalists—prevention, screening, noninvasive testing, treatment of angina—are considered in this chapter; issues regarding angiography and revascularization are mentioned, but in-depth discussion is beyond the scope of this chapter.

II. **The Theory**

   A. **Hyperlipidemia** (see Chapter 100) is major factor in development of CAD
      1. Overall, women are protected, especially in premenopausal years, because estrogen promotes high-density lipoproteins (HDLs) and HDL protects against development of CAD
   B. **Atherosclerosis is complicated, multistage process**
      1. Fatty streaks occur in most arterial vessels, in both sexes, by age 15
         a. At young age, almost certainly represents cholesterol production *in situ* more than deposition of circulating cholesterol
         b. Fatty streaks do not directly correlate with eventual development of clinically evident atherosclerosis
      2. Cholesterol deposition in coronary artery wall, at site of prior injury, results in fibrous plaque which is relatively stable
         a. Injury may occur from hypercholesterolemia, infection by microorganisms, hypertension, autoimmune disorders, hyperglycemia, or other medical conditions

     b. Disruption of endothelium provides nidus for deposition of cholesterol; injury and repair leads to complex plaque of extracellular lipid, macrophages, other cellular elements, and necrotic cell material

     c. Plaque bulges into vessel lumen, producing stenosis

  3. Fibrous plaque is further complicated by ulceration

     a. Exposed collagen attracts platelets and thrombin, leading to healing/injury cycle and plaque growth

       i. Stenosis of vessel progresses, sometimes rapidly

     b. Creates platelet/thrombin aggregates that may break off and embolize downstream

  4. Ulcerated plaque stimulates release of vasoactive agents

     a. Vasoconstrictors released at ulcerated plaque contribute to vasospasm

     b. Natural vasodilators may be inhibited by complicated plaque

  5. Once a cholesterol plaque becomes "active," i.e., ulcerated with production of thrombus and vasoactive agents, rapid changes may occur

     a. Development of thrombus on ulceration, producing greater stenosis even obstruction

     b. Clot is unstable, growing under stimulus of platelet aggregation and coagulation and decreasing under stimulus of lysis (and embolization)

       i. This very active period may explain why symptoms wax and wane

       ii. Because of the pro-stenosis effects of platelet and coagulation clot growth, emergent clinical efforts to reverse this process employ combination of blockers of platelet aggretation (e.g., aspirin); thrombolytic agents (e.g., streptokinase); anti-vasospastic drugs (e.g., calcium channel blockers)

C. Risk factors

  1. Many risk factors well established and accepted (see Chapter 100, especially Table 2). However, active controversy surrounds several issues:

  2. Lipoprotein (a) [Lp(a)]

     a. This carrier of lipids is strongly associated with a positive family history of premature cardiac death

     b. Estrogen is one of few interventions demonstrated to lower elevated Lp(a); may lower by as much as 25%

       i. Few common therapies, such as diet, exercise, weight loss, or statins, lower Lp(a) as much as estrogen

       ii. Only medications that seem effective include nicotinic acid, neomycin, and androgens, none of which are first-line drugs for women

     c. Lp(a) should perhaps be measured with appropriate family history—and might be strong recommendation for HRT in postmenopausal women

  3. *Chlamydia pneumoniae*

     a. Developing data demonstrate higher antibody titers of *C. Pneumoniae* in patients with CAD; cellular particles in atherosclerotic plaques; animal data implicating *C. pneumoniae* in plaques and reporting reduced MI in animals treated with antibiotics

     b. Felt that inflammation from infection may initiate accelerated atherosclerosis process (described above)

       i. Interruption of infectious inflammation might prevent plaque growth

       ii. Animal data consistent with hypothesis

     c. Intervention studies in humans at the earliest stages and results conflicting

       i. Early data support antibiotic treatment post-MI with hopes of preventing second MI

       ii. Primary prevention studies planned but results not forthcoming

     d. Treatment protocols and guidelines far from established; random therapy may actually do more harm than good

  4. Homocysteine

     a. High levels associated with increased risk of CAD (and stroke, peripheral vascular disease) and seems to be an independent risk factor not associated with other risk factors

     b. Magnitude may be as great as for smoking, hypertension

    c. High levels may compound adverse effects of hypertension, especially in women
        i. Measurement of homocysteine, at $60–80, is expensive
    d. Treatment is relatively simple and inexpensive
        i. Folic acid 0.4–1.0 mg/day (perhaps along with vitamins B_6 and B_{12} frequently normalizes homocysteine level
    e. As additional data become available, guidelines will most certainly incorporate folic acid at some dose
  5. Iron
    a. Intriguing association between low iron stores and protection against CAD
        i. Mechanism unknown but initial interest stemmed from observation of high CAD rates in iron-overload states
    b. Noted initially when studying CAD rates in men who donate blood; association extrapolated to menstruating women
    c. Remains an interesting observation (with beneficial consequence of encouraging blood donation) in men but with no specific recommendation

D. **Symptoms**
  1. Difference in symptoms and MI association between men and women
    a. MI first symptom of CAD in almost half of men; in women, MI is first symptom in less than 30%
    b. Conversely, angina/MI symptoms in women ar much more likely to be misinterpreted and significance ignored
        i. First MI more likely fatal in women than men
        ii. Delayed diagnosis accounts for more advanced CAD when angina diagnosed and diagnostic studies performed
  2. Angina in women more commonly atypical
    a. Classic presentation of chest tightness, gripping, viselike with radiation to neck or shoulder frequently replaced by symptoms listed in Table 1
    b. Not always associated with exertion; may occur at sleep
  3. Lack of association with exertion, atypical presentation, and complaints of vague discomfort, fear, or anxiety results in misdiagnosis—attributing symptoms to psychological disorders
  4. No evidence that women physicians diagnose or evaluate symptomatic women earlier or more accurately than men physicians; missed diagnosis seems to be gender-neutral

E. **Evaluation**
  1. EKG should be done, but interpreted with caution
    a. Non–Q-wave infarct more common in women
  2. Exercise testing
    a. Women, especially premenopausal women, have poor diagnostic accuracy with exercise EKG testing
        i. Sensitivity of test only 61%; specificity not much better at 69%
        ii. Leads to almost unacceptably high false-positive testing, necessitating further expensive, and possibly invasive, testing
        iii. In premenopausal women, related to low pretest probability (i.e., there is less CAD in premenopausal women, so likelihood of false-positive test higher)
    b. Thallium exercise testing not much better (sensitivity 78%, specificity 64%)
        i. Difficulties with reading due to breast attenuation artifact

TABLE 1. Atypical Symptoms of Coronary Artery Disease in Women

Dyspnea	Neck, shoulder, upper back pain
Nausea or vomiting	Perspiration
Fatigue or weakness	Acute chest pain, but interpreted
Indigestion	as anxiety or stress disorder
Abdominal pain	

      c. Sestamibi isotope has higher energy than thallium and generally gives better results, as it is not as likely to be attenuated by breast tissue
         i. Use of EKG gating also improves reading
      d. Echocardiography exercise testing gives better results (sensitivity 86%, specificity 79%) but is limited by availability of expertise and by body habitus (including large breasts)
   3. Pharmacologic testing
      a. Dobutamine or dipyridamole testing possibly indicated in women who cannot exercise
      b. Usually less functional data forthcoming
      c. Not widely studied in women
   4. Radiographic
      a. Electron-beam computed tomography has capability of detecting calcium deposition in atherosclerosis, which occurs virtually only in complicated plaques
      b. Age and gender differences in patterns of calcification—imperative to apply gender-specific data to interpretation
      c. Although electron-beam CT holds promise as noninvasive "screening" test in future, cost limits application to investigative sites at present
   5. Angiography
      a. Multiple studies, almost up to the present, show that women are many more times less likely than men to be referred for coronary angiography (still considered the "gold standard" for detection and eventual intervention)
      b. Still not certain whether women are *under*-referred or men are *over*-referred
      c. Reasons for difference not known but probably reflects underdiagnosis of angina, misinterpretation of severity of symptoms in women, misguided belief that women are less likely surgical/intervention candidates
      d. Of interest, once angiography is performed, "anatomy is destiny"—that is, once anatomy of coronary vessels indicates likelihood for successful intervention (CABG, PTCA, etc.) the rates for men and women are identical

III. **An Approach**
  A. **Risk factors**—typically identified during general examination, presence of multiple risk factors leads to further evaluation for CAD (see also Table 2, Chapter 100)
    1. Family history
      a. Especially important in early-onset CAD, i.e., onset in parent or sibling before age 55.
         i. Should prompt consideration of lipid profile, Lp(a), homocysteine level
    2. Hyperlipidemia
      a. In premenopausal women, or on HRT, strongly consider obtaining HDL along with total cholesterol
      b. Controversy about age range and interval to screen (see chapter 100)
    3. Cigarette smoking
      a. Any smoking greater than ½ pack per day
      b. Smoking actually increasing in younger women; since addiction so strong, predicts many women smokers for years to come
    4. Hypertension
    5. Diabetes mellitus
    6. History of cerebrovascular or peripheral vascular disease
    7. Severe obesity (> 30% overweight)
    8. Less established factors: sedentary lifestyle, stress, premature menopause, absence of estrogen replacement after menopause, other illnesses (e.g., hypothyroidism, renal disease, Cushing's disease), glucocorticoid use, alcohol abuse
  B. **Symptoms**
    1. Although classic symptoms of angina occur in women, atypical symptoms are present more often than in men
      a. Instead of chest discomfort, women often have abdominal distress readily confused with esophagitis or reflux symptoms, i.e., fullness, bloating, gagging
         i. Also confused with gallbladder symptoms, i.e., right upper quadrant discomfort, even through to back

      b. Dyspnea with or without exertion

      c. Fatigue, especially with modest exertion

      d. Anxiety, tachycardia, chest discomfort

      e. Shoulder, neck, upper back pain

  2. Women also more likely to have atypical symptoms of MI

      a. Even without diabetes, more commonly have "silent" MI

      b. Symptoms of fatigue, indigestion, nausea

  3. Still common to dismiss symptoms as anxiety/panic disorder

  4. High index of suspicion needed to differentiate cardiac from other chest or abdominal discomforts

C. **Evaluation**

  1. Laboratory tests

      a. Measure and follow creatine phosphokinase (CPK) and lactate dehydrogenase (LDH) isoenzymes

         i. Typical pattern of elevation and fall not different between sexes

      b. Cardiac troponins (proteins involved in interaction of myosin and actin) useful as one-time indication of cardiac injury; troponin T specific to cardiac muscle damage

         i. Rise in troponins reported to be more rapid then CPK or LDH, making this a useful test in emergency department evaluation

      c. Lipids should be measured but stress of ischemia often leads to artifactual elevation of cholesterol

  2. Electrocardiogram

      a. Patterns (Q-wave, non–Q-wave, ST depression, etc.) not different from men

      b. Women may have more Prinzmetal angina (coronary spasm, often at night, resolving on its own or in response to nitrates and/or calcium channel blockers

         i. Means that EKG will be abnormal only when spasm occurs—if suspected, indication for 24-hour EKG monitor test

      c. Women also tend to have more non–Q-wave infarcts

  3. Admission to hospital should be based on appropriate clinical history, physical signs of cardiac compromise, EKG and blood tests—with the exception of higher index of suspicion regarding clinical presentation, no different from decision making in men

D. **Stress testing**

  1. As noted above, exercise EKG testing has poor sensitivity and specificity (athough figures improve if pretest probability is high)

      a. May be considered in postmenopausal women with strong compatible presentation

      b. In premenopausal women, or those with atypical presentation, likelihood of false-positive high enough to skip to other noninvasive test

  2. Nuclear isotope scanning exercise testing

      a. Thallium or sestamibi should be considered

      b. Decision as to which test to use based on availability of local expertise

  3. Exercise echo a reasonable alternative if noninvasive cardiologist trained in this technique available

  4. If patient unable to do exercise test, appropriate to proceed to dobutamine or dipyridamole test, again based on local expertise

E. **Radiographic studies**

  1. Many fewer angiograms performed in women, although once angiography performed, likelihood of proceeding to angioplasty or surgery similar to men

      a. Studies vary but as recently as early 1990s men were being referred for angiograms 15–25% more often than women

  2. Most common reason given for lower angiogram rate is a minimizing of symptoms in women

  3. Proper evaluation, using combination of high index of suspicion, blood test corroboration, and exercise or pharmacologic stress testing should lead logically to angiography, if indicated

F. **Treatment (noninvasive)**

  1. Reduction of risk factors

      a. Cessation of smoking

      b. Cessation of alcohol abuse

      c. Weight loss (if > 30% overweight)

      d. Control

      e. Treatment of hyperlipidemia

      f. Initiation of exercise program

  2. Medications

      a. Standard angina therapy: nitrates, beta blockers, calcium channel blockers

      b. Aspirin

          i. Early studies in men document improved survival and fewer infarcts as both primary protection and as treatment after onset of symptomatic CAD (angina, unstable angina, infarct)

         ii. Although data not readily available for women, daily use of aspirin (80–325 mg/day) felt to be safe and probably efficacious

      c. Hormone replacement therapy (HRT)

          i. Known improvement in lipid profile

         ii. No evidence for increased CAD risk from use of HRT

        iii. Although specific figures for cardiac protection unavailable, if no contraindications exist would consider initiation of HRT

  3. Thrombolytic therapy for MI

      a. Currently, more often use tissue plasminogen activator (t-PA) somewhat more often than streptokinase

      b. Both therapies carry more morbidity than in men

          i. Mortality and stroke about twice the rates in men

         ii. Cardiac mortality and rate for intracerebral hemorrhage higher

      c. In studies including enough women for analysis, women tended to be older, more likely to have hypertension, diabetes, and hyperlipidemia

          i. Even when corrected for these factors, female gender carried some added risk

      d. However, use of thrombolytic therapy still carries better prognosis than nontreatment

G. **Treatment (invasive)**

  1. PTCA (percutaneous transluminal coronary angioplasty)

      a. No apparent differences in outcome between sexes

  2. Coronary artery bypass grafting

      a. Because of women's smaller size, early studies showed poorer outcomes

          i. Smaller coronary vessels and smaller saphenous veins led to longer operative time, slower vessel blood flow, more complications

         ii. Also, smaller vessels more likely to restenose with higher rate of second infarctions

      b. Prompted use of internal mammary artery

          i. High success rate caused adoption of this procedure in both sexes when possible

SUGGESTED READING

1. Blasi F, Cosentini R: A possible association of *Chlamydia pneumoniae* infection and acute myocardial infarction in patients younger than 65 years of age. Chest 112:309–312, 1997.
2. Grodstein F, Stampfer MJ: Postmenopausal estrogen and progestin use and the risk of cardiovascular disease. N Engl J Med 335:453–461, 1996.
3. Gurwitz JH, Col NF, Avorn J: The exclusion of the elderly and women from clinical trials in acute myocardial infarction. JAMA 268:1417–1422, 1992.
4. Hsia JA: Cardiovascular diseases in women. Med Clin North Am 82:1–19, 1998.
5. Kugn FE, Rackley CE: Coronary artery disease in women: Risk factors, evaluation, treatment and prevention. Arch Intern Med 153:2626–2636, 1993.
6. Meyers DG, Stickland D: Possible association of a reduction in cardiovascular events with blood donation. Heart 78:188–193, 1997.
7. Moghadasian MG, McManus BM: Homocyst(e)ine and coronary artery disease. Arch Intern Med 147:2299–2308, 1997.
8. Nobulsi AA, Folsom AR, White A, et al: Association of hormone replacement therapy with various cardiovascular risk factors in postmenopausal women. N Engl J Med 328:1069–1075, 1993.

9. Redberg RF: Diagnostic testing for coronary artery disease in women and gender differences in referral for revascularization. Cardiol Coin 16:52–62, 1998.
10. Weaver WD, White HD: Comparisons orf characteristics and outcomes among women and men with acute myocardial infarction treated with thrombolytic therapy. JAMA 275:777–782, 1996.
11. Wenger NK, Speroff L, Packard B: Cardiovascular health and disease in women. N Engl J Med 329:247–256, 1993.

98. Hypertension

Bruce E. Johnson, M.D.

I. **The Issues**

Hypertension is an extremely common condition, afflicting perhaps 30% of adult Americans. In certain subgroups, especially blacks and the elderly, hypertension is a greater concern for women than for men. Blacks, including black women, suffer a disproportionately high incidence of hypertension-related chronic renal failure. Most hypertension is essential, though it is clear that there are different physiologies within this large grouping. Some presentations of hypertension are almost exclusively found in women (although hypertension in pregnancy is not considered in this chapter). Although the pathophysiology may not differ markedly between the sexes, certain effects are prominent in women, especially at menopause. Treatment presents special issues for women. Until recent years, there was a relative lack of data specifically related to hypertension and women. Currently, epidemiology studies and intervention trials strive to include women in analysis.

II. **The Theory**

A. **Demographics**
   1. White women
      a. Essential hypertension not common before menopause
      b. Affects up to 40% with advancing age
   2. Black women
      a. Hypertension seen in up to 60% of black women over age 65
   3. Asian/Hispanic demographics more closely resemble whites

B. **Natural history of essential hypertension**
   1. Typical age of onset for essential hypertension varies with gender and racial makeup
      a. White men—40s–mid 50s
      b. Black men—30s–40s
      c. White women—50s
      d. Black women—mid 40s–50s
   2. Early in course of hypertension, recorded blood pressures tend to be labile, which causes caution in making a diagnosis and difficulty in determining whether adequate control is attained with treatment
   3. Progressive rise in blood pressure with age
      a. Industrialized countries
         i. Diastolic pressure tends to peak in mid to late 50s, then plateaus; systolic pressure often rises with age
         ii. Results in increased prevalence of all hypertension with advancing age, especially isolated systolic hypertension (i.e., elevated systolic BP with "normal" diastolic BP)
      b. Developing countries may not have progressive blood pressure rise with age
         i. Uncertain explanation but speculation involves diet, pollutants, "stress"

C. **Pathophysiology of hypertension**
   1. **Secondary causes of hypertension in women**
      a. Account for 5–8% of hypertension
         i. Important to recognize since these causes are generally assumed to be treatable

      b. Renal artery fibromuscular hyperplasia: unilateral renal artery stenosis due to overgrowth of muscular layer of artery

         i. Rapid-onset hypertension in young females

         ii. Female:male ratio—8:1

         iii. Strong suspicion in women < age 25

      c. Oral contraceptive pills (OCPs)

         i. Initial concerns raised when OCPs contained high doses of estrogen and progesterone; current pills have much lower doses and, consequently, OCP-induced hypertension not common

      d. Diseases with higher incidence in women in which hypertension is a sign: systemic lupus erythematosus, hyperthyroidism, Cushing's disease

  2. **Menopause**

      a. Estrogens generally are protective against usual causes of hypertension; incidence of hypertension rises with menopause, especially in white women

      b. With loss of estrogen, women with hypertension tend to have increased peripheral resistance, low or normal plasma volumes and low plasma renin—similar to men with hypertension; these observations along with echocardiograhic evidence suggests a loss of "elasticity"

      c. Women on ERT demonstrate modest return to premenopausal physiology

         i. women on hormones have slightly greater plasma volume and lower peripheral resistance along with return of premenopausal circadian rhythm of blood pressure

         ii. Some studies e.g., Postmenopausal Estrogen/Progesterone Intervention trial (PEPI), suggest decrease in expected rise in hypertension

      d. Uncommon to have ERT-induced hypertension

  3. **Essential hypertension**

      a. White women

         i. No single theory, but profile suggests hyperdynamic system, i.e., higher catecholamines with higher cardiac output, heart beat, and pulse pressure

         ii. Usually normal-to-high renin hypertensives with somewhat diminished peripheral resistance

      b. Black women

         i. Normal-to-low renin hypertensives with increased blood volume, and salt sensitivity

      c. Elderly women (not on ERT)

         i. Pathophysiology similar to elderly men, i.e., increased peripheral resistance, low plasma volume, low renin

      d. Isolated systolic hypertension becomes more common, especially in women; after age 65, accounts for > 10% of all hypertension

         i. Increased peripheral resistance and loss of elasticity in arterial vessels

      e. Although not a precise predictor, the pathophysiology can help with initial choice of therapeutics in many cases

D. **Pathologic consequences of inadequately treated hypertension**

  1. Coronary artery disease

      a. Increased, but hypertension not as significant a risk factor as elevated lipids

  2. Left ventricular hypertrophy (LVH)

      a. More common in women than men

      b. More LVH in women at all ages—poorly controlled hypertension adds to discrepancy

      c. May be related to overall smaller size heart and tendency, under pressure gradient (i.e., hypertension) to concentric enlargement

  3. Congestive heart failure:

      a. Consequence of LVH

      b. Treatment of hypertension more likely to have beneficial effect in this modality than in men

  4. Stroke

      a. Incidence closely related to uncontrolled hypertension

         i. Incidence higher in women than men

    b. Major end-organ effect of isolated systolic hypertension
    c. Considerable decline in stroke since 1960s directly attributed to improved control of hypertension
  5. Renal failure
    a. More common in black than white women
    b. Suspect factors other than simple BP control contributes to increased renal failure

III. An Approach
A. Diagnosis
  1. **General measures**
    a. Obtain several measurements over time, preferably not all in office; eliminates early diagnosis due to labile blood pressure
    b. Patient should be quiet, not anxious
    c. Room should be warm
    d. Full bladder, recent coffee or cigarettes may raise blood pressure
  2. **Do not overdiagnose hypertension**
    a. Beware "white-coat" hypertension
      i. Refers to elevated blood pressures when taken by doctor; not necessarily elevated in other settings
      ii. Prevalence may as high as 20%; more common in early-onset hypertensives with labile readings, young females
    b. Beware pseudohypertension in elderly
      i. Persistently elevated blood pressures without evidence of end-organ effects
        (a) Due to rigid arteries
        (b) Common in elderly women
      ii. Should be suspected with long-standing elevated blood pressure but no evidence of retinal changes, cardiac S4 sound, renal insufficiency
      iii. Osler's maneuver: palpate radial artery and inflate sphygmomanometer above systolic; if radial artery still palpable, rigid artery suggested
        (a) Unfortunately, Osler's maneuver is of more historic than accurate, clinical interest
    c. Consequences for insurance ratings if inaccurate diagnosis
    d. "Labeling": after receiving diagnosis, otherwise healthy, asymptomatic person may adopt "ill" self-image
      i. Increased absenteeism and sick leave
      ii. Self-denial of certain activities, jobs, hobbies
    e. Potential usefulness of 24-hour blood pressure monitoring is that total time hypertensive can be measured, obviating "white-coat" concerns
      i. Drawback—standards not agreed upon, predictive value not clear, costly and often not covered by insurance
  3. **Guidelines for diagnosis**
    a. JNC VI guidelines (1997) in Table 1 are more precise, but somewhat more complicated, than earlier guidelines

TABLE 1. Classification of Blood Pressure in Adults*

Category	Systolic (mmHg)		Diastolic (mmHg)
Optimal	< 120	and	< 80
Normal	≤ 130	and	< 85
High-normal	130–139	or	85–89
Hypertension			
Stage 1	140–159	or	90–99
Stage 2	160–179	or	100–109
Stage 3	≥ 180	or	> 110

* Age 18 and older, based on average of 2 or more readings taken at 2 or more visits
Adapted from Black HR, Cohen JD: The sixth report of the Joint National Committee on Detection, Evaluation, and Treatment of High Blood Pressure (JNC VI). Arch Intern Med 157:2413–2145, 1997.

        i. More in line with actual risk factor analysis from multiple epidemiologic and intervention studies

        ii. Earlier BP readings that suggest intervention

    b. Isolated systolic hypertension diagnosed with consistent readings > 160–165 despite diastolic < 90

4. Diagnosis of hypertension, once made, does not automatically result in medication, especially for lower stages

B. **Nonpharmacologic therapies**

1. Patient should be instructed and strongly encouraged to use appropriate nonpharmacologic therapies at all stages

    a. For high-normal, and even stage 1 hypertension, often possible to return BP to normal with nonpharmacologic therapy alone

2. **Weight loss**

    a. Possibly single most effective intervention

    b. In obese, loss of 10–20% body weight almost invariably brings labile blood pressure under control or makes control with medications easier

    c. Effect due, in part, to improvement in diet and exercise

3. **Exercise**

    a. May be helpful in short term; many studies in already hypertensive subjects, typically overweight, suggest blood pressure returns to (elevated) baseline after 6–12 months, even with continued exercise

    b. Excellent adjunct to weight loss

    c. Hypertension not contraindication to most exercise; counseling should emphasize orthopedic caution rather than worry about elevated BP, stroke, heart attack, etc.

    d. Women who exercise continually from youth have less prevalence of hypertension

4. **Salt reduction**

    a. Typical daily American diet contains up to 10–15 g salt; a diet of no added salt has 4–5 g

    b. No added salt diet of value to salt-sensitive hypertensives, typically blacks, elderly

    c. Greatest use as adjunct; high salt intake can overwhelm benefit of low doses of many medications, especially diuretics

5. **Calcium supplementation**

    a. Advocates claim calcium lowers blood pressure but evidence sketchy; doubtful as single intervention

6. **Potassium supplementation**

    a. Studies suggest high potassium diet, possibly in association with other minerals such as magnesium and calcium, can modify BP in borderline or labile hypertensives

    b. Diuretic induced hypokalemia should be corrected

        i. Risk of hypokalemia-induced arrhythmias, including ventricular tachyarrhythmias

        ii. Most antihypertensive medications are less effective if hypokalemic

7. **Estrogen replacement therapy** (ERT)

    a. Observation that ERT limits expected rise in BP at menopause leads some to suggest ERT should be used to treat hypertension

        i. Incomplete evidence of efficacy

    b. Occasionally hypertension exacerbated by ERT

        i. Attempt reduction in estrogen/progesterone dose

        ii. May choose to use antihypertensives in addition to ERT as ERT has overall beneficial effect on risk for cardiovascular disease

8. **Biofeedback**

    a. Little evidence for long-term effectiveness though participants do report overall well-being

9. **Other therapies**, including garlic, fish oil, "natural" treatments, unproven

C. **Drug therapy**

1. **General principles** (outlined by JNC VI)

    a. Single-agent medicines control most mild hypertension

b. Unless hypertension is moderate-to-severe, start with low dose and increase gradually

c. Some controversy whether better to use one drug up to maximal tolerated or effective dose, or to use two drugs at low dose

    i. Almost always less expensive to use one drug

d. When the patient is taking two drugs, one of the drugs should almost always be a diuretic

e. All things equal, choose once-daily formulations

f. Cost is major factor; newer drugs invariably cost $\geq$ $1–3/day for lowest dose

    i. Take into account total cost of drug; for example, thiazide diuretic may be inexpensive, but potassium supplement and testing drives up total costs

g. Each class of drugs has "me-too" choices; familiarize and use one or two drugs per class

h. Choose agent on basis of presumed effectiveness for patient's subgroup, interactions with other disease states, acceptable side effects

i. When adding second or third agent, avoid classes with similar or overlapping mechanisms of action

    i. For example, beta blockers, angiotensin-converting enzyme inhibitors and angiotensin II blockers all lower blood pressure by interfering with renin/angiotensin/aldosterone cycle

j. JNC VI considers first-line agents to be diuretics or beta blockers

    i. Based on large, outcome-based, randomized, controlled intervention studies which have consistently demonstrated less morbidity/mortality with diuretics or beta blockers

    ii. Controversial recommendation because side effects may be greater with these classes of drugs

2. **Diuretics**

a. Thiazides effective and inexpensive but require regular follow-up to avoid hypokalemia

b. Indicated for low-renin, salt-sensitive blacks and elderly, especially with isolated systolic hypertension

c. Thiazide effective dose relatively low

    i. Hydrochlorothiazine (HCTZ) dosed at 12.5–25 mg/day

    ii. Thiazides in fixed combination with potassium-sparing agent (triamterene, e.g., Dyazide, Maxzide; amiloride, e.g., Moduretic) more expensive than HCTZ alone but reduces need for potassium monitoring

d. Indapamide (Lozol): thiazide diuretic with little effect on lipids and less potassium wastage than other thiazides

e. Loop diuretics (e.g., furosemide, bumetamide) indicated for mild-to-moderate renal insufficiency (e.g., creatinine > 1.5)

    i. Difficult-to-control blood pressure in mild renal insufficiency greatly improved by adequate diuretic

    ii. Rarely used as first-line or single-agent therapy

f. Many diuretics alter lipid profile

    i. Caution in supplanting one risk factor (hypertension) by another (lipids)

    ii. Not major consideration in patients with normal lipids

3. **Centrally acting alpha-agonists**

a. Function in brain by decreasing autonomic stimulation, lowering peripheral resistance

b. Mechanism suggests efficacy in white women, elderly

c. Examples: reserpine, methyldopa (Aldomet), clonidine (Catapres), guanadril (Wytensin)

d. Reserpine long-acting; others require multiple dosing

    i. Exception is clonidine skin patch (Catapres TTS), effective constant release of clonidine for 7 days

e. Available as single agents or combined with diuretic

f. Special concern with reserpine

        i. Poor reputation derives from 25–30 years ago when higher doses used

        ii. With modest dosing (0.1–0.2 mg), side effects generally not excessive

        iii. Low cost, once-daily dosing deserves consideration

  g. Side-effect profile of this class not ideal

        i. Central, autonomic action leads to problems with: drowsiness, lethargy, mild confusion; decreased salivation, dry mouth; urinary retention (worse in men); decreased libido in both sexes (impotence in men)

  h. Side effects reduced with clonidine patch

        i. May be related to constant release

        ii. Major side effect at site of patch: "contact dermatitis" leaves skin inflamed for 1–2 days after removal and may even result in prolonged hyperpigmentation

4. **Beta blockers**

  a. Mechanism of action: combination of decreased chronotropy (heart rate), decreased inotropy (force of contraction), and decreased release of renin from kidney

        i. Pharmacology also includes blockade of peripheral vascular relaxation—actually increases peripheral vascular resistance

        ii. Most significant component of BP decrease is renin blockade

  b. Important differences in pharmacology

        i. Lipid/water solubility

           (a) Lipid-soluble beta blockers tend to cross blood–brain barrier, with more central effects and side effects

           (b) Lipid-soluble beta blockers tend to have greater variability in blood levels, shorter half-life

        ii. Cardioselectivity

           (a) More cardioselective agents have less bronchospastic and peripheral vascular side effects

           (b) Atenolol (Tenormin) and metoprolol (Lopressor) most cardioselective

  c. Often considered in middle-aged white women, who frequently are anxious and hard-driving

        i. Agent with central effects may provide bit of anxiolytic effect

  d. Although intervention studies demonstrate reduced morbidity/mortality, need to think twice before using for blacks or elderly

        i. Frequently have low-renin, salt-sensitive hypertension; less likely to respond maximally to beta blockers

  e. Major side effects include lethargy, fatigue, vivid dreams, decreased libido, occasional orthostatic hypotension

  f. Contraindicated in asthma and chronic obstructive pulmonary disease

  g. Many beta blockers adversely alter lipid profile, especially noncardioselective agents

5. **Angiotensin-converting enzyme inhibitors** (ACE inhibitors)

  a. Block conversion of renin to angiotensin, decreasing quantity of powerful vasoconstrictor (angiotensin) and sodium-retaining aldosterone

        i. First developed for high renin states, such as unilateral renal stenosis

  b. Indicated in essential hypertension subgroups with presumed high renin states, e.g., white women and men

        i. Less likely to be effective in blacks and elderly

  c. Strong evidence for efficacy in congestive heart failure—separate indication for ACE inhibitor

  d. Direct relaxation effect on afferent glomerular arterioles; protective in multiple types of renal damage

        i. Documented decrease in progression of diabetic microalbuminuria; hence indicated in diabetics at virtually any stage of disease

  e. Pharmacology varies primarily in half-life

        i. Captopril (Capoten) requires multiple dosing; others (e.g., enalapril [Vasotec], lisinopril [Zestril]) once daily

        ii. Little adverse effect on lipids

f. Side effects generally mild and infrequent
   i. Widely used without side effects seen in other antihypertensives (e.g., ortho-static hypertension, decreased libido, lethargy)
   ii. Because of wide acceptance, ACE inhibitors often used as benchmark agents in quality-of-life studies
g. Important side effects which limit use
   i. Idiosyncratic angioedema (often of face; rarely compromises larynx)
   ii. Cough (dry, nonproductive, insidious onset without bronchospasm)—may be present to some degree in as many as 15–20% of patients though not that many need to discontinue ACE inhibitors for this reason
      (a) This side effect seems much more likely to occur in women than men
   iii. Increased creatinine (may worsen mild renal insufficiency; important con-traindication with bilateral renal artery stenosis)
   iv. Hyperkalemia (usually occurs with underlying renal insufficiency)
6. **Angiotensin II blockers**
   a. Mechanism of action occurs at the next biochemical step after ACE inhibitors, i.e., by blocking the action of angiotensin II (formed by angiotensin converting enzyme) at the angiotensin II receptor
   b. Developed for circumstances in which ACE inhibitors effective but side effects, primarily cough, limit use
   c. Similar indications to ACE inhibitors, i.e., high-renin hypertensives (frequently middle-aged women)
      i. Although studies not yet complete, expect that angiotensin II blockers will also be efficacious in CHF and diabetes
   d. Side effect profile similar to ACE inhibitors except that cough rarely seen
7. **Calcium channel blockers** (CCBs)
   a. Mechanism involves interference with influx of calcium into cells, primarily af-fecting vascular cells, reducing contraction and resulting in decreased peripheral vascular resistance
      i. Additional major effect on renal afferent arterioles, reducing glomerular pressure and possibly renin release
      ii. Despite mechanism, generally not affected (adversely or otherwise) by cal-cium supplements
   b. Pharmacology revolves around differences in major CCB groups, usually simply designate as dihydropyridines (nifedipine and others) and nondihydropyridines (diltiazem, verapamil, and others)
      i. Differences involve cardiac conduction, side effects (edema, headache) with remarkably similar efficacy on BP control
      ii. Most native drugs require multiple dosing; drug companies have formulated sustained-release forms (e.g., Procardia XL, Cardizem CD, Calan SR)
   c. Important uses in all hypertensives, especially effective in blacks and, in lower doses, elderly
      i. Also valuable in moderate-to-severe hypertension, renal insufficiency, and as cardiac remodeling agent in left ventricular hypertrophy
   d. Side effects vary and may be important
      i. Reduction in cardiac conductivity (especially verapamil); orthostatic hy-potension; peripheral edema (especially nifedipine); constipation (especially verapamil)
8. **Peripheral alpha blockers**
   a. Mechanism involves blockade of peripheral vascular alpha1 receptors, reducing vascular resistance
   b. Pharmacology differences include half-life, side effects
      i. Prazosin (Minipress) requires multiple dosing; terazosin (Hytrin), doxazosin (Cardura) generally once daily
      ii. Orthostatic hypotension somewhat more common with prazosin
      iii. Little adverse effect on lipids
   c. Effective in most hypertensive subgroups

      i. Doxazosin often used in moderate-to-severe hypertension and renal insufficiency

    d. Side effects include orthostatic hypotension (prominent in first dose; hence recommendation to give first dose just before bedtime), mild edema, lethargy

9. **Vasodilators**
   a. Mechanism includes direct vasodilation of peripheral vasculature
   b. Hydralazine (Apresoline) and minoxidil (Lonitin) effective but largely supplanted by newer agents
   c. Side effects
      i. Hydralazine: orthostatic hypotension, reflex tachycardia requiring beta blocker, occasional drug-induced lupus syndrome
         (a) Because of favorable use over many years, still used in hypertension in pregnancy
      ii. Minoxidil: profound fluid retention requiring loop diuretic, hypertrichosis
      iii. Minoxidil occasionally used in men with resistant hypertension but hypertrichosis universally resented by women

10. **Ganglionic blockers**
    a. Examples: phentolamine, phenoxybenzamine
    b. Virtually never used except occasionally in preoperative treatment of pheochromocytoma

11. **Special considerations**
    a. Elderly
       i. Isolated systolic hypertension, with important effect being stroke, more likely in women
       ii. Recommend diuretics, clonidine patch, long-acting calcium channel blockers
       iii. Very important to avoid orthostatic hypotension; antihypertensives strongly implicated in falls and hip fracture
    b. Quality of life
       i. Many side effects of antihypertensives adversely affect quality of life
          (a) Lethargy, fatigue, edema, constipation, alteration in dreams, decreased concentration
    c. Sexual dysfunction
       i. In women, manifested by decreased libido
       ii. Centrally acting alpha agonists and some beta blockers more often implicated than other classes of antihypertensives, though no class immune to this side effect
       iii. Questionnaires seeking altered sexual dysfunction with antihypertensive agents rarely ask if drugs diminish frequency of intercourse, interfere with orgasm, affect lubrication etc.
    d. Breast disease
       i. Occasionally reports of breast enlargement, galactorrhea with methyldopa, spironolactone
    e. Osteoporosis
       i. Thiazide diuretics block calcium excretion; used in women with hypercalciuria

D. **Special uses of antihypertensive drugs**
   1. There are circumstances in which judicious use of antihypertensives may effectively address two problems with one drug, making choice of drug important in patients with more than one diagnosis
   2. Osteoporosis—thiazide diuretics decrease excretion of calcium, making more calcium available for bone metabolism
   3. Menopausal symptoms, e.g., hot flashes—if estrogens cannot be used, consider an antihypertensive such as the clonidine patch which may decrease effects of hot flashes
   4. Migraine headaches—both beta blockers and calcium channel blockers effective in prophylactic treatment of migraine headaches
   5. Excess hair growth, especially face, chest and abdomen—use of spironolactone often used for antiandrogen effect, diminishing hair growth

6. Mastalgia—if cyclic around menstrual periods, thiazide diuretics and spironolactone occasionally helpful
7. Premenstrual syndrome—diuretics and spironolactone occasionally helpful

SUGGESTED READING

1. Anastos K, Charney P: Hypertension in women: What is really known? Ann Intern Med 115:287–293, 1991.
2. Black HR, Cohen JD: The sixth report of the Joint National Committee on Detection, Evaluation, and Treatment of High Blood Pressure (JNC VI). Arch Intern Med 157:2413–2145, 1997.
3. Brunner E, White I: Can dietary interventions change diet and cardiovascular risk factors? A meta-analysis of randomized controlled trials. Am J Public Health 87:1415–1422, 1997.
4. Garavaglia GE, Messerli FH: Sex differences in cardiac adaptation to essential hypertension. Eur Heart J 10:1110–1114, 1989.
5. Hayes SN, Taler SJ: Hypertension in women: Current understanding of gender differences. Mayo Clin Proc 73:157–165, 1998.
6. Hodge RH, Howard MP: Sexual function of women taking antihypertensive agents: A comparative study. J Gen Intern Med 6:290–294, 1991.
7. Kaplan NM: The treatment of hypertension in women. Arch Intern Med 155:563–567, 1995.
8. Lewis C, Duncan LE: Is sexual dysfunction in hypertensive women uncommon or understudied? Am J Hypertens 11:733–735, 1998.
9. Mulrow CD, Cornell JA: Hypertension in the elderly: Implications and generalizability of randomized trials. JAMA 272:1932–1938, 1994.
10. Neaton JD, Grimm RH Jr: Treatment of Mild Hypertension Study: Final results JAMA 270:713–724, 1993.
11. National High Blood Pressure Education Program Working Group: National High Blood Pressure Education Program Working Group Report on Primary Prevention of Hypertension. Arch Intern Med 153:186–208, 1993.
12. Weinberger MH: Lowering blood pressure in patients without affecting quality of life. Am J Med 86(Suppl 1B):S94–S97, 1989.
13. Writing Group for the PEPI Trial: Effects of estrogen or estrogen/progestin regimens on heart disease risk factors in postmenopausal women: The Postmenopausal Estrogen/Progestin Interventions (PEPI) Trial. JAMA 273:199–208, 1995.

99. Obesity

Bruce S. Liese, Ph.D., and Bruce E. Johnson, M.D.

I. The Issues
Obesity is a multifaceted problem that affects the medical, social, and psychological health of many women. Obese women are likely to develop medical complications due to obesity. Overweight people face social stigma in a society that emphasizes thinness. Losing weight can be a difficult and frustrating task, and the psychological toll can be considerable. Recidivism (regaining of weight) is widespread and common leading to a "yo-yo" pattern of weight gain/weight loss which itself may carry medical consequences. Adequate intervention by the physician with the enthusiastic involvement of the patient can result in both medical and psychological gains.

II. The Theory
A. Definition
1. Obese women have excessive amount of body fat or adipose tissue
2. Previous weight tables (the most quoted was the Metropolitan Life Insurance Co. tables) had been based on actuarial information, standardized for both males and females, and were widely accepted. These tables listed a range of weights according to small, medium, or large "body frames," a difficult measurement
3. Current practice is to calculate the body mass index (BMI) which implicitly includes body frame in the calculation.

TABLE 1. Body Weights Corresponding to Height and Body Mass Index

Height (in)	Body Mass Index					
	20	25	30	35	40	45
58	96	119	143	167	181	214
59	99	124	148	173	189	223
60	102	128	153	179	204	229
61	109	136	164	197	225	254
62	113	141	169	197	225	254
64	116	145	174	204	232	262
65	120	150	180	210	240	270
66	124	155	186	216	247	279
67	127	159	191	223	255	286
68	131	164	197	230	263	296
69	135	169	203	237	270	304
70	139	174	209	243	278	313
71	143	179	215	250	286	321
72	147	184	221	258	294	321
73	151	189	227	265	303	340
74	155	194	233	272	311	350

a. $BMI = \dfrac{weight\ (kg)}{[height\ (m)]^2}$

b. Because most people in the U.S. use pounds and inches, this formula can be adapted with a correction factor:

$BMI = \dfrac{weight\ (lb) \times 705}{[height\ (in)]^2}$

4. A table of BMI with representative weights is included in Table 1
5. Using BMI, definitions of weight include:
   a. BMI 19–25—normal
   b. BMI 26–29—overweight
   c. BMI 30–39—obese
   d. BMI > 40—extreme obesity
6. Overweight does not always mean too much fat; physically fit persons may have BMI> 25 due to increased muscle weight

B. **Epidemiology**
   1. Obesity increasing—almost epidemic
   2. According to National Health and Nutrition Examination Survey (NHANES III) data, 55% of adult Americans are overweight (BMI > 26)
      a. Compared to as recently as 1960s when "only" 43% of adult Americans were overweight
      b. Among middle aged women, 53–64% are overweight
   3. Prevalence of obesity begins to increase around ages 20–24 years and only plateaus (at 64%) in mid-60s
   4. Higher prevalence of obesity in black, Hispanic, American Indian women than white women, regardless of education level
   5. International statistics
      a. In comparative study of France, U.K., and U.S., prevalence of obesity was highest in U.S., followed by U.K. and France
   6. Prevalence of obesity greater in people with lower level of education and income
   7. Smoking: inverse relationship between obesity and smoking was observed in France, U.K., and U.S.

TABLE 2. Partial List of Consequences of Obesity

Diabetes	Osteoarthritis	Urinary stress incontinence
Hypertension	Cholelithiasis	Infertility
Dyslipidemia	Sleep apnea	Menstrual disorders
Atherosclerotic vascular	Gastroesophageal reflux	Cancer (especially endometrium,
disease	Venous stasis	breast, ovary, colon, gallbladder)

C. **Consequences**
   1. Table 2 presents a partial list of major consequences of obesity
   2. Obesity not sole cause of listed consequences, but contributes
   3. Obesity often makes management of conditions more difficult (e.g., diabetes, hypertension, osteoarthritis of weight bearing joints)
   4. Often, minimal weight loss can help management considerably
D. **Childbearing**
   1. Estrogen and progesterone promote production of adipose tissue
      a. Enables body to prepare physiologically for childbirth
   2. Weight gained during childbearing is often difficult to lose—average weight 1 year following pregnancy is 2 kg greater
E. **Physicians' attitudes toward obesity**
   1. In one study, only 42% of patients who met criteria for obesity had diagnosis listed in chart; only one-third of those had been advised to lose weight, even when a concomitant disease known to be exacerbated by obesity was present
   2. Other surveys suggest that many doctors believe obesity is a "lack of will-power" and weight loss quite resistant to intervention
   3. Physicians who feel skilled in counseling and directing weight management programs achieve relatively high proportions of patient losing weight
F. **Eating disorders** (see Chapter 81)
   1. Binge eating and bulimia nervosa represent lack of control over eating behavior, excessive concern with body image and weight
   2. Characterized by excessive eating; often in private (embarrassed by what others may think of eating); rapid, large quantities, even to point of discomfort; often without set mealtimes
      a. Woman with bulimia nervosa additionally engages in self-induced vomiting, laxative or diuretic use, periods of fasting or vigorous exercise
   3. "Yo-yo" pattern with weight loss followed by regain of weight
G. **Causes of obesity**
   1. **Altered regulation of body weight**
      a. Metabolic theory
         i. Excess fat intake is preferentially directed to storage in adipose tissue
            (a) Protein, rather than being saved for use as structural protein and enzymes, oxidized for energy
            (b) Carbohydrates used for current energy needs before being stored as glycogen
         ii. Fats mobilized from adipose tissue only after other circulating energy sources (protein, carbohydrates) are gone
      b. Set point theory
         i. Body weight set point is predetermined biologic weight for individual
         ii. Because culture and society affect perception of desirable weight for individual, it is possible that individual's set point may be higher than societal norm, making attempts to change weight by dieting difficult
      c. Fat cell theory
         i. Adipose tissue increases by either hyperplasia (increased number of fat cells) or hypertrophy (increase in size of fat cells)
         ii. If excess fat results in hyperplasia, it is more difficult to lose weight since cells will not be allowed to die and once excess calories return, the increased number of atrophied cells ingest and store the calories

      iii. Hypertrophied cells can be allowed to atrophy, though when excess calories present, storage will result

      iv. Many obese persons, actually, probably use both mechanisms

2. **Genetic component of obesity**

   a. Anthropologic explanation

      i. Throughout the millennia, humans were far more vulnerable to famine and starvation than abundance and obesity

      ii. Natural selection favored those with ability to store excess fat—giving obesity a survival value

      iii. In current America, with excess food and limited physical exertion, obesity flourishes

   b. Family studies

      i. Heritability ranges from 0.40 to 0.60, suggesting genetics are responsible for approximately one-half of total phenotype variation in obesity

   c. Adoption studies

      i. Adoption studies suggest that environment is less important factor in determining body weight than genetics

      ii. Data also show no significant correlation between adoptees and adoptive parents

   d. Twin studies

      i. Correlation between twins reared together is similar to correlation of twins reared apart

   e. Molecular genetics has identified as many as 6 genes having some role in energy metabolism

      i. Best known is ob gene which produces leptin

      ii. Leptin appears to derive from adipose tissue and signals brain how much fat is stored

      iii. Resistance to leptin is one factor in development of extreme obesity in so-called Zucker rat

         (a) Only one, highly consanguinous family has defect similar to Zucker rat

      iv. Partial resistance to leptin, however, may be factor in some mechanisms of obesity

3. **Altered eating patterns**

   a. A new observation is evident in U.S.: people may be adjusting fat intake (which has fallen over past decade), but replacing fat with more calories from other sources.

      i. For example, a serving of fat-free ice cream actually has more calories than a similar serving of regular ice cream

   b. In attempt to follow "healthy diet," people get more calories, gain weight, and become frustrated

H. **Weight modification**

1. Very-low-calorie diets

   a. Provide < 800 kcal/day

   b. Designed to provide rapid weight loss but maintain lean body mass by providing adequate dietary protein

2. Low-calorie diets

   a. Provide nutritional needs but restrict caloric intake below caloric output

   b. Individual draws on fat stores for energy

3. Behavior modification

   a. Examines factors that contribute to weight gain, such as eating behaviors and lack of exercise

   b. Once relationship between factors is clear, maximize behaviors that contribute to weight loss

   c. Following components can help patients to self-manage weight loss

      i. Set reasonable short-term goals

      ii. Formulate specific plans to achieve goals

      iii. Develop reinforcement and social support for carrying out each element of plan

      iv. Assess progress by keeping records, including food diaries, and graphs indicating weight change

      v. Modify action plan regularly by using self-management records

I. **Yo-yo dieting**

  1. Defined as repeated weight gain and weight loss

  2. Some experts believe that repeated cycles of weight loss and weight gain may make subsequent attempts to lose weight more difficult

  3. Medical complications to yo-yo dieting as yet unspecified but concerns vary from osteoporosis (bone loss during weight loss) to heart disease (lipid deposition during weight gain)

J. **Commercial weight loss programs**

  1. **Nutrient-balanced hypocaloric diets**

    a. **Weight Watchers**

      i. Nutritionally balanced program restricting caloric intake to 1000–1500 calories/day using an exchange list of food choices

      ii. Weekly meetings include behavior modification and exercise tips; weekly "weigh-in" a major focus through peer pressure

      iii. Average cost is $1.50–$2.50/kg over 12 weeks

    b. **Nutri/System**

      i. Prepackaged foods must be purchased from program though fruits, vegetables, and beverages not included and must be purchased at extra cost

      ii. Weekly nutrition and behavior modification sessions included

      iii. Cost determined by amount of weight lost to achieve goal body weight

        (a) Ranges from $12–19/kg with higher costs to those with less weight to lose

    c. **Diet Center**

      i. Patients check in daily for weigh-in, counseling

      ii. Dairy products eliminated; supplement by soy protein to ensure adequate macronutrients

      iii. Foods purchased outside clinic

      iv. Cost varies according to current weight and goal weight

      v. Five-phase program

        (a) Conditioning reduces caloric intake and changes current eating patterns

        (b) Reducing involves nutritionally balanced diet in combination with individual supervision

        (c) Sta-b-ilite involves greater variety of foods in combination with continued supervision

        (d) Maintenance involves establishing nutritional eating habits for lifelong weight maintenance, including weekly consultation

        (e) Image-One classes provided throughout all phases, teaching behavior modification, nutrition, self-direction, stress management, and sensible exercise

    d. **Jenny Craig Weight Loss Centers**

      i. Prepackaged foods must be purchased from program; fruits, vegetables, and beverages not included and are purchased at extra cost

      ii. Cost determined by amount of weight lost to achieve ideal body weight

      iii. Weekly nutrition and behavior modification sessions included

      iv. Flat rate according to current weight and goal weight

  2. **Self-help support groups**

    a. Take Off Pounds Sensibly (TOPS)

    b. Overeaters Anonymous (OA)

III. **An Approach**

A. **Weight history**

  1. Chubbiness in childhood correlates with obesity in adulthood

    a. Combination of heredity and environment

      i. Habits start which interact with heredity to lead to lifelong struggle with weight

2. Adulthood
   a. Multiple attempts to lose weight are common
   b. Previous attempts to lose weight can give insight into unsuccessful methods
   c. Common history is weight gain with pregnancy followed by only partial loss, never completely regaining pre-pregnancy weight
B. **Behavioral intervention**
   1. The **LEARN program** for weight loss (acronym for **L**ifestyle, **E**xercise, **A**ttitudes, **R**elationships, and **N**utrition) supports systematic behavior modification approach useful for understanding and intervening in process of weight reduction
   2. **Lifestyle**
      a. Significant factor in weight reduction involves changing current eating behaviors
         i. Food diary
            (a) Keep track of what foods are eaten, assess amount and type of calories consumed
            (b) Record should be filled out immediately after eating, noting what is eaten, including snacks, as well as calories of each item
            (c) Later, more comprehensive diary records feelings, exercise, and time; goal is to record changes in behavior
         ii. Weight record to graph weekly changes
   3. **Exercise**
      a. Type of exercise prescribed based on current health condition and medical/orthopedic risk
      b. Exercise combined with dieting loses adipose tissue but preserves lean body mass
         i. Lean body mass provides increased basal metabolic demands with increased basal caloric use
      c. Walking is preferred method of exercise for most obese individuals
         i. Water aerobics an increasing option due to low impact, joint preservation
      d. Goal is exercise 5 days/week
         i. Increasing time commitment to each exercise session but eventually aim for 20–30 minutes
      e. Simple exercise actions such as walk dog, park at far end of parking lot, climb stairs, walk (don't sit) during lunch, etc.
   4. **Attitudes**
      a. Combat common view that individual is either perfect or terrible, good or bad
         i. Such beliefs contribute to distress since any lapse (weight gain) indicates that she is terrible or bad, leading to sadness and hopelessness
      b. As coping mechanism, many individuals facing such emotions turn to eating more food to feel better
   5. **Relationships**
      a. Social support can be important in weight loss
      b. Dieters also may benefit from partnership in process of weight loss
         i. Partner may be fellow dieter or nondieting participant to provide support and encouragement
      c. Spouses, relatives, and friends are candidates for partners
      d. Health care providers and counselors can be support but must avoid being sole partner
   6. **Nutrition**
      a. Many dieters unconcerned with nutritional needs
         i. So anxious to lose weight that neglect proper balanced nutritional intake
      b. Skipped meals are common but misguided effort
      c. Information about nutrition can be provided so that dieters are aware of and adhere to nutritional goals
         i. Highlights importance of trained dietitians or adequate dietary input into meal plans (e.g., commercial programs)
      d. Vitamins and supplements occasionally useful, especially in very-low-calorie diets but should not be considered a substitute for nutritionally sound program

C. **Diets**
   1. **Low-calorie diets** (LCDs)
      a. Restricted diet should provide approximately 100 g of carbohydrate and 0.8–1.2 g protein/kg ideal body weight
      b. Fat should be restricted to 25–30% total calories
      c. For adults, calories for weight loss are typically 1000–1200 kcal/day; sometimes 1500–1800 kcal/day are used if individual is active or has large frame
      d. Supplementation for vitamins and minerals recommended for diets of 1200 kcal or less
      e. Weight loss goal should be 0.25–1 kg/week
   2. **Very-low-calorie diets** (VLCDs)
      a. Developed to provide rapid weight loss
      b. Must be medically supervised
         i. May be unexpected shifts in plasma components, especially electrolytes
         ii. Early sudden death associated with hypokalemia; other blood chemistry abnormalities include serum proteins, calcium, phosphorus
         iii. Common side effects include fatigue, dizziness, constipation, irregular menses, brittle nails
         iv. Gallstones may occur in up to 11% of patients though majority remain asymptomatic
      c. Liquid formula diets allow 450–800 kcal/day, given as 3–5 shakes per day
      d. Protein-sparing modified fast (PSMF)
         i. Provides 70–120 g of protein daily along with vitamins, minerals, electrolytes and essential fatty acids but very little carbohydrate or fat
         ii. Relatively safe when done under close medical supervision
         iii. Average weight loss ranges from 2–5 kg in first week, with subsequent losses of 1–2 kg/wk for women
            (a) Average weight loss of 20 kg in 12-week programs
      e. Along with medical supervision, must have intensive counseling and support; even so, attrition rate is 33–50%
      f. Of those who persist to weight goal, 1/4 to 1/2 maintain weight loss after 1–3 years
      g. VLCDs are high in cost; patients represented in studies are of high socioeconomic status
D. **Maintenance of weight loss**
   1. Most studies of long-term maintenance show that few individuals maintain weight loss beyond 2 years
   2. Keys to maintaining weight loss
      a. Continued self-monitoring after weight loss
      b. Continued meetings with client-therapist
      c. Active participation in support groups
   3. Maintainers ($\geq$ 2 yr) reported regular exercise
   4. Dieters in therapist-supported maintenance program more likely to maintain weight loss than those with minimal support (mailings and phone calls)
E. **Pharmacologic therapy**
   1. Drug therapy of obesity has been spurred by acceptance of at least two factors:
      a. Recognition that obesity is a chronic disorder with high morbidity/mortality and needs long-term intervention (frequent analogy is with therapy of another asymptomatic condition—hypertension)
      b. Development of safer, effective medications
   2. Initially, use of amphetamine-based appetite suppressants resulted in addictive behavior and high side effect profile
      a. Use of similar agents, such as phentermine (as single agent), diethylpropion, or phendimetrazine had fewer side effects but little investigational support
   3. Though technically not a drug, Olean is a fat substitute designed to decrease saturated fats, especially in snacks, while maintaining desired cooking properties
      a. Nonabsorbed in intestines and, in large quantities, may result in occasional fecal incontinence

4. Orlistat (Xenical) an inhibitor of pancreatic lipase resulting in fat malabsorption and reduced caloric intake
   a. Weight reduction resulted in initial studies along with lipid profile change toward less LDL, slightly increased HDL
   b. Indigestion and occasional fecal incontinence occurs early in treatment
   c. Mild reduction in fat-soluble vitamin D; supplement encouraged
5. **Fen-phen**
   a. Included fenfluramine, phentermine, dexfenfluramine— popularized as "fen-phen"
   b. Side effects had included anxiousness, sleeplessness
   c. Initial concerns raised about increase in pulmonary hypertension, altered uptake at neural serotonergic receptors
   d. Most seriously, reports of cardiac valvular abnormalities, occasionally requiring replacement
      i. Pathology bore some resemblance to carcinoid-induced valvular changes
      ii. Subsequent studies have failed to develop an hypothesis, nor to detect continued changes in others than the initial proband
   e. Fenfluramine (Pondimin) and dexfenfluramine (Redux) withdrawn from market
6. Sibutramine (Meridia)
   a. Norepinephrine and serotonin reuptake inhibitor originally developed as antidepressant but subsequently noted to have weight-reduction properties
   b. Long-term studies (> 1 year) confirm weight loss in range of 5–10% body weight on dose of 15 mg/day
      i. In addition to weight loss, noted improvement in lipids, glucose tolerance
      ii. Occasional rise in BP from drug often offset by decrease in BP from weight reduction
   c. Side effects include dry mouth, constipation, insomnia, dizziness, nausea
   d. No other long-term effects noted, including heart valves
   e. Other serotonin reuptake inhibitors, such as fluoxetine and sertraline are not as effective in long-term studies
7. **Future weight loss drugs**
   a. Leptin congeners, which at present require injection
      i. May be more useful in weight maintenance
   b. Beta-agonists, acting selectively on muscle or adipose tissue, to increase metabolic rate and lipolysis
   c. Corticotropin-releasing agents
8. Adjuvant therapies in diabetics
   a. In diabetics, and, according to some experts, in obese patients with presumed Syndrome X, consider drugs to reduce insulin resistance
      i. Metformin (Glucophage) frequently ameliorates the weight gain often seen with insulin or sulfonylurea treatment of type 2 diabetics
      ii. Troglitazone (Rezulin) reduces insulin sensitivity, perhaps decreasing rebound appetite often seen in insulin-users
   b. Weight reduction improves diabetes control resulting in less medication use overall
F. **Surgery**
1. Infrequently done due to high complication rate, high cost
2. Consider for individuals with BMI > 35–40 and repeatedly unsuccessful with other means of weight loss
3. Should consider method permanent with permanent change in lives
4. Additional counseling for women of child-bearing age
   a. Metabolic consequences during rapid weight loss could be injurious to fetus
   b. May make adequate nutritional intake during pregnancy difficult
   c. Recommend contraception during rapid weight loss and intensive nutritional advice during any subsequent pregnancy
5. **Jejunoileal (intestinal) bypass**
   a. Involves bypassing most of absorptive capacity of intestine by connecting jejunum directly to terminal ileum

    b. Stomach and large intestine remain intact and bypassed portion of small intestine is left in place

    c. Weight loss substantial, ranging from 60–100 lb or more within 1 year after surgery

    d. Weight stabilizes after 2 years to a point 20–25% above ideal body weight

    e. Complications and early side effects include surgical morbidity and mortality, electrolyte imbalances, diarrhea, and abdominal discomfort

        i. Long-term complications include vitamin B_{12} and fat-soluble vitamin deficiency

        ii. Serious, irreversible liver disease (a form of fatty-liver cirrhosis) common and may be fatal

    f. Surgical and metabolic complications have virtually halted this procedure

  6. **Gastric partitioning**

    a. Closes part of stomach, reducing its reservoir capacity

    b. Gastric bypass

        i. Creates gastroenterostomy

        ii. Bypassed portion of stomach can be restored to continuity again if necessary

        iii. Complications include dumping syndrome, nausea, gallstones, and steatorrhea

    c. Gastroplasty or gastric stapling

        i. Involves partitioning stomach to allow small opening into distal stomach

        ii. Induces sensation of satiety, reduced intake

        iii. Unfortunately, pouch can be "stretched"

        iv. Complications reduced compared with bypass

        v. Weight loss is considerable, although less than from bypass

G. **Dietitian**

  1. Should be included in any comprehensive approach to weight reduction

  2. Dietitians provide knowledge and care that physicians cannot provide

  3. Dietitians are only health care professionals trained primarily to provide nutritional information

SUGGESTED READING

1. Aronne LJ: Obesity. Med Clin No Am 82:161–181, 1998.
2. Baum JG, Clark HB: Preventing relapse in obesity through posttreatment maintenance systems: Comparing the relative efficacy of two levels of therapist support. J Behav Med 14:287–302, 1992.
3. Brownell KD: The LEARN Program for Weight Control. Dallas, American Health, 1991.
4. Burke GL, Savage PJ: Correlates of obesity in young black and white women: The CARDIA study. Am J Public Health 82:1621–1625, 1992.
5. Grubbs L: The critical role of exercise in weight control. Nurse Pract 18:20–29, 1993.
6. Kayman S, Bruvold W: Maintenance and relapse after weight loss in women: Behavioral aspects. Am J Clin Nutr 52:800–807, 1992.
7. Kuczmarski RJ, Flegel KM: Increasing prevalence of overweight among U.S. adults: The National Health and Nutrition Surveys, 1960–2001. JAMA 272:205–211, 1994.
8. Laurier D, Guiguet M: Prevalence of obesity: A comparative survey in France, the United Kingdom, and the United States. Int J Obesity 16:565–572, 1991.
9. McBride AB: Fat: A women's issue in search of holistic approach to treatment. Hol Nurs Pract, Nov 9–15, 1988.
10. National Task Force on the Prevention and Treatment of Obesity: Long-term pharmacotherapy in the management of obesity. JAMA 276:1907–1911, 1996.
11. Spielman AB, Kanders B: The cost of losing: An analysis of commercial weight loss programs in a metropolitan area. J Am Coll Nutr 11:36–41, 1992.
12. Spitzer RL, Devlin M: Binge eating disorder: A multisite field trial of the diagnostic criteria. Int J Eating Disord 11:191–203, 1992.
13. Wadden TA: Treatment of obesity by moderate and severe caloric restriction: Results of clinical research trials. Ann Intern Med 119:688–693, 1993.
14. Weinsier RL, Hunter GR: The etiology of obesity: Relative contribution of metabolic factors, diet, and physical activity. Am J Med 105:145–150, 1998.

100. Hyperlipidemia

Bruce E. Johnson, M.D.

I. The Issues

There is no escaping the impact of hyperlipidemia in the U.S. Hyperlipidemia is purported to have an etiologic role in coronary artery disease (CAD), stroke, peripheral vascular disease and other vascular conditions. Heart disease kills more women than any other cause—more women die of heart disease than of all cancers combined. Although not all heart disease is related to hyperlipidemia, the complicated plaque that results in coronary narrowing has its genesis in cholesterol deposition. In women, the impact of CAD is greatest after menopause. Rates of heart disease for premenopausal women are one-fourth those for men of the same age, whereas incidence rates equalize with advancing age, reaching parity in the mid 70s. Estrogen clearly has a protective role. Even so, premature death from heart disease is a health concern for all women. Much effort is expended to identify, evaluate, and, if necessary, intervene in the processes associated with hyperlipidemia. However, recommendations made in women, especially older women, are frequently not based on the same quality data as similar recommendations in men—and all guidelines are under attack from a reconsideration of risks and costs associated with treatment of hyperlipidemia.

II. The Theory

A. Lipid metabolism

1. Cholesterol crucial to structure of cell membranes
   a. 93% of all body cholesterol in cell membranes
   b. Remaining 7% circulates and is measured in blood
   c. Cholesterol also used by liver to make bile salts and by adrenal glands and gonads in synthesis of steroid hormones
2. Total body cholesterol from two sources
   a. Intracellular production, regulated in part by 3-hydroxy-3-methylglutaryl-coenzyme A (HMG-CoA) reductase
   b. Extracellular (dietary) sources
3. **Triglycerides** transported to adipose tissue and stored until used as free fatty acids for energy
4. **Lipoproteins** transport lipids in blood
   a. Five major lipoprotein families; chylomicrons, very-low-density lipoprotein (VLDL), intermediate-density lipoprotein (IDL), low-density lipoprotein (LDL), high-density lipoprotein (HDL)
   b. Chylomicrons and VLDL transport mostly triglycerides; LDL and HDL transport mostly cholesterol
5. **Apoproteins** (also called apolipoproteins) control interactions and metabolism of lipoproteins
   a. Activate enzymes that modify composition and structure of lipoproteins
   b. Assist in exchange of lipids between lipoprotein classes
   c. Apoproteins generally under genetic control and have proved difficult to modify
6. LDL transports cholesterol to cells, where it binds to LDL receptors
   a. Once internalized, cholesterol is released
   b. Rising free intracellular cholesterol levels inhibits HMG-CoA reductase, suppressing cell's intrinsic cholesterol production
7. **HDL** functions in part as scavenger of cholesterol and triglyceride particles
   a. Scavenger role helps to remove atherogenic particles
8. **Lipid profile** altered secondarily by certain diseases or medications (Table 1)
   a. Effect may be modest (e.g., antihypertensive alpha blockers) or rather profound (e.g., some cases of uncontrolled diabetes)
   b. Any evaluation of hyperlipidemia should include appropriate search for treatable secondary condition

TABLE 1. Effect of Certain Diseases or Medications on the Lipid Profile

	LDL	HDL	Triglycerides
Hypothyroidism	↑		
Nephrotic syndrome	↑	↓	
Uncontrolled diabetes		↓	↑
Cholestatic liver disease	↑		
Chronic renal disease			↑
Obesity		↓	↑
Medications			
Alcohol		↑	↑
Anabolic steroids	↑		
Alpha blockers		↑	
Antiepileptics		↑	
Beta blockers		↓	↑
Estrogen		↑	↑
Glucocorticoids		↑	↑
Isoretinoin		↓	↑
Progestins	↑	↓	
Thiazides	↑	↓	↑

B. **Lipids and lipid-related cardiovascular risk**
   1. LDL oxidation apparent final common pathway in development of atherosclerosis
      a. LDL strongly associated with CAD
   2. HDL protective against CAD
      a. Low HDL seen as risk for CAD
   3. Apolipoprotein E (apoE) phenotype
      a. Isotype E4 codes for LDL/HDL ratio with high risk for CAD, especially in women
      b. Cannot change phenotype but intervention to lower LDL lowers risk
   4. Apolipoprotein C-III lipoprotein positive risk factor
   5. Lipoprotein a [Lp(a)] yet another identified risk for CAD
      a. Attaches to apolipoprotein (a) and leads to accumulation of apo(a) in vessel wall
      b. Also decreases fibrinolytic activity of plasminogen
   6. Not all cardiovascular risk factors are lipids
      a. Increasing interest in abnormal coagulation factors, inflammatory processes, even altered cell repair and growth factors
      b. Table 2 lists only some of the traditional and newly recognized CAD risk factors though abnormal lipids are among the most important
      c. Not all risk factors are established or modifiable

TABLE 2. Traditional and Recently Identified Cardiovascular Risk Factors

Family history of premature CAD	Apolipoprotein E
Female > 55 or premature menopause without HRT	Apolipoprotein C-III
Male > age 45	Lipoprotein (a)
Obesity (> 35% ideal body weight)	Plasminogen activator inhibitor
Diabetes mellitus	Tissue plasminogen activator
Sedentary lifestyle	Cell adhesion molecules
Hypertension	Homocysteine
Smoking	Ferritin
High total cholesterol	Transforming growth factor
High LDL	Vitamin D
Low HDL	*Chlamydia pneumoniae* antibodies

7. Recommendations for "normal" and "abnormal" cholesterol noted below; measurement of individual's cholesterol and intervention with certain risk factors is strongly advocated by National Cholesterol Education Program (NCEP)
   a. Group including both government and private organizations
   b. Proposes studies and interprets results
   c. Develops guidelines and recommendations, then widely disseminates conclusions
   d. Strong advocate for multimodality approach to lowering CAD risk through combination of identification of risk factors (primarily lipids), modification of lifestyle concerns, and drug intervention if necessary

C. **Clinical manifestations of hyperlipidemia**
   1. **Cholesterol**
      a. Vascular disease including: coronary artery disease with myocardial infarction: cerebrovascular disease with stroke; peripheral vascular disease with claudication, renal artery stenosis, mesenteric stenosis
      b. Certain familial hypercholesterol syndromes, in addition to blood cholesterol levels > 300 mg/dl and premature vascular disease, also present with tendon xanthomas
   2. **Triglycerides**
      a. Hypertriglyceridemia may be isolated finding or in combination with hypercholesterolemia
         i. Elevated triglyceride poses independent risk for premature vascular disease, especially peripheral
      b. Very high levels of triglyceride (i.e., > 1500–2000 mg/dl) associated with pancreatitis, eruptive xanthomas, and vascular "sludging"

D. **Role of estrogen**
   1. Lipid profile before and after menopause changes
      a. Total cholesterol rises after menopause
         i. HDL tends to fall
         ii. LDL tends to rise
      b. Triglyceride varies but may rise
   2. Postmenopausal women given estrogen replacement show trend toward premenopausal lipid profile
      a. Estrogen lowers LDL and raises HDL
   3. Progesterone as single agent tends to raise LDL in premenopausal females
   4. In postmenopausal women, combined estrogen and progesterone therapy has no adverse effects on lipid profile
   5. Estrogen lowers Lp(a) levels

E. **Evidence of treatment efficacy**
   1. **Epidemiology**
      a. Reduction of CAD mortality in persons on HRT 35–45%
      b. Observational (e.g., Nurses Health Study); multiple other factors not taken into account
   2. **Primary prevention** (i.e., studies in which selection based on risk factors, primarily cholesterol level)
      a. AFCAPS/TexCAPS one of few primary prevention studies to include women
         i. Used lovastatin to raise low HDL levels
         ii. Reported 36% reduction in acute coronary events and 33% reduction in unstable angina
         iii. Unusual study in that total cholesterol normal but HDL low—supporting role of low HDL as risk factor (and that interventions to raise HDL protective)
   3. Secondary prevention (i.e., studies in which selection based on known presence of CAD, either by documented infarct, unstable angina or angiographic evidence)
      a. At least 5 large scale studies, all including a statin, with somewhat different entrance criteria, have included enough women to conclude that lowering total or LDL cholesterol effective in reducing subsequent events (or in reducing the size of an angiographic lesion)
      b. Some suggestions that secondary prevention may have more impact in women than men

      i. May be related to smaller size of coronary arteries in women; even modest reduction in plaque size improves blood flow by greater degree

F. **Controversy**

1. Skepticism persists regarding scope of NCEP recommendations and current practice
2. Skepticism focuses on groups addressed in this book—women, especially post-menopausal and older women
3. Data for men solid, both primary and secondary prevention. This seems to extend to older men as well (though number > 65 included in studies limited)
4. For women, virtually no data for:
   a. Screening
      i. Different groups have developed screening guidelines but these vary widely, e.g., for women with no risk factors initial screening exam ranges from age 20–45
   b. Primary prevention, with recent APCAPS/TexCAPS only study including women (to be fair, with positive results)
   c. Level of cholesterol for intervention
      i. Many women, especially premenopausal, may exceed NCEP levels for total cholesterol but have disproportionate elevation of HDL
      ii. NCEP has been downplaying the HDL/LDL ratio which corrects for high HDL (though, to be fair, NCEP states that HDL> 60 negates another risk factor)
5. Controversy raised regarding cost/benefit of cholesterol intervention, especially in normal or low-risk persons
   a. Prevalence of CAD in premenopausal women is hard to know is studies could even demonstrate a cost/benefit advantage
   b. Costs can be high: for example, estimated it may cost from $25,000/life year for men age 55–64 with risk factors and cholesterol > 300, to $520,000/life year for men age 35–44 with cholesterol > 300 but no other risk factors
      i. Estimates can barely be attempted in women due to much lower prevalence in similar age groups
6. Finally, in the older age group where prevalence of CAD does increase, there is virtually no data that intervention in women (or men) carries an advantage without prior CAD disease (i.e., secondary intervention)

III. **An Approach**

A. **Screening**

1. Recommendations on frequency vary (Table 3)

TABLE 3. Recommendations by Selected Organizations Regarding Lipid Screening*

Organization	Total Cholesterol	HDL Cholesterol	Age Range	Interval
USPSTF (1996)	Yes	No	Male 35–65 Female 45–65	Every 5 years
NCEP/AHA (1994)	Yes	Yes	20+ (no upper limit)	Every 5 years (low risk)
				Every 1–2 years (mild elevations)
ACP (1996)	Yes	No	Male 35–65 Female 45–65	Every 5 years
AAFP (1994)	Yes	No	19+ (no upper limit)	Every 5 years
ACOG (1993)	Yes	No	Female 20+ (no upper limit)	Periodic

USPSTF, U.S. Preventive Services Task Force; NCEP/AHA, National Cholesterol Education Program/American Heart Association; ACP, American College of Physicians; AAFP, American Academy of Family Physicians; ACOG, American College of Obstetricians and Gynecologists.
* All groups assume no additional risk factors and do not include recommendations for other lipid-related measurements (e.g., Lp(a), homocysteine). Furthermore, if the screening value falls outside recommended levels, a full lipid profile including HDL and LDL should be performed.

a. Controversy heated on both ends of age scale (i.e., age of onset of screening, age at cessation of screening)
b. Only one group recommends HDL as part of initial screen
   i. Controversy because HDL difficult to modify through diet, exercise and most medications
c. All groups say that if risk factors are present (smoking, hypertension, diabetes, etc.) screening should be more comprehensive
2. Issue regarding HDL of particular concern to women
a. HDL > 60 frequent in premenopausal women, especially if on OC, postmenopausal women on HRT
b. Elevated HDL contributes to total cholesterol and may give "false positive" total cholesterol measurement
   i. Some experts suggest automatically including HDL in screen test in women liable to have baseline elevation
3. If total cholesterol > 200 mg/dl and/or HDL < 35 mg/dl, fasting triglycerides should be assessed
B. **Diagnosis**
1. Lipid measurement
a. Total cholesterol and HDL accurate (± 11%) for nonfasting specimen; triglycerides and LDL require 9–12 hour fast
b. When triglycerides < 400 mg/dl, can calculate LDL
   i. LDL = Total cholesterol – (HDL) – (TG/5)
c. Lipid levels termed desirable, borderline, and high
   i. Note: values are given for adult men and women; some sources believe that low HDL cholesterol for women should be < 40 mg/dl
2. **Assessment of risk factors**
a. Definite CAD
   i. Definite prior myocardial infarction
   ii. Definite myocardial ischemia (e.g., angina)
b. Other risk factors
   i. See Table 2 (some also include previous cerebrovascular and peripheral vascular disease)
   ii. The risk factors that "count" are the traditional risk factors in the left column
3. **Interpretation of values**
a. No intervention (other than general guidance regarding diet, weight control, and exercise) needed if
   i. Total cholesterol < 200 mg/dl
   ii. LDL < 130 mg/dl
   iii. HDL > 40 mg/dl in females
   iv. No definite risk factor
   v. Not more than one other risk factor

TABLE 4. Lipid Level Definitions (Men and Women)

Total cholesterol		Triglycerides	
Desirable	< 200 mg/dl	Normal	< 200 mg/dl
Borderline high	200–239 mg/dl	Borderline high	200–400 mg/dl
High	> 240 mg/dl	High	400–1000 mg/dl
LDL cholesterol		Very high	> 1000 mg/dl
Desirable	< 130 mg/dl		
Borderline high	130–159 mg/dl		
High	> 160 mg/dl		
HDL cholesterol			
Low	< 35 (or 40) mg/dl		

From Expert Panel on Detection, Evaluation and Treatment of High Blood Cholesterol in Adults: Summary of the Second Report of the National Cholesterol Evaluation Program (NCEP) Expert Panel on Detection, Evaluation and Treatment of High Blood Cholesterol in Adults (Adult Treatment Panel II). JAMA 269:3015–3023, 1991.

   b. Borderline high total cholesterol, HDL < 40 mg/dl with fewer than two other risk factors requires diet, weight, and exercise intervention and reevaluation within 1–2 years

   c. Borderline high values with two or more risk factors may require more intensive treatment, including drug therapy

   d. Total cholesterol > 240 mg/dl and/or LDL > 160 mg/dl requires intervention, including consideration of drug therapy

   e. Triglycerides
     i. Risk for CAD may be increased in > 400 mg/dl range

C. **Interventions and treatments**
  1. **Diet**
   a. "Typical" American diet consists of approximately 40% total calories from fat, 30–40% from carbohydrates, and 20–30% from protein
     i. Fats include too much saturated fatty acid and dietary cholesterol
   b. American Heart Association has proposed a two-step dietary intervention for persons with elevated cholesterol
     i. Step-one diet (reasonable goal for entire U.S. population)
       (a) Total calories to maintain desirable weight
       (b) Fat < 30% total calories (10% from saturated fat)
       (c) Carbohydrates 50–60% total calories
       (d) Protein 10–20% total calories
       (e) Cholesterol < 300 mg/day
     ii. Step-two diet (hyperlipidemia persists despite step-one diet)
       (a) Same as step-one diet except fat < 20% total calories (saturated fat < 7%) and cholesterol < 200 mg/day
   c. Special dietary consideration in patients with very high triglycerides
     i. For values > 1000 mg/dl, immediately institute very low fat diet
     ii. Rapid lowering of triglyceride important to prevent pancreatitis
   d. Dietary guidance can be difficult
     i. Education to identify types of foods, learn how to read side labels, encourage lean portions of meats, etc.
     ii. Special shopping and preparation, not just smaller portions of meals
     iii. Instruction and frequent reinforcement by dietitian/nutritionist
     vi. For best results, requires cooperation of spouse and other household members; impractical to prepare separate meals
   e. Alcohol
     i. To excess, elevates total cholesterol and triglycerides
     ii. In moderation, may increase HDL
   f. Calcium
     i. Purported to reduce total and LDL cholesterol
     ii. Interferes with fat absorption
   g. Fiber
     i. Soluble dietary fibers lower total and LDL cholesterol (e.g., oat bran/oatmeal, wheat bran)
   h. Coffee
     i. Filtered coffee has no effect on lipid levels
     ii. Boiled coffee may raise total and LDL cholesterol

  2. **Exercise**
   a. Independent factor in alteration of lipid profile
   b. In men, exercise lowers triglycerides and raises HDL; in women, effect not as pronounced and exercise may lower HDL and increase triglycerides modestly (in postmenopausal women)
   c. Even with no alteration in lipid profile, exercise associated with fewer cardiac events

  3. **Weight control**
   a. Almost always lowers triglyceride levels
   b. Effect on cholesterols varies in women

       i. LDL lowered or unchanged

       ii. HDL may not be improved with weight control

  c. Differences in response to weight control may relate to body weight distribution

       i. High waist-to-hip ratio correlated with coronary events; this is typical weight distribution in men and some postmenopausal women

4. **Exogenous hormones**

  a. Effects on lipids

       i. In general, estrogens raise HDL, lower LDL, and may raise triglycerides

       ii. In general, progestins raise LDL, lower HDL, and somewhat lower triglycerides

  b. Effects on vessel walls

       i. Estrogen may decrease LDL uptake by arterial wall, decrease arterial spasm, and decrease platelet adhesiveness in areas of plaque

       ii. Even without positive alteration of lipid profile by progestins, net effect from combined administration of hormones is favorable

  c. Oral contraceptives (OCs)

       i. Current choices use more lipid neutral progestins, may be even more advantageous

       ii. Use of OCs with 15-year follow-up shows no increase in CAD events

       iii. Any beneficial effect negated for older women on OC who smoke

  d. Postmenopausal hormone replacement therapy

       i. No intervention studies of unopposed estrogen

         (a) Cohort (observational) studies show decline in risk of coronary events (primary prevention)

         (b) Other studies in women with established coronary disease show increased survival (secondary prevention)

       ii. Most women with intact uterus are given progestin to prevent endometrial hyperplasia; cross-sectional studies suggest added progestin does not adversely affect CAD protection

       iii. Recent evidence concludes both oral and percutaneous estrogen has beneficial effect on lipids

       iv. In treatment of hyperlipidemia, especially in postmenopausal female, estrogens should be considered if not contraindicated

5. **Nicotinic acid** (niacin)

  a. Mechanism involves reduced lipolysis, inhibition of synthesis of lipoproteins, and shift in HDL subtypes

  b. In patients with combined hyperlipidemias, nicotinic acid can lower LDL by 20–35% and triglycerides by 20–40%, and raise HDL by 10–20%

  c. Effective dose: 3–6 g/day given in divided doses

       i. Typically start 100–200 mg/day with meals

  d. Side effects numerous

       i. Most noticeable is flushing, especially with higher doses; may be inhibited with aspirin or nonsteroidal anti-inflammatory drugs taken prior to nicotinic acid dose

       ii. Other side effects include nausea, abdominal bloating, skin dryness, visual changes

       iii. Laboratory abnormalities include glucose, uric acid, aminotransferases, alkaline phosphatase

  e. Preparations developed to minimize side effects

       i. Sustained-release formulations differ in efficacy and side effects

       ii. Derivatives have less flushing but poorer lipid-lowering effects and continue to carry risk to liver

  f. Non–sustained-release formulations relatively inexpensive

6. **Bile acid sequestrants**

  a. Cholestyramine and colestipol

  b. Bind bile acids in intestinal lumen and excrete in stool

       i. Stimulate hepatic production of bile acids from cholesterol, lowering hepatic levels of cholesterol and recruiting LDL from blood

    c. Lowers LDL by 15–30% with modest increase in HDL and triglycerides

    d. Usual dose: cholestyramine, 8–16 g/day (2–4 scoops); colestipol, 10–20 g/day (2–4 packets)

        i. Because it is a resin binder, sequestrants should be taken with meals, and most other drugs (especially beta blockers, digitalis, thyroxin, warfarin) should be taken well apart from sequestrants

        ii. May also interfere with absorption of folic acid and vitamin K

    e. Side effects

        i. Greatest difficulty is bowel function, including constipation, bloating, nausea, flatulence, indigestion, anorexia, and exacerbation of hemorrhoids—frequently leads to medication failure

        ii. Transient changes in liver enzymes

    f. Costly

7. **HMG-CoA reductase inhibitors** (the "statins")

    a. At least 6 currently FDA-approved and marketed

    b. Interfere with synthesis of cholesterol by inhibiting HMG-CoA reductase enzyme

    c. Reduce LDL by 30–40% and triglycerides by 10–30%, and increase HDL by up to 15%

    d. Several features currently make statins a frequent, first-choice medication

        i. Effectiveness as demonstrated in both primary and secondary prevention trials

        ii. Ease of use (pill, often taken only once daily), few side effects, patient acceptance

    e. Usual doses: lovastatin, 10–80 mg/day; pravastatin, 10–40 mg/day; simvastatin, 10–40 mg/day, etc.

    f. Side effects

        i. Generally well-tolerated; mild nausea, fatigue, myalgias, change in bowel function, skin rashes

        ii. Less common but more serious includes elevation in liver enzymes and myopathy (especially when combined with cyclosporine, nicotinic acid, or gemfibrozil)

        iii. Recommend monitoring liver enzymes and creatine phosphokinase (CPK) first and third month and 6–12 months thereafter

    g. Relatively expensive

8. **Fibrates**

    a. Clofibrate and gemfibrozil

    b. Lower LDL by 5–10%; virtually no effect on HDL; may have significant (up to 30%) effect on triglycerides

        i. Gemfibrozil especially indicated in severe hypertriglyceridemia

    c. Usual dose: clofibrate, 2 g/day; gemfibrozil, 1200 mg/day

    d. Side effects

        i. Generally well-tolerated; most side effects gastrointestinal, with other complaints being headache, rash, urticaria

        ii. Increase bile acid lithogenicity and may cause gallstones

        iii. Increase liver enzymes; monitoring appropriate

    e. Relatively expensive

9. **Other treatments**

    a. Neomycin

        i. May lower LDL by 10% but infrequently recommended because of impairment in renal function and ototoxicity

    b. Fish oils

        i. May lower triglycerides more than cholesterols; also effective in decreasing platelet adhesiveness

        ii. Large doses—up to 12 capsules/day

        iii. Side effects include changes in bowel function, "fishy" taste but no adverse liver effects

        iv. At 12 capsules/day, relatively expensive

    c. Garlic
        i. Typically comes as concentrated garlic extract
        ii. Anecdotal effectiveness: placebo-controlled and/or cross-over studies lacking
        iii. Probably safe, might be considered in patients with mild hyperlipidemia

D. **Other issues**
  1. **Xanthelasma**
    a. Usually associated with hypercholesterolemia
      i. May occur in persons with normal cholesterol levels
    b. Raised fleshy/yellow-colored lesions located near eyes
    c. May occur early in life
    d. Usually persist despite cholesterol control
  2. **Xanthoma**
    a. Over tendons (tendinous xanthoma), especially Achilles, dorsum of hand, knee, elbow
      i. Modified by control of cholesterol
    b. Eruptive xanthoma
      i. Dramatic, sudden appearance of pinkish, raised plaques on trunk and back
      ii. Associated with very high levels of cholesterol and usually disappear with treatment
  3. **Arcus corneae**
    a. Circular, whitish deposits in pupil
    b. Not always associated with hypercholesterolemia
  4. **Pancreatitis**
    a. Occurs in hypertriglyceridemia, usually with levels > 1000 mg/dl
    b. Occasionally severe, life-threatening
    c. Requires immediate dietary intervention
      i. Very low saturated fat, low cholesterol diet
    d. Drug therapy includes atorvastatin, nicotinic acid, gemfibrozil
      i. If these drugs used together, heightened awareness of liver enzyme elevations
  5. **Pregnancy**
    a. Typically raises cholesterol by as much as 50%
      i. Peaks in second trimester
    b. Triglycerides increase significantly
      i. Peak in third trimester
      ii. With prepregnancy hypertriglyceridemia, elevation may be dangerous—risk of pancreatitis without dietary intervention
    c. In women without underlying lipid abnormality, rarely of clinical significance
    d. Lipids decline rapidly after delivery
      i. Reach baseline within 6 weeks
    e. Transient elevations not associated with increased CAD risk
  6. **Cholesterol and violence**
    a. Persistent reports and meta-analysis suggest increased violent death by homicide, suicide or accident in men with low cholesterol
      i. Studies including women show similar trend but not statistical significance
    b. Most frequent cut-off is total cholesterol < 160
    c. In studies including both men and women, odds ratio 1.17–1.55
    d. Purported reason—lower cholesterol could lead to lower serotonin and low serotonin as a causal link to violence has some support, especially in nonhuman primates
    e. Data not solid enough to deny treatment but disquieting

SUGGESTED READING

1. American College of Physicians: Clinical Guideline Part 1: Guidelines for using serum cholesterol, high-density lipoprotein cholesterol and triglyceride levels as screening tests for preventing coronary heart disease in adults. Ann Intern Med 124:515–517, 1996.
2. Ballantyne CM: Current thinking in lipid lowering. Am J Med 104:33S–41S, 1998.
3. Downs JR, Clearfield M: Primary prevention of acute coronary events with lovastatin in men and women with average cholesterol levels: Results of AFCAPS/TexCAPS. JAMA 279:1615–1622, 1998.

4. Expert Panel on Detection, Evaluation and Treatment of High Blood Cholesterol in Adults: Summary of the Second Report of the National Cholesterol Evaluation Program (NCEP) Expert Panel on Detection, Evaluation and Treatment of High Blood Cholesterol in Adults (Adult Treatment Panel II). JAMA 269: 3015–3023, 1993.

5. Golomb BA: Cholesterol and violence: Is there a connection? Ann Intern Med 128:478–487, 1998.

6. Hunninghake DB (ed): Lipid Disorders. Med Clin North Am 78:1–266, 1994.

7. Ory SJ, Field CS: Effects of long-term transdermal administration of estradiol on serum lipids. Mayo Clin Proc 73:735–738, 1998.

8. Pearson TA: Lipid lowering therapy in low-risk patients. JAMA 279:1659–1660, 1998.

9. Stampfer MJ, Coldtiz GA: Postmenopausal estrogen therapy and cardiovascular disease. N Engl J Med 325:756–762, 1991.

10. Taylor PA, Ward A: Women, high-density lipoprotein cholesterol, and exercise. Arch Intern Med 153:1178–1184, 1993.

11. Vaziri SM, Evans JC, Larson MG, et al: The impact of female hormone usage on the lipid profile. Arch Intern Med 153:2200–2206, 1993.

12. Wood PD, Stefanick MC, Williams PT, et al: The effects on plasma lipoproteins of a prudent weight-reducing diet, with and without exercise, in overweight men and women. N Engl J Med 325:461–466, 1991.

PART XIII
CANCERS

101. Breast Cancer

Bruce E. Johnson, M.D.

I. **The Issues**

Few diseases carry as heavy an emotional burden for women as breast cancer. The breasts are such an integral aspect of femininity that most women feel an intimate violation when confronted with disease of the breasts. Even beyond the symbolic significance, the surgery required to treat breast cancer was, until recent years, particularly disfiguring. Finally, the fear and dread of breast cancer is well placed. Many women face this disease; perhaps as many as 1 in 9 of all women develop breast cancer at some time in their lives. Breast cancer is the second leading cause of cancer death in the U.S. For these reasons and more, the interest in breast cancer is intense, and the patient may confront the primary care physician with concerns well beyond the scope of this book. However, three areas germane to primary care practice will be addressed: (1) the issue of risk factors for breast cancer and whether, or even if, these risk factors are modifiable; (2) practices regarding screening, with special emphasis on mammography; and (3) interactions with specialists (surgeons, oncologists) regarding breast cancer. Issues of counseling, within the expected knowledge base of the primary care practitioner, are also considered.

II. **The Theory**

A. **Epidemiology**

1. Too simplistic to state that 1 in 9 American women develop breast cancer
    a. Stratify by age
        i. For example, the risk of a 35-year-old woman developing cancer over the next 10 years is only 0.9%
        ii. By contrast, the risk of a 65-year-old woman developing cancer over the next 10 years jumps to 3.17%
    b. Only when considering all women over a lifetime is the cumulative risk of developing breast cancer 10.2% (or 1 in 9)
    c. Risk of dying of breast cancer over a lifetime is 3.6% (or 1 in 28)
2. Annually, 182,000 new cases of breast cancer (1997 data)
    a. After skin cancer, leading site of cancer detection in women
3. Annually, 46,000 deaths from breast cancer
    a. Second leading cause of cancer death behind lung cancer
4. Concern regarding "epidemic" of breast cancer may be overblown
    a. Recent cancer data show leveling of incidence (new diagnosis) since early 1990s
        i. Number of deaths from cancer has not appreciably changed since 1930s; since there is a greatly increased population of women, this means better detection and treatment is improving survival
    b. Data fueling "epidemic" fears may be related to detection bias, especially in older women who otherwise might die "with" rather than "of" cancer
5. Intense media coverage of breast cancer seems to focus on younger women (< 50 years); an apparent increase in numbers of young women with breast cancer actually reflects not greater incidence but greater total numbers due to more women at risk in their 40s and 50s ("baby-boomers")

B. **Risk factors**

1. Majority of women with breast cancer (60–75%) had no risk factor beyond advancing age
    a. This fact puts risk factors in some perspective

TABLE 1.   Risk Factors for Breast Cancer

Advancing age	Previous breast biopsy?	Hormonal manipulation
Over age 40	Atypical hyperplasia	Postmenopausal hormone
	Lobular neoplasia	replacement
Breast cancer in relative	Menstruation and	Oral contraceptives
Premenopausal status	pregnancy	
Previous breast cancer	Menarche before age 12	Obesity
	Menopause after age 55	Android distribution
BRCA-1 and 2 genes	Nulliparity	
	First pregnancy after	Environmental factors
Other cancers	age 30	Fats in diet
Previous endometrial or colon cancer		Heavy alcohol use
Colon cancer in first-degree relative		Radiation exposure

2. Consensus of risk factors (Table 1)
   a. Risk begins to rise about age 40
      i. Increased incidence after menopause
      ii. No plateau of risk, although stage of disease at detection may decrease after age 75
   b. Breast cancer in relative
      i. Odds ratio for woman who has first-degree relative with breast cancer—2.45; second-degree relative—1.8; third-degree relative—1.35
      ii. Risk may be negligible if relative developed cancer after age 70
      iii. Difficult to quantify, but risk increased if mother developed breast cancer before menopause
   c. BRCA-1 and 2 genes identified as conferring increased risk for both breast and ovarian cancer
      i. Alarmingly, as high as 50–60% risk of breast cancer by age 80
      ii. Gene is seen in frequency as high as 2.5% in Ashkenazi Jews, < 1% in overall population
      iii. Guidelines for screening have not been developed; neither have guidelines for interventions such as preventive measures or prophylactic surgery (mastectomy)
         (a) Concern regarding discrimination by employer and/or insurer
   d. Time interval between early menarche and later age at first pregnancy supports view that cancer development can be altered by pregnancy
   e. Postmenopausal hormone replacement
      i. Complicated, controversial issue with studies varying in design and conclusions
      ii. Variables include type of estrogen used, e.g., Swedish study, suggesting increased risk, looked largely at estradiol while in U.S., conjugated estrogens are more commonly used as replacement therapy and definitive studies not published
      iii. Developing consensus that estrogens used alone may have modest increased risk (relative risk: 1.2–1.7); possibility that combination with progestogens may confer modest protection
   f. Role of fat in diet and other environmental toxins unclear
      i. Some evidence that polyunsaturated fats associated with increased risk but many confounders; modification of fat in diet is valued for many reasons, but decreasing risk of breast cancer not yet confirmed
      ii. Heavy alcohol use and previous exposure to therapeutic radiation both increase risk
   g. Xenoestrogens (chemicals in environment such as organochlorides having weak estrogenic activity) have not been supported in recent studies as breast cancer risk factors
3. A negative risk factor is breastfeeding
   a. Longer length of time breastfeeding, and multiple breastfed children reduces overall risk
C. **Screening**
   1. No question that screening (breast self-exam, clinical breast exam, mammography) detects cancers at earlier stage

    a. Earlier stage translates into more conservative treatment options, better outcomes

    b. Also clear that mammography fulfills ideal criteria for screening test

        i. Test applied to general population that has both high sensitivity and specificity and for which early detection results in better outcome

    c. Question and concern arise in trying to balance appropriate intervals for screening test against costs of performing test

2. Several organizations have made recommendations for screening

    a. Recommendations not identical, reflecting differing interpretations of available data, differing screening approaches

    b. Most commonly cited recommendations from U.S. Preventive Services Task Force (USPSTF), National Cancer Institute (NCI), American Cancer Society (ACS), American College of Physicians (ACP), Canadian Task Force on Periodic Health Examination (CTFPHE)

3. **Breast self-exam** (BSE)

    a. Little controversy; most organizations recommend all women begin BSE at age 20

    b. BSE should be performed monthly and should occur at the end of menstrual period when hormonally sensitive glandular tissue likely to be smaller and softer, and less likely to be interpreted as a "lump"

    c. Patient must be taught and physician willing to perform reexamination when patient feels change during BSE

    d. Although sensitivity and specificity of BSE is poor, it has low cost and encourages involvement by patient

    e. See Chapter 122 (Breast Examination)

4. **Clinical breast exam**

    a. Examination performed by physician or specially trained provider

        i. Numerous studies unfortunately suggest that exam performed rather poorly by physicians, if at all

        ii. Exam by specially trained provider often more comprehensive and more likely to be accompanied by teaching of BSE

    b. Done properly, requires a time commitment of 3–11 minutes for this exam alone

    c. Clinical breast exam should start at age 20 and be performed every 3 years until age 40; after age 40 yearly clinical breast exam recommended

    d. Current study in Canada contrasts mammography with clinical breast exam against clinical breast exam alone

        i. Initial reports suggest clinical breast exam may be substituted for mammography for some subgroups of women but study has been criticized for design and interpretation biases

    e. See Chapter 122 (Breast Examination)

5. **Mammography**

    a. Difficult issue to advise women since recommendations are modified frequently

    b. Most controversy involves women younger than 50 and women older than 70–75

        i. Age 50 chosen as typical age of menopause

        ii. After age 70–75, data becomes unclear regarding survival outcome even after detection

            (a) Probably represents more indolent tumor biology and mortality from causes other than breast cancer

    c. Premenopausal breast more difficult to examine by mammogram

        i. Premenopausal breast has more glandular tissue which is dense, retarding passage of x-rays

        ii. Before microcalcification occurs, early changes of cancer growth gives dense appearance on mammogram; early cancer growth hidden by denser glandular tissue

        iii. Postmenopausal breast has relatively more fat; denser cancer tissue stands out better

        iv. Difficulties in interpretation may mean more false-positive mammograms

(a) Results in more additional testing (e.g., sonography) and more biopsies—all increasing costs without increasing detection or changing mortality
(b) False-positive test also causes fear and worry

d. Other issues of importance in implementing recommendations
   i. Quality of mammogram facility with up-to-date equipment and well-trained radiology technicians
   ii. Skills of interpreter
     (a) Even among skilled radiologists, interpretation varies in 8–10% of cases
   iii. Concern for excessive radiation
     (a) New equipment and high sensitivity screen-film reduces radiation exposure to virtually inconsequential amounts
     (b) One estimate puts the risk of lifetime of mammograms at less than pack of cigarettes

e. Problems with false-positive screening very real
   i. 6-year study, women age 40–69, with median 4 mammograms and 5 clinical exams showed almost 24% with at least one false-positive mammogram and 13% with one false-positive clinical breast exam
   ii. Lead to unnecessary procedures: over 20% of participants in study had biopsy without breast cancer
   iii. For every $100 spent on screening mammograms, $33 spent on evaluating false-positive results

f. Screening recommendations for women less than age 50 (premenopause)
   i. Because of problems with adequate screening, it has been difficult to document improvement in outcome (i.e., improved mortality rate) by screening mammogram in 40–49 age group, which makes this a controversial group for establishing guidelines
     (a) Only recently, with pooled data by meta-analysis has data come forth with small survival benefit from screening younger women
   ii. Most organizations no longer recommend baseline mammogram at age 35
   iii. ACS and NCI suggest screening mammogram at 1–2 year intervals, beginning age 40, for all women
   iv. ACP, USPSTF, CTFPHE do not recommend screening mammogram for age 40–49 for low risk women
   v. All groups recommend screening mammogram every 1–2 years for women at high risk (primarily on basis of first-degree relative) beginning age 40

g. Screening recommendations for women aged 50–59
   i. All organizations recommend screening mammogram every 1–2 years

h. Screening recommendations for women aged 60–70/75
   i. Some divergence, largely based on mortality outcomes for older women
   ii. ACS and NCI do not specifically address question and let stand recommendation for yearly mammogram age > 50
   iii. USPHTF and ACP continue recommendation for yearly (or every other year) mammogram to age 69
   iv. CTFPHE makes no specific recommendation for screening mammogram after age 59

i. Screening recommendations for women age > 70/75
   i. ACS and NCI imply continued yearly mammogram (unless woman "in good health"); other organizations drop screening recommendation

j. There is another source of "recommendation"
   i. Medicare regulations restrict payment for screening mammograms to no more than every 2 years; since Medicare generally covers population older than 65, this is a de facto recommendation (that has not been seriously challenged by other organizations)

k. All organizations acknowledge that certain circumstances require enhanced awareness and screening
   i. Women at high risk on basis of previous breast cancer, strong family history, previous colon, uterine or ovarian cancer, etc.

      ii. Research in other detection strategies for high-risk women, including more frequent mammogram or even periodic breast needle aspiration and cytologic examination for dysplastic cells

D. **Prevention of breast cancer**
1. Spurred by considerable research and lay interest
2. Investigative efforts have focused on lifestyle modifications
3. **Fat intake**
   a. Several epidemiologic studies suggest increased fat intake increases risk for breast cancer; subsequent investigation has tried to identify the fat component of diet which may reduce risk
      i. In Western societies, much of increased fat intake due to animal dietary sources; vegetarians in all societies have reduced, but not absent, breast cancer
   b. Any modification of fat type, short of total reduction, difficult to support though recent indication that reduced polyunsaturated fats may be associated with slightly lower risk than reduced monounsaturated fats
   c. Entire issue may be surrogate for obesity (i.e., diet higher in fats more likely to result in obesity) and obesity relatively strong risk factor—and the reason may relate more to higher estrogen levels in overweight women rather than the components of an obese person's diet
4. **Micro- and macronutrient supplements**
   a. Suggestions that beta-carotene, calcium and vitamin E may have some protective effect in younger women difficult to demonstrate as women age
      i. Little support for megavitamin supplements nor for supplements other than those listed
   b. High fiber diet (which tends to be low in fat) associated with reduced risk
   c. Soy protein–based diets have laboratory (both rat and human breast cancer cell line) support of inhibited cancer growth
5. **Exercise**
   a. Despite multiple efforts to find a reduction in breast cancer in women who exercise vigorously, the data cannot support such a recommendation
   b. Exercise known effective to prevent other conditions (e.g., cardiovascular disease, osteoporosis) and is important in weight control, but not yet an independent factor in risk reduction for breast cancer
6. **Vitamin D**
   a. Vitamin D may inhibit breast cancer cell proliferation
   b. In U.S., some stratification of breast cancer incidence between northern and southern states (with slightly less breast cancer in southern states)
   c. Some protection may be present from casual exposure to sunlight—though only applies to white women, not black women
7. **Oral contraceptives**
   a. Long-standing recognition that oral contraceptive use, even for short period of time as young adult, associated with reduced cancer risk
   b. May be related to progesterone component which is antiproliferative to breast cells
8. **Tamoxifen**
   a. When given to women with cancer of one breast, tamoxifen significantly reduced recurrence in that breast or development of cancer in contralateral breast.
   b. Use as primary prevention, in women with higher than normal risk, resulted in reduced breast cancer by 26% or more in all age groups when compared to placebo
      i. Also resulted in reduced osteoporotic fractures
   c. Tamoxifen has increased rate of vascular events and endometrial cancer
   d. Study of reloxifen in osteoporosis had unexpected, but welcome, result of decreased breast cancer, without increased endometrial cancer
   e. Hope that other selective estrogen receptor modulators (SERMs), fenretinide (a retinoid) or even bisphosphonates may have beneficial effects of tamoxifen without adverse effects

TABLE 2.   Breast Cancer Screening

Breast self-exam (BSE)	Screening mammogram (average breast cancer risk)
Should be taught to all women	No baseline mammogram
Should be practiced monthly	Age 40–49—every 1–2 years (at physician discretion)
	Age 50–65—yearly
Clinical breast examination	Above age 65—every 2–3 years (at physician discretion)
Age 20–40—every 2–3 years	
Above age 40—yearly	Screening mammogram (high risk)
	Age 40–65—yearly
	Above age 65—every 1–3 years (at physician discretion)

III. **An Approach**
  A. **Counseling about risk for breast cancer**
    1. Review of Table 1 suggests that only a few risks can be modified
    2. Encourage breastfeeding
    3. Control obesity
      a. Not unreasonable to suggest low fat, high fiber diet
    4. Modify alcohol intake
    5. Continue to be aware of advances in other risk-lowering areas
      a. Oral contraceptives
      b. Postmenopausal hormone replacement
      c. Tamoxifen in certain high-risk circumstances
      d. Putative protective effects of antioxidants
  B. **Counseling about screening**
    1. Table 2 represents a reasonable consensus, especially in light of cost pressures on primary care providers
    2. Physicians need to remain sensitive to patient needs and demands but to modify them when appropriate with reasoned, scientifically based responses
  C. **Counseling about treatment and follow-up** once cancer has been detected
    1. A primary care physician who has rapport with patient is often asked to direct further care or at least to advise on recommendations, once diagnosis of breast cancer has been made
    2. Treatment of breast cancer is highly complex, frequently changing field of oncology
    3. Recent trends include more conservative surgery, use of radiation, timing and type of chemotherapy, secondary chemoprevention, breast reconstruction—all issues with conflicting data
    4. Best counsel—seek experienced physicians or treatment centers, become as informed as possible, ask lots of questions
      a. Important role of primary care physician is to identify questions to be asked
      b. Rarely is there extreme urgency, allowing some time for reflection and fact finding
    5. Following sections outline issues likely to be raised, attempting to identify important questions
    6. **Prognosis**
      a. Highly variable and can be best answered only in conjunction with surgeon, radiation oncologist and medical oncologist after surgery and pathology report
    7. **Breast conservation**
      a. Most data show lumpectomy and radiation comparable to mastectomy
        i. True for stage I or II breast cancer, most likely stages after detection of cancer through routine screening
      b. This permits preservation of breast contour with modest alteration following radiation
      c. May not be appropriate in certain circumstances
        i. Early pregnancy (risks of radiation)
        ii. Multicentric tumors
        iii. Extensive ductal carcinoma
        iv. Previous radiotherapy
        v. For her own reasons, patient insists on mastectomy or refuses radiation

8. **Lymph node exploration**
   a. Procedure previously associated with considerable morbidity
      i. Swelling in affected arm ranged from transient to persistent and mild, significant and requiring treatment, or disabling
      ii. Also occasional occurrence of painful, disabling reflex sympathetic dystrophy
   b. Currently may not even perform lymph node sampling or use "sentinel-node biopsy" technique
      i. Small amount of dye or radioisotope injected at site of lumpectomy and node which takes up dye or radioisotope removed somewhat later through small incision
      ii. Predictive value very high and morbidity associated with lymph node dissection eliminated
9. **Radiation**
   a. Typical choice is external beam to affected breast 2–4 weeks after lumpectomy
      i. Occasionally use interstitial approach to provide radiation boost to tumor bed
   b. Reduces local recurrence significantly and enhances breast conservation techniques
   c. When combined with chemotherapy, results in enhanced survival
   d. Patients with certain collagen vascular diseases (e.g., scleroderma, systemic lupus) may not tolerate radiation well
10. **Chemotherapy**
    a. Highly dependent on number of circumstances variable to each woman
       i. Menopausal state
       ii. Pregnancy
       iii. Size of tumor
       iv. Presence of positive lymph nodes
       v. Estrogen and progesterone receptor status of tumor
       vi. Histology, flow cytometry, ploidy, and oncogenes
       vii. Choice of radiation
       viii. Presence of known metastases
       ix. Others
    b. Increasing trend toward offering adjuvant chemotherapy to most if not all women
    c. Chemotherapy may be combined with radiation
    d. Tamoxifen used widely, especially among postmenopausal women, regardless of cancer stage
    e. Interventions available to limit nausea and hair loss
11. **Breast reconstruction** (see Chapter 67)
    a. Counsel women to speak with surgeon about this issue well before surgery
       i. Techniques vary, according to amount of breast tissue removed
       ii. May involve relatively simple plastic procedure to implants to extensive flap development and construction of nipple
       iii. May be possible even after radiation
    b. Depending on circumstances, may be possible to perform reconstruction at time of lumpectomy or mastectomy
       i. May be performed by breast surgeon or in conjunction with plastic surgeon
    c. Women of any age may wish to consider these options
12. **Sexuality**
    a. Breast surgery and possible disfigurement major blows to self-image
    b. Fear of loss of sexuality to partner
    c. Counseling should at least raise the issue, preferably preoperatively
       i. Can honestly counsel that most couples retain full loving and sexual relationship
    d. Caution about difficulties with intercourse
       i. Most therapy for breast cancer induces hypoestrogen state, which may lead to hot flashes, emotional lability, vaginal dryness
       ii. Issues of estrogen use need to be discussed with medical oncologist
          (a) In general, estrogen replacement contraindicated after breast cancer though vaginal estrogen cream occasionally used

13. **Follow-up**
   a. May find patient returning for frequent visits to surgeon, radiation oncologist, and medical oncologist for prolonged time
      i. Unless patient involved in sponsored investigation, this means multiple visits often with overlapping exams and tests
   b. Primary care physician should communicate with consultants about appropriate relationship
   c. Typically, medical oncologist follows closely while patient undergoing chemotherapy
   d. After radiation and chemotherapy protocols and reasonable follow-up period, may be desirable for primary care physician to provide continuity care
      i. Coordinate follow-up tests (blood tests, radiographs, scans, mammograms) with consultant
      ii. Episodic care
      iii. Evaluation of risk for osteoporosis, cardiovascular disease, other tumors (ovarian, uterine, colorectal)

14. **Support groups**
   a. Communities often have multiple resources for women following breast cancer
   b. Organized through hospitals, mastectomy support groups, cancer survivor groups
   c. National examples include: American Cancer Society (800-ACS-2345, www.cancer.org); National Cancer Institute (800-4-CANCER, www.nci.nih.gov); American Health Foundation (212-551-2501)

SUGGESTED READING

1. Cady B, Steele GD: Evaluation of common breast problems: Guidance for primary care providers. CA Cancer J Clin 48:49–63, 1998.
2. Council on Scientific Affairs: Management of patients with node-negative breast cancer. Arch Intern Med 153:58–67, 1993.
3. Dodd GD: American Cancer Society guidelines on screening for breast cancer: An overview. CA Cancer J Clin 42:177–180, 1992.
4. Early Breast Cancer Trialists' Collaborative Group: Tamoxifen for early breast cancer: An overview of the randomised trials. Lancet 351:1451–1457, 1998.
5. Elmore JG, Barton MB: Ten-year risk of false-positive screening mammograms and clinical breast examinations. N Engl J Med 338:1089–1096, 1998.
6. Hortobagyi GN: Treatment of breast cancer. N Engl J Med 339:974–984, 1998.
7. Kattlove H, Liberati A, Keeler E, et al: Benefits and costs of screening and treatment for early breast cancer: Development of a basic benefit package. JAMA 273:142–148, 1995.
8. Kerlikowske K, Grady D, Rubin SM, et al: Efficacy of screening mammography: A meta-analysis. JAMA 273:149–154, 1995.
9. Stoll BA: Macronutrient supplements may reduce breast cancer: How, when and which? Eur J Clin Nutr 51:573–577, 1997.
10. Winchester DP, Cox JD: Standards for breast-conservation treatment. CA Cancer J Clin 42:134–162, 1992.

102. Cervical, Vulvar, and Vaginal Cancer

Gary R. Newkirk, M.D.

I. The Issues

Gynecologic cancers account for approximately 23,000 deaths annually in the U.S. The genital organs are among the most common sites of cancer in women. Screening efforts to prevent mortality due to gynecologic malignancy are productive, because 90% of cervical, vulvar, and vaginal cancers are curable if discovered early and confined to the primary site of origin. The decline in mortality due to cervical cancer is related to the success of Papanicolaou smear screening. Detection of vulvar and vaginal premalignant lesions and cancer require special attention on the part of the clinician, because cervical Papanicolaou screening misses the majority of lesions. Careful inspection of the vagina and vulva with attention to palpatory abnormalities are critical components of the screening system. Furthermore, precancer at any one site, cervix, vagina, or vulva, mandates careful examination of the other sites. Primary care providers are in an excellent position to facilitate cancer screening with women in their practice.

II. *Cervical Cancer*
 A. **The Theory**
  1. Over 6,000 deaths/year caused by cervical cancer in the U.S. with approximately 14,000 new cases of cervical cancer and over 45,000 new cases/year of carcinoma *in situ* of cervix.
  2. Leading cause of death in young women in developing countries
  3. Early detection is key to reducing mortality rates; an antiviral vaccine is currently under investigation
  4. 85% of cervical cancers are squamous cell carcinomas with approximately 15% adenocarcinomas or mixed types
  5. Epidemiology
   a. Over 90% related to human papillomavirus (HPV)-infection which is mostly transmitted through sexual contact. There are over 15 genital subtypes of HPV; subtypes 16 and 18 are especially virulent.
   b. Risk factors
    i. Onset of sexual activity before age 20 years, multiple sexual partners, low socioeconomic status
   c. Cofactors include: other sexually transmitted diseases (STDs), infection with human immunodeficiency virus (HIV), smoking, and nutritional deficiencies
   d. Not advanced by exogenous hormones, pregnancy
   e. Peak incidence of carcinoma *in situ* between ages 35–45 years and invasive cancer between age 45–55 years
   f. Increasing incidence in younger women
   g. Time between initial exposure and carcinoma *in situ* traditionally considered to be 5–10 years. However, there are documented cases occurring < 1 year after exposure, especially in teenagers.
 B. **An Approach**
  1. Diagnosis
   a. Papanicolaou smear primary mode of detection
    i. Only a screening test, nondiagnostic, cervical biopsy diagnostic
    ii. Annual Papanicolaou recommended with onset of sex or by age 18
    iii. Persistent atypia or dysplasia are indications for colposcopy
   b. Abnormal-appearing cervix indication for colposcopy and biopsy
   c. Rarely, postcoital bleeding is primary sign of cervical cancer
  2. Staging
   a. Important for selecting therapy and helping with prognosis
   b. Often performed as separate work-up by gynecologic oncologist, requiring referral
   c. International Federation of Gynecology and Obstetrics (FIGO) system of staging recommended
  3. Management approaches
   a. Precancer (dysplasia including carcinoma *in situ*)
    i. Treatment options include: cryotherapy, loop electrosurgery, laser, cervical cold cone, hysterectomy
   b. Invasive cancer
    i. Depends on staging, clinical setting
     (a) Stromal invasion to < 1 mm is treated by therapeutic conization or total hysterectomy
     (b) Invasion to < 3 mm treated by conventional hysterectomy
     (c) Stromal invasion > 3 mm requires radical hysterectomy with pelvic node dissection and aortic node assessment
    ii. Highly individual and complex treatment strategies have evolved

        iii. Combination of radical surgery and radiation; chemotherapy rarely used

        iv. Staging ultimately determines choice of treatment

           (a) Requires careful preoperative evaluation, including physical/pelvic exam, chest radiograph

           (b) Intravenous pyelography, barium enema, cystoscopy, sigmoidoscopy may be necessary

           (c) Special tests, such as computed tomography, retrograde pyelography, electromagnetic imaging, may be desired in special instances

III. *Vulvar Cancers*

  A. **The Theory**

    1. Vulvar cancer accounts for approximately 1–2% of all gynecologic cancer deaths per year with 5-year survival rates of 46%. Squamous cell carcinoma accounts for 90–95% of primary vulvar tumors. It is more common in older women, but may occur even in teenagers. Its incidence is rising, especially in younger women. Lesions usually occur on labia majora, clitoris, periurethral areas and often ulcerate as they enlarge. Cancer is often multifocal with more than one area of simultaneous focal invasion. A causal link between HPV infection and vulvar squamous cell carcinoma is suspected. Vulvar cancer spreads primarily by lymphatic dissemination.

  B. **An Approach**

    1. Differential diagnoses

      a. Vulvar dystrophies

        i. Often appear as leukoplakia and thick white plaques

        ii. Hyperplastic dystrophy with and without atypia

        iii. Lichen sclerosis

        iv. Mixed dystrophy

        v. Paget's disease

          (a) Redness

          (b) May appear as yeast eruption

          (c) Treated by wide local excision

      b. Vulvar intraepithelial neoplasia

        i. Preinvasive disease

        ii. Previously known as Bowen's disease or vulvar carcinoma *in situ*

        iii. Most patients experience pruritus; one-third may have no symptoms

        iv. Lesions may be white, red, or dark

        v. Increasing incidence

        vi. Half of patients under age 50 years

        vii. Older women more likely to progress to cancer

        viii. Treatment must be individualized, including local excision, cryosurgery, laser evaporation, vulvectomy, chemical agents

      c. Bowenoid papulosis

        i. Benign, self-limited

        ii. Usually pigmented

        iii. Treated with local excision or local destructive methods

      d. Vulvar condyloma

        i. HPV-related

        ii. May mimic vulvar preneoplasia

        iii. Associated with later development of vulvar dysplasia, especially in women who smoke

      e. Pigmented lesions

        i. Simple freckles

        ii. Lentigo

        iii. Nevi

        iv. Melanomas

    2. Diagnosis of vulvar cancer

      a. Simple punch biopsy of suspicious areas warranted

        i. Less crush artifact and easier to orient than punch biopsy

        ii. Must be full-thickness biopsy

        iii. Accurately measure diameter of lesion

   b. Toluidine blue may be applied to vulva to guide biopsy sites

        i. Vital nuclear stain, nonspecific, suspicious areas stain blue

   c. Acetic acid may be used to highlight areas to biopsy (acetowhite)

   d. All areas of persistent ulceration require biopsy

   e. Biopsy pigmented areas

        i. Two-thirds of cancers appear ulcerated, acetowhite

        ii. One-third are pigmented

   f. Diagnostic workup with confirmed cancer warranted

        i. Cystoscopy, sigmoidoscopy, chest radiograph

        ii. Advanced disease requires liver and bone scan, skeletal radiographs, CT scan

   g. Important for initial staging process

  3. Treatment

   a. Precancerous areas can be treated with local destructive methods, including laser vaporization, loop electrosurgery, cryotherapy, topical chemodestruction, e.g., 5-fluorouracil

   b. Cancerous areas

        i. Staging important

        ii. Surgery primary mode of therapy, individualized

        iii. Irradiation may supplement therapy

        iv. Recurrence in 30–50% of cases

        v. Referral to gynecologic oncologist often warranted

IV. *Vaginal Cancers*

  A. **The Theory**

Vaginal cancer accounts for less than 2% of all gynecologic cancers. Most affected women are over age 50 (sixth and seventh decades). The vagina is frequently involved from local spread of cervical or endometrial cancer. Most vaginal cancers are found in proximal one-third of posterior vagina. Women with hysterectomy for cervical carcinoma are at higher risk for developing vaginal cancer. Squamous cell carcinoma represents 95% of histology. Other vaginal cancer types include: adenocarcinoma, verrucous carcinoma, diethylstilbestrol (DES)–associated clear-cell adenocarcinoma, sarcoma, melanoma, metastatic cancer.

There is a correlation between vaginal squamous cell carcinoma and HPV and it should be carefully sought in all cases of high-grade cervical or vulvar dysplasias or cancers.

  B. **An Approach**

  1. Diagnosis

   a. High index of suspicion in DES-exposed patients

   b. Carefully palpate vagina for firm or rough areas

   c. Inspect vaginal fornices with speculum in place

   d. Use dilute Lugol's solution to demonstrate iodine-negative areas (Schiller's test)

   e. All abnormal areas should be biopsied

        i. 2–3 mm depth usually adequate

        ii. Each abnormal area should be biopsied

   f. Colposcopy for abnormal Papanicolaou smear requires inspection of vagina and vulva

  2. Treatment

   a. Therapy depends on stage and location of tumor, patient's age

   b. Laser vaporization, cryosurgery, electrosurgery, intravaginal chemotherapeutic creams

   c. Local excision for unifocal lesions

   d. Multifocal recurrences usually require addition of radiotherapy

   e. In some instances, radical hysterectomy, vaginectomy, and pelvic lymphadenectomy are required

   f. Referral to gynecologic oncologist often required

SUGGESTED READING

1. Cancer links:http://www.cancerlinks. org
2. American College of Obstetricians and Gynecologists, Diagnosis and management of invasive cervical carcinomas. Techn Bull 138:1–6, 1989.
3. Boring CC, Squires TS, Tong T: Cancer statistics, 1993. CA Cancer J Clin 43:7–26, 1993.
4. Dewar MA, Hall K, Perchalski J: Cervical cancer screening: Past success and future challenge. Prim Care 191:589–606, 1992.
5. Fahs MC, Mandelblatt J, Schecter C, et al: Cost-effectiveness of cervical cancer screening for the elderly. Ann Intern Med 117:520–527, 1992.
6. Friedrick EG: Vulvar Disease, 2nd ed. Philadelphia, W.B. Saunders, 1983.
7. Gusberg SB, Runowicz CD: Gynecologic cancers. In Holleb AI, Fink DJ, Murphy GP (eds): American Cancer Society Textbook of Clinical Oncology. Atlanta, American Cancer Society, 1991, pp 481–497.
8. Koutsky LA, Holmes KK, Critchlow CW, et al: A cohort study of the risk of cervical intraepithelial neoplasia grade 2 or 3 in relation to papillomavirus infection. N Engl J Med 327:1272–1278, 1992.
9. Nelson JH, Averette HE, Richart RM: Cervical intraepithelial neoplasia (dysplasia and carcinoma in situ) and early invasive cervical carcinoma. CA Cancer J Clin 39:157–178, 1990.
10. Spitzer M, Krumholz B, Selter V: The multicentric nature of disease related to human papillomavirus infection of the female lower genital tract. Obstet Gynecol 73:303–307, 1989.
11. Vontver LA: Management of vulvar diseases. In Stenchever MA (ed): Office Gynecology. St. Louis, Mosby, 1992, pp 284–292.

103. Endometrial Cancer

Bruce E. Johnson, M.D.

I. The Issues

Concern about endometrial cancer is still influenced by a relatively brief increase in incidence in the 1960s and 1970s. At the time, this concern was appropriate because a connection between continuous estrogen administration, a pattern of estrogen use begun in the 1950s, and endometrial cancer was fairly strong. Despite considerable change in prescribing habits and a substantial drop in the incidence of endometrial cancer, many women still harbor a dread of the disease; this dread almost certainly influences a willingness to accept hormone replacement therapy in circumstances in which the benefit of such therapy might be substantial. The outlook is not all bad regarding this cancer. With current methods of surveillance, detection and treatment, the prognosis for endometrial cancer is optimistic.

II. The Theory

A. Epidemiology

1. Incidence rather high—about 36,000 women each year, accounting for about 8% of all cancers in women
   a. Incidence rate higher in African-Americans and Hispanics than whites and Asians—a difference not explained by delayed detection or access to care
2. Deaths from endometrial cancer about 6,000/year
3. Almost 80% of cancers detected in localized stages
   a. For those detected in stage 1 (low grade), 5-year survival rate is 85–95%
4. Most uterine cancers are adenocarcinoma of endometrium—other cell types, including papillary, clear cell, choriocarcinoma and sarcoma, are rare

B. Risk factors (Table 1)

1. Age
   a. Occurrence rate of 12/100,000 in women < age 50, rising to 160/100,000 for age > 65; 25% of cases in premenopausal women and only 5% in women < age 40
2. Obesity
   a. Mechanism probably reflects hyperestrogen state
   b. For women > 50 lb overweight, relative risk up to 10.0
3. Hyperestrogen state

TABLE 1. Risk Factors for Endometrial Cancer

Advancing age	Hyperestrogen states
Obesity*	Polycystic ovary syndrome
Nulliparity	Granulosa cell tumors of ovary
Early menarche	Chronic liver disease
Late menopause	Previous pelvic irradiation
Infertility	Previous breast or colon cancer
Unopposed exogenous estrogen	(possibly Lynch syndrome type II[§])
administration	Tamoxifen
	Atypical endometrial hyperplasia

* Diabetes mellitus and hypertension are often listed as risk factors, but this may be due to high incidence of obesity in these disorders
[§] Lynch syndrome type II is a genetic disorder resulting in increased likelihood of developing colon, breast, ovarian, and uterine cancer

    a. During 1960s and 1970s there was a dramatic increase in incidence of endometrial cancer
        i. For women age 50–65, incidence rose 90% between 1960 and 1975
    b. Epidemiologic studies quickly pointed to use of unopposed (continuous) estrogen replacement therapy (ERT), which was the standard means of administration after the introduction of HRT in late 1940s
    c. Additional studies suggested link between estrogen, premalignant lesions, and early stage (stages I, II) endometrial cancer, though not between estrogen and later stage cancer (stages III, IV)
    d. At the time, there was controversy as to whether studies suggesting estrogen–cancer link were biased, i.e., detection bias, exclusion bias, or methodologic bias
        i. Those critics who contended that bias existed admitted an almost certain increased risk with hyperestrogen state—their concern was that any bias, by overestimating the risk, actually flamed the intensity of media hysteria and would lead to future caution regarding any estrogen use
    e. Recognition of the role of a hyperestrogen state led to other associated risk factors
        i. Polycystic ovary syndrome: state of increased estrogen stimulation and increased endometrial cancer risk
        ii. Early menarche
        iii. Late menopause
        iv. Chronic liver disease
        v. Obesity
    f. Obesity results in increased estrogen due to a secondary sex steroid production mechanism
        i. Production of androstenedione by adrenal gland persists in postmenopausal women
        ii. Adipocytes convert androstenedione to estrone, a weak estrogen
        iii. Large numbers of adipocytes, in obese women, leads to increased production of estrone, resulting in relative hyperestrogen state
4. Atypical endometrial hyperplasia and endometrial polyps
    a. Pathologic diagnosis after endometrium sampled for another reason, often abnormal endometrial bleeding
    b. Atypical endometrial hyperplasia associated with as high as 30% likelihood of finding endometrial cancer elsewhere in uterus
    c. This finding should result in increased surveillance for endometrial cancer (or as another indication for hysterectomy)—however, should not conclude that all women have endometrial sampling to find this relatively rare diagnosis
5. Tamoxifen
    a. Used as treatment or adjuvant therapy in breast cancer
        i. Ironically, while it has unquestioned estrogen-blocking activity in breast tissue, this agent also has weak estrogen-agonist activity in endometrial cells
    b. As weak estrogen, tamoxifen contributes to endometrial stimulation

    c. Several studies show increased incidence of endometrial cancer; similar association not yet established for other selective estrogen receptor modulators (SERMs)

  6. Other risk factors (strength of these associations not clear)

    a. Pelvic irradiation for benign disease

    b. Previous breast cancer

    c. Previous colon cancer

    d. Lynch syndrome, type II

    e. Infertility

C. Protective factors

  1. Progesterone

    a. Studies of association of ERT and endometrial cancer indicated that incidence of cancer dropped with use of progesterone

    b. Progesterone use suppresses hyperplasia of endometrium whether administered in cycling regimen or continuously

    c. Progesterone use, even with ERT, lowers risk of endometrial cancer below non-hormonally treated postmenopausal women

  2. Oral contraceptives (OCs)

    a. Protective benefit related to progesterone in OCs

    b. Relative risk for endometrial cancer in women using OCs for more than 3 years may be as low as 0.5

    c. Effect lasts up to 15 years—consequently, use of OCs in women late in reproductive life (40s) may have long-term protective effect

  3. Hysterectomy

    a. When performed for benign disease, obviously removes organ from risk of cancer

  4. Endometrial ablation

    a. Usually done for benign disease, e.g., dysfunctional uterine bleeding

    b. Various techniques to remove all, or almost all, endometrium down to myometrium

      i. However, endometrium may regenerate at some point and endometrial cancer has been reported even after ablation

  5. Cigarette smoking

    a. Relative risk as low as 0.7 for postmenopausal women currently smoking

    b. Probably due to decreased luteal phase estrogen production as well as, perhaps, to observation that smokers tend to be less obese

    c. Overall risks of smoking enormously outweigh protective effect on development of endometrial cancer

D. Screening

  1. **Techniques**

    a. No reliable blood tests

    b. Papanicolaou smear insensitive

      i. Detects only about 25% of endometrial cancers

      ii. Presence of endometrial cells on Papanicolaou smear does not mean that endometrial sampling needs to be performed, except in postmenopausal woman not on HRT

    c. Pelvic exam

      i. Poor sensitivity; detects only stage II and greater cancer

    d. Pelvic ultrasound and CT of pelvis

      i. Effective in determining cavitary lesions from benign conditions (e.g., fibroids)

      ii. Typically used after symptom of abnormal uterine bleeding; consequently, not truly screening methods

    e. Endometrial sampling

      i. Methods include catheter (cytology) or pipette (histology) inserted into uterine cavity, typically without anesthesia

      ii. While described as simple outpatient procedures, they are not without discomfort

      iii. Not a screening test

    f. Dilatation and curettage

      i. The gold standard for diagnosis but not a screening test

2. **Selection of patients**
  a. No recognized authoritative body recommends screening all women for endometrial cancer
    i. Prominent groups refusing to endorse screening process include Canadian Task Force, U.S. Preventive Services Task Force
  b. American College of Obstetricians and Gynecologists suggests screening women at high risk
    i. Women at high risk may include postmenopausal, aged, obese, estrogen replacement (including, under some definitions, those using progesterone as well), hyperestrogen states, radiation therapy for benign disease
      (a) By some estimates, this places at "high risk" almost 70% of adult female population
    ii. Even if all "high-risk" women are screened, only about 50% of endometrial cancers would be detected in this manner
3. Whole concept of screening needs considerable refinement and advances before broad acceptance can be realized

III. **An Approach**
  A. **Prevention**
    1. Weight loss
      a. Theoretical benefit; no demonstration of reduced cancer risk in obese women who lost weight
    2. Hysterectomy
      a. Multiple practical problems with implementation
    3. Oral contraceptives (OCs)
      a. Use by older reproductive women may result in protection into postmenopausal years
      b. Many women feel OCs less desirable than sterilization as contraception
    4. Progesterone
      a. Used in hormone replacement therapies, either cycling or continuous
        i. Protective effect renders hormonally treated women at lower risk than women never having taken hormones
      b. Seems to be no difference between continuous and cycled regimens
  B. **Screening**
    1. No single technique meets ideal of ease of use, accuracy, detection at early stage, and cost-effectiveness
    2. Endometrial sampling has been proposed in certain high-risk women
      a. Estrogen replacement therapy (ERT)
        i. Protective benefit of progesterone, which is used in virtually all regimens, makes screening less necessary
      b. Tamoxifen therapy
        i. Cost/benefit analysis did not support use of endometrial sampling in this high-risk group
      c. Other cancers (colon, breast, Lynch syndrome II)
      d. Pelvic irradiation for benign disease
      e. Obesity?
    3. No consensus on what constitutes high risk for endometrial cancer—no effective screening strategy has yet been developed
  C. **Clinical presentation**
    1. Abnormal uterine bleeding in postmenopausal woman
    2. Menstrual abnormalities in premenopausal woman
      a. Increased menstrual flow; decreased menstrual interval; intermenstrual bleeding
    3. Abnormal Papanicolaou smear
      a. Atypical endometrial cells at any age
      b. "Normal" endometrial cells in postmenopausal woman not on ERT
  D. **Staging and evaluation**
    1. Consensus that most accurate staging is done at time of initial surgical procedure and that preoperative staging adds little

      a. Surgical staging includes involvement of uterus, para-aortic nodes, widespread metastases, abdominal cytology

2. Staging usually correlates with prognosis
      a. Stage I—tumor limited to endometrium
         i. 5-year survival 85–95%
      b. Stage II—endocervical tumor (primary or invasion)
         i. 5-year survival up to 60%
      c. Stage III—invasion of serosa, adnexa, vagina, pelvic/para-aortic lymph nodes, or positive peritoneal cytology
         i. 5-year survival about 30%
      d. Stage IV—invasion of bladder or bowel, distant metastases
         i. 5-year survival only 10%

3. Preoperative evaluation
      a. Physical exam
         i. Clinical evaluation of external genitalia, vagina, cervix; bimanual exam for pelvic nodules, induration, immobility
      b. Office procedures
         i. Papanicolaou smear, including endocervical; endometrial biopsy and/or endocervical curettage; stool for occult blood
      c. Laboratory
         i. Usual preoperative tests—none specific for endometrial cancer
      d. Transvaginal ultrasound
         i. Quite sensitive for cystic vs. solid mass, and for depth of endometrial lining—but excessive if endometrial sampling already positive
      e. Consider other tests as age and circumstances warrant
         i. CA-125 blood test not useful for diagnosis—only in rare circumstances of extensive disease at initial presentation and CA-125 to be used for periodic surveillance
         ii. Intravenous pyelography
         iii. Abdominal and pelvic CT exam
         iv. Sigmoidoscopy and colonoscopy or barium enema

4. In surgically removed specimen, determination of estrogen and progesterone receptors

E. **Treatment**

1. Almost always includes surgery (only exception might be aged or very poor operative risk)
      a. Stage I: total abdominal hysterectomy and bilateral salpingo-oophorectomy
         i. True stage 1 endometrial cancer almost always curative without adjuvant therapy
         ii. Aggressive cell types, e.g., papillary serous, may warrant adjuvant external beam radiation
      b. Stage II, involving endocervix, may require radical hysterectomy
      c. Stages III and IV requires radical hysterectomy with possible debulking and omentectomy

2. Radiation therapy
      a. Occasionally use external beam radiation for stage I and stage II with gross endocervical disease; poor surgical candidates as primary treatment; rare circumstances of aggressive cell type even without evidence of spread
      b. External beam radiation in stage III disease
      c. Recurrences often treated locally with radiation

3. Chemotherapy and hormonal therapy
      a. Used in distant metastases, peritoneal spread, sometimes in bowel or bladder disease
      b. Hormonal therapy consists of medroxyprogesterone acetate or megestrol acetate
      c. Chemotherapy consists of combinations of medicine, including doxorubicin, cisplatin, carboplatin, paclitaxel and, ironically, the occasional use of tamoxifen
      d. Combinations of chemotherapy and hormonal therapy have better results than either alone

F. **Long-term treatments**
   1. Recurrences may be treated with surgery, radiation, chemotherapy, or hormonal therapy
      a. Hormonal therapy often well tolerated and provides excellent long-term control
   2. ERT is occasionally considered, even with history of endometrial cancer
      a. Protective effect of estrogen on atrophic vaginitis, osteoporosis, cardiac disease
      b. Only realistic to consider in stage I disease with low-grade histology
         i. Imperative to inform patient of risks of disease recurrence
         ii. Some estimates (no studies) suggest risk of recurrence of cancer at 5%

SUGGESTED READINGS

1. American College of Obstetricians and Gynecologists: Carcinoma of the endometrium. ACOG Technical Bulletin No. 162, 1991.
2. American College of Obstetricians and Gynecologists: Estrogen replacement therapy and endometrial cancer. ACOG Committee on Gynecologic Practice, Committee Opinion No. 126, 1993.
3. Barakat RR: Contemporary issues in the management of endometrial cancer. CA Cancer J Clin 48:299–314, 1998.
4. Fisher B, Costantino JP: Endometrial cancer in tamoxifen treated breast cancer patients: Finding from the National Surgical Adjuvant Breast and Bowel Project (NSABP) B-14. J Natl Cancer Inst 86:527–537, 1994.
5. McGonigle KF, Karlan BY: Development of endometrial cancer in women on estrogen and progestin hormone replacement therapy. Gynecol Oncol 55:126–132, 1994.
6. Pritchard KI: Screening for endometrial cancer: Is it effective? Ann Intern Med 110:177–179, 1989.
7. Rose PG: Endometrial carcinoma. N Engl J Med 335:640–649, 1996.

104. Ovarian Cancer

Bruce E. Johnson, M.D.

I. **The Issues**
Ovarian cancer is the fifth most common malignancy in women in the U.S. It is especially deadly, with a mortality rate of over 50%. Also distressing is the fact that it develops with so few symptoms; the typical presentation is with advanced disease. Thus, efforts to develop effective screening tests have been ongoing for some time, with several different approaches investigated. Preliminary results for each test are often magnified by the lay media. Unfortunately, no screening test is really acceptable, and screening remains a viable option for a small minority of women. Data suggest a protective effect for therapies in which many women already engage—namely, oral contraceptives and tubal sterilization. Such data, if confirmed, promise modest hope for an insidious disease.
II. **The Theory**
   A. **Epidemiology**
      1. In the U.S. approximately 27,000 new cases of ovarian cancer each year (1997 data)
         a. Affects about 1 in 70 women
         b. About 14,000 ovarian cancer deaths each year
            i. 60% death rate virtually unchanged over past several decades
      2. Incidence increases with advancing age peaking in 55–65 age group
      3. Some variation by cell type
         a. Epithelial cell type more common in white, postmenopausal women
         b. Germ cell lines more common in young, nonwhite women
         c. An uncommon syndrome, called borderline ovarian tumor, is may present with either serous or mucinous but has a less aggressive course
      4. Higher incidence in western, industrialized countries; lower rate in Mediterranean countries, Japan
         a. Pattern similar to breast cancer
         b. Japanese who immigrate to U.S. have rate similar to U.S., not Japan

      c. Suggests environmental influence but no apparent association with coffee, tobacco, alcohol, or occupational group

B. **Risk factors**
1. Most cases of ovarian cancer do not have identifiable risk factor
2. Parity
    a. Higher rates in nulliparous and first pregnancy after age 35
    b. Higher rates in women with infertility, anovulation
    c. Lower rates with first pregnancy before age 25 and with multiple pregnancies
3. Environmental
    a. Association with high dietary intake of meat/animal fat
4. Association with other diseases
    a. Women with breast cancer have 2- to 4-fold increased risk of ovary cancer
    b. Peutz-Jeghers contributes 5-fold increased risk
    c. Some types of gonadal dysgenesis increase risk of developing ovary cancer
5. Family history
    a. Strongest risk factor
       i. Woman with one first-degree relative with ovarian cancer has 10% chance of developing cancer
       ii. If two first-degree relatives with ovarian cancer, risk increases to 50%
6. Genetic ovarian cancer syndromes (despite the strong penetrance in families with these syndromes, these only account for 3–5% of all ovarian cancer)
    a. Familial breast-ovary cancer syndrome
       i. Careful, extensive family history shows either breast or ovarian cancers (occasionally both) in female members
       ii. Autosomal dominant pattern means that cancer develops from either maternal or paternal genes but, since neither ovary (obviously) nor male breast cancer develops in fathers, this syndrome very difficult to identify
    b. Lynch syndrome type II
       i. Family cancer syndrome giving increased incidence of cancer of colon (without polyposis), lung, prostate, uterus, and ovary
       ii. Possible linkage to abnormalities on long arm of chromosome 17
    c. BRCA 1 and 2
       i. Although better known for association with breast cancer, the BRCA 1 and 2 defects also confer heightened risk for ovarian cancer
       ii. Largely found in Ashkenazi Jewish women
       iii. In families with suggestion of genetic trait, can test for these genetic defects—though issues of ethics, management (e.g., prophylactic oophorectomy?), and insurability not fully explored
       iv. Early suggestion that oral contraceptives might reduce risk of development (in this highly selected group) by 20–60% depending on length of use of OCs

C. **Protective measures**
1. High parity
2. Breastfeeding
    a. At least once for more than 6 months
3. Oral contraceptives (OCs)
    a. Five years of OC use by nulliparous woman reduces risk to that of parous woman who never used OC
    b. Mechanism not known, although lack of hormonal stimulation suspected (i.e., OCs suppress stimulation of follicle-stimulating hormone and luteinizing hormone)
4. Hysterectomy
    a. Reduction in risk associated with hysterectomy even when ovaries preserved
    b. In one study, reduced relative risk to 0.66 compared with women with uterus
5. Tubal sterilization
    a. Reduction in risk with tubal sterilization, regardless of procedure performed
    b. One study reports reduction in risk ratio to 0.33
    c. Mechanism unknown, although suspicion includes interruption of ovarian blood supply with subsequent changes in steroid production

6. Oophorectomy
   a. Discussion of oophorectomy should be undertaken with any patient anticipating hysterectomy or surgery for benign ovarian disease after age 35–40
   b. Unclear whether predictability accurate enough with familial ovarian cancer syndromes to recommend prophylactic oophorectomy

D. **Screening methods**
   1. Perspective
      a. One rule of thumb suggests that, when an invasive procedure (e.g., laparotomy, laparoscopy) is performed to rule out or confirm ovarian cancer, 1 case of cancer for every 9 cases of benign disease is "acceptable"
         i. Even so, for every 1000 tests, 996 (99.6% sensitivity) would have to be true negatives to achieve a positive predictive value resulting in 1 to 9 ratio
         ii. No test discussed below comes even close to this accuracy
   2. Bimanual pelvic exam
      a. Most available and least expensive (assuming it is done at same time as Papanicolaou smear and general exam)
      b. Also, least sensitive and least specific
      c. Estimated to take 10,000 pelvic exams on asymptomatic women to detect 1 cancer of ovary
      d. No one suggests that bimanual pelvic exam should not be done simply because it is not a sensitive test for ovarian cancer, but limitations of exam should be recalled by provider
   3. Blood tests
      a. CA-125 is a monoclonal antibody against antigen expressed by serous ovarian adenocarcinoma
      b. In 90% of advanced epithelial ovarian cancer, CA-125 > 35 U/ml; however, only 50% of women with stage I disease have CA-125 > 30 U/ml.
      c. Population studies suggest sensitivity as screening test only 55% and specificity > 95%
      d. CA-125 may be elevated in endometriosis and pelvic inflammatory disease
      e. Evaluation with other tests (see below) improves both sensitivity and specificity; CA-125 is not accurate enough to warrant use by itself as general screening test though may have limited use in women at high risk
   4. Abdominal ultrasonography
      a. Little improvement over CA-125
      b. Sensitivity about 90%, but specificity < 90%
         i. Detects pelvic masses but poor differentiation of cancer vs. benign disease
      c. Relatively expensive, time-consuming, and requires patient preparation
   5. Transvaginal sonography
      a. Fairly good interobserver interpretation
      b. Improves sensitivity of test to > 90% with specificity up to 98%
      c. Combination with Doppler color blood flow imaging improves accuracy considerably
   6. One study combined CA-125 with sonography to achieve sensitivity of 95% and specificity > 99%
      a. Unfortunately, this approach not cost-effective is proposed as screening test for general population
         i. Strategy increased theoretical life expectancy by < 1 day
         ii. One estimate gives expenditure of close to $1 million per single stage I cancer detected
         iii. Cost of screening all U.S. women > age 45 one time is $14 billion—and clearly more than one life-time screening would be necessary
   7. None of these strategies can be recommended as screening test for general population despite impassioned urging of celebrities, politicians, advocates

III. **An Approach**
A. **Prevention**
   1. As public health measure, discounting other risks/benefits, physicians may wish to consider recommending certain measures

      a. Multiple pregnancies do confer some protection but such a recommendation is unlikely to be followed for risk reduction alone

      b. Breastfeeding

         i. Another reason to advocate this valued practice

      c. Oral contraceptives

      d. Tubal sterilization once childbearing completed

      e. Oophorectomy at time of hysterectomy or benign ovarian disease in women over age 35–40 could prevent up to 10% of all ovarian cancers

  2. Prophylactic oophorectomy for high-risk women

      a. Consideration for women with identified genetic ovarian cancer syndrome

         i. Strong argument for surgery once childbearing completed in breast-ovary cancer, familial ovary cancer, BRCA-1 and 2, and Lynch II syndromes

      b. For women with two or more first-degree relatives who had ovarian cancer, even without "diagnosis" of genetic ovarian cancer syndrome, opinion now leaning toward prophylactic surgery

         i. For women with one first-degree relative with ovarian cancer, current practice makes it difficult to recommend prophylactic oophorectomy though more aggressive monitoring may be indicated

B. Screening

  1. Current technology does not support recommending screening of asymptomatic, average-risk women with CA-125 and/or sonography

  2. When performing Papanicolaou smear for cervical cancer (for which screening of asymptomatic women is established), bimanual pelvic exam should accompany speculum exam

  3. High-risk women (familial cancer syndromes; prior breast, colon, uterine cancer; first-degree relative with ovarian cancer)

      a. Follow strategy of periodic evaluations, including yearly pelvic exam, CA-125 and transvaginal sonography with Doppler color blood flow if available

      b. Specificity of combined tests > 99%, with sensitivity just below 95%

      c. Expense considerable with this approach, but possibly 30% increase in early stage detection

C. Clinical presentation

  1. Clues to early diagnosis

      a. Woman > 1 year after menopause should not have follicular or corpus luteum cysts; consequently cystic ovary in this setting requires evaluation

      b. Palpable ovary in postmenopausal woman should be evaluated; a palpable ovary in postmenopausal women is not usual

      c. Women on oral contraceptives who develop cysts are a particular problem

         i. Benign cysts do develop in patients on low-dose OCs, making indication for laparoscopy more problematic

  2. 70% of women present with advanced disease

      a. Common symptoms include abdominal fullness and early satiety

         i. Ascites typically present—a common aphorism states that ascites in postmenopausal woman is ovarian cancer until proved otherwise

      b. Tumor implants on omentum or small bowel may cause symptoms of bowel obstruction

         i. Occasional tumor implant near umbilicus (Sister Mary Joseph node)

      c. Distant metastases may lead to development of pleural effusion or axillary or inguinal lymph nodes

  3. Minority of women with limited disease have pelvic pain due to ovarian torsion

      a. However, most limited stage tumors are detected serendipitously during routine exams or evaluation for other symptoms

  4. Uncommon presentation includes paraneoplastic conditions

      a. Hypercalcemia; cerebellar degeneration; sudden, multiple seborrheic keratoses (sign of Leser-Trélat); migratory thrombophlebitis (Trousseau's sign)

  5. Initial evaluation includes pelvic exam, CA-125, transvaginal ultrasonography with Doppler color blood flow

      a. Laparoscopy used when cancer diagnosis not strongly suspected

6. Laparotomy almost always performed for staging purposes and initial debulking
7. **Staging of ovarian cancer**
   a. Stage I—cancer confined to ovaries
      i. Rarely with ascites
   b. Stage II—cancer confined to pelvis
      i. Occasionally with ascites
   c. Stage III—cancer spread throughout peritoneal cavity
      i. Typically with ascites
      ii. Implants on surface of liver but not in parenchyma
   d. Stage IV—cancer involves liver parenchyma or has spread outside peritoneal cavity
8. Prognosis at time of staging
   a. Stage I—up to 75% 5-year survival
   b. Stage II—about 60% 5-year survival
   c. Stage III—less than 35% 5-year survival
   d. Stage IV—less than 10% 5-year survival

D. **Treatment**
   1. Best results occur with aggressive surgical debulking and chemotherapy
      a. Surgical approach includes removal of pelvic organs, omentum, and most large masses of tumor
   2. Stage I, and often stage II, ovarian cancer frequently found serendipitously when operation done for other reasons
      a. Surgical removal, with lymph node sampling, probably adequate therapy though role of adjuvant chemotherapy actively debated
   3. Current first-line chemotherapy, for all stage III and IV patients, uses platinum-based agents (cisplatin, carboplatin) and paclitaxel (Taxol)
      a. Response rates considerably improved over non-paclitaxel therapies—as much as double life-expectancy compared to 15 years ago
      b. Toxicity high but current dosing regimens limits this as much as possible
   4. Other issues
      a. **Second-look surgery**
         i. Refers to laparotomy done after chemotherapy to seek remaining or recurrent disease
         ii. Once common, but fell into disfavor as CT and other imaging tests detect recurrence without surgical morbidity
      b. Newer chemotherapy agents include Topotecan and Doxil
      c. Intraperitoneal chemotherapy
         i. Capable of delivering high-dose chemotherapy to residual peritoneal disease, but high morbidity with unclear therapeutic advantages
      d. **Whole-abdomen radiation**
         i. Not commonly chosen, but alternative to chemotherapy
         ii. Likelihood of severe gastrointestinal, liver and bladder complications
      e. High-dose chemotherapy with autologous bone marrow transplantation
         i. Still under investigation
   5. **Terminal concerns**
      a. Likely to have ascites, often massive and uncomfortable
         i. Repeated paracentesis helpful; peritoneal-subclavian catheters not often used but may be considered
      b. Lower extremity edema
         i. Lymphatic blockage from tumor invasion of retroperitoneal nodes or from massive obstructing ascites
         ii. Diuretics rarely of value; consider compression stockings or automated compression devices
      c. Bowel obstruction, usually small bowel, a frequent complication
         i. May be possible to maintain patient for some time with total obstruction, using decompression with gastrostomy tube or long intestinal tube
         ii. If bowel obstructed and surgical intervention not planned, consider parenteral nutrition needed

    d. Tumor pain not common without bony metastases or involvement of nerve plexus and adequate pain management a necessity

SUGGESTED READING

1. Barnes MN, Deshane JS: Gene therapy and ovarian cancer: A review. Obstet Gynecol 89:145–155, 1997.
2. Cannistra SA: Cancer of the ovary. N Engl J Med 329:1550–1559, 1993.
3. Carlson KJ, Skates SJ: Screening for ovarian cancer. Ann Intern Med 121:124–128, 1994.
4. Grimes DA: Primary prevention of ovarian cancer. JAMA 270:2855–2856, 1993.
5. Hankinson SE, Hunter DJ: Tubal ligation, hysterectomy, and risk of ovarian cancer: A prospective study. JAMA 270:2813–2818, 1993.
6. Helzlsouer KJ, Bush TL: Prospective study of serum CA-125 levels as markers of ovarian cancer. JAMA 269:1123–1126, 1993.
7. Kerlikowske K, Brown JS: Should women with familial ovarian cancer undergo prophylactic oophorectomy? Obstet Gynecol 80:700–707, 1992.
8. McGuire WP, Hoskins WJ: Cyclophosphamide and cisplatin compared with paclitaxel and cisplatin in patients with stage III and stage IV ovarian cancer. N Engl J Med 335:1950–1955, 1996.

105. Other Cancers (Lung, Colorectal, Skin)

Bruce E. Johnson, M.D.

Several cancers, not exclusive to female reproductive organs, are of particular importance to women's health. Cancers of the lung, colorectum, and skin are included here because of recent changes in incidence, diagnosis, or treatment. The reader is referred to other sources for more in-depth consideration.

Lung Cancer in Women

  I. **The Issues**

Lung cancer is increasing at an alarming rate in women. Just a century ago it was a medical curiosity in either sex. But now it is the leading cause of cancer death in women. (Breast cancer is the most common cancer site in women but, because of improved treatment, contributes less to cancer mortality rates.) There are several possible environmental reasons for this increase in incidence, but by far the most important is cigarette smoking. Diagnosis and treatment of lung cancer hold little promise for lowering the death rate; prevention is the only intervention likely to affect this disease.

  II. **The Theory**

    A. **Epidemiology**

      1. About 80,000 new cases of lung cancer in women each year (1998 data)

        a. 13% of all new cancer cases

      2. Kills 67,000 women each year

        a. 25% of all cancer deaths

        b. In late 1980s, lung cancer overtook breast cancer as number-one cause of cancer death in women in U.S.

      3. From 1950–1990, age-related death rate increased sevenfold for lung cancer in women

      4. Uncommon cancer before age 35, but most common cancer death after age 55

    B. **Cigarette smoking in women**

      1. Cigarette smoking is the cause of 80–85% of all lung cancers in women

        a. Other purported causes in women include:

          i. Indoor radon gas

          ii. Exposure to ionizing radiation (previous cancer treatment, e.g., Hodgkin's disease)

          iii. Industrial exposure (nickel, cadmium, asbestos, chloromethyl ether)

          iv. Passive smoking from partner or household member

   2. Cigarette smoking virtually absent in women in 1900; substantial increase during 1920s and 1930s with major jump in 1940s
   3. Prevalence of smoking peaked in women in 1960s at 44%
      a. Decline in percentage of female population smoking until 1990 (25.6%)
      b. Slight increase in percentage of smokers since then (around 27%)
         i. Increase believed due to targeting of young female population by cigarette manufacturer advertising
      c. If current trends in U.S. continue, by 2000 there will be more women smokers than men
   4. Smoking proportionately higher in nonwhite women (especially African-Americans) and women of lower socioeconomic status and lower level of education
      a. Recent data suggest that incidence of new teenage smokers is dropping among African-Americans while stabilizing in white teenagers
         i. Speculation is that smoking among African-American women is not used as much for weight control or social status as in whites
   5. "Passive," "second-hand," or environmental smoke
      a. Most studies examine female spouses and children of male smokers
      b. Several effects noted, especially in children, including throat and chest irritation, increased pulmonary disease ("colds," asthma)
      c. Surgeon General determined lung cancer to be medical effect of passive smoking
         i. Studies vary in quality and conclusions, but at least 25% increase in lung cancer among women exposed to passive smoking over nonsmoking, nonexposed population
   6. Cigarette smoking also strongly linked to cancers of oral cavity, larynx, pharynx, esophagus, stomach, bladder, cervix and to chronic obstructive pulmonary disease, coronary artery disease, cerebro- and peripheral vascular disease
      a. Estimated that > 420,000 deaths/year in U.S. are related to smoking
   7. After smoking cessation, increased risk of cardiovascular disease drops rapidly toward nonsmoker levels; in contrast, 10–15 years estimated for risk of lung cancer to approach that of nonsmoker
C. **Screening**
   1. No effective screening programs demonstrated
   2. Periodic chest radiographs
      a. Studied in high-risk persons—smokers, miners, certain occupations, including factory workers in chemical, paper, textile industries
      b. Performed in several countries (including Germany, England, Japan, Czechoslovakia, U.S.)
         i. Variable intervals between radiographs from 4 months to 3 years
      c. No controlled or noncontrolled study demonstrated improved outcome, i.e., lower death rate, for screened population
   3. Sputum cytology also evaluated in large populations at risk for lung cancer
      a. Most studies in U.S. and Europe
      b. No study could demonstrate improved outcome, i.e., lower death rate, for screened population
   4. No organization (e.g., U.S. Preventive Services Task Force, American Cancer Society) recommends either screening chest radiograph or sputum cytology for persons at risk for lung cancer
III. **An Approach**
   A. **Clinical presentation**
      1. Only 10–20% of lung cancers are asymptomatic
      2. Most common symptoms, including cough, hemoptysis, dyspnea, chest pain, are caused by interference of cancer with patency of major bronchi
      3. Other symptoms relate to local effects of primary cancer, to metastases, or to paraneoplastic effects
         a. Fever—obstructing pneumonia
         b. Hoarseness—involvement of recurrent laryngeal nerve
         c. Bone pain—bony metastasis, hypertrophic osteoarthropathy

    d. Headache, paralysis—brain metastases
    e. Horner's syndrome (myosis, ptosis, loss of sweating)—apical tumor
    f. Pancoast syndrome—apical tumor invading neurovascular bundle to arm
    g. Superior vena cava syndrome—large, central tumor obstructing venous return
    h. Confusion—paraneoplastic syndromes of inappropriate secretion of antidiuretic hormone (SIADH) or hypercalcemia
    i. Weakness—myasthenia (Eaton-Lambert syndrome)
    j. Ataxia—cerebellar degeneration
4. Chest radiograph is still most likely means by which lung cancer initially discovered
    a. Smallest lesion can be detected at 2–3-mm diameter
    b. Positive predictive value > 90% once lesion > 8 mm

B. Evaluation

1. Chest radiograph is first step in diagnosis
    a. Nodule detected with > 85% accuracy; hilar adenopathy detected with 65% accuracy; mediastinal adenopathy detected with 55% accuracy on plain-film radiograph
    b. False-negative rate for chest radiograph is higher in women than men; explanation unclear
2. Tomography and fluoroscopy important in past; current use supplanted by computed tomography (CT)
3. CT is second diagnostic procedure of choice
    a. Evaluates chest parenchyma, hilum, mediastinum, chest wall, liver, and adrenal glands
    b. More sensitive at detecting calcification than conventional radiography
        i. Calcification more likely seen in benign lesions such as granuloma, hamartoma
    c. Evaluation important in determining presence of hilar or mediastinal adenopathy
        i. Presence of adenopathy denotes metastatic disease, removing patient from limited disease category
    d. CT-guided biopsy can be valuable
4. Magnetic resonance imaging (MRI)
    a. Can be useful but mostly as adjunct to CT
        i. Deficiencies include poor definition in aerated lung, motion artifacts, poor detection of calcification
    b. Most useful for superior sulcus tumor, detection of residual or scar tumor, invasion of chest wall
5. Sputum cytology
    a. If present, confirms diagnosis and cell type
        i. Cytology more likely positive with central, bronchial lesions than with peripheral lesions
    b. Obviates need for extensive invasive evaluation when taken with compatible chest radiograph
        i. Presence of extensive disease on radiograph and positive cytology completes work-up
6. Pleural fluid cytology
    a. Pleural effusion confirms metastatic spread; cytology can give firm diagnosis, cell type
7. Transthoracic needle aspiration
    a. Using CT- or sonogram-guided needle, can obtain tissue sample
    b. Not always definitive—benign tissue does not rule out malignancy in compatible radiograph
8. Bronchoscopy
    a. Visualization and biopsy of large, central tumor is definitive
        i. Patient is not a surgical candidate if tumor is positioned near carina
    b. Cytology brushings or lavage help to detect peripheral lesions
9. Lymph node biopsy, mediastinoscopy
    a. Used both for diagnosis and for staging
        i. Peripheral lymph node biopsy relatively benign procedure and with compatible radiograph can avoid additional, invasive tests

C. **Treatment**
   1. Depends in large part on staging
      a. Stage I—isolated tumor without evident metastasis at least 2 cm from carina
      b. Stage II—metastatic tumor to ipsilateral peribronchial or hilar lymph node
      c. Stage III—metastatic tumor to mediastinal or subcarinal lymph nodes or contralateral side
      d. Stage IV—distant metastases (including pleura)
   2. Survival ranges from about 50% for stage I to 10% for stage III
   3. Treatment also depends on cell type
      a. Small-cell carcinoma characterized by rapid growth and early metastasis
      b. Non–small-cell carcinomas (squamous, large cell, adenomatous) have similar natural history and treatments
   4. Up to 50% of non–small-cell tumors are stage IV at detection
      a. Treatment consists of supportive care only
         i. Conservative, palliative radiation therapy for selected complications
         ii. Life expectancy for stage IV often only months
   5. For stage I and II patients, surgical therapy provides best chance for prolonged survival
      a. Surgical techniques now attempt removal of lesion and mediastinal nodes. Although these patients represent only 10% of cases, 5-year survival may approach 30%
      b. On occasion, limited chemotherapy used to reduce tumor bulk and improve operative chance for cure
   6. Radiation therapy for cure offered in stage III, but usually not successful
      a. Radiation therapy useful for palliation
         i. Obstructing bronchus with pneumonia, dyspnea
         ii. Local brain, bone metastases
   7. Chemotherapy has only limited role
      a. Any modest benefit limited by overall mortality (very high) and toxicity of cisplatin-based therapies
      b. Use of adjunct chemotherapy following possible surgical cure unclear
   8. Small-cell lung cancers are staged as limited or extensive disease
      a. Not very useful distinction therapeutically since almost all patients are recommended for chemotherapy
         i. Very high metastatic rate makes surgery and radiation for cure almost useless
      b. Chemotherapy has extended survival to 12–16 months but overall 5-year survival rate is still only 10%, even for limited disease
      c. In contrast to previous, highly toxic therapies, current two-drug regimen of etoposide and cisplatin better tolerated with equal, or perhaps better, survival
D. **Solitary pulmonary nodule**
   1. Defined as opacity on chest radiograph of 1–4-cm diameter, not associated with hilar enlargement or atelectasis
      a. Patients typically asymptomatic
      b. Almost all solitary nodules detected serendipitously
   2. Diagnostic thrust is to differentiate cancer (bronchogenic, metastatic, carcinoid or sarcoma) from benign lesions
      a. Common benign causes of pulmonary nodules include infection (coccidioidomycosis, histoplasmosis, tuberculosis, echinococcal cyst), hamartoma, pneumonitis, Wegener's granulomatosis, rheumatoid nodule, atrioventricular malformation, lipoma, fibroma, bronchogenic cyst
      b. 90% of benign nodules caused by coccidioidomycosis, histoplasmosis, tuberculosis, and hamartoma
   3. Solitary nodules are more often benign than malignant (up to 95%)
      a. Benign nodules more likely found during widespread screening programs of asymptomatic persons
   4. Evaluation
      a. Since almost all solitary pulmonary nodules are detected by plain-film chest radiograph, very important to locate any prior radiographs

        i. If size unchanged for 2 years, nodule usually benign and may be followed-up with periodic chest radiograph

   b. Presence of calcification

        i. Reliable indicator of benign lesion

          (a) Not all benign lesions are calcified

   c. Tomography, fluoroscopy

        i. Supplanted by CT

   d. CT examination of nodule

        i. More sensitive for detecting calcium than plain film or tomography

        ii. Calcification present in small percentage of carcinomas but pattern is different from most benign causes

   e. Sputum cytology

        i. Noninvasive but negative result does not rule out malignancy

   f. Skin tests and serology

        i. Useful for possible TB, cocci

  5. Growth of nodule

   a. Even benign nodules can grow (e.g., hamartomas, histoplasmomas) but at slower rate than malignancies

   b. Growth of lesion in weeks to months likely to be malignant

  6. Observation

   a. Includes repeat chest radiograph every 3–4 months for 1–2 years, then periodically thereafter

   b. If size of nodule stable or diminishing, likely benign; increasing size should prompt removal

   c. Decision not to intervene depends on patient risk factors

        i. Smoking, older age, prior malignancy should prompt resection

        ii. If woman is nonsmoker and younger than 35, nodule may be observed

   d. If a nodule that has been observed is eventually determined to be malignant, outcome/survival is not changed

  7. If further evaluation believed to be indicated, proceed with invasive tests

   a. Bronchoscopy, transthoracic needle biopsy, thoracoscopy, thoracotomy

E. Smoking cessation

  1. Only real advances in lung cancer will come from prevention, not improvement in detection or therapy

  2. Smoking cessation should be raised at every office visit and time taken to discuss steps covered in Chapter 82

Colorectal Cancer in Women

  I. **The Issues**

While the incidence of colorectal cancer has remained steady for the entire population over the past decades, there has been a modest decline in women Guidelines for detection of polyps is important, as further declines in cancer occurrence may be accomplished through effective screening. Finally, treatment of colorectal cancer involves issues of significance to women, especially in the context of sexual relations.

  II. **The Theory**

   A. **Epidemiology**

    1. Accounts for about 69,000 new cases of cancer per year in women (1998 data)

      a. 11% of all new cancers in women

    2. Causes about 29,000 deaths per year (11% of cancer deaths)

    3. Colorectal cancer much more prevalent in developed countries than in developing countries

    4. Incidence rates peaked in 1985 (at 45/100,000 women) and have fallen by > 10% since then

      a. Mortality rate has also fallen, more rapidly for white than African-American women, and more rapidly for women than men

      b. Reason for fall unclear but may represent changes in diet and removal of adenomatous polyps

5. As age increases, right-sided colon cancer (e.g., cecum, ascending colon) becomes more common; referred to as "rightward" shift

B. **Risk factors**
1. Age
   a. Increases sharply after age 40, with > 90% of colorectal cancers occurring after age 50; most common cancer in women over age 75 (more than breast and lung)
2. Previous cancer
   a. Previous colon cancer
   b. Other gynecologic cancer such as uterine, ovarian
3. Previous adenomatous polyp in colon
   a. Regarded as precursor to colorectal cancer
   b. Untreated adenoma > 1 cm progresses to cancer at rate of 2.5% at 5 years, 25% at 20 years
   c. Finding of one adenomatous polyp increases possibility of development of additional polyps in future; not true for hyperplastic polyps
4. Family history
   a. Incidence increases 2- to 3-fold with first-degree relatives with colorectal cancer
   b. Hereditary nonpolyposis colorectal cancer syndromes
      i. Family history, especially if cancer developed at early age
      ii. Cancers often mucinous, multicentric and located on right side of colon
         (a) Lynch syndrome I and II also includes risk for cancer of breast, ovary, uterus
5. Familial polyposis syndromes
   a. Gardner's syndrome, Peutz-Jeghers syndrome, familial juvenile polyposis
   b. Seem to share similar defective genes
6. Inflammatory bowel disease
   a. Long-standing active disease; higher risk for cancer in ulcerative colitis than Crohn's disease
   b. Cumulative risk > 10% after 25 years of inflammatory disease
7. Diet
   a. Dietary fat, alcohol consumption associated with colorectal cancer
8. Cholecystectomy
   a. Possible increased risk with prior removal of gallbladder

C. **Protective factors**
1. Diet
   a. Dietary fiber, especially insoluble fiber
      i. Probably protects by combination of diluting, trapping, or accelerating transit of fat and/or other carcinogens
      ii. Long-standing explanation for decreased incidence of colorectal cancer in developing countries
   b. Protective benefits of folate, vitamin E, calcium, vitamin C, other antioxidants strongly suspected but as yet unproved
2. NSAIDs
   a. Early reports suggest modest decline in colorectal cancer by regular use of NSAIDs, typically aspirin
3. Estrogen hormones
   a. Early reports suggest that estrogen hormones, as either oral contraceptives or postmenopausal hormone replacement, confer some protection against colorectal cancer
   b. Relative risk (RR) from 0.62–0.72
4. Removal of adenomatous polyps
   a. Removal prevents polyp from developing into cancer
   b. Constitutes primary prevention

D. **Screening** (also see Chapter 2)
1. Four available techniques—biomarkers, digital rectal examination, fecal occult blood test (FOBT), screening sigmoidoscopy

2. **Biomarkers**
   a. Best known is carcinoembryonic antigen (CEA); others include sialic acid, CA19-9, tissue polypeptide antigen, DNA tumor-cell ploidy by flow cytometry
   b. Although CEA can be useful for following colorectal cancer after resection, none of mentioned tests combines adequate sensitivity and specificity to function as effective screening test

3. **Digital rectal examination**
   a. Effective at detecting rectal cancer (10–15% of all colorectal cancer)
   b. Also used to obtain sample of stool for FOBT
   c. Only reaches 10 cm or less
      i. Decreasing number of cancers detectable at this depth (epidemiologic observation of "rightward" shift of colorectal cancer)
   d. Can be performed during rectovaginal portion of pelvic examination

4. **Fecal occult blood test** (FOBT)
   a. False-positive rate is 2–3%; false-negative rate is 20–30%; positive predictive value for adenoma and cancer is 25–55%
      i. False-positive rate higher for hydrated FOBT; false-negative rate lower for hydrated FOBT: perform hydrated FOBT whenever possible
   b. In one study, performing at least one FOBT in preceding 5 years lowered RR of developing colorectal cancer to 0.69
      i. Presumably by detecting and removing adenomas
   c. Many contend that virtually any rate of adenoma detection by FOBT is result of serendipity, unrelated to results of FOBT
   d. Cost of evaluation of false-positives makes this an expensive test for relatively modest gains in cancer prevention
      i. Costs of false-negative tests also considerable but more difficult to measure
   e. Nonetheless, FOBT recommended yearly for women age > 50 by American Cancer Society, U.S. Preventive Services Task Force

5. **Flexible sigmoidoscopy**
   a. In contrast to rigid sigmoidoscopy, flexible reaches one half of colon, encompassing two-thirds of polyps and cancers
   b. Poorly accepted by public and physicians
      i. Public perception is of painful, prolonged procedure
      ii. Even with recent training, majority of primary care physicians do not perform flexible sigmoidoscopy
   c. Detection rate is high—in some series as many as one-third of asymptomatic persons undergoing screening have polyps
      i. Small portion of adenomatous polyps develop into cancer (maybe 5%); natural history of hyperplastic polyps less clear but risk considerably lower
   d. Consensus is developing that full colonoscopy not uniformly needed even if adenoma detected on sigmoidoscopy
      i. Large adenoma, multiple adenomas, high-risk status still should prompt full colonoscopy
   e. Costs for screening flexible sigmoidoscopy of entire population high; for colonoscopy (if indicated), even higher
   f. Screening sigmoidoscopy recommended by American Cancer Society for all women over age 50 every 3–5 years; U.S. Preventive Services Task Force concludes screening flexible sigmoidoscopy recommended but interval unclear—perhaps every 10 years?
   g. For persons at high risk (first-degree family members), screening colonoscopy should be initiated at age 35–40

III. **An Approach**
   A. **Screening and prevention** (see above)
   B. **Clinical presentation**
      1. Many cancers are detected by screening
      2. Initial presentation

        a. Rectal bleeding—usually low lying tumor of rectum or blood streaking by sigmoid tumor

          i. Rectal tumors may also result in tenesmus, urgency

        b. Anemia—due to chronic blood loss from tumor

          i. Often, but not always, microcytic, hypochromic anemia reflecting iron deficiency

          ii. Frequently associated with thrombocytosis

        c. Obstruction—sigmoid or rectal tumors

        d. Jaundice/hepatomegaly—metastatic disease

        e. Sepsis/bacterial endocarditis—if organism is *Streptococcus bovis*, strong association with colorectal cancer of cecum

  3. Diagnosis not difficult

        a. Colonoscopy or barium enema routinely performed

          i. Tissue for definitive diagnosis

          ii. Important to search for second primary colorectal cancer

        b. Computed tomography to detect liver metastases

        c. Measurement of CEA level valuable

          i. Disappearance of titer postoperatively suggests no metastatic disease

          ii. Reappearance of CEA concerning, but not diagnostic of recurrence or metastatic cancer

          iii. CEA level can also be elevated in smoking, inflammatory bowel disease, pancreatitis, renal disease, hepatic disease, cancer of breast, stomach, or lung

C. Treatment

  1. Over 85% of colorectal cancers are amenable to surgical resection

        a. Resection offers best chance for cure

        b. Resection may be carried out to prevent complications (obstruction, bleeding) even if cure not anticipated

        c. Cancers not resected under special circumstances

          i. Low-lying rectal cancer in debilitated older woman who is not surgical candidate

          ii. Far advanced liver metastases with shortened life expectancy

          iii. Overwhelming medical problems that shorten life expectancy

        d. Most colonic cancers can be managed with en bloc resection and anastomosis

          i. Primary anastomosis in > 80% of rectal cancers, reducing need for colostomy

  2. In postmenopausal woman with curable colon cancer, prophylactic oophorectomy should be strongly considered

        a. Colon cancer is a risk for ovarian cancer; possibility of occult colon metastases to ovary

  3. Maintenance of intact colon without colostomy makes acceptance of surgery greater

        a. Although modern colostomy care greatly reduces likelihood of discomfort and "accidents," many women fear colostomy

          i. Concern about cleanliness, clothing, sexuality

         b. Except in cases of complete colectomy (e.g., familial polyposis), anastomosis can usually be accomplished or even "continent colostomy" constructed

  4. Adjuvant therapy

        a. Radiation therapy

          i. Controversial but may be valuable in preoperative reduction in size of bulky tumor

          ii. Occasionally primary treatment modality in rectal cancer in women who are poor surgical risk

          iii. May also be useful in controlling local metastases, especially in pelvis

        b. Chemotherapy

          i. Often offered postoperatively for patients with liver metastases to prolong life by several months

          ii. Major advance is reduction in cancer death by 32% using 5-FU and levamisole in Dukes stage C disease (regional lymph node metastases)

5. **Follow-up**
   a. Yearly chest radiograph
   b. If CEA falls to undetectable range, should periodically measure (every 4 months first year, yearly thereafter)
      i. Elevation not always definitive for recurrence but suggestive
   c. Detection of solitary hepatic metastasis—not infrequent occurrence
      i. Patient may be candidate for resection with improved survival
   d. Colonoscopy should be performed regularly (perhaps every 3–5 years)

Skin Cancer in Women
I. **The Issues**

Skin cancer is by far the most common cancer in the U.S., and the incidence is rising rapidly. Fortunately, the vast majority of skin cancers are either basal cell or squamous cell, cancers that are only infrequently invasive. Malignant melanoma, which can be widely and aggressively metastatic, is also increasing. Recognition of these lesions is important as this is the only means of diagnosing the cancer in a curable stage. Important, however, is recognition of preventive steps that can be taken at many office visits. (Most of this section refers to malignant.)

II. **The Theory**
   A. **Epidemiology**
      1. Basal cell and squamous cell cancers number more than 800,000 new cases per year
         a. Incidence twice as high in men as in women, reflecting greater occupational sun exposure
         b. Basal cell cancer almost never results in death; but estimated almost 1,500 deaths from squamous cell cancer per year, mostly in men
      2. Melanoma accounts for > 17,000 new cases of cancer in women per year (1998 data)
         a. Almost 2700 deaths from melanoma in women each year
         b. Both incidence and death rates approximately two-thirds the rate in men
      3. Most ominous is rapid increase in incidence
         a. Between 1950s and 1990s, incidence of melanoma in women has increased almost 200%
      4. Melanoma affects all age groups
         a. Median age 53
         b. If incidence continues, prevalence rate will approach 1% all females by year 2000
   B. **Risk factors**
      1. Of risk factors, only two may respond to intervention (pigmented lesions, sun exposure)
         a. Age > 15
         b. Family history of cutaneous melanoma
         c. Pigmented lesions (see below)
            i. Dysplastic moles
            ii. Lentigo maligna
            iii. Congenital mole (?)
         d. White (vs. black) race
         e. Previous cutaneous melanoma
         f. Immunosuppression
         g. Excessive exposure to sun (see below)
         h. Sun sensitivity
      2. **Pigmented lesions**
         a. In past decades, increasing recognition that both acquired and congenital lesions associated with degeneration into melanoma
            i. Raises possibility of removal (even by laser in case of congenital nevus) or close observation and frequent biopsy
         b. Acquired dysplastic nevi typically measure 5–12 mm in diameter, have macular and papular components, and irregular, ill-defined borders
            i. Variegated color (tan to dark brown)
            ii. Especially on trunk, also buttock, breast, scalp
            iii. More numerous than common nevi, often > 100
            iv. Appear in youth, but also in adult years up to age 35

      c. Congenital nevi present at birth or develop in infancy
         i. Vary in size from 1–20 cm
         ii. Irregular surface, increased pigmentation
         iii. Hypertrichosis
  3. **Excessive exposure to sun and sun sensitivity**
      a. Increase relative risk to as high as 3.0–5.0
      b. Originally thought to be associated with ultraviolet B range (280–320 nm); now suspected that exposure to ultraviolet A range also predisposes to melanoma
      c. Early exposure to large quantities of sun
         i. Early, frequent blistering sunburn
         ii. Highest frequency in persons of light skin living near equator
      d. Sun sensitivity refers to red-haired persons with freckled skin who typically have difficulty tanning
      e. Melanoma not highly associated with occupation; melanoma not unduly common on face (part of the body most exposed to sun)
         i. Emphasizes significance of sunburn at young age
  4. Growing association with increased radiating light through "holes" in earth's ozone layer, i.e., depletion of ozone layer
C. **Protective factors**
  1. Interest in possible agents that correct DNA breakage, which is thought to be one mechanism of damage by sun radiation on skin
  2. For congenital nevi and dysplastic nevi, regular physician visits and frequent biopsy detect melanoma at early, curable stage
      a. Many recommend early treatment of congenital nevi by excision or laser depigmentation
  3. Avoidance of sunburn
      a. Avoidance of direct, overhead sun
      b. Skin-protective clothing, including hats, long-sleeved shirts, long skirts Sunscreens
         i. Controversy due to one organization's implied lack of support for use of sunscreens to prevent skin cancer; in fact, the recommendation cautions against the concept that sunscreen use can allow even more prolonged sun exposure
      c. Change societal dictum that strong tan equates with health
      d. Preliminary evidence links melanoma to sun beds and tanning parlors
III. **An Approach**
A. **Prevention and screening**
  1. Example taken from Darwin, Australia
      a. Tropical location with almost constant sun
      b. Social activities in Darwin involve sun exposure
      c. In 1980s, incidence of basal cell cancers and melanoma reached alarming levels
         i. Almost 2% of population had been treated for melanoma
      d. Culture has changed
         i. Virtually the only people on beaches in swimsuits are tourists; locals now routinely dress in wide-brimmed hats, long-sleeved blouses, and loose skirts
      e. Too early to tell if incidence is declining
         i. Again, melanoma associated with blistering sunburn at young ages; changes in melanoma in Darwin will be apparent in future decades
  2. Encourage protective clothing, sunscreens (SPF > 15) for young children as well as adults, avoid prolonged sun exposure during hours of 10 AM to 4 PM
  3. Support efforts to develop alternatives to chlorofluorocarbons to allow restoration of ozone layer
  4. Discourage use of sun beds and tanning salons
  5. Primary care physicians should include skin examination in routine health care
      a. Look for premalignant lesions
         i. Actinic keratoses as precursor for squamous cell
         ii. Dysplastic nevi and congenital nevi as precursors for melanoma

B. **Clinical presentation**
  1. Refer to Suggested Reading for pictures of basal cell, squamous cell, and melanoma along with frequently confusing, similar lesions
  2. Melanoma suspected by ABCD rule
     a. A—asymmetry of borders or surface
     b. B—border irregularity
     c. C—color variegation or dark black color
     d. D—diameter > 0.6 cm
  3. Melanoma often found on back, buttocks, trunk, feet, and other sites not often examined by patient
  4. Actinic keratoses typically in sun-exposed areas of head, face, neck, arms, and back of hands
  5. Basal cell cancer often pearly appearing with telangiectasia
  6. Nonhealing lesion after scratching or picking by patient also suspicious
  7. Melanoma may present with local or distant metastases
     a. Especially true if primary lesion large or amelanotic
     b. Metastasizes to almost any organ or site
     c. Occasionally true that metastasis identified and biopsied without ever finding primary lesion
C. **Treatment**
  1. At initial presentation, may perform biopsy
     a. Useful for determining depth of melanoma (Clark stages)
        i. Clark stage I, with depth < 0.75 mm, has good prognosis with excision
        ii. Other Clark stages accompanied by increased likelihood of metastasis
     b. Biopsy may remove entire lesion by elliptical excision, if appropriate
     c. Biopsy may also sample representative portion of lesion
        i. Key to biopsy is to obtain enough depth for pathologist to measure
        ii. Consequently, shave biopsy, curettage, or needle biopsy may be contraindicated
  2. Primary treatment is surgical
     a. Traditionally was done with wide margins (up to 5 cm)
        i. Now apparent that results similar for margins as narrow as 1 cm when removing tumors < 2 mm thick
        ii. For tumors > 2 mm, recommend 3 cm margins
     b. Local recurrence can be treated surgically
     c. Metastases almost always present at time of original removal; wide excision decreases local recurrence but not metastatic disease
     d. Local lymph node disease treated with lymph node dissection
        i. Purpose is not to halt further metastatic disease (although that would be desirable), but to prevent local destructive erosion by tumor
  3. Adjuvant and chemotherapy
     a. Metastatic disease is generally incurable; treatment largely palliative
     b. Chemotherapy often used first
        i. Combinations of dacarbazine, nitrosoureas, cisplatin
        ii. Tends to halt growth more than shrink tumor size
     c. Melanoma largely resistant to radiation therapy
        i. May be useful for treating CNS metastases
     d. More aggressive surgery for destructive lesions
     e. Because of dismal prognosis, innovative efforts are being tried
        i. High-dose chemotherapy with autologous bone marrow transplant; interferon; tamoxifen; adoptive immunotherapy (plasmapheresis to collect and stimulate lymphokine-activated killer cells)

SUGGESTED READING

Lung Cancer
1. Fielding JE: Smoking and women: Tragedy of the majority. N Engl J Med 317:1343–1345, 1987.
2. Fiore MC (ed): Cigarette smoking: A clinical guide to assessment and treatment. Med Clin North Am 76:289–539, 1992.

3. Johnson BE: Tobacco and lung cancer. Prim Care 25:279–292, 1998.
4. Midthun DE, Swensen SJ: Approach to the solitary pulmonary nodule. Mayo Clin Proc 68:378–385, 1993.
5. Richert-Boe KE, Humphrey LL: Screening for cancers of the lung and colon. Arch Intern Med 152:2398–2404, 1992.

Colorectal Cancer
1. DeCosse JJ, Tsioulias GJ: Colorectal cancer: Detection, treatment and rehabilitation. CA Cancer J Clin 44:27–42, 1994.
2. Giovannucci E, Stampfer MJ: Multivitamin use, folate, and colon cancer in women in the Nurses' Health Study. Ann Intern Med 129:517–524, 1998.
3. Grodstein F, Martinez E: Postmenopausal hormone use and risk for colorectal cancer and adenoma. Ann Intern Med 128:705–712, 1998.
4. Midgley R, Kerr D: Colorectal cancer. Lancet 353:391–398, 1999.
5. Ransohoff DF, Lang CA: Sigmoidoscope screening in the 1990s. JAMA 269:1278–1281, 1993.
6. Willett WC, Stampfer MJ, Colditz GA, et al: Relation of meat, fat, and fiber intake to the risk of colon cancer in a prospective study among women. N Engl J Med 323:1664–1672, 1990.

Skin Cancer
1. Chanda JJ: The clinical recognition and prognostic factors of primary cutaneous malignant melanoma. Med Clin North Am 70:39–55, 1986.
2. Consensus Conference, National Cancer Institute: Precursors to malignant melanoma. JAMA 251:1864–1883, 1984.
3. Koh HK: Cutaneous melanoma. N Engl J Med 325:171–182, 1991.
4. McDonald CJ: American Cancer Society perspective on skin cancer prevention and screening. CA Cancer J Clin 48:229–231, 1998.
5. Preston DS, Stern RS: Nonmelanoma cancers of the skin. N Engl J Med 327:1649–1661, 1992.

PART XIV
SPECIAL TESTS AND PROCEDURES

106. Pregnancy Testing

Cynda Ann Johnson, M.D., M.B.A.

Thirty years ago if a woman presented with a missed period, the physician usually recommended expectant waiting for the next period. After two missed periods, a positive physical exam, and typical symptoms, the woman was determined to be pregnant. Now with pregnancy test kits that are inexpensive and highly sensitive, the diagnosis of pregnancy may be made even before the first missed period. Patients then have the opportunity to begin more timely prenatal and self-care appropriate to the pregnant state.

I. **History and Physical Exam**
   A. Not to be forgotten in era of technology
   B. Opportunity to carry out pelvic exam in first trimester should not be missed
      1. Early ultrasound is indicated if size and dates do not correlate
      2. Accurate dating is imperative
         a. Allows prenatal testing to be carried out at appropriate times
         b. Results in less intervention at term

II. **Principles of Pregnancy Testing**
   A. Currently used pregnancy tests are based on amount of human chorionic gonadotropin (hCG) in blood or urine
   B. hCG is detectable in serum as early as 7–9 days after ovulation, that is, within days after implantation
   C. During first 3–4 weeks after implantation, hCG level doubles every 2 days
   D. Level is 50–250 mIU/ml at time of first missed menstrual period
   E. Level peaks at 60–70 days after fertilization, then declines over remainder of first half of pregnancy
   F. During second half of pregnancy level remains constant

III. **Types of Pregnancy Tests**
   A. **Immunometric tests**
      1. Performed on blood or urine samples
         a. Concentrated urine improves pregnancy detection rate of urine test to equal that of serum test
         b. Use first morning void when possible
      2. Based on ELISA (enzyme-linked immunosorbent assay) design
      3. Specific for β-subunit of hCG, eliminating cross-reactivity with other hormones
      4. Depending on specific test used, level of hCG as low as 5–50 mIU/ml may be detected
         a. May be positive as early as 3–4 days after implantation
         b. Test results are positive for 98% of women within 7 days after implantation
      5. Qualitative tests, i.e., results are read as positive or negative
      6. Rare false-positive tests—usually laboratory error or mislabeling
      7. Most useful routine pregnancy tests
   B. **Agglutination inhibition slide tests**
      1. Performed on urine sample
      2. Not specific for β-subunit of hCG; cross-reactivity possible
      3. Detect levels of hCG only as low as 1000–2500 mIU/ml
      4. Positive between 6 and 16 weeks of pregnancy
      5. May be performed rapidly (2 minutes) and inexpensively, but are not sensitive or specific and must always be confirmed by different test if accuracy is in doubt

C. **Quantitative β-hCG radioimmunoassay**
   1. Performed on blood sample
   2. Radioisotope test
   3. Results are quantitative
   4. Detect levels as low as 5 mIU/ml
   5. Test processing usually requires 1–2 hours
   6. Most useful when serial testing is desired or with confusing or variable results among other tests, physical exam, and/or ultrasound
   7. Possible reasons for serial testing
      a. Suspected ectopic pregnancy to follow doubling time or disappearance rate
      b. Impending spontaneous abortion when dilatation and curettage not desired
   8. Very high levels help to make diagnosis of molar pregnancy
   9. Specify "quantitative β-hCG" when ordering test
D. **Home pregnancy testing**
   1. Very popular, used by a third of pregnant women and others to rule out pregnancy
   2. Variable accuracy
   3. Results should still be confirmed by health care provider

SUGGESTED READING

1. Braunstein GD: HCG Testing: A Clinical Guide for the Testing of Human Chorionic Gonadotropin [monograph]. Abbott Park, IL, Abbott Diagnostics, 1992.
2. Hatcher RA, Trussell J, Stewart F, et al: Contraceptive Technology, 17th ed. New York, Ardent Media, Inc., 1998.

107. Wet Smear

Barbara S. Apgar, M.D., M.S.

The wet smear is an important tool for the office diagnosis of vaginitis. It should be performed on each patient presenting with vaginal symptoms even if the diagnosis seems obvious. The wet smear is an accessory tool to the history, inspection of the vulvar and vaginal mucosa, and determination of the pH of the vaginal secretions in women with a presumptive diagnosis of vaginitis. To make an accurate diagnosis, it is necessary to examine the patient rather than to rely on history alone.

I. **Indications**
   A. Vaginal discharge
   B. Malodorous vaginal secretions
   C. Vulvar or vaginal pruritus
   D. Vulvar or vaginal pain
II. **Precautions**
   A. Excessive vaginal bleeding that precludes accurate wet smear
III. **Patient Evaluation and Preparation**
   A. Explain procedure to patient; no written consent needed
   B. Patient should not have used vaginal medication, douched, or had coitus for 24 hours before wet smear
   C. For optimal wet smear interpretation, excessive vaginal bleeding should not be present
IV. **Equipment**
   A. Vaginal speculum
   B. Cotton-tipped applicators
   C. Small test tubes
   D. Normal saline
   E. 10% solution of potassium hydroxide (KOH)

    F. Glass slides and coverslips

    G. Microscope

    H. pH test tape (Nitrazine)

V. **Technique**

    A. Patient is placed in lithotomy position and vaginal speculum is placed

    B. Cotton-tipped applicator is rubbed along lateral vaginal walls and lateral fornices to collect specimen

      1. Cotton-tipped applicator is then placed in small test tube (3–4 inches long) that contains approximately 1 ml of normal saline

      2. Applicator is left in test tube until wet smear is prepared

    C. Speculum is removed from vagina

    D. Test tube is taken to laboratory for preparation of wet smear

      1. Cotton-tipped applicator is removed from test tube and drop is placed on left side of glass slide

      2. Coverslip is immediately placed over drop

    E. Another drop from cotton applicator is placed on right side of slide

      1. Drop of KOH solution is added to drop from applicator

      2. Coverslip is immediately placed over drop

    F. Saline- and KOH-prepared samples are examined under low and high power of microscope

      1. KOH drop is smelled ("sniffed") to detect amine odor

    G. Saline preparation is examined for:

      1. *Lactobacillus* sp. (normal vaginal flora)

      2. Leukocytes (> 10 per HPF may indicate infection)

      3. Parabasal/basal cells (may indicate low estrogenic state)

      4. Trichomonads

      5. Clue cells (bacterial vaginosis)

    H. At least five different microscopic fields should be surveyed to observe representative number of cells and organisms

    I. KOH-prepared sample is scanned for hyphae or buds (indicates candidiasis)

    J. pH tape may be used to diagnose specific types of vaginitis

      1. Piece of pH test tape may be directly applied to vaginal wall or tape may be applied to vaginal secretions adhering to speculum when it is removed from vagina

      2. Test tape color that results from application of secretions is compared with color meter guide on tape dispenser

      3. Range of values determined by color of tape

        a. Normal flora—pH 4

        b. Candidiasis—pH 4–5

        c. Trichomoniasis—pH 6–7

        d. Bacterial vaginosis—pH 4.5–6

      4. Correlation of pH reading and microscopic impression assists in making accurate diagnosis

    K. At same time vaginitis evaluation is performed, cervical cultures may also be obtained for *Chlamydia* sp. and gonorrhea

      1. Depending on type of test, selection of proper sampling devices and proper preparation are important

      2. To obtain cervical sample with cotton-tipped applicator, cervix does not need to be wiped clean

      3. Insert applicator directly into cervical os

      4. Gently twirl device several times in os

      5. Withdraw device and place it in proper container

      6. Lab should provide specific directions for obtaining samples

VI. **Diagnostic Criteria for Specific Vaginal Infections**

    A. **Bacterial vaginosis** (3 of 4 must be present)

      1. pH > 4.5

      2. Positive whiff test

      3. Clue cells

      4. White or gray discharge

B. *Trichomonas* **vaginitis**
 1. pH in upper ranges
 2. Motile trichomonads on saline smear
 3. Culture positive for *Trichomonas vaginalis*
 4. Thin, colored discharge
C. *Candida* **vaginitis**
 1. Hyphae or budding spores on KOH smear
 2. Culture positive for *Candida* sp.
 3. Thick, white adherent discharge
 4. Non–hyphae-forming *Candida* sp. (non-*albicans* sp.)
 5. Buds only seen on wet smear
VII. **Postprocedure Care**
 A. Patient is instructed about use of medication
 B. Follow-up appointment is made if necessary

SUGGESTED READING

1. American College of Obstetricians and Gynecologists (ACOG) Technical Bulletin: Vaginitis. No 221, March 1996.
2. Bertholf ME, Stafford MJ: An office laboratory panel to assess vaginal problems. Am Fam Physician 32:113–125, 1985.
3. Eschenbach DA, Hiller SL: Advances in diagnostic testing for vaginitis and cervicitis. J Reprod Med 34:555–564, 1989.
4. Schaaf VM, Perez-Stable EJ, Borchardo K: The limited value of symptoms and signs in the diagnosis of vaginal infections. Arch Intern Med 150:1929–1933, 1990.
5. Shesser R: Common vaginal infections—a concise work-up guide. Female Patient 15:53–60, 1990.
6. Sobel JD: Treating resistant vaginal infections. Female Patient 20:32–36, 1995.

108. Papanicolaou Smear

Cynda Ann Johnson, M.D., M.B.A.

The incidence of cervical cancer has declined from 44 cases per 100,000 women in 1947, when Papanicolaou testing became routinely available, to under 8 cases per 100,000 in the 1990s. Although the perceived need for their "annual Pap" brings many women to the physician, 65% of invasive cervical cancer in the 40–69-year-old age group and 15% in the 20–39-year-old age group in the U.S. results from failure to screen.

Issues surrounding the use of the Papanicolaou (Pap) smear—its role as a screening tool, sensitivity, frequency of testing, and follow-up of abnormal results—are in the forefront of medical literature. The generalist physician must understand—and help patients to understand—that guidelines are in flux. The doctor and patient can then work together to modify their approach as new information becomes available.

I. **Goals of Pap Smear Testing**
 A. To decrease morbidity and mortality from cervical cancer
 B. To identify by cytologic evaluation of cervical cells, precancerous (dysplastic) changes that may be treated so that they do not progress to invasive cancer
 C. To describe other cellular changes that result in diagnosis of such processes as cervical or vaginal infections or cancer of other organs
II. **Classification System**
 A. Reporting system for the Pap smear has undergone serial changes over past 40 years
 B. Table 1 summarizes comparative nomenclature among systems
 C. All pathology laboratories should now use Bethesda system, which was updated most recently in 1991 (Table 2)
 D. Bethesda system introduced significant change in reporting of squamous cell abnormalities

TABLE 1. Pap Smear Nomenclature

Pap Class System 1954	Descriptive 1968	CIN 1978	Bethesda System 1988
Class I	Negative for malignant cells	Negative	Within normal limits
Class II	Atypical cells of squamous type		Atypical squamous cells
Class III	Slight dysplasia	CIN I	Low-grade SIL; includes condyloma
	Moderate dysplasia	CIN II	High-grade SIL
Class IV	Severe dysplasia Carcinoma *in situ*	CIN III	High-grade SIL
Class V	Invasive carcinoma	Invasive carcinoma	Invasive carcinoma

CIN = cervical intraepithelial neoplasia; SIL = squamous intraepithelial lesion.

1. **Bethesda system** replaces three categories of cervical intraepithelial neoplasia (CIN) with two categories of squamous intraepithelial lesions (SIL)
   a. Justification for term intraepithelial lesion
      i. High spontaneous regression rate of all degrees of dysplasia; even moderate dysplasia regresses in 50% of cases
      ii. Lack of predictable progression to invasive carcinoma, even from carcinoma *in situ* (CIS)
   b. Justification for two categories
      i. Lack of reproducibility of interpreting lesions in CIN system among different laboratories and even by same cytologist
      ii. Putting CIN II, CIN III, and CIS into one category reduces discordance between interpretation of cytologic (Pap smear) and pathologic (biopsy) specimens

TABLE 2. Revised Bethesda System for Reporting Cervical and Vaginal Cytologic Diagnoses

Specimen adequacy
  Satisfactory for evaluation
  Satisfactory for evaluation but limited [reason specified]
  Unsatisfactory for evaluation [reason specified]
General categorization (optional)
  Within normal limits
  Benign cellular changes: see descriptive diagnoses
  Epithelial cell abnormality: see descriptive diagnoses
Descriptive diagnoses
  Benign cellular changes
    Infection
      Trichomonas vaginalis
      Fungal organisms morphologically consistent with *Candida* sp.
      Predominance of coccobacilli consistent with shift in vaginal flora
      Bacteria morphologically consistent with *Actinomyces* sp.
      Cellular changes consistent with herpes simplex virus
      Other
    Reactive changes
      Reactive cellular changes associated with:
        Inflammation (includes typical repair)
        Atrophy with inflammation (atrophic vaginitis)
        Radiation
        Intrauterine device (IUD)
        Other

Descriptive diagnoses (*cont.*)
  Epithelial cell abnormalities
    Squamous cell
    Atypical squamous cell of undetermined significance (ASCUS)
    Low-grade squamous intraepithelial lesion (LGSIL) encompassing human papillomavirus (HPV)/mild dysplasia/CIN 1
    High-grade squamous intraepithelial lesion (HGSIL) encompassing moderate and severe dysplasia/CIN 2 and CIN 3/CIS
  Squamous cell carcinoma
  Glandular cell
    Endometrial cells, cytologically benign in postmenopausal women
    Atypical glandular cells of undetermined significance (AGUS)
    Endocervical adenocarcinoma
    Endometrial adenocarcinoma
    Extrauterine adenocarcinoma
    Adenocarcinoma NOS (not otherwise specified)
  Other malignant neoplasms
  Hormonal evaluation (vaginal smears only)
    Hormonal pattern compatible with age and history
    Hormonal pattern incompatible with age and history [reason specified]
    Hormonal evaluation not possible due to [reason specified]

CIN = cervical intraepithelial neoplasia; CIS = carcinoma *in situ*.

TABLE 3. Suggestions to Reduce False-Negative Rate of Pap Smears

Generalist physician	Cytologist
Obtaining sample	Processing sample
Do not obtain sample during menses	Log in correctly
Use optimal technique for specific sampling	Wash before staining
device	Use fresh or filtered solution
Collect sufficient cells	Use glass coverslip, not liquid plastic
Collect endocervical cells	Forward results of previous smears and biopsies
Sample must be firmly smeared on clear glass	Screening smears
slide	Hire well-trained cytologists
Fix slide quickly to avoid air-drying artifact	Allow adequate screening time
Identify sample clearly	Limit number of slides screened according to
Give history and findings to assist pathologist/	national guidelines
cytologist	Incorporate quality control

      iii. All abnormalities within category of high-grade SIL may be treated in similar manner

III. **Reliability of Pap Smear Results**
   A. High false-negative rate
     1. Usually reported in 10–20% range
     2. May be as high as 70%, depending on level of cervical abnormality and criteria for false-negativity
     3. Characteristics of cancers most likely to be missed by Pap smear testing:
       a. Cancer outside large eversion
       b. Small cancerous lesions
       c. Advanced, invasive cancer with inflammation obscuring cytology
       d. Rapidly progressive tumors
       e. Cancers deep in cervical canal
     4. Table 3 offers suggestions to reduce false-negative rate of Pap smear
     5. New technologies may reduce false-negative results
       a. Computer-assisted inspection systems are costly
       b. Slide preparation system resulting in fewer overlapping cells and less debris (e.g., ThinPrep®) may be useful
   B. Rare false-positive results—when the degree of abnormality is greater on Pap smear than from histologic specimen, conflict is usually resolved when the pathologist reviews both specimens together

IV. **Frequency of Pap Smear Testing**
   A. Increased frequency of screening results in reduced rate of cervical cancer (Table 4) but greater cost and personnel needs
   B. According to 1988 joint statement from the American Cancer Society and American College of Obstetricians and Gynecologists, "All women who are, or have been, sexually active, or have reached age 18, should have an annual Pap test and pelvic examination. After a woman has had three or more consecutive satisfactory examinations, the Pap test may be performed less frequently at the discretion of her physician."

TABLE 4. Percentage Reduction in Cumulative Rate of Invasive Cervical Cancer over the Age Range 35–65 with Different Frequencies of Screening

Screening Frequency	% Reduction in Cumulative Rate*	No. of Tests
1 year	93.3	30
2 years	92.5	15
3 years	91.4	10
5 years	83.9	6
10 years	64.2	3

* Assuming a screen occurs at age 35 and that a previous screen had been performed.
From IARC Working Group: Screening for Cancer of the Uterine Cervix, 1986, p 141, with permission.

TABLE 5. Characteristics of Patients at High Risk for Abnormal Pap Smear

Exposure to diethylstilbestrol (DES) in utero	Partner with history of human papillomavirus
History of abnormal Pap smear	infection
Coitus before age 18	Promiscuous male partner
More than one sexual partner (ever)	Illicit drug use
History of sexually transmitted disease	Smoker
History of human papillomavirus infection	Infection with human immunodeficiency virus

1. Patients at high risk (Table 5) for cervical cancer should continue to have yearly Pap testing; possibly every 6 months in women with HIV infection
2. Patients at low risk for cervical cancer may decrease frequency of screening to every 3 years
3. Many physicians in U.S. still ask patients to return yearly for Pap testing; many women are comfortable with yearly testing
4. Studies show that 33–40% of women with invasive cancer apparently had Pap smear in previous 1–3 years that was read as "normal" or showing "mild atypia"
5. It remains controversial whether celibate women need to undergo Pap testing, despite recommendations of joint statement
6. Hysterectomized women
   a. Canadian Task Force recommends no further Pap smears if:
      i. Hysterectomy was for nonmalignant condition
      ii. Cervix was totally removed
      iii. No history of abnormal Pap smears
   b. Recent studies in the American literature conclude that low incidence of vaginal dysplasia and carcinoma, combined with the high false-positive rate, supports decreasing or eliminating Pap smears after hysterectomy for benign disease
   c. Reservations in implementing these recommendations
      i. Few patients in U.S. have comprehensive, life-time medical records
      ii. Patient may have had abnormal Pap smear and information was either not shared with her or forgotten
      iii. Recommendations are based on data collected before the epidemic of HPV, which has resulted in greatly increased incidence of vaginal intraepithelial neoplasia that may be picked up on Pap smear
   d. Compromise may be to perform Pap smear every 3 years
   e. Hysterectomy for premalignant or malignant disease should result in yearly Pap testing
7. Women exposed to DES *in utero*—begin testing at menarche, age 14 or after first coitus
8. Elderly/postmenopausal women
   a. If patient does not adopt higher-risk lifestyle, and especially if she remains with one partner, frequency can be decreased to every 2–3 years after age 60–65
   b. Some concede that Pap testing can be discontinued altogether after age 65 if 3 previous Pap smears had been negative

V. **Follow-up for Various Findings on Pap Smear**
   A. Metaplasia is a normal finding
   B. Inflammation
      1. No intervention if mild inflammation
      2. Various studies indicate that more severe inflammation may be predictive of cervicovaginal infection, HPV, and/or dysplasia
   C. Follow-up of atypia, or atypical squamous cell of undetermined significance (ASCUS), is controversial
      1. One approach is colposcopy and biopsy after initial finding
      2. Alternate approach: repeat Pap smear in a few months
      3. Most studies emphasize the importance of colposcopic examination in patients with ASCUS because all degrees of dysplasia and high rates of infection with human papillomavirus (HPV) are demonstrated in patients with this finding

D. Similar approaches can be used to follow up hyperkeratosis, leukoplakia, and koilocytosis but repeat Pap smear may be preferred

E. LGSIL, HGSIL—colposcopy and biopsy

F. Invasive carcinoma—colposcopy and biopsy: oncology consult for staging and definitive therapy

G. No endocervical component—repeat Pap in 3–12 months depending on risk

H. Atypical glandular cells of undetermined significance—colposcopy and biopsy
   1. Many of these patients actually have squamous abnormalities found on biopsy
   2. Risk of premalignant, and even malignant lesion is high with glandular disease; includes adenocarcinoma and endometrial carcinoma
   3. Endometrial biopsy should be performed unless the cytologic report states: AGUS—favor reactive; and the patient is young

I. Endometrial cells
   1. Low risk finding if woman is perimenopausal or postmenopausal on HRT—routine follow up
   2. High-risk finding if woman is postmenopausal and not on HRT—proceed to endometrial biopsy

VI. **Collection Techniques**
   A. **Sampling devices**
      1. Goal is sample that includes cervical squamous epithelial cells and generous sampling of cells from within transformation zone
         a. Cells within transformation zone that are undergoing change are called "metaplastic"
         b. Cells still in native state are called "columnar" and are original cells from endocervical canal—reported on Pap smear as "endocervical cells"
         c. Presence of adequate number of endocervical cells is thought to decrease percentage of false-negative results
      2. In multiple studies, use of "broom" or combination of "brush" and "spatula" results in best yield of endocervical cells (Figs. 1 and 2)
         a. Broom
            i. Preferred technique: place middle and longest bristles into cervical canal, allowing other bristles to maintain contact with ectocervix, and rotate broom 180° (5 rotations)
               (a) Results in satisfactory yield of endocervical cells without excessive bleeding
               (b) Both surfaces are then spread across slide and slide is placed in fixative
            ii. May be used in pregnancy
         b. Combination of brush and spatula (see Figs. 1 and 2)
            i. Gives best yield of endocervical cells in most comparative studies
            ii. Spatula—should be used before the brush
               (a) Place contoured end, which best conforms to cervical anatomy, at os
               (b) Rotate 360° about circumference of cervical os, maintaining contact with ectocervix
               (c) Counterclockwise rotation begun at 3:00 or clockwise rotation at 9:00 so that sample will be retained on upright horizontal surface as it is withdrawn from the vagina

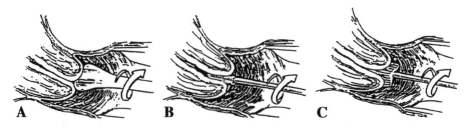

FIGURE 1.   Adequate cervical sampling may require 1–2 instruments, including a spatula (*A*), brush (*B*), or broom (*C*).

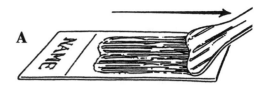

FIGURE 2. To transfer cervical material to the slide from a spatula (*A*), smear the sample with a single stroke using moderate pressure to thin out clumps of cells and mucus. Excessive force or manipulation will damage cells. To transfer material from a brush (*B*), roll the bristles across the slide by twirling the brush handle. To transfer material from a broom (*C*), use a painting action, and use both sides of the broom.

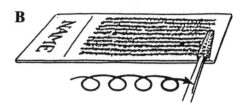

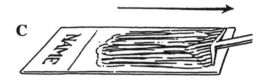

      (d) Sample is held and smeared on slide after endocervical sample is collected because slide must be fixed immediately; only a single slide is needed for both samples

   iii. Brush

      (a) Insert into os and rotate no more than 180°, maintaining contact with cervical canal—if canal is narrow, sufficient cells are collected by simply inserting and removing brush or rotating it one-fourth of turn (90°)

      (b) Sample is unrolled onto slide in opposite direction from which it was collected by twirling handle of brush

      (c) Although blood is often seen macroscopically on brush, it rarely interferes with interpretation of specimen

      (d) Manufacturer recommends that brush not be used during pregnancy, although no evidence indicates that use is detrimental

B. Procedural details

  1. Timing of collection

    a. Optimally in middle of cycle, but such timing is unrealistic in most settings and adequate smears may be obtained at other times

    b. Sample should not be taken during menstrual period

    c. Patient should avoid vaginal medications, vaginal contraceptives, or douches during 48 hours prior to appointment

    d. If patient is postmenopausal and previous smears have lacked endocervical cells, cervix may be primed with 3 weeks of estrogen cream used intravaginally (for example, 0.625 mg of conjugated estrogen daily), which will drive squamocolumnar junction onto ectocervix

    e. Intercourse not recommended on the night before or the day of exam

    f. Postpartum Pap smears should be avoided until 6 or even 8 weeks after delivery, by which time cervix has undergone reparative changes, less inflammation is present, and fewer smears will be uninterpretable

  2. Observe universal precautions: cytologic specimens should be considered infectious until fixed with germicidal fixative

3. Choose appropriate speculum
   a. Long virginal speculum is excellent choice for small women with tight introitus
   b. Whenever possible, use narrow Pederson's speculum rather than wider-blade Graves speculum
   c. If long or large speculum is needed for a particular patient, note is needed in chart and patient told to remind health care provider at next exam so that multiple attempts to expose cervix need not be made
4. Use warm water as lubricant for speculum—test against patient's thigh if speculum may be too hot
5. Inserting speculum and collecting specimen
   a. When inserting speculum, spread labia, then apply pressure posteriorly at introitus so that blades do not press on periurethral area, which can be quite painful
   b. Position speculum so that entire face of cervix can be viewed, but open speculum blades no wider than necessary
   c. Wipe away only large amounts of mucus obscuring cervical os, but do so gently
   d. Do not wash cervix with water or saline
   e. Note squamous epithelium of ectocervix by pink, smooth appearance; columnar epithelium is red with cobblestone appearance
      i. Red appearance has been mistakenly thought to be cervical "erosion" or evidence of cervicitis
   f. After evaluating gross appearance of cervix, collect needed samples for diagnosing infectious diseases, then proceed with cytologic specimen collection, sampling ectocervix and endocervix as described above
   g. Spread specimen evenly on clean glass slide, avoiding frosted portion
   h. Specimen from vaginal pool may be useful to detect endometrial cells in postmenopausal women
   i. Vaginal side wall sample should be collected on separate slide if maturation index is warranted
   j. Some clinicians apply acetic acid to cervix after performing Pap smear
      i. Women with abnormal acetowhite areas then undergo colposcopy
      ii. This approach has not been thoroughly studied and is not part of routine screening
   k. Speculum is removed gently, slowly closing blades and taking care not to catch and pinch any tissue in process
   l. Bimanual examination then carried out

SUGGESTED READING

1. Boon ME, Kok LP: Neural network processing can provide means to catch errors that slip through human screening of Pap smears. Diagn Cytopathol 9:411–416, 1993.
2. Eddy GL, Strumpf KB: Biopsy findings in five hundred thirty-one patients with atypical glandular cells of uncertain significance as defined by the Bethesda system. Am J Obstet Gynecol 177:1188–1195, 1997.
3. Fetters MD, Fischer G: Effectiveness of vaginal Papanicolaou smear screening after total hysterectomy for benign disease. JAMA 275:940–947, 1996.
4. Johnson CA, Lorenzetti LA, Liese BS, Ruble RA: Clinical significance of hyperkeratosis on otherwise normal Papanicolaou smears. J Fam Pract 33:354–358, 1991.
5. Kerpsack JT, Finan MA: Correlation between endometrial cells on Papanicolaou smear and endometrial carcinoma South Med J 91:749–752, 1998.
6. Kinney WK, Manos MM: Where's the high-grade cervical neoplasia? The importance of minimally abnormal Papanicolaou diagnoses. Obstet Gynecol 91:973–976, 1998.
7. Kobelin MH, Kobelin CG: Incidence and predictors of cervical dysplasia in patients with minimally abnormal Papanicolaou smears. Obstet Gynecol 92:356–359, 1998.
8. Koss LG: The new Bethesda system for reporting results of smears of the uterine cervix. J Natl Cancer Inst 82:988–990, 1990.
9. Pearce KF, Haefner HK: Cytopathological findings on vaginal Papanicolaou smears after hysterectomy for benign gynecologic disease. N Engl J Med 335:1559–1562, 1996.
10. Tezuka F, Oikawa H: Diagnostic efficacy and validity of the ThinPrep method in cervical cytology. Acta Cytol 40:513–518, 1996.

109. Vaginal Hormonal Cytology Testing (Maturation Index)

Cynda Ann Johnson, M.D., M.B.A.

Vaginal hormonal cytology is an infrequently ordered test that can be of value in assessing relative estrogen effect, particularly in local tissues. No prospective studies have demonstrated a direct relationship between overall estrogen status and maturation index; therefore, the maturation index should not be used alone to determine whether to offer a woman hormonal replacement therapy during menopause.

I. **Definition of Maturation Index** (MI)
   A. Cytologic assessment of estrogenic effect of vaginal squamous epithelial cells
II. **Principles of MI Assessment**
   A. Vaginal hormonal cytology is based on specific response of vaginal epithelium to stimulation by steroid hormones, mainly of ovarian origin
   B. Estrogen induces maturation of vaginal squamous epithelium
   C. Maturation is manifested by increase in number of cellular layers and by differentiation of squamous cells toward their most evolved forms, from parabasal to intermediate to superficial cells (Fig. 1)
      1. Smear is prepared with hematoxylin and eosin (H&E) staining
         a. Parabasal cells are small cells with large nuclei and sparse blue cytoplasm
         b. Intermediate cells have smaller nuclei and pink-colored cytoplasm
         c. Superficial cells have even smaller nuclei and more abundant pink cytoplasm
   D. MI indicates relative number of each of these cells per hundred cells counted and is expressed as ratio of parabasal to intermediate to superficial cells (known as "being read from left to right")
   E. Several hormonal agents affect ratio
      1. Estrogen stimulation results in increase in number of layers of superficial cells and shift to right
      2. Progesterone stimulation causes shift to mid-zone
      3. Corticosteroid stimulation also causes shift to mid-zone
   F. Typical MI patterns over life span are shown in Table 1
      1. Postmenopausal women with MI of 0:100:0 (intermediate cell atrophy) usually have minimal symptoms of atrophic vaginitis, whereas MI of 100:0:0 (parabasal cell atrophy) results in significant symptoms
   G. Inflammation on smear makes MI determination impossible, because it causes spreading of all three types in unpredictable and irreproducible manner
   H. Estrogen effect vs. MI
      1. Some laboratories note "estrogen effect" routinely on Papanicolaou smear report
      2. "Estrogen effect" is estimate of squamous maturation seen on cervical smear under low magnification on quick evaluation and should not be considered equivalent to MI
III. **Collection of Samples**
   A. Using long side of oblong end of wooden spatula, both vaginal side walls are firmly scraped and sample spread on clean, labeled glass slide
   B. If Papanicolaou smear sample is also collected, separate slide must be prepared for vaginal hormonal cytology
   C. Sample is placed immediately in fixative
IV. **Value of MI**
   A. To reassure young patient that she is premenopausal
   B. To reassure premenopausal patient that perceived vaginal dryness is not from lack of estrogen
   C. To help assess whether vaginal dryness in postmenopausal patient (particularly one already on estrogen replacement) is result of inadequate local estrogen
      1. 5–10% superficial cells usually correlates with adequate estrogen effect

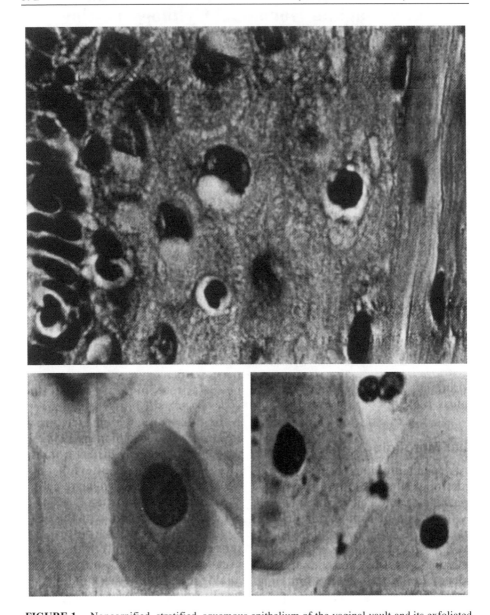

FIGURE 1. Noncornified, stratified, squamous epithelium of the vaginal vault and its exfoliated cells. *Upper section, from left to right*, basement membrane, true basal cells, parabasal cells, intermediate cells, superficial cells (× 1500). *Lower left*, parabasal cell (exfoliated, in vaginal smear); cytoplasm is thick from nucleus to cell border (× 1500). *Lower right*, intermediate cell (*left*) and superficial cell (exfoliated, in vaginal smear); cytoplasm of both is uniformly "wafer-thin" from nucleus to cell border. The intermediate cell nucleus is vesicular and retains chromatin pattern. The nucleus of the superficial cell is pyknotic, measuring less than 6 μ, hyperchromatic, and has lost chromatin pattern. For size reference, a neutrophil is in upper midfield (× 1500).

    D. To assess vaginal estrogen status in postmenopausal woman with mildly atypical Papanicolaou smear
    E. To assess woman who had hysterectomy, without oophorectomy, as adjunct to other assessment of ovarian failure

TABLE 1. Normal Maturation Index Averages

Age or Physiologic State	Variability	Maturation Index
At birth (first week)	Slight	0/95/5
Childhood (to 6 years)	Moderate	90/10/0
Perimenarche	Great	
Childbearing age		
Ovulation	Moderate	0/40/60
Menstruation	Moderate	0/70/30
Pregnancy	Slight	0/95/5
Postpartum	Moderate	90/10/0
Perimenopausal		
"Estratrophy" (lack of estrogen)	Moderate	0/100/0
"Teleatrophy" (lack of all hormones or agent)	Moderate	100/0/0

SUGGESTED READING

1. Gomel V, Munro MG, Rowe T: Gynecology: A Practical Approach. Baltimore, Williams & Wilkins, 1990.
2. Jones HW Jr, Jones GS: Novak's Textbook of Gynecology, 10th ed. Baltimore, Williams & Wilkins, 1981.

110. Colposcopy

Barbara S. Apgar, M.D., M.S.

Colposcopy has largely replaced conization for evaluation of the abnormal Pap smear. Colposcopic-directed biopsies are a dramatic improvement over random biopsies of the past. Colposcopy defines the abnormalities of the epithelium and blood vessels that are the hallmark of preinvasive and invasive disease of the cervix. The colposcopist should follow a systematic protocol to avoid missing important steps of the colposcopic examination. Preparation of the patient and the examination room are part of a systematic approach. If steps are skipped or proper equipment is not available, the information obtained may be insufficient to ensure an accurate diagnosis. The prediction of the histopathologic diagnosis based on colposcopic patterns requires experience and practice. At each colposcopic examination, the clinician should try to predict each diagnosis based on the principles of accurate assessment. Every colposcopist should know:

- Whether or not the colposcopic examination is satisfactory
- How to recognize whether the tissue is normal or abnormal
- How to appropriately biopsy the abnormal lesion
- How to rationally triage the histopathology and treat and manage the lesion

I. **Indications and Contraindications**
- A. Indications
    1. Abnormal Pap smear
    2. Presence of obvious lesion with normal Pap smear
    3. Undiagnosed vaginal discharge or bleeding
- B. Contraindications
    1. Any condition that precludes vaginal speculum placement and inspection of lower genital tract

II. **Preoperative Evaluation and Preparation**
- A. **Appropriate history** should include the following information
    1. Obstetric and gynecologic history
        - a. Menstrual pattern; method of contraception; sexually transmitted disease; previous abnormal cytology and treatment; symptoms of malignant disease; diethylstilbestrol exposure; previous obstetric complications; gynecologic surgery;

Consent for Colposcopic Examination

Date_____
Time_____

I hereby authorize Dr._____ and his/her assistants to perform a colposcopic examination upon me. I understand that this examination involves the use of a colposcope, which is a magnifying instrument with a strong light which can be focused on my cervix and other parts of the genitals. It allows for detailed study of these organs. I understand that this exam will be done in the same position as used for a Pap smear.

I understand that a vinegar solution will be used for this examination and that it may cause a slight burning sensation.

I understand that samples of tissue (biopsies) may need to be removed from any abnormal areas in order for a pathologist to examine that tissue under a microscope. I authorize my doctor to take whatever biopsies are necessary to properly investigate my condition. I understand that I may have some discomfort and cramping at the time of the biopsies. I understand that I may also have some bleeding, which can be controlled with pressure against the bleeding site, along with one of several chemicals that help coagulate blood. I understand there is a very slight chance that I could get an infection at a biopsy site, and if so, it would be treated with antibiotics.

I understand that I will likely have a bloody vaginal discharge for the next couple of days and that I should not douche, use a tampon, or have vaginal intercourse during that period of time.

I have/have not had the opportunity to view the patient education video on the colposcopic examination. I understand the risks and benefits of the exam and have had the opportunity to have my questions answered.

_____   _____
Signature of witness   Patient's signature

                                          _____
                                          Current telephone number

FIGURE 1.   Consent form for colposcopic examination.

      number of sexual partners in the past year; social history; cigarette smoking or substance abuse
2. Medical history
   a. Immunosuppression, prescription drug use, allergies, current medical problems

B. **Preparation of examination room**
1. Supplies should be available and equipment in good working condition, extra supplies for procedure and extra bulbs for colposcope should be available in near vicinity

C. **Patient preparation** for colposcopic examination
1. Colposcopy is optimal when performed on days 10–14 of menstrual cycle when cervical mucus is clear and not tenacious. Informed consent should be obtained (Fig. 1). A pregnancy test should be performed if there is question of inadequate contraception.

D. **Equipment arrangements**
1. Must occur months before first patient arrives for colposcopic examination. Attending to details prior to start-up makes actual colposcopic evaluation more successful. If instruments and equipment are not purchased with quality assurance in mind, results will be disappointing and both patient and clinician will be less than satisfied
2. To decide what equipment and supplies should be purchased, the following steps should be performed:
   a. **Arrange for representatives from several companies to visit office and demonstrate equipment.** The visit should include survey of existing examination space and limitations of space. The following issues should be considered:

      i. Purchase price of colposcope and what ancillary equipment is included in primary cost

     ii. Whether teaching head or TV monitor is desired

   iii. Guarantee on equipment

   iv. How easy it is to receive service on equipment and whether equipment can be serviced in office or must be sent back to company

    v. Whether equipment can be upgraded if new parts become available

   vi. Possibility of leasing equipment with option to buy at later date

  vii. What type of service contract is available

b. **Assess number of colposcopies to be performed each month.** This approximate number helps decide what price of scope can be afforded and what payment plan should be. Clinicians performing < 10 colposcopies each month may not have adequate number to maintain quality skills.

c. **Ask the following questions about patient visit:**

      i. Would it be possible to group patients on half days? If not, how will flow of patients be affected by performance of colposcopy at odd times during the day? Is dedicated nursing assistance appropriate?

d. **Estimate number of biopsy instruments needed for procedure.** Biopsy instruments must be sharpened on regular basis to ensure clean and less painful biopsy sampling. Cervical biopsy punch and endocervical curette must be sharpened about every 20 uses. Determine how many biopsy instruments are needed based on ability to autoclave them quickly after each patient or at end of day

      i. Care of instruments

        (a) Where will instruments be sharpened? How often will they need to be sharpened? How many biopsy instruments will be necessary to ensure smooth operation? Who will be in charge of instruments and anticipate need for sharpening or repair? How will instruments be cleaned and maintained? What is the procedure for repairing instrument and returning it quickly?

e. **Contact laboratory that interprets pathology specimens**

      i. Clinician and pathologist should agree on accurate reporting system and language. Clinician and pathologist should talk before procedure is set up. Clinician who cannot trust pathology report and is constantly worried that report is not accurate will not be successful. Treatment based on colposcopic-directed biopsy, not on cytology report. Histology must be analyzed by best available pathologist

     ii. Consider following regarding pathology:

        (a) How should samples be prepared for pathology? Are correct containers and solutions available? What is turn-around time for reports? How available is pathologist to consult on difficult cases? Are correct lab forms available? Does cytopathologist use the Bethesda system? Does pathologist know current data about human papillomavirus-associated disease?

f. **Begin training of nursing personnel early in operational preparation**

      i. Competent assistant makes colposcopy seem more successful and lowers frustration level of everyone involved. Assistant should be placed in charge of checking equipment before colposcopy and replacing supplies after procedure completed. A checklist should be completed each time procedure is initiated. It will be frustrating to begin colposcopy and realize that instruments or equipment are not working or absent. Spare parts should be available at time of each colposcopic examination

     ii. Consider following issues:

        (a) Is checklist of equipment and supplies available? Has check of equipment been performed prior to colposcopy? Does assistant understand expectations for stocking examination room after colposcopy? Does assistant share clinician's concern for care of equipment and take responsibility for adopting excellence in performance of procedure?

COLPOSCOPIC EVALUATION

Date_____   Referring Doctor_____
BP_____ P_____   WT_____ Age_____
G_____ P_____ Ab_____ LMP_____ Pregnant? Y_____ N_____
Type of Contraception_____
Age first intercourse_____ # of sex partners (lifetime)_____
Smoker? Y_____ N_____ Do you use tampons? Y_____ N_____
Reason for Colpo_____
_____

Last Pap smear: Date_____ Result_____
Previous abnormal Pap smear? Y_____ N_____
    If yes, Date_____ Diagnosis_____ Treatment_____
Previous Colposcopy? Y_____ N_____
    If yes, Date_____ Diagnosis_____ Treatment_____
History of Chlamydia? Y_____ N_____   Gonorrhea? Y_____ N_____
          Herpes?   Y_____ N_____   Condyloma? Y_____ N_____
Any vaginal or pelvic infections in last 3 months? Y_____ N_____
    If yes, which ones?_____
Date of last exam: Bimanual_____ Breast_____

Exam: Border   Surface Pattern Vascular Pattern Intercapillary Distance
        Indistinct Flat   Normal   Normal
        Distinct   Raised   Punctate   Slight increase
                                     Mosaic   Marked increase
                                     Atypical

Key: Columnar Epithelium = /////
        White =
        Whiter = XXX
        Whitest = ###
        Mosaic = M
        Punctation = P
        Abnormal Vessels = AV
        Biopsy = B

Additional History

Bimanual?   Y_____ N_____
      If yes, describe

Pap today?   Y_____ N_____
ECC done?   Y_____ N_____
SCJ seen?   Y_____ N_____
CRYO candidate? Y_____ N_____
Cultures today? Y_____ N_____
      Which ones?

Assessment:

Plan:

                                                        Colposcopist_____
Colposcopy Aftercare Instructions given? Y_____ N_____

FIGURE 2.   Form for primary colposcopic evaluation.

g. **Prepare documentation and informed consent forms before start of procedure**
   i. Standard forms may be reproduced from available sources. Clinician may
      adapt or develop personal forms but they should contain basic medicolegal
      documentation format. Demographic and clinical information may be con-
      tained on same form or separate forms (Figs. 2 and 3). It will be necessary to
      maintain "tickler" file or computer database so that patients may be recalled
      if they fail to show up for specified appointments. A simple card file will

REPEAT COLPOSCOPIC EXAM

Date_____ Referring Doctor_____
BP_____ P_____ T_____ Wt_____ Age_____ LMP_____
Pregnant? Y____ N____ Type of contraception _____
Reason for repeat colpo_____
_____
_____

Date of last Pap_____ Result_____
Date of last Colpo_____ Result_____
Vaginal or pelvic infections in last 3 months? Y____ N____
  If yes, which ones?_____
Date of last exam: Bimanual _____ Breast _____

Exam: | Border | Surface Pattern | Vascular Pattern | Intercapillary Distance |
| --- | --- | --- | --- |
| Indistinct | Flat | Normal | Normal |
| Distinct | Raised | Punctate | Slight increase |
| | | Mosaic | Marked increase |
| | | Atypical | |

Key: Columnar Epithelium = /////
     White =
     Whiter = XXX
     Whitest = ###
     Mosaic = M
     Punctation = P
     Abnormal Vessels = AV
     Biopsy = B

Additional History

Bimanual? Y____ N____
  If yes, describe

Pap today? Y____ N____
ECC done? Y____ N____
SCJ seen? Y____ N____
CRYO candidate? Y____ N____
Cultures today? Y____ N____
  Which ones?

Assessment:

Plan:

Colposcopist_____
Colposcopy Aftercare Instructions given? Y____ N____

FIGURE 3. Form for repeat colposcopic examination.

suffice, but optimal to have data on computer. It should be decided who will maintain recall file and how patients will be contacted

ii. Consider following issues about reporting:

(a) How will forms be developed and printed? Are forms available for informed consent and clinical documentation? Are patient education materials purchased or developed? What is procedure for recalling patients? Who will be in charge of giving patients their reports? What is system for notifying patients of their report? In what time frame will reports be given and how will they be communicated to patient? Is letter or card for patient recall available? Who will handle patient calls about results or follow-up?

    h. **Ensure that colposcopist has adequate training and experience** to perform responsible and competent examination

        i. Preceptorship following didactic training is suggested. To learn under watchful eye of experienced colposcopist is ideal.

3. **General equipment**

    a. Examination room adequate for performing colposcopy, Examination table (with adjustable height preferred) with stirrups, Examination gloves for clinician and assistant, Mayo stand or table for surgical supplies, Rubber container for placement of the surgical instruments after use, Specula of various sizes (Graves—short and long, Peterson—short and long, Plastic disposable—Graves and Peterson), Autoclave equipment, Solution for disinfection (containing 2% glutaraldehyde)

4. **General supplies**

    a. Lugol's (dilute iodine) solution
    b. Monsel's solution (ferric subsulfate) dehydrated to thick paste
    c. Silver nitrate sticks
    d. Acetic acid or household vinegar (4–5%)
    e. Topical 20% benzocaine (Hurricaine)
    f. Urine cups for individual solutions
    g. Blue pads to place under patient's buttocks
    h. Nonsteroidal anti-inflammatory samples for postoperative discomfort
    i. Scopettes and cotton-tipped applicators
    j. Gauze pads (4 × 4)

5. **Equipment for Papanicolaou smear**

    a. Cervical sampling devices: wooden spatulas, cervix broom, cytobrushes
    b. Glass slides
    c. Fixative (specially designated lab spray)
    d. Transport container
    e. Laboratory forms

6. **Colposcopy equipment**

    a. Colposcope
    b. Extra light bulbs for colposcope
    c. Lens paper to clean binocular lenses
    d. Cervical biopsy forceps
    e. Endocervical curette (without basket)
    f. Toothpicks
    g. Endocervical specula (two sizes of tips)
    h. Cervical hook
    i. Ringed or sponge forceps
    j. Anoscopy specula, clear plastic
    k. Teaching head or TV monitor (optional)
    l. Camera for colposcope (optional)
    m. Video attachments (optional)
    n. Specimen bottles with formalin or other fixative requested by pathology
    o. Patient educational material

7. **Paper and forms** (stamped with patient identification card before procedure)

    a. Colposcopy form
    b. Demographic form
    c. Informed consent form
    d. Laboratory forms for surgical pathology and cytology
    e. Laboratory form for human chorionic gonadotropin, if needed
    f. Pre- and postcolposcopy information sheets with office telephone number
    g. Card for "tickler" file or computer database
    h. Patient reminder card

III. **Specific Equipment and Supply Information**
  A. **Colposcope**
    1. Colposcopes are as varied as colposcopists performing procedure. The colposcope provides magnification and illumination. By varying magnification, clinician can identify patterns indicating normal or abnormal tissue
    2. The colposcope is a binocular microscope with built-in light source and converging objective lens attached to support stand. The lens has fixed focal distance which determines working distance between lens and patient. If focal distance is too short, room to maneuver instruments in front of colposcope is limited. The most practical lens has focal length of 300 mm, which allows exam of cervix, vagina, vulva, and anal region. New video colposcopes have no binocular lenses and are viewed on a video screen
    3. Cost varies according to capability of lenses, mounting support, desired video components, and type of light. Range: $4,000–20,000. Although purchasing less expensive scope may seem prudent initially, colposcopist must consider comfort and future needs. A scope with limited capability can be frustrating when colposcopist becomes more experienced.
    4. Focus capability may include fine, coarse, or zoom focus knobs. Coarse focus can be achieved by moving head of colposcope closer or farther away from patient. Zoom provides for continuous focusing throughout all magnifications. Most scopes without zoom can be set for par-focal capability so focus remains throughout all magnification levels
    5. Magnification varies among colposcopes. Colposcopists will be most satisfied with capability for variable magnification. Although less expensive scopes with single magnification (4–12 ×) are available, they have limited capability for complete examination of entire lower genital system. It is useful to be able to scan at low (5–6x), medium (10–16 ×), and high (20 × +) magnification: Lower power used for examination of vulva and male genitalia, medium power used to examine vulva and cervix and high power used to detect finer detail of vascular patterns. Changing magnification changes diameter of field of view. The higher the magnification, the smaller the surface area of target tissue that can be visualized
    6. Green filter enhances vascular patterns. Green filters usually within easy reach to facilitate switching from white light to green filter. Green filter absorbs certain wavelengths of light, making red color of vessels appear blacker and easier to see
    7. Light sources vary. Colposcope can be fitted with incandescent bulb or halogen light. Halogen light provides brighter light that is excellent for photography. Light may be provided through fiberoptic cable that reduces heat during procedure
    8. Mounting of colposcope varies according to individual preference. Can be mounted by swivel arm on wall or examination table or on stand attached to colposcope. Size of exam room must be considered. Colposcope with wide stand may not fit in limited space and wall swivel mount may be preferable. Some clinicians prefer a colposcope that does not have the stand directly in front of them. Several different types of mountings should be evaluated to ensure that comfortable position is achievable
    9. Setting up colposcopic equipment requires experimentation and patience. Preferable to have supplies situated next to dominant hand of clinician. If supplies are administered by the assistant, it is necessary that he or she be positioned comfortably next to colposcope and supply tray. It is not impossible to perform colposcopy without assistant but more difficult. If colposcopist individually retrieves instruments and supplies, it is important to place only enough supplies for current procedure to avoid contamination of whole supply of solutions or swabs. After colposcopic exam is completed, instruments are placed in disinfectant solution before autoclaving
  B. **Biopsy instruments**
    1. **Biopsy forceps**
      a. Must be sharp and in good working condition to obtain good biopsy sample
      b. Composed of handle grip mechanism with anchoring edge and cutting edge on distal head. There are many types (Tischler, Burke, Kevorkian, and Eppendorfer); each

produces slightly different sample. Each must be selected carefully because each has distinctive properties. Some biopsy forceps have shank that can be rotated 360°

    c. Must be sharpened frequently to ensure sharp, clean, and precise sample. Sharp instrument produces less discomfort when biopsy is obtained

    d. Put instruments in rubber rather than a stainless steel container so heads will not be dulled by rough handling

    e. Should be cleaned in disinfectant solution and then autoclaved

    f. Tischler, Burke and Eppendorfer instruments have anchoring tooth to immobilize tissue and sharp edge for cutting so crushing of tissue prevented

       i. Baby Tischler produces smaller sample but less bleeding at biopsy site

      ii. Kevorkian forceps has row of teeth instead of single tooth. Teeth can easily tear tissue

2. **Endocervical curettes**

    a. Samples of endocervical canal are obtained at time of colposcopy with endocervical curettes which must be sharp to obtain adequate sample of endocervix

    b. Characteristics of curettes

       i. Kevorkian curette without basket is preferred. Toothpicks are used to remove sample from curette. If basket is used, sample collects in basket and proves difficult to remove

      ii. Curettes are available with disposable tips or entire curette may be disposable. Stainless steel curettes are reusable, but must be sharpened frequently. They are designed with finger grip that aids in holding but also indicates that cutting edge faces up when finger grip is on upper surface

3. **Skin hooks**

    a. Used to pucker tissue so sample can be obtained

       i. May also be used to visualize vaginal rugae

    b. If surface is flat, tooth of biopsy forceps cannot anchor properly. Skin hook can fix area of tissue so it will not slip away from biopsy forceps

    c. Tip of hook should not be too sharp; tissue may be torn in process of sampling

4. **Endocervical canal specula**

    a. Used to visualize endocervical canal to determine position of squamocolumnar junction or to view endocervical structures

    b. May be placed in canal and gradually opened to aid visualization

    c. Speculum blades come in various lengths and have different tips for nulliparous, parous, or stenotic cervices

5. **Vaginal sidewall retractors**

    a. Used to aid visualization of cervix if obscured by vaginal sidewalls

    b. May be placed inside speculum

    c. Condom or index finger of exam glove also may be placed over blades of speculum in place of retractor to keep sidewalls out of viewing path

C. **Chemicals used during colposcopy**

1. **Acetic acid or vinegar**

    a. Used to enhance colposcopic image by process called "acetowhitening." Tissue does not turn white until vinegar is applied

    b. Household vinegar (4–5%) or acetic acid (4–5%) is used to produce acetowhite reaction

    c. Solution applied with sponges, large swabs, or spray bottle then left in contact with tissue for at least 1 minute or until pattern emerges

2. **Aqueous Lugol's solution**

    a. Aids in assessment of cervix and vagina

       i. Normal glycogenated squamous epithelium is stained dark mahogany brown

    b. Must be diluted to one-fourth to one-half strength

       i. Diluted solution produces good stain and does not cause irritation like full-strength solution

    c. Unstable; should be replaced every 3–6 months

3. **Monsel's solution**

    a. Ferric subsulfate solution used for hemostasis after biopsy

      b. Comes as dark brown suspension
         i. Should be quickly shaken and then poured into smaller container. It is allowed to dehydrate until it becomes thick paste which usually occurs when about one-third of volume is evaporated
         ii. To prevent hardening, thin layer of Monsel's solution should be kept on surface of paste. In some humid areas, may take up to 1 month to evaporate 1 urine cup of solution. Several containers of solution evaporating at different times should be available so supply is not exhausted. Monsel's paste can be purchased already dehydrated
         iii. It is important to remember that Monsel's paste interferes with biopsy interpretation for even a month after it is applied. Monsel's should be applied only after all biopsies are obtained.
      c. Patient should be warned that Monsel's may produce charcoal-appearing vaginal discharge for first several days after colposcopy
      d. Monsel's interferes with biopsy interpretation
    4. **Silver nitrate sticks**
      a. May be used for hemostasis, but patient may notice more irritation or burning than with use of Monsel's
      b. Silver interferes with biopsy interpretation
IV. **Technique of Colposcopy**
  A. Clinician sits comfortably at end of examination table and sets magnification and illumination on colposcope
  B. Patient is placed in dorsal lithotomy position and properly draped
  C. **Anal area and vulva** are inspected with colposcope
    1. 5% vinegar or acetic acid may be used to enhance tissue
    2. Appropriate cultures are obtained, if indicated
    3. If abnormal areas are identified, vulvar and anal biopsies can be deferred until exam of cervix is completed
  D. **Speculum inserted into vagina**
    1. Good visualization is important part of colposcopic routine
    2. Vaginal sidewalls should be out of field of view
      a. If they obstruct viewing area, they can be displaced by use of vaginal retractor or finger of exam glove placed over speculum blades
      b. Active bleeding and mucus may hinder visualization of cervix and should be removed if possible
  E. **Papanicolaou smear is obtained** before applying 3–5% acetic acid or vinegar to cervix
    1. Bleeding after cytologic sampling usually stopped by gently placing cotton-tipped applicator into endocervical canal
    2. Monsel's solution should not be applied at this time; may hinder biopsy interpretation
  F. **Cervix is soaked with normal saline** and viewed with low power (4–10×)
    1. Gross lesions and leukoplakia are identified
  G. **Vascular pattern examined** with green filter
    1. Vessels are examined in detail from low to high power
    2. Acetic acid should not be applied until after vascular pattern is detailed
  H. **Acetic acid (3–5%) or vinegar applied to cervix** with saturated cotton balls on ringed forceps, large cotton swabs, or spray bottle
    1. Rubbing or patting cervix should be avoided
    2. Placing cotton balls or swabs on cervix and allowing acetic acid to soak tissue thoroughly avoids unnecessary abrasions
    3. Second application of acetic acid should follow to ensure proper acetowhite reaction
      a. Mucus easily removed after application of acetic acid and gently wiped away with swabs or removed with ring forceps
    4. Abnormal epithelium turns white after application of acetic acid (acetowhite reaction)
      a. Acetowhite reaction begins to fade after few minutes
      b. As it fades, vascular patterns become more distinct
         i. Red color of vascular patterns (mosaic and punctation) becomes more apparent
         ii. Vascular patterns should be examined with high power

       iii. As acetowhite reaction resolves, atypical vessels can again be viewed with green filter

I. **Cervical landmarks** and any accompanying atypical areas should be mentally mapped because it will be necessary to recall details later when documentation forms are completed

J. **Staining of cervix** can be accomplished with dilute Lugol's iodine solution
    1. Iodine staining of various tissue types depends on interaction between glycogen and iodine
    2. Normal mature squamous epithelium of cervix and vagina contain glycogen and stain mahogany brown after application of Lugol's iodine
    3. Columnar and immature squamous metaplasia do not contain glycogen and do not take up stain
    4. Precancerous lesions of cervix produce varying responses to Lugol's iodine, ranging from normal mahogany to mustard yellow
       a. Mustard yellow color is produced and easily washed away with saline

K. **Endocervical curettage** (ECC) is performed to evaluate status of endocervical canal and to rule out the presence of cancer
    1. Curette without basket facilitates removal of sample from curette
       a. Curette is held like pencil and the index finger can be placed in finger hold indentation on shaft of curette
    2. Technique of endocervical curettage
       a. Curette inserted into endocervical canal under colposcopic guidance
       b. Entire canal is sampled with short definitive strokes as cutting edge of curette is rotated 360°
       c. Care should be taken not to contaminate ECC with ectocervical tissue
       d. Curette should remain in endocervical canal until curettage is completed
       e. Sample is spun onto end of curette and curette is removed straight from endocervical canal
       f. Cytobrush or ringed forceps may be used to remove remaining sample
       g. Entire specimen placed into tissue fixative, and specimen bottle labeled with patient identification
    3. Special considerations of endocervical sampling
       a. ECC not performed if patient is pregnant
       b. Comparison of ECC and endocervical brush (ECB) sampling indicates that the ECB is more sensitive but less specific than the ECC
          i. If the colposcopy is satisfactory, ECB can be used to select those patients on whom the ECC should be performed; glandular lesions should be evaluated with ECC
          ii. If the colposcopy is unsatisfactory, ECC should be performed and if HGSIL is present, conization should be considered

L. **Ectocervical biopsies** are performed as necessary under colposcopic guidance
    1. Colposcopic-directed biopsies have replaced blind or four-quadrant biopsies
    2. Biopsies are best obtained after careful inspection of entire cervix
       a. Critical element for successful colposcopy is determination of proper site for biopsy. Entire transformation zone must be visible to determine proper biopsy site
       b. Use of cotton-tipped applicators or endocervical speculum may aid in visualization of entire transformation zone
       c. Biopsy instrument placed at site of lesion and anchoring piece allowed to hold tissue firmly so lesion will not slip away as biopsy is performed
          i. If cervix cannot be anchored by use of tooth on biopsy instrument, skin hook can be used to create fold of tissue so jaws of biopsy instrument can close around it
          ii. Posterior surface of cervix should be biopsied first to avoid dripping blood that obscures remaining biopsy sites
          iii. Biopsy punch should be sharp. Actual biopsy obtained with definitive snap of jaws of instrument. Tissue should not be pulled from biopsy site
       d. After biopsy, cervix should be inspected to ensure that correct sites have been sampled

      e. Biopsy specimens are removed from biopsy instrument with toothpicks and placed in fixative

      f. Bottles of fixative are labeled with patient identification

  3. Colposcopically directed biopsies should be obtained after careful inspection and assessment and use of colposcopic grading systems

    a. Biopsies obtained from appearance of acetowhite reaction alone should be discouraged

M. Hemostasis

  1. Monsel's paste should be applied to biopsy site to promote hemostasis only after all biopsies have been taken; premature application may make histologic samples unreadable

    b. Monsel's paste should contact actual tissue rather than blood oozing from biopsy site

  2. Silver nitrate sticks also may be used to achieve hemostasis

  3. Blood should be cleaned from fornices with cotton swab before removing speculum

  4. Patient should be warned that black charcoal-appearing discharge may be present for several days after colposcopic exam

N. Inspect vagina as speculum is removed

  1. Application of Lugol's iodine solution is helpful for delineating suspicious tissue

  2. Skin hook can be used to see between vaginal rugae if lesion is obscured

O. Biopsies of vulva and anal area are obtained after speculum is removed

P. Bimanual examination is performed to assess presence of pelvic masses

Q. Colposcopic findings are recorded on documentation forms

  1. Records should be documented as soon as possible after procedure is completed

  2. Normal landmarks and location of abnormal areas should be clearly recorded

  3. Each abnormal area is designated as if present on clock face

  4. The following should always be documented: Whether exam was satisfactory, whether signs of invasive cancer were present, and where biopsies were taken

V. Postprocedure Care

  A. Allow patient to recover from procedure

    1. Inform patient about preliminary impression and mechanism for reporting results

    2. Discharge patient with educational material about her condition

  B. Clean colposcope and replenish supplies

SUGGESTED READING

1. Barrasso R, Guillemotonia A: Cervix and vagina: Diagnosis. In Gross GE, Barrasso R (eds): Human Papillomavirus Infection: A Clinical Atlas. Berlin, Ullstein Mosby, 1997, pp 147–274.
2. Burghardt E (ed): Colposcopy Cervical Pathology: Textbook and Atlas. Stuttgart, Georg Thieme, 1984.
3. Cartier R: Practical Colposcopy, 3rd ed. Karger Basel, Laboratoire Cartier, Paris, 1993.
4. Campion MJ, Sedlacek TV: Colposcopy in pregnancy. Obstet Gynecol Clin North Am 20:153–163, 1993.
5. Campion MJ, Greenberg MD, Kazamil TEG: Clinical Manifestations and Natural History of Genital Human Papillomavirus Infections. Obstet Gynecol Clin North Am 23:783–809, 1996.
6. Cox JT and ASCCP Practice Guidelines Committee: Endocervical curettage. J Lower Genital Dis 1:251–256, 1997.
7. Ferenczy A: Anatomy and histology of the uterine corpus. In Kurman RJ (ed): Blaustein's Pathology of the Female Genital Tract. New York, Springer Verlag, 1994, pp 327–366.
8. Giuntoli RL, Atkinson BF, Ernst CS, et al: Malignant lesions of the cervix. In Atkinson's Correlative Atlas of Colposcopy, Cytology and Histopathology. Philadelphia, J.B. Lippincott, 1987, pp 161–195.
9. Reid R, Scalzi P: Genital warts and cervical cancer. VII. An improved colposcopic index for differentiating benign papillomaviral infections from high-grade cervical intraepithelial neoplasia. Am J Obstet Gynecol 153:611–618, 1985.
10. Stafl A, Wilbanks GD: An international terminology of colposcopy: Report of the Nomenclature Committee of the International Federation of Cervical Pathology and Colposcopy. Obstet Gynecol 77:313–314, 1991.
11. Wright TC, Kurman RJ, Ferenczy A: Precancerous lesions of the cervix. In Kurman RF (ed): Blaustein's Pathology of the Female Genital Tract. New York, Springer Verlag, 1994, pp 229–277.
12. Wright TC, Ferenczy A, Kurman RJ: Carcinoma and other tumors of the cervix. In Kurman RF (ed): Blaustein's Pathology of the Female Genital Tract. New York, Springer Verlag, 1994, pp 279–326.

111. Cervical Polypectomy

Cynda Ann Johnson, M.D., M.B.A.

Cervical polyps are a common phenomenon, and as the number of women in whom the cervix is evaluated colposcopically has increased, so has the number of diagnoses of cervical polyps. The importance of cervical polypectomy lies not in the malignant potential of a cervical polyp, but in confusion with other polypoid masses found in the same location.

I. **Description of Cervical Polyps**
   A. Pedunculated growths from mucous surface of cervix
   B. Represent overgrowth of one of cervical folds
   C. More often single than multiple (88% vs. 12%)
   D. Associated with, but not caused by, chronic cervicitis
   E. Microscopic to 2 cm or more
   F. Soft, shotty if associated with Nabothian cysts
   G. Pink to red in color
   H. May be ulcerated
   I. Microscopic characteristics
      1. Loose vascular connective tissue
      2. Surface covered by endocervical epithelium
      3. Occasional cervical glands
      4. Stroma usually very inflamed
      5. Squamous metaplasia in 8–31%
   J. Location
      1. Portio vaginalis
      2. Squamocolumnar junction
      3. Lower endocervix (most common)
   K. Lower potential for malignancy than any other portion of cervical anatomy (0.2–0.4%)

II. **Clinical Setting**
   A. Most commonly in parous women in fifth decade
   B. Incidence may be as high as 6%
   C. Presentation
      1. Abnormal vaginal bleeding
         a. Postcoital bleeding is common
      2. Most are asymptomatic

III. **Differential Diagnosis of Cervical Polypoid Mass**
   A. Cervical polyp
   B. Endometrial polyp
   C. Endocervical hyperplasia
   D. Chronic cervicitis
   E. Condyloma acuminata
   F. Squamous cell carcinoma
   G. Adenocarcinoma
   H. Prolapsed myoma

IV. **Cervical Polypectomy**
   A. Why perform cervical polypectomy?
      1. Prevent complications of bleeding
      2. Polyps often obscure cervical and endocervical exam
      3. Need for pathologic diagnosis
   B. **Procedure**
      1. Office-based
      2. Simplified with aid of colposcopy
      3. Determine site of origin
         a. Remove only polyps believed to be cervical in origin

    b. Refer to gynecologist if location of base cannot be determined—high risk of bleeding if base within uterine cavity
4. Use tonsil snare or cervical biopsy forceps
5. Remove at base
6. Perform endocervical curettage if base is in canal
7. Hemostasis with Monsel's solution or silver nitrate
8. Send specimen to pathology
    a. Perform endometrial biopsy if pathology consistent with endometrial polyp

SUGGESTED READING

1. Caroti S, Siliotti F: Cervical polyps: A colpo-cyto-histological study. Clin Exp Obstet Gynecol 15:108–115, 1988.
2. Farrar HK Jr, Nedoss BR: Benign tumors of the uterine cervix. Am J Obstet Gynecol 81:134–137, 1986.
3. Golan A, Ber A, Wolman I, David MP: Cervical polyp: Evaluation of current treatment. Gynecol Obstet Invest 37:56–58, 1994.
4. Rupke S, Luber TJ: Evaluation and management of cervical polyps. Hosp Pract 33:81–82, 1998.
5. Selim MA, Shalodi AD: Benign diseases of the uterine cervix: Ruling out neoplasia a diagnostic priority. Postgrad Med 78:141–150, 1985.

112. Biopsy of the Vulva

Barbara S. Apgar, M.D., M.S.

Assessment of vulvar disease requires knowledge of dermatologic conditions affecting this area and skill with diagnostic procedures. Whether the conditions are straightforward or more complex, accurate differential diagnosis is important if the evaluation of vulvar disease is to be successful. Office biopsy techniques for the evaluation of the vulva should be mastered by any clinician who examines the lower genital system. Many of the changes that occur on the vulva can be confirmed by a simple visual examination. Inspection with the colposcope, however, enhances the gross visual impression. The majority of vulvar lesions exhibit striking variation and are often multicentric. The same pathologic process may exhibit different visual patterns at a single examination or on consecutive visits. To add to the confusion, similar clinical presentations may be initiated by very different pathologic conditions. An adequate and accurate interpretation may be difficult when two or more diseases present with a combination of findings such as dystrophy, infection or neoplasia. Often, biopsy of the vulva is the only answer to this dilemma.

Vulvar lesions that do not disappear within several weeks either spontaneously or therapeutically or that tend to have a chronic course must be followed closely. If a decision is made to follow a lesion with observation, a baseline histologic determination should be made. Histologic documentation of the findings is important. A subjective diagnosis without histologic confirmation of a chronic or progressive lesion is not sufficient. Decisive distinctions of benign vs. malignant disease are often impossible without biopsy confirmation. Vulvar biopsy is a rapid and simple office procedure and is the hallmark of successful management of vulvar disease.

  I. **Indications**
    A. Evaluation of lesions on the vulva and surrounding tissues
  II. **Contraindications**
    A. None
  III. **Patient Evaluation and Preparation**
    A. Informed consent should be obtained for vulvar biopsy
    B. Explanation to patient
      1. Vulvar biopsy is often necessary to differentiate benign and malignant conditions that cannot be determined by visual inspection alone
      2. Gross appearance of a lesion is not always indicative of its histologic character; biopsy confirmation is important before therapy can be initiated

IV. **Equipment**
   A. Depending on whether punch or excisional biopsy is to be performed, instrument set-up is slightly different; instruments may be sterilized and packaged as a kit
   B. **Punch biopsy of vulva**
      1. Anesthetic agent (epinephrine usually not necessary)
      2. Syringe: 5 ml
      3. Needles: 30 gauge
      4. Biopsy punch (disposable or reusable)
      5. Iris forceps
      6. Scissors
      7. Small needle holder if sutures required
      8. Monsel's paste
      9. Gauze sponges
     10. Bottles of formalin or other preservative
   C. **Excisional biopsy of vulva**
      1. Anesthetic agent
      2. Syringe: 5 ml
      3. Needles: 30 gauge
      4. Scalpel blades # 11 and 15
      5. Pick-up forceps
      6. Iris scissors
      7. Small needle holder
      8. Suture material
         a. 4-0 vicryl
         b. 4-0 chromic
      9. Gauze sponges
     10. Bottles of formalin
V. **Technique for Punch Biopsy**
   A. Keyes cutaneous biopsy punch is a dermatologic instrument used to core out small circular plug of tissue on skin
      1. Punches are manufactured in diameters ranging from 2–12 mm
      2. 4 mm and 5 mm diameters are the most practical size for vulvar use and result in a pellet-shaped specimen that is easily oriented and has sufficient surface to allow adequate histologic sectioning
      3. Types of punch biopsy instruments
         a. Stainless steel punch can be obtained from most surgical supply companies
         b. Disposable variety also available
      4. If sharp, instruments cleanly incise the tissue with only light pressure and a simple twisting motion
   B. Hair is clipped over lesion if necessary and skin is prepped with antiseptic solution
   C. Circular biopsy incision is made by maintaining pressure and rotation of biopsy punch until subcutaneous tissue is reached
      1. Depth of biopsy varies with lesion, depending on thickness of epidermis
      2. Subtle sensation of decreased resistance when dermis is reached
         a. Making incision too deep results in cutting deeper and larger blood vessels and inviting more blood loss than necessary
         b. Too shallow a cut, however, results in fragmented specimen, which impairs accurate diagnosis
   D. Once incision is made, punch is laid aside
   E. Specimen is grasped beneath epithelium with iris forceps, and dermal tissue is cut transversely with small scissors
   F. Clean circular defect produced is usually fairly avascular
   G. In presence of slight bleeding, drop of Monsel's paste applied to surgical defect is sufficient for hemostasis; remove any Monsel's not directly over punch, because it will pigment
   H. Stubborn bleeding sites are best handled with single suture using 4-0 vicryl or chromic
   I. Wound is covered with Telfa pad, which in turn is covered with sanitary napkin

VI. **Technique for Excisional Biopsy**
    A. Generally used for larger lesions that require more complete excision
    B. Incision should be made with scalpel blade held at right angles to vulvar surface
        1. Ellipse or diamond should be inscribed in wedge down to subcutaneous tissue
        2. Long axis of excision should be performed in 12 to 6 o'clock direction if lesion is located on labia
        3. On perineum, horizontal axis 3 to 9 o'clock is preferred
        4. Attention to placement of long axis of ellipse results in linear scar under minimal tension. After completion of healing process, such excision sites are virtually invisible
    C. Subcutaneous sutures of 4-0 chromic should be placed if defect is large or deep bleeding is encountered
        1. Skin edges of defect should be closed without tension in linear fashion, using interrupted sutures of 4-0 vicryl
    D. Proper handling of specimen is important
        1. Biopsy specimen is worthless if it fails to yield accurate pathologic diagnosis
        2. May not be possible for pathologist to give precise interpretation if sample is dehydrated, distorted, or oriented tangentially
        3. Tissue sample is gently placed in formalin and container properly labeled
        4. Place biopsies from different sites in separate bottles
VII. **Anesthesia of Vulva**
    A. Vulva differs from cervix and endometrium in that anesthesia is necessary before biopsy can be performed
    B. Anesthesia may be accomplished by local infiltration, which is quite sufficient to make patient comfortable during procedure
    C. Anesthesia may be administered at single site or in field block technique. Either mode of infiltration depends on size of lesion, location, type of biopsy contemplated
        1. Most diagnostic biopsies of vulva require single infiltration at biopsy site
        2. For lesions < 1 cm, 1% xylocaine without epinephrine is ideal
        3. For larger lesions, field block method may be necessary
            a. Placing small amount of topical anesthetic such as Hurricaine over puncture site minimizes needle stick
            b. Anesthetic solution is injected subepidermally with fine 30-gauge needle
            c. Because of rich vascular and lymphatic supply of vulva, small amounts of anesthetic may be quickly dissipated. This can be avoided by using adequate amount at onset (1–3 ml per site)
            d. Wheal created by infiltration actually facilitates biopsy by raising lesion and producing some local vasoconstriction, thus minimizing blood loss
        4. For larger lesions, 1% xylocaine with epinephrine may help to prolong anesthetic effect and promote vasoconstriction
            a. Without addition of epinephrine, excessive amounts of solution may be needed to produce anesthesia in larger lesions
            b. Xylocaine is infiltrated subepidermally in clover-leaf fashion; 1–1.5 ml is placed at each clover leaf under lesion
            c. Wheal facilitates performance of biopsy by lifting tissue toward scalpel blade
VIII. **Postprocedure Care**
    A. If large excisional biopsy is performed, secondary edema may result
        1. Minimized by postoperative use of ice pack
        2. Patient should be instructed to fill plastic sandwich bag with crushed ice when she arrives home and to wear it like pad for rest of day
    B. Daily sitz baths help to ensure complete absorption of suture material along with rapid and uncomplicated healing
    C. Little if any scarring results from this procedure, and biopsy site is practically invisible within 2–3 weeks
        1. Discomfort during healing period usually minimal and generally requires nothing more than simple analgesics (e.g., acetaminophen, ibuprofen)
    D. Patient should keep the incision site clean and dry

E. Patient should be scheduled for follow-up discussion to outline results of biopsy and to detail management plan

IX. **Complications**
   A. Hematoma formation, infection and scarring
   B. **Patient should report**
      1. Persistent bleeding
      2. Increasing discomfort
      3. Redness
      4. Unusual local reaction such as pus formation

SUGGESTED READING

1. Apgar BS, Cox JT: Differentiating normal and abnormal findings of the vulva. Am Fam Physician 53:1171–1180, 1996.
2. Wilkinson EJ, Hardt NS: Histology of the vulva. In Sternberg SS (ed): Histology for Pathologists. New York, Raven Press, pp 865–879, 1991.
3. Wilkinson EJ, Stone IK: Atlas of Vulvar Disease. Baltimore, Williams & Wilkins, 1995.
4. Wilkinson EJ: Premalignant and malignant tumors of the vulva. In Kurman RJ (ed): Blaustein's Pathology of the Female Genital Tract, New York, Springer Verlag, 1994, pp 87–129.

113. Biopsy of the Vagina

Barbara S. Apgar, M.D., M.S.

Diagnosis and evaluation of the vagina is especially challenging. The area is a closed, topographically complex space, and inspection is impossible unless distention is accomplished with a vaginal speculum. The speculum examination presents a problem in itself; unless the speculum is rotated 180°, only half of the vagina is visible at any one time. Transparent plastic speculums are helpful but tend to be more uncomfortable for the patient. Most lesions of the vagina are not located perpendicular to the plane of view, and because the vaginal rugae are often contracted, it is necessary to engage the lesion into good view before examination and biopsy can be performed. The location of the biopsy area is aided by the use of Lugol's solution or acetic acid.

I. **Indications**
   A. Lesions in vagina
   B. Undiagnosed bleeding of vaginal wall
   C. Undiagnosed chronic vaginal pruritus or pain
   D. Palpable but invisible vaginal lesions

II. **Contraindications**
   A. Inability to place vaginal speculum

III. **Patient Evaluation and Preparation**
   A. Obtain informed consent
   B. Adequate inspection of vagina requires 360° panoramic view that cannot be obtained by opening bivalved speculum and inspecting only lateral vagina walls
      1. Closing speculum and rotating it from its usual 12–6 o'clock position to 3–9 o'clock position allows thorough exam. Dental mirror is helpful in visualizing entire surface
   C. Vinegar may be used in vagina to delineate acetowhite tissue; however, it is not as useful as Lugol's solution
   D. Lugol's solution does not stain abnormal tissue; no mahogany color at sites of tissue warranting further inspection and possible biopsy
      1. Absence of staining with Lugol's solution indicates lack of glycogen in affected tissue and is generally indicative of abnormality

IV. **Equipment**
   A. Size and position of vaginal lesion dictate whether punch or excisional biopsy is necessary
   B. **Equipment needed for vaginal punch biopsy**

1. Cervical biopsy punch
2. Skin hook
3. Needle holder (optional)
4. Suture: 4-0 vicryl (optional)
5. 1% xylocaine
6. Syringe—3 ml; 30-gauge needle
7. Needle extender (optional)
8. Monsel's paste
9. Formalin bottles
10. Large cotton swabs

C. **Equipment needed for vaginal excisional biopsy**
1. Scalpel and blade
2. Skin hook or Allis clamp
3. Toothed forceps
4. Long-handled needle holder
5. 30-gauge needle
6. Suture—4-0 vicryl
7. 1% xylocaine
8. Syringe—3 ml
9. Needle extender (optional)
10. Formalin bottles
11. Large cotton swabs

V. **Anesthesia**
A. Vaginal fornices, like cervix, may not require anesthesia for biopsy because of relatively less sensitive nature of mucosa
B. Mucosa approaching mid-vagina and hymenal ring is more sensitive to painful stimuli and usually requires anesthesia. The pain threshold of patient at any level of vagina should be tested before biopsy is performed
C. Unless lesion is located close to introitus, most needles and syringes do not reach upper limits of vagina
1. Needle extender placed on Luer-Lok tip of syringe greatly aids in administering anesthesia
2. Small amount of topical anesthetic (Hurricaine) decreases discomfort of needle stick
3. Small amount (1–3 ml) of 1% xylocaine may be injected submucosally with 30-gauge needle
   a. Necessary to make only a wheal under lesion so it is lifted out of rugae and exposed for proper examination
4. Sometimes helpful to use skin hook to pull lesion out from rugae and create better exposure
   a. If skin hook is used in nondominant hand, it is preferable to use dental type syringe in dominant hand
   b. May be awkward to operate regular syringe that requires use of two hands
5. Another alternative is Potocky needle (Cooper Surgical) used in electrosurgical excision on cervix

VI. **Technique of Punch Biopsy**
A. Biopsy instruments
1. Dermatologic punch biopsy instrument not practical for use in vagina because of the inadequate length
2. Most commonly used instrument is cervical punch biopsy instrument
   a. Long shaft makes it easier to biopsy lesions located higher than mid-vagina
3. Tischler punch instrument works well because biopsy tooth can be used to stabilize mucosa while performing biopsy
B. Mucosa is infiltrated with 1% xylocaine to create wheal
C. Skin hook, Allis clamp, or toothed forceps is used to gently pull rugae out from vaginal wall
D. Lesion is biopsied with quick, sharp cut
1. 5-mm sample is sufficient for pathologic analysis
2. Sample is placed in bottle of formalin

    E. Cotton swab held on biopsy site facilitates hemostasis of minor bleeding
      1. If bleeding is moderate, Monsel's paste is applied with Q-tip or large cotton swab
      2. If bleeding is brisk and cannot be controlled with Monsel's paste, it may be necessary to place 1–2 mucosal sutures of 4-0 vicryl
        a. Sutures do not need to be excessively deep to achieve hemostasis
      3. Rarely is any other intervention other than pressure or use of Monsel's needed

VII. **Technique of Excisional Biopsy**
    A. Necessary if cervical biopsy punch instrument not available
    B. "Pull and snip" technique is used
    C. Anesthesia is infiltrated as described for vaginal punch biopsy
    D. Lesion is mobilized with a hook, Allis clamp, or toothed forceps and pulled away from vaginal wall
      1. Scalpel excises the lesion
        a. Care should be taken not to enter mucosa too deeply. Usually a 5-mm sample is sufficient
    E. Hemostasis is achieved as described for vaginal punch biopsy or placement of sutures as required

VIII. **Complications**
    A. Excessive blood loss
      1. Rarely should biopsy go deeper than 5 mm
      2. Cutting too deep invites excessive blood loss
    B. Inadequate anesthesia
      1. Vaginal mucosa should be tested before biopsy is obtained to ascertain whether anesthesia is required

SUGGESTED READING

1. Heller DS: Benign and malignant diseases of the vagina. In Heller DS (ed): The Lower Female Genital Tract: A Clinicopathologic Approach. Baltimore. Williams & Wilkins 1998, pp 165–195.
2. Barrasso R, Guillemotonia A: Cervix and vagina: Diagnosis. In Gross GE, Barrasso R (eds): Human Papilloma Virus Infection: A Clinical Atlas. Berlin, Ullstein Mosby, 1998, pp 147–274.
3. Zaino RJ, Bobboy SJ, Bentley R, Kurman RJ: Diseases of the vagina. In Kerman RJ (ed): Blaunstein's Pathology of the Female Genital Tract. New York, Springer Verlag, 1994, pp 131–183.

114. Treatment Options for Human Papillomavirus and Cervical Dysplasia

Cynda Ann Johnson, M.D., M.B.A.

I. **Human Papillomavirus** (HPV)
    A. **Cervix**
      1. Cauliflower condyloma can be treated with cryotherapy or loop electrosurgical excision procedure (LEEP)
      2. Flat condyloma and subclinical HPV generally do not require treatment. If patient is extremely concerned and prefers treatment, a rational approach is to consider treatment if there are localized lesions near or within the transformation zone. The goal of treatment is destruction of the T-zone on the ectocervix. Cryotherapy is preferred because it is effective and is safer and costs much less than LEEP
      3. Pathologists cannot reliably make a distinction between HPV only and mild dysplasia. Clinicians face a dilemma when the biopsy is interpreted as HPV/mild dysplasia because they usually tell the patient that they are looking for cancer or precancer (dysplasia) of the cervix and must explain why treatment for mild dysplasia is not indicated

B. **Endocervix**
1. When HPV is found on endocervical curettage (ECC), treatment is rarely indicated if colposcopy was deemed adequate. However, if colposcopic follow-up is otherwise indicated, a repeat ECC may be carried out at that time
2. If LEEP is to be performed, a LEEP cone may be done at the time of the procedure

C. **Vagina**
1. Treatment of flat HPV of the vagina is almost never indicated. Rarely can a case be made that symptoms are present. If so, laser is the treatment of choice
2. Cauliflower condyloma of the vagina may be treated with liquid nitrogen (cryoprobe not recommended by CDC), trichloracetic acid (TCA), or podophyllin
3. Pregnant women who have extensive lesions in line with the usual location for episiotomy may benefit from local treatment. Tissues with extensive HPV do not hold suture well and bleed easily

D. **Vulva**
1. Exophytic lesions on the vulva can be treated by many modalities. Although they are almost never precancerous, most patients prefer to have them treated. The viral load will also be cut greatly. Local chemical therapy including podophyllin or TCA, or cryotherapy are the first-line treatment options. It is unpredictable how well the lesions will respond. Sometimes large lesions dissolve after a single treatment; other times small lesions are very resistant to therapy. If one therapeutic modality fails repeatedly, try another. Reliable patients may use podofilox solution or gel or imiquinod at home; otherwise, it may be applied in the office. Larger lesions may be treated initially with local therapy, but LEEP, surgical excision, and/or laser may be necessary. This is an excellent indication for interferon therapy as well
2. Subclinical lesions of the vulva rarely require treatment. Women with subclinical HPV at the introitus may occasionally be symptomatic, particularly with new onset dyspareunia. Laser is usually the treatment of choice

E. **Perianal area**
1. Perianal lesions generally respond to local therapy. Treatment options are the same as described for exophytic vulvar lesions
2. If at the anal verge, lesions are more likely to be symptomatic

F. **Rectum**
1. Rectal lesions are recognized by their acetowhite appearance after swabbing with acetic acid, usually viewed through the anoscope
2. They may be treated with nitrous oxide cryogun or by local application of liquid nitrogen. A small amount of rectal bleeding may result. Occasionally, there will be some transient rectal pain. However, treatment is usually surprisingly well tolerated

TABLE 1. Recommended Chemical Treatment Regimens for Genital Warts

	Location	Treatment
Patient-applied	External genital/ perianal	Podofilox 0.5% solution or gel. Apply twice daily for 3 days, then off for 4 days. May repeat cycle a total of 4 times.
		Imiquinod 5% cream. Apply nightly 3 times per week. Wash off after 6–10 hours; may use up to 16 weeks. May expect clearing in 8–10 weeks or less.
Provider-applied	External genital/perianal	Podophyllin 10–25% in compound tincture of benzoin. Wash off thoroughly 1–4 hours after application. Repeat weekly as necessary.
	Vaginal	Podophyllin 10–25%—apply to affected areas which must be dry before removing speculum. Treat < 2 cm per session. Repeat weekly.
	External genital/perianal/ vaginal	Trichloracetic acid (TCA) 80–90%. Apply only to warts. Powder with talc or baking soda to remove unreacted acid. Repeat weekly if necessary.

    3. If lesions persist, they should be biopsied; rectal dysplasia can be a precursor to rectal cancer. If resistant, dysplastic lesions may require interferon, laser therapy, or, rarely, surgery

  G. See Table 1 for treatment recommendations

II. Cervical Dysplasia

A. On Papanicolaou smear

    1. LEEP has been overused at the time of initial colposcopy. This approach, called "one-stop shopping," may result in overtreatment of low-grade or benign lesions. It is also a very expensive approach

    2. For the patient in whom compliance with follow-up examinations and treatment is problematic, however, LEEP may be indicated during the initial colposcopic exam, if lesions grossly consistent with cervical dysplasia are present or if the Pap smear indicates that high-grade dysplasia is present

B. Biopsy findings from colposcopic examination

  1. Mild dysplasia

    a. The need for any treatment for mild dysplasia of the cervix is controversial. The trend is toward no treatment

    b. Arguments for treatment are the same as those in favor of treatment for HPV of the cervix

    c. Treatment for any degree of dysplasia is indicated whenever there is significant doubt that the patient will follow-up reliably

  2. Moderate and severe dysplasia

    a. With all degrees of dysplasia, the accessibility of the lesion to the type of therapy chosen is an important consideration

    b. As the degree of dysplasia becomes greater, the success rate of cryotherapy of the cervix decreases. However, the success rate is greater than 80% even with the highest grade of dysplasia, so clinicians not performing LEEP should not hesitate to treat the patient with cryotherapy (carried out as carefully and optimally as possible)

    c. Physicians performing LEEP should discuss both options (cryotherapy and LEEP) with the patient, weighing all factors, including cost of the procedure and cost and frequency of follow-up with either procedure. Studies find that the LEEP specimen often contains a portion with higher-grade dysplasia than the known biopsy—but whether this is clinically relevant is unknown

    d. Some patients and physicians may choose not to treat moderate dysplasia of the cervix, because spontaneous regression is still possible (whether it is "likely" depends on the literature one reads). Careful follow-up is mandatory if no treatment is carried out initially.

    e. If glandular invasion of the dysplasia is present, LEEP therapy is preferred. Cryotherapy is still an option, but the cryoprobe must be optimally fitted to the lesion and lesions at 9:00 and 3:00 are especially hard to treat because of the "heat sink," as the blood vessels traverse this area

    f. Laser is not superior to cryotherapy, especially if the lesion is of moderate dysplasia or lower grade, and it is only slightly superior in severe dysplasia. It is not superior in either case to LEEP and has the disadvantage of no resultant tissue specimen.

  3. Carcinoma *in situ* (CIS)

    a. Most family physicians prefer to obtain consultation in this setting. A supportive consultant, however, may encourage the family physician to carry out the therapy

    b. Other considerations are the same as discussed regarding moderate and severe dysplasia. LEEP becomes an increasingly attractive option in the setting of CIS.

  4. Endocervical dysplasia

    a. Cryotherapy is **not** an option. According to the argument that mild dysplasia need not be treated, a case could be made for close follow-up. Most clinicians, however, would not be comfortable following a lesion that could not be well seen in the endocervical canal.

    b. LEEP cone therapy has put treatment of endocervical dysplasia in the realm of the family physician. A cold knife cone is now rarely necessary. Laser therapy offers no advantage

    c. Hysterectomy is always a consideration in any high-grade lesion or with endo-cervical canal disease when other clinical considerations make that option attractive (as in perimenopausal patients with significant dysfunctional uterine bleeding)

5. **Vaginal and vulvar intraepithelial neoplasia** (VAIN and VIN)
    a. Vaginal and vulvar intraepithelial neoplasia are best treated by laser therapy. Low dose 5-FU may be used in selected cases
    b. Close follow-up only may be indicated in some instances of low-grade VIN or VAIN. The trend is toward this conservative approach

SUGGESTED READING

1. Felmar E: Primary care office procedures: Treatment of genital lesions via cryocautery. Prim Care Cancer 6:1–7, 1988.
2. Krebs HB: Treatment of vaginal intraepithelial neoplasia with laser and topical 5-fluorouracil. Obstet Gynecol 73:657–660, 1989.
3. Richart P: Ways of using LEEP for external lesions. Contemp Obstet Gynecol 5:138–152, 1992.

115. Cryotherapy of Cervical Intraepithelial Neoplasia

Barbara S. Apgar, M.D., M.S.

Cryotherapy is a proven, effective treatment for all grades of cervical intraepithelial neoplasia (CIN) that does not involve the cervical glands. Freezing the tissue followed by thawing leads to the formation of intracellular ice crystals, expansion of intracellular material, and rupture of the cells with subsequent denaturation of cell proteins. Cure rates diminish as the size of the lesion increases, especially if more than two quadrants of the cervix are involved. The grade of the lesion (CIN I–III) is not in itself a factor, but usually higher grades of CIN are represented by larger lesions. Lesions located at the 3 and 9 o'clock positions on the cervix have a higher degree of inadequate destruction of tissue from cryotherapy, presumably because of the increased blood supply to these areas from the cervical branches of the uterine arteries. If endocervical disease is present, an excisional method of treatment is preferred, because cryotherapy failure rates are high in this situation.

I. **Indications**
    A. Ablative therapy of cervical intraepithelial neoplasia
    B. Cure rates
        1. CIN I—94%
        2. CIN II—93%
        3. CIN III—86%

II. **Guidelines for Ablative Therapy of the Cervix**
    A. Goal of ablative therapy: to destroy lesional tissue and entire transformation zone
        1. Mean depth of involved crypts: 1.24 mm
        2. Destruction to depth of 7 mm should eradicate involved crypts in over 99% of cases
        3. At least 7-mm depth of destruction is recommended for appropriate treatment of CIN
    B. Prerequisites for cryotherapy ablation
        1. Involvement of two quadrants or less of lesional tissue
        2. Endocervical canal free of disease
        3. Satisfactory colposcopy
        4. Good correlation between cytology, colposcopy, and histology
        5. No evidence of microinvasive or invasive disease by cytology, colposcopy, or histology
        6. Compliant patient who agrees to return for follow-up visits

III. **Contraindications**
- A. Presence of microinvasive or invasive cancer
- B. Cryoglobulinemia
- C. Presence of menstrual period
- D. Pregnancy

IV. **Equipment**
- A. Cryogun
- B. Large nitrous oxide tank, 20 lbs at least, with pressure gauge
- C. Various sizes of cryotips
- D. Lubricating gel, water-soluble
- E. Vaginal speculum
- F. Colposcope
- G. 3–5% acetic acid or vinegar
- H. Vaginal wall retractors
- I. Disinfectant for cryoprobes

V. **Choice of Cryoprobe**
- A. Depends on size of lesion and transformation zone
  1. Flat probe without nipple
     - a. Diminishes possibility of cervical stenosis to approximately 1%
     - b. Less likely to cause squamocolumnar junction to recess into endocervical canal and result in unsatisfactory colposcopy at future examinations
  2. Large probes
     - a. Should be avoided on cervices with portio diameter < 3.0–3.5 cm
- B. Cryonecrosis produced by cryotherapy results after formation of iceball
  1. Temperatures at cryotip during NO_2 therapy: –65°C to –85°C
  2. Margin of iceball equals 0°C
  3. Cell death occurs at –20°C
  4. Recovery zone is area of iceball between 0°C and –20°C
     - a. Recovery zone represents area 2 mm proximal to iceball margin
     - b. Lethal zone during cryotherapy occupies area beginning at 2 mm proximal to iceball margin

VI. **Preoperative Care**
- A. Patient is asked to return for cryosurgery 1 week after start of menses
  1. Ensures patient is not pregnant
  2. Allows cervical healing before next menses
- B. If there is question about reliability of menses, a pregnancy test should be performed before procedure
- C. Informed consent should be obtained
- D. Patient must be reliable and agree to return for follow-up visits
- E. Administration of nonsteroidal anti-inflammatory agent 1 hour before procedure reduces pain associated with procedure

VII. **Technique for Cryosurgery**
- A. Patient is placed in dorsal lithotomy position
- B. Vaginal speculum is placed and vaginal retractor is used if vaginal sidewalls prevent adequate visualization of cervix
- C. Colposcopy is performed with 3–5% acetic acid to determine if signs of invasive disease are present
- D. Nitrous oxide tank is activated and sufficient pressure documented (indicator should be in green zone)
  1. Inadequate pressure = inadequate treatment
  2. Allow time for gas regeneration and filling of cylinder
- E. Cryoprobe is placed on cryogun and screwed in place until tight
  1. Gun is activated and O-ring is checked
  2. If gas escapes around contact area between probe and stem of cryogun, replace O-ring
- F. Cryogun with probe attached is inserted in vagina
  1. Size of probe is checked by applying it onto transformation zone

2. Probe should cover transformation zone but not touch vaginal sidewalls
3. After correct size of probe is determined, cryogun is removed from vagina
4. Thin layer of lubricating gel is applied to cryoprobe to effect sufficient seal with cervix
5. Cryogun is placed on cervix again

G. Cryogun is activated to allow gas to flow into unit
   1. Patient should be warned she will hear a pop and hiss as cryogun is activated

H. Freeze continues until at least 7–10 mm iceball is present outside probe
   1. Time is not as critical as formation of iceball
   2. Each cervix requires different time to reach 7–10 mm iceball formation
   3. Care should be taken during the freeze to ensure that cryogun or probe is not touching the vaginal sidewalls
   4. Total iceball lateral spread of freeze of 7–10 mm is necessary to ensure freeze depth of 5 mm
      a. Cervical glands destroyed at this depth

I. After iceball is formed, cryogun is deactivated and cervix is allowed to thaw for approximately 4–5 minutes
   1. Central zone gets mushy during thawing time
   2. Do not remove probe from cervix until it is defrosted
      a. Pulling probe off cervix before it is defrosted produces pain and bleeding

J. Cryoprobe is again placed on cervix and another freeze is performed
   1. Freeze until 7-mm iceball forms again
      a. 10-mm iceball is ideal but rarely achieved

K. Cryoprobe is removed from cervix after it is thawed
   1. Cryogun is removed from vagina
   2. Speculum is removed from vagina

L. Process of reepithelialization
   1. On day of procedure, tissue demonstrates erythema and hyperemia
   2. Within next 24–48 hours, bullae or vesicle forms with associated edema
   3. Tissue then sloughs
   4. Eschar equates to denuding to 5-mm depth of epithelium
   5. Reepithelialization and neovascularization subsequently occur as eschar fills in

M. Reepithelialization is complete at 6 weeks in 47% of patients

VIII. **Postprocedure Care**

A. Patient is allowed to recover until stable, usually about 15 minutes
B. Patient is observed for any vasovagal symptoms during recovery time
C. Patient is given sanitary pad because discharge begins immediately after procedure
   1. Expect profuse, watery discharge for 2–3 weeks
D. Patient is instructed to call if she experiences:
   1. Excessive bleeding
   2. Purulent or foul-smelling discharge
   3. Fever or abdominal pain
   4. Absence of menses at next expected date
E. Patient returns for follow-up visits at 4, 8, 12, 18, and 24 months
   1. Majority of treatment failures detected by end of first year
   2. Evidence of 5 negative cytologic smears and normal colposcopy equates with adequate therapy
F. Patient should refrain from tampon use or intercourse during vaginal discharge phase of recovery process, usually 3 weeks

IX. **Complications**

A. **Menstrual cramps**
   1. Produced by release of prostaglandins
   2. Relieved by nonsteroidal anti-inflammatory agents
   3. 5% of patients experience cramps severe enough to warrant stronger drugs

B. **Vasomotor symptoms**
   1. 20% of patients experience flushing and lightheadedness
   2. Patients should get up slowly from examination table

C. **Cervical stenosis**
   1. External os should be probed at each follow-up visit
   2. Cervical stenosis sufficient to not allow passage of cytobrush is rare
D. **Pregnancy complications**
   1. No indications that cryosurgery produces pregnancy complications or adverse peri-
      natal outcome if guidelines are followed during procedure

SUGGESTED READING

1. Berget A, Andreasson B, Bock J: Laser and cryosurgery for intraepithelial neoplasia: A randomized trial
   with long-term follow-up. Acta Obstet Gynecol 70:231–235, 1991.
2. Boonstra H, Aalders J, Koudstaal J, et al: Minimum extension and appropriate topographic position of
   tissue destruction for treatment of cervical intraepithelial neoplasia. Obstet Gynecol 75:227–231,
   1990.
3. Boonstra H, Koudstaal J, Oosterhuis J, et al: Analysis of cryolesions in the uterine cervix: Application
   techniques, extension, and failures. Obstet Gynecol 75:232–239, 1990.
4. Creasman W, Hinshaw W, Clarke-Pearson D: Cryosurgery in the management of cervical intraepithelial
   neoplasia. Obstet Gynecol 63:145–149, 1984.
5. Einerth Y: Cryosurgical treatment of CIN I–III: A long-term study. Acta Obstet Gynecol Scand 67:627–630,
   1988.
6. Ferency A: Comparison of cryo- and carbon dioxide laser therapy for cervical intraepithelial neoplasia.
   Obstet Gynecol 66:793–798, 1985.
7. Ferris D, Crawley G, Baxley E, et al: Cryosurgery precision: Clinician's estimate of cryosurgical iceball
   lateral spread of freeze. Arch Fam Med 2:269–275, 1993.
8. Hillard P, Biro F, Wildey L: Complications of cervical cryotherapy in adolescents. J Reprod Med
   36:711–716, 1991.

116. Loop Electrosurgical Excision

Barbara S. Apgar, M.D., M.S.

The loop electrosurgical excision procedure (LEEP), also referred to as large loop excision of the
transformation zone (LLETZ), is gaining acceptance in the United States as a method for treating
cervical intraepithelial neoplasia (CIN) and other lower genital tract lesions. Loop excision is accomplished by using a high-frequency, alternating current (radiofrequency) and thin wire-loop
electrodes. Advantages of loop excision include reduced risk of inadvertently missing invasive
cervical cancer and high rates of successful therapy after a single treatment. Disadvantages include the potential of excising too much stroma leading to cervical incompetence. On the cervix,
loop excision may be in the form of a simple excision of the transformation zone or a conization
procedure. The specimens obtained with this technique are submitted for histologic evaluation.
Loop excision is an outpatient procedure performed under local anesthesia with minimal short-
term or long-term morbidity. Patient acceptance of the procedure is high. The majority of the excised cervical beds heal with minimal scarring or complications.

   I. **Indications for Loop Excision of Transformation Zone or Conization**
      A. Cervical intraepithelial neoplasia with satisfactory colposcopy and negative endocervical
         curettage
      B. Positive endocervical curettage
      C. Lack of correlation of cytology, histology, and colposcopy
      D. Unsatisfactory colposcopy
  II. **Contraindications**
      A. Active cervicitis, vaginitis or pelvic infection
      B. Pregnancy
      C. Bleeding disorder
      D. Known invasive cervical carcinoma

Consent for LEEP

Date _____

Time _____

I hereby authorize Dr. _____ and his/her assistants to perform LEEP (loop excision electrosurgical procedure) on my cervix. This is going to be done to remove abnormalities of my cervix, which have been discussed with me.

The instrument consists of a thin wire loop, small ball-like electrode and electric power source. I understand that this procedure requires acetic acid and/or iodine application to the cervix and local anesthesia of the areas to be treated. To my knowledge, I am not allergic to either xylocaine or iodine.

I understand that this is just one of a number of ways which are used to treat human papillomavirus (HPV) and/or pre-cancer (dysplasia) of the cervix. I understand that LEEP involves removal of diseased tissue of the cervix. I understand that some vaginal discharge mixed with blood and other compounds used to help control bleeding from the cervix will result and may last up to six weeks. I understand that I should not douche, use a tampon, or have vaginal intercourse until that discharge goes away.

I understand that I will most likely have cramping during LEEP and, perhaps, for a few days afterwards. I may also get light-headed during the procedure. I understand that bleeding is an occasional complication of the treatment that can be controlled. I understand that infection of the cervix is another uncommon complication of the procedure and that cervical infection would require treatment with antibiotics. I understand that cervical stenosis (narrowing of the cervical opening) is a rare complication that would require dilating (enlarging) the canal of the cervix. Rarely hospitalization and/or surgery may be required in the event of a serious complication.

I understand that LEEP may not totally cure my diseased cervix and that further examinations of my cervix will be necessary in the future to be sure that the disease stays under control.

I have/have not had the opportunity to view the patient education video on LEEP. I understand the risks and benefits of the exam and have had the opportunity to have my questions answered.

_____   _____
Signature of witness   Patient's signature

                                          _____
                                          Current telephone number

FIGURE 1.   Consent form for loop electrosurgical excision procedure.

III. **Equipment**
   A. All equipment should be assembled before actual procedure
       1. Informed consent forms (Fig. 1)
       2. Electrosurgical generator (ESU)
       3. Patient grounding pad
       4. Loop electrodes
       5. Ball electrodes
       6. Insulated electrode holder
       7. Nonconductive speculum with smoke-evacuator port
       8. Endocervical curette
       9. Nonconductive vaginal retractor
      10. Smoke evacuator and filter system
      11. Colposcope
      12. 3–5% acetic acid or vinegar
      13. Aqueous Lugol's solution (half-strength)
      14. Large cotton swabs
      15. Dental type syringe with four 1.8-ml ampules of 2% xylocaine with 1:100,000 epinephrine

16. 27 gauge needles, 1.5 inches in length
17. Monsel's paste
18. Specimen bottles with 10% neutral-buffered formalin
19. 12-inch needle holder and 2-0 vicryl suture material
20. Vaginal pack
21. Postprocedure instruction sheet

B. **Description**
   1. **Electrodes**
      a. Wire-loop electrode is connected to insulated transverse bar fixed into pencil-type holder
         i. Some styles of electrode holders have buttons for activation of cutting and coagulation current
      b. Various sizes of loop electrodes
         i. For loop excisions, standard loop is 20 mm wide by 8 mm deep or 15 mm wide by 8 mm deep
         ii. With larger loops there is tendency to excise more tissue than necessary
         iii. Dimensions of loop are selected according to size of transformation zone to allow removal of entire transformation zone
      c. Ball electrode required for fulgurating crater base and any bleeders
         i. Ball electrodes usually measure 5 mm or 3 mm in diameter and fit into electrode handle in same manner as loop electrode
      d. Ball and loop electrodes can be obtained in either reusable or disposable forms
         i. Reusable type must be carefully cleaned of carbonized material with electrode cleaning pad and sterilized before reuse
   2. **Electrosurgical generator units** (ESUs)
      a. Loop excision procedure uses low-voltage, high-frequency alternating current to excise tissue and produce hemostasis
      b. Most electrosurgical generators produce currents in frequency range of 350,000 cycles/second or 350 KHz to 4,000,000 cycles/second or 4 mHz
      c. Current referred to as radiofrequency current because it is same frequency range as AM radio
         i. Neuromuscular excitation that induces muscle contraction and pain is usually not produced during electrosurgery because alternating current used for loop excision is above frequency range to which nerve and muscle cells respond
      d. To achieve waveform of alternating current that both cuts and produces hemostasis, it is necessary to convert 60-cycle alternating current to high-frequency alternating current by using modern ESU
      e. Most modern ESUs are actually variations of original Bovie type
         i. Early, nonsolid state generators used spark-gap (discontinuous, asymmetric) waveform to achieve coagulation and sinewave (continuous, symmetric) waveform to achieve electrosurgical cutting
      f. Modern ESUs use undamped pure, sinewave current of low peak voltage to produce pure cutting effects
      g. Pure coagulation effects are achieved by short, intermittent bursts of high-peak voltage sinewave current
         i. Pauses between current flow and high-peak voltage are responsible for hemostatic effects
      h. Modern ESUs produce blended current with both cutting and coagulating effects
         i. Blended current is interrupted sinewave current
         ii. Amount of hemostasis achieved during cutting is not affected by actual power setting of coagulation mode
   3. **Ancillary equipment**
      a. Insulated, nonconductive speculum
         i. Does not allow transmission of current from loop electrode to unanesthetized vagina

b. Smoke evacuator
    i. Speculum must have outlet for smoke evacuation
    ii. Smoke evacuator should have adequate filter and be of size that fits compactly into exam room
c. Additional equipment includes:
    i. Return electrode placed on the patient's thigh
    ii. Dental syringes with 27-gauge needles and ampules of anesthetic
    iii. 3–5% acetic acid or vinegar
    iv. Half-strength aqueous Lugol's solution
    v. Monsel's paste for packing crater base to obtain hemostasis
        (a) Ancillary equipment may be purchased in kit form for convenient use
d. Kevorkian endocervical curette
    i. Endocervical curettage performed at end of procedure
e. 10% neutral buffered formalin in containers is used for sample fixation
f. Long-handled needle holder and 2-0 absorbable suture should be available should hemostasis be impossible to achieve with Monsel's paste

IV. **Electrosurgical Effects on Tissue**
  A. Electrosurgical cutting occurs when temperature within tissue rises rapidly enough to cause explosive vaporization of water
    1. This condition is met when the temperature rises above 100°C and superheating of water within tissue occurs, resulting in shock waves within tissue and disruption of tissue architecture. Only very high current density can cause rapid enough rise in temperature to cause explosive vaporization of water
       a. Such high current densities occur only when current arcs between active electrode and tissue
       b. Arcing is facilitated by presence of steam envelope around electrode, which becomes ionized in electric field
       c. Steam envelope is generated by vaporization of water within tissue during active cutting
       d. Cutting is achieved only if electrode is moved slowly and continuously through tissue
          i. Allows electrosurgical cutting as arc travels through steam envelope between electrode and tissue
          ii. If electrode is moved too quickly, steam envelope is collapsed, electrode is placed in direct contact with tissue, cutting is inhibited and thermal damage occurs
  B. In contrast to electrosurgical cutting current, coagulation current can result in either fulguration or desiccation of tissues
    1. Fulguration occurs when high-voltage intermittent current travels between electrodes and tissue in arc
       a. Due to high voltage and intermittent nature of current
       b. Extensive tissue destruction and charring occurs
    2. Desiccation occurs under conditions of low current density, as when electrode is placed in direct contact with tissue
       a. Under such conditions, temperature within cells is slowly raised to less than 100°C and cellular proteins coagulate as water evaporates from cells
    3. Both electrosurgical fulguration and desiccation result in hemostasis as small vessels contract

V. **Anesthesia**
  A. To minimize discomfort from loop excision, local anesthesia is required
  B. Technique of administering anesthesia
    1. Superficial (2–5 mm deep) submucosal injection 3 mm beyond transformation zone of 2% xylocaine with a 1:100,000 solution of epinephrine
       a. For cervical excisions, a vasoconstrictive agent is always used, preferably epinephrine or a dilute strength of vasopressin
       b. Anesthesia is easily administered with dental syringes and 27-gauge needles
          i. 1–3 cartridges of 1.8 ml each usually sufficient (1.8–5.4 ml total)

    2. Anesthesia injected into 12, 3, 6, and 9 o'clock positions

    3. Patients report minimal discomfort with local anesthesia

    4. Paracervical block is not necessary

VI. **Technique of Loop Electrosurgical Excision**

  A. Loop excision requires good colposcopic skills:

    1. Transformation zone is adequately identified

    2. The presence or absence of significant cervical disease is confirmed

    3. Complications can be managed quickly and effectively

  B. Options for treatment are discussed with patient and informed consent is obtained

  C. Health care assistant familiar with procedure should be in treatment room during surgery

  D. Patient is placed in dorsal lithotomy position

    1. It may be preferable for patient's comfort to use leg stirrups

      a. Insulation for stirrups should be provided to prevent alternate site burn

  E. Ground electrode pad is attached to patient's medial thigh

  F. Insulated speculum with smoke evacuation port is inserted in vagina and smoke evacuation tubing is connected to smoke evacuator

    1. Speculum must be placed to allow complete, unobstructed view of cervix

  G. If vaginal walls obscure view, insulated vaginal retractor should be used

  H. Routine colposcopy of cervix is performed with 3–5% acetic acid to identify abnormal transformation zone followed by application of half-strength aqueous Lugol's solution

  I. Cervix is infiltrated with 2% xylocaine with 1:100,000 epinephrine

    1. Approximately 0.5–1.4 ml is injected at the 12, 3, 6, and 9 o'clock positions for a total of 1.8–5.6 ml

    2. Infiltration should be superficial, not more than 5 mm deep, and placed approximately 3 mm outside margin of transformation zone

  J. Correct choice of loop size should be based on size of transformation zone and ability to perform excision in 1 or 2 passes

    1. For simple ectocervical excision, 20 mm wide by 8 mm deep loop is usually sufficient

    2. For conization, additional 10 mm wide by 10 mm deep loop is necessary

  K. Power settings on generator depend on ESU and diameter of loop

    1. 20 mm × 8 mm loop requires approximately 30–40 watts of power

    2. 10 mm × 10 mm loop requires approximately 20–30 watts of power; goal is to cut effectively with as little power as possible to avoid tissue damage

    3. Loop electrode is fitted into electrode handle

    4. Blend or cut mode on generator should be selected

  L. **Three different types of excisions** can be performed depending on size of lesion and extension into endocervix

    1. Small lesions on ectocervix

      a. 20 mm × 8 mm loop electrode normally selected

      b. Test pass (without generating power) is made over lesion to ensure loop size is correct and that vaginal walls remain clear of loop

      c. Tissue is moistened with saline prior to activation of ESU

      d. Loop electrode is activated in blend mode

      e. Loop is positioned 3 mm outside transformation zone at 12, 3, 6, or 9 o'clock position, depending on shape of transformation zone

      f. By applying slight pressure on shaft, loop is pushed into cervix until insulated crossbar is reached

      g. Loop is not pushed to depth greater than 5 mm at the 3 and 9 o'clock positions since these are sites of cervical branches of uterine artery

        i. Significant bleeding can develop if these arteries are cut

      h. Loop is then drawn across and underneath transformation zone to position 3 mm outside transformation zone on opposite side where loop exits

        i. If loop stalls during pass, procedure should be stopped by deactivating ESU, removing loop, and cleaning it

        ii. Loop is repositioned where exit site would have been and excision is performed back to original area

      i. This single-pass procedure produces donut-shaped specimen with endocervical canal in center

2. **Larger transformation zones**
    a. If single pass was not wide enough to remove entire transformation zone, additional 1 or 2 passes may be performed with loop electrode of same size or slightly smaller

3. **Conization loop excision**
    a. If lesions extend into endocervical canal for short distance (usually < 7 mm), cone biopsy procedure can be performed with loop electrodes in two-step procedure
        i. 20 mm × 8 mm and 10 mm × 10 mm loop or rectangular electrode are used to produce a "cowboy hat" type excision
        ii. Exocervix is anesthetized in usual fashion but additional 0.5 ml of xylocaine with epinephrine is infiltrated around cervical canal for depth of 10 mm at 12 and 6 o'clock positions
        iii. 10 mm × 10 mm loop or square electrode is then used to excise the endocervical portion of lesion to depth of 9–10 mm
        iv. Exocervical portion of lesion can then be excised using 20 mm × 8 mm electrode
        v. Canal is then examined colposcopically, using 5% acetic acid to determine extent of disease; endocervical spreader facilitates exam

M. Completion of loop excision procedure is same for all three types
    1. After specimen or specimens are excised, they are removed from cervix
    2. Specimens are opened with scissors along one side and placed in plastic cassette so proper orientation is maintained during processing
      a. Cassette is placed in 10% neutral-buffered formalin
    3. Endocervical curettage is performed
    4. Loop electrode is replaced by ball electrode and ESU is set on coagulation mode
      a. If 5-mm ball electrode is used, power setting of 50 watts is usually sufficient
      b. Bleeding points are lightly fulgurated by allowing spark to arc between electrode and tissue along crater rim
      c. Do not fulgurate inside external os or crater base
    5. A layer of Monsel's paste is packed into base
    6. After bleeding has stopped, speculum is removed from vagina and patient is recovered

VII. **Postprocedure Care**
    A. Brownish discharge expected for up to 3 weeks after procedure
      1. If discharge becomes malodorous, patient should call physician's office
    B. Bleeding that persists more than 1 week should be reported
    C. Patient is to avoid heavy lifting, vaginal tampons, douching, or intercourse for 4 weeks
    D. Follow-up visits
      1. Patient returns at 6 months for colposcopy, cytology, and endocervical curettage
      2. If all results are negative, patient returns at 1 year for repeat cytology
      3. If results are negative at 1 year, patient may be seen for annual routine examinations with cytologic screening
      4. If 6- or 12-month exam is positive, biopsies should be performed and therapy reassessed
    E. **Cure rates**
      1. 92% of SIL successfully treated after a single loop excision
      2. 95% of SIL successfully treated after a repeat loop excision

VIII. **Complications**
    A. **Bleeding**
      1. Perioperative bleeding uncommon, but clinician should be prepared to manage it quickly
        a. Avoid inserting loop too deep at 3 and 9 o'clock
        b. Much more common in patients with cervicitis, patients using oral contraceptive pills, and patients < 5 months postpartum

    c. Diffuse type of bleeding from crater base

    d. Nonarterial bleeding that is difficult to control with coagulation

    e. Usually responds to copious amounts of Monsel's paste packed in crater

    f. Vagina may also be packed with iodoform gauze that is left in place for 2–3 hours while patient remains at bed rest

    g. More extensive after conization but usually controlled with fulguration and Monsel's paste

    h. Percentages vary from 0–1% for exocervical excisions

  2. Postoperative bleeding occurs 4 days to 3 weeks after procedure and is usually controlled with fulguration or application of Monsel's paste

    a. Percentages range from 0.7–9%

    b. Patient may need hospitalization for treatment of severe bleeding

      i. Severe postoperative bleeding rarely requires transfusion, suturing, or hospitalization

      ii. Such patients may have clots in crater base

    c. Mild postoperative bleeding more frequent

      i. Crater base can usually be cauterized with ball electrode or Monsel's paste can be packed in crater

      ii. If blood clots are present, they should be removed and crater packed with Monsel's paste

B. Squamocolumnar junction is preserved after majority of loop excision procedures

C. Postmenopausal patients treated with loop excision have highest probability of cervical stenosis

D. **Secondary infection:** rare

  1. Usually occurs 8–21 days after procedure

  2. All reported cases have responded to broad-spectrum antibiotics

E. **Positive margins**

  1. Up to 64% spontaneous regression rate of positive margins after loop excision

  2. Similar to rate following cold knife conization

  3. Follow-up with colposcopy and cytologic sampling every 4 months for first year

F. Pregnancy outcome rates following loop excision do not significantly differ from non-pregnancy rates

IX. **Safety**

A. All equipment should be checked prior to actual procedure

B. All supplies should be checked for adequacy and performance capability

C. Clinician should understand electrode-power (watt) capability of the equipment

  1. Power settings should be checked on beef tongue (or other source) before first use

D. All electrodes should be clean and free of charred remnants

E. Clinician should understand types of energy produced by each waveform and how patient is affected as appropriate energy accomplishes surgical effect

  1. Depth of coagulation during procedure

    a. Pure cut—least

    b. Blend cut—more

    c. Coagulation—most

  2. Clinician should have tried each range to understand how cervix will react

F. Clinician should understand effect of impedance (electrical resistance) on tissue

  1. Larger loops = lower impedance (less power required)

  2. Smaller loops = higher impedance (more power required)

  3. Wet tissue = lower impedance

  4. Dry tissue = higher impedance

G. Safety guidelines for current flow to avoid unintended burns

  1. Grounding pad: return electrode (grounding pad) can be source of unintended burns

    a. Burns can occur because of defect in manufacturing or pad not being in close contact with skin of patient

    b. If close contact is not maintained, current can increase under pad and burn patient

    c. ESU should be equipped with alarm system that indicates to clinician if return electrode is not properly grounded

  2. Active electrode: if patient or clinician comes in contact with active electrode at other than intended site, burn can occur

    a. ESU should be equipped with safety feature so that audible signal occurs when electrode is activated

    b. Great care should be taken to anesthetize tissue properly so unexpected movement by patient is avoided

  3. Alternate current paths: alternate site burns can occur with alternate path from patient to ground

    a. May occur at any site other than ground electrode

    b. May include noninsulated speculum site or earring touching metal on exam table

    c. Isolated circuitry should be built into ESU so that ESU inactivates if significant amount of current is not returning to grounding pad

  H. Vaporization of tissue with LEEP has potential to disseminate viral particles

    1. Clinician should follow universal precautions

    2. At minimum, viral protection mask should be worn during procedure

X. **Documentation**

  A. Informed consent

  B. Operative note

    1. Safety check (connections, grounding pad)

    2. Infiltration of anesthesia

    3. Full visualization, test pass performed

    4. Size of electrodes—power setting

    5. Cut and coagulation settings

    6. Monsel's paste applied

    7. Management of complications

  C. Postoperative instructions

    1. Goals

      a. Avoid postoperative bleeding

      b. Be aware of complications

      c. Reassure patient

      d. Expect the unexpected

    2. Guidelines

      a. No intercourse, tampons, or douching for 4 weeks

      b. No strenuous exercise or heavy lifting for 4 weeks

      c. Expect reddish-black discharge for 1–2 weeks

      d. Call if bleeding is heavier than menses during first week

      e. Call if malodorous discharge is present

      f. Call if bleeding lasts more than 1 week

SUGGESTED READING

1. Apgar BS, Wright TC, Pfenninger JL: Loop electrosurgical excision procedure for CIN. Am Fam Physician 46:505–518, 1992.
2. Eduardo AM, Ding TV, Hannigan EV, et al: Outpatient loop electrosurgical excision procedure for cervical intraepithelial neoplasia: Can it replace cold knife conization? J Reprod Med 41:729–732, 1996.
3. Dinh TA, Garcia MN, Waag IM, et al: Conservative management of positive resection margins after loop electrosurgical excision procedure. J Lower Gen Tract Dis 2:141–143, 1998.
4. Ferenczy A, Choukroun D, Arseneau J: Loop electrosurgical excision procedure for squamous intraepithelial lesions of the cervix: Advantages and potential pitfalls. Obstet Gynecol 87:332–337, 1996.
5. Ferenczy A, Choukroun D, Falcone T, Franco E: The effect of cervical loop electrosurgical excision procedure on subsequent pregnancy outcome: North American experience. Am J Obstet Gynecol 172:1246–1250, 1995.
6. McLucas B, Emens M, Hamou J, Rothenberg R: Diathermy loop treatment of CIN: International perspectives. Female Patient 15:79–91, 1990.

7. Monk A, Pushkin SF, Nelson Al, Gunning JE: Conservative management of options for patients with CIN involving endocervical margins of cervical cone biopsy samples. Am J Obstet Gynecol 174:1695–7000, 1996.
8. Mor-Yosef S, Lopes A, Pearson S, Monagham JM: Loop diathermy cone biopsy. Obstet Gynecol 75:884–886, 1990.
9. Prendiville W, Cullimore J, Norman S: Large loop excision of the transformation zone (LLETZ): A new method of management for women with cervical intraepithelial neoplasia. Br J Obstet Gynaecol 96:1054–1060, 1989.
10. Randall T: Loop electrosurgical excision procedures gaining acceptance for cervical intraepithelial neoplasia. JAMA 266:460–462, 1991.
11. Seltzer MS, Habermehl DA, Julian TM: A comparison of loop electrosurgical excision, laser ablation, and cold-knife conization in relation to precise specimen removal in an inanimate model. J Lower Gen Tract Dis 1:67–72, 1997.
12. Shafi MI, Chernoy R, Buxton EJ, Luesley DM: Invasive cervical disease following large loop excision of the transformation zone. Br J Obstet Gynaecol 99:614–621, 1992.
13. Wright TC, Ferenczy AF, Richart R, Koulos J: Comparison of specimens removed by CO_2 laser conization and the loop electrosurgical excision procedure. Obstet Gynecol 79:147–153, 1992.
14. Wright TC, Ferenczy AF, Richart R: Electrosurgery for HPV-Related Diseases of the Anogenital Tract. New York, Arthur Vision, 1992.
15. Wright TC, Gagnon S, Richart R, Ferenczy AF: Loop excision procedure for treating CIN. Obstet Gynecol 79:173–178, 1992.
16. Wright TC, Gagnon S, Ferenczy A, Richart R: Excising CIN lesions by loop electrosurgical procedure. Contemp Obstet Gynecol 3:57–73, 1991.

117. Endometrial Biopsy

Cynda Ann Johnson, M.D., M.B.A.

I. **Definition of Terms**
   A. **Endometrial sample**
      1. Generic term
      2. Depending on collection method, may be acceptable for histologic and/or cytologic evaluation
   B. **Endometrial aspirate**
      1. Usually acceptable for cytologic evaluation; may be acceptable for histologic evaluation
   C. **Endometrial biopsy**
      1. Acceptable for histologic evaluation
II. **Indications**
   A. Dysfunctional uterine bleeding; other menstrual disorders
      1. Biopsy on day 24–25 in apparently anovulatory patient; within 5–6 days after ovulation in others
      2. Information obtained from biopsy
         a. Pathology
         b. Evidence of ovulation
         c. Endometrial thickness
   B. Postmenopausal bleeding
   C. Abnormal cytology
      1. If abnormal endometrial cells present on Papanicolaou smear in premenopausal women
      2. If any endometrial cells present on Papanicolaou smear in postmenopausal women not on hormone replacement
   D. Evaluation for hormonal therapy
   E. Follow-up of hormonal therapy
   F. Infertility evaluation

   1. Before day 14
      a. Nonendocrine abnormalities
      b. Response to estrogen
   2. 5–6 days after ovulation
      a. Prior to implantation
      b. Maximal development of glands
   3. 2–3 days before menstruation
      a. Optimal timing for detection of luteal phase defect
         i. Luteal phase defect is defined as a lag of more than 2 days in the histologic development of the endometrium compared to the day of the cycle
      b. Disadvantage is possible disruption of pregnancy
   4. During menstruation
      a. Too much tissue destruction
      b. Cannot quantitate glandular, stromal, or blood vessel responses occurring earlier
G. Adjuvant hormonal therapy (tamoxifen citrate)
H. Spontaneous abortion
   1. May be used as follow-up of probably complete abortion
I. Screening for endometrial malignancy
   1. Not considered routine
   2. Consider endometrial biopsy before beginning tamoxifen therapy and periodically thereafter; not considered standard of care
J. Follow-up of abnormal pelvic ultrasound
   1. If total endometrial thickness > 5 mm in a postmenopausal woman
   2. Fluid in the endometrial cavity of a postmenopausal woman

III. **Contraindications**
   A. **Absolute**
      1. Pregnancy
   B. **Relative**
      1. Uterine infection or acute pelvic inflammatory disease
      2. Cervical infection (e.g., chlamydia cervicitis)
      3. Coagulopathy

IV. **Risks**
   A. Uterine cramping
      1. Minimal in most patients
      2. Increased markedly with stenotic cervix
   B. Vasovagal syncope
   C. Vaginal bleeding
      1. Usually minimal
   D. Infection
      1. Uncommon
      2. Minimized by using sterile technique
      3. 0–4 cases reported per 1000 patient
   E. Uterine perforation
      1. Rare with plastic biopsy instrument
      2. Advantage over dilatation and curettage

V. **Choosing an Endometrial Sampling Device**
   A. Must result in histologic, not only cytologic, sample
   B. Recommend small, plastic unit
      1. Less traumatic than stainless steel
      2. Greater patient acceptance
      3. Inexpensive
      4. No wall suction required
      5. No anesthesia
      6. Easy to use
      7. Disposable
      8. **Choice of instrument**
         a. GynoSampler (GynoPharma)—external diameter 2.92 mm; internal diameter 2.6 mm

    b. Pipelle (Unimar)—external diameter 3.1 mm; internal diameter 2.6 mm; $3–6 each, depending on quantity ordered

    c. Pipette (Milex Products)—available with external diameter of 3 mm or 4 mm; $3.50–6 each depending on quantity ordered

    d. Z-Sampler (Zinnanti Surgical Instruments)—external diameter 3.0 mm; internal diameter 2.4 mm; box of 25 at $120

    e. Endometrial sampler (BEI Medical Systems)—external diameter 3.0 mm

    f. Endocell (Wallach)—box of 20 at $73.20

    g. Endorette (Medscand Co.)—box of 25 at $73.75

VI. Equipment

A. Mayo stand covered with sterile towel
    1. Sterile items to be placed on stand
        a. Endometrial biopsy samplers
        b. Graves vaginal speculum; wider-blade Graves results in improved procedural exposure
        c. Tenaculum
        d. Uterine sound (optional)
            i. Recommended for use with endometrial samplers by most manufacturers
                (a) Metal sound increases risk of perforation
                (b) May use biopsy instrument to estimate depth of uterus; avoid overestimate by bending
                (c) Diameter of most samplers is less than diameter of metal sound
        e. Ringed forceps
        f. Cup of povidone/iodine solution with three sponges placed in it
            i. Ask about iodine allergy
        g. Small package of dry sponges
        h. Suture scissors

B. Bottle of antiseptic spray (povidone/iodine)

C. Specimen bottle containing preservative

D. One pair nonsterile gloves

E. One pair sterile gloves

F. Nonsterile towel
    1. For examiners lap

G. Nonsterile cloth or Chux
    1. Place on floor directly below patient's thighs

VII. Technique

A. May premedicate with nonsteroidal anti-inflammatory drug

B. Obtain consent (Fig. 1)

C. Patient placed in lithotomy position

D. Bimanual examination to determine uterine size and position, use nonsterile gloves, water for lubricant

E. Spray perineum and speculum with antiseptic spray
    1. Insert speculum, lock into position as widely as possible, keeping patient's comfort in mind

F. Grasp povidone/iodine-soaked sponges one at a time with ringed forceps
    1. Less drippage if grasped after moistening
    2. Cleanse cervix and surrounding vaginal tissue
    3. Repeat with remaining sponges

G. Grasp upper lip of cervix with tenaculum
    1. Warn patient of cramp or pinch

H. Clamp tenaculum quickly and firmly
    1. Cervix has stretch receptors and discomfort ensues if grasped slowly
    2. May use topical anesthetic before this step

I. Sound uterus with metal sound (optional)
    1. When placing sound or sampler into uterus, place fourth and fifth fingers on lateral perineum for stabilization to control advance of instrument should internal cervical os suddenly open

Consent for Endometrial Biopsy

Date _____
Time_____

I hereby authorize Dr. _____ and his/her assistants to perform an endometrial biopsy on me.

I understand that this is one method to obtain a sample of tissue from the inside of the uterus (womb). It will be done in the doctor's office. I will not be put to sleep, nor will any anesthesia be used during the procedure.

An endometrial biopsy is a procedure that can be done to look for answers to many different medical problems. I understand that the reason that it is being done on me today is

_____

_____

I understand that I may have cramping while the endometrial biopsy is being done and, perhaps, for a few days afterwards. I may also get light-headed during the procedure. I understand that I may have some vaginal bleeding after the endometrial biopsy. I understand that infection of the uterus is an uncommon complication of the procedure and that infection would require treatment with antibiotics. I understand that a very rare complication of an endometrial biopsy is perforation of the uterus (the biopsy instrument can make a tiny hole in the uterus) and that surgery might be necessary to close the hole.

I understand that an endometrial biopsy must not be done during pregnancy, and I am not pregnant.

I understand that an endometrial biopsy is used to find out answers to problems and does not usually cure medical problems.

I understand the risks and benefits of the procedure and have had the opportunity to have my questions answered.

_____   _____
Signature of witness   Patient's signature

                                _____
                                Patient's phone number

FIGURE 1.   Consent form for endometrial biopsy.

   J. Insert endometrial sampler
     1. Guide sampler gently from external os, through canal, and beyond internal os to top of uterine fundus
     2. Pull tenaculum gently forward to straighten uterus and provide countertraction for smooth insertion of sampler
     3. Sampler will be moist to length equal to depth of uterine cavity, obviating need to formally sound uterus
   K. Stabilize sheath of sampler
     1. If assistant available, she can now hold tenaculum up and out of way
     2. While holding sheath of sampling device with one hand, firmly withdraw plunger with other
       a. Withdraw plunger until stop near end of sheath is reached, creating vacuum

        b. It is possible to pull plunger out of sheath entirely if pulling too vigorously; this destroys vacuum and instrument must be withdrawn

   L. Rotate sheath several times while slowly withdrawing from endometrial cavity

        1. Ribbon of tissue is created from circumference of endometrial lining

        2. Vacuum may be broken at any point after sampler is withdrawn beyond internal os

        3. When entirely out, sheath will contain endometrial sample

   M. Place tissue sample in bottle of fixative

        1. Push plunger down, being careful that sampler does not touch fixative unless no further samples needed

        2. Plunger is thin and flexible; must be grasped close to end of sheath to replace it within sheath

        3. If sample of tissue remains in tip of sheath, snip it off and send it with sample

        4. Send specimen to pathology

   N. Remove tenaculum

        1. Press dry sponge against teeth marks if there is bleeding; silver nitrate sticks may be used if necessary

   O. Remove speculum

   P. Ask patient to get up slowly, to avoid vasovagal reaction

VIII. **Postprocedure Care**

   A. Advise patient to use pad rather than tampon until vaginal bleeding stops

   B. Advise patient to call if she bleeds excessively with clots or continues to bleed or spot over several days

   C. Advise patient to call if she continues to experience cramping over next few days or if she becomes febrile

   D. Prepare follow-up plan

 IX. **Pearls**

   A. To perform Papanicolaou smear at time of endometrial biopsy

        1. Perform initial bimanual examination

        2. Begin sterile procedure

           a. Spray perineum and speculum with antiseptic solution

           b. Place speculum in vagina

        3. Before cleansing cervix, collect specimens for Papanicolaou smear; grasp nonsterile Pap smear collection devices with a sterile 4 × 4 gauze

   B. **Cervical stenosis**

        1. Prime cervix with vaginal estrogen cream (in postmenopausal women) several weeks before procedure

        2. Partial cervical dilation

           a. Disassemble biopsy instrument and grasp tiny plunger with ringed forceps

           b. Advance plunger into cervical canal and through internal os, using tenaculum to provide countertraction

           c. Leave plunger in canal when opening second instrument pack

           d. Slowly remove plunger from canal and quickly place intact sampler within; some force often required

        3. Keep an endometrial sampler in the freezer; stiffer sample may penetrate internal os

        4. Use plastic endocervical dilator to dilate endocervical canal and internal os

   C. **Elusive cervical canal**

        1. Usually in multiparous patient

        2. External cervical os visible; sampler tip cannot be threaded into canal

        3. Methodically, begin at one corner of mouth of external os

        4. Serially search in all directions for canal with gentle pressure, moving carefully across length of os

        5. Canal is usually found along the way, frequently in one of the corners

   D. **Sampler cannot be threaded beyond internal os**

        1. Place tenaculum on other lip of cervix (e.g., remove from anterior lip and place on posterior lip)

           a. Solves problems created by highly flexed uterus

E. **Inadequate tissue sample**
   1. Obtain second sample
      a. Be sure sampler is threaded beyond internal os and to top of uterine fundus
      b. Note depth of placement of sampler—internal os may be several cm into canal
      c. Increase number of rotations of sampler while withdrawing slowly from uterine cavity
      d. If sampling carried out appropriately, minimal tissue indicates atrophic or minimal growth of endometrium; not suggestive of cancer of uterus

SUGGESTED READING

1. Apgar BS, Newkirk GR: Office procedures: Endometrial biopsy. Prim Care 2:303–326, 1997.
2. Barakat RR : Benign and hyperplastic endometrial changes associated with tamoxifen use. Oncology Huntingt 11:35–37, 1997.
3. Chambers JT, Chambers SK: Endometrial sampling: When? Where? Why? With what? Clin Obstet Gynecol 35:28–39, 1992.
4. Shelly MS: Endometrial biopsy. Am Fam Physician 55:1731–1736, 1997.
5. Stoval TG, Solomon SK: Endometrial sampling prior to hysterectomy. Obstet Gynecol 73:405–409, 1989.

118. Insertion of Word Catheter for Bartholin Cyst or Abscess

Barbara S. Apgar, M.D., M.S.

Simple incision and drainage of a Bartholin duct cyst or abscess may produce immediate and dramatic symptom resolution, but the recurrence rate after such a procedure is unacceptably high. Total excision of the gland and duct is rarely required unless the gland and duct have been previously scarred due to incision and drainage. It is preferable to create an epithelialized tract from the vulvar vestibule to the cyst that will allow continued functioning of the Bartholin's gland, proper drainage, and minimal recurrence. Use of a Word catheter creates a fistulous tract that preserves the gland and allows for adequate drainage. The Word catheter is a short latex stem with an inflatable bulb at the distal end (Fig. 1).

I. **Indications**
   A. Treatment of symptomatic Bartholin's gland cyst
   B. Treatment of Bartholin's gland abscess

II. **Contraindications**
   A. Any condition that precludes normal incision and drainage of vulvar cyst or abscess

III. **Preoperative evaluation and preparation**
   A. Explain procedure to patient and obtain informed consent
   B. Non-narcotic oral analgesic may be administered before procedure. Narcotic analgesia is not usually necessary.

IV. **Equipment**
   A. Bartholin gland (Word) catheter
   B. 3-ml syringe (for catheter inflation)
   C. 22-gauge needle (for catheter inflation)
   D. 1% xylocaine without epinephrine
   E. 27-gauge needle (for anesthesia)
   F. 5-ml syringe (for anesthesia)
   G. Scalpel with no. 11 blade
   H. Small hemostats
   I. 4 × 4 gauze pads
   J. Normal saline
   K. Antiseptic solution (question about allergies before using iodine)

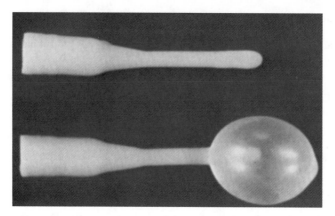

FIGURE 1. Word catheters before and after inflation. (From Friedrich EG: Vulvar Disease, 2nd ed. Philadelphia, W.B. Saunders, 1983, with permission.)

V. **Technique**
A. Vestibule is prepped with antiseptic and wheal is made by infiltration of 1% xylocaine approximately in area of original duct orifice external but immediately adjacent to hymenal ring
B. Vulvar epithelium is incised and underlying fascia is dissected with hemostats until cyst wall is identified
    1. Careful dissection will prevent inadvertent premature incision of cyst wall before wall is grasped with hemostats
C. Anterior cyst wall is grasped with 2 hemostats placed 5 mm apart
    1. Enables stabilization of cyst wall while catheter is inserted
    2. Prevents creation of false tracts outside cyst
D. Cyst wall is lanced or incised between 2 hemostats with scalpel blade
    1. Essential that stab wound penetrates cyst wall as evidenced by free flow of pus or mucus
    2. Stab wound must be large enough for catheter to be inserted, usually 1–1.5 cm long
    3. It should not be difficult to find cyst lumen after incision is made if walls are held by hemostats
E. Insert small hemostat into stab wound and break away any loculations while still grasping cyst walls
F. Instill 25–50 ml of normal saline to wash out cyst cavity
G. Insert sterile Word catheter into incision and inflate bulb with 2–3 ml of saline through sealed-stopper end
    1. Use exact quantity of saline necessary to ensure that catheter will not fall out with normal activity
    2. Do not air inflate catheter
H. The two edges of the cyst wall should be sutured to the edges of the vulvar excision
I. Catheter stem is tucked into vagina, where catheter rests perpendicular to perineum to avoid tension on tissue due to bending of catheter stem
    1. Catheter in vagina allows freedom of movement and activity without added awareness of protrusion of the catheter stem
VI. **Postprocedure Care**
A. Patient should be instructed to expect discharge since catheter allows drainage of cyst fluid
B. Catheter is left in place for 4–6 weeks until epithelialization of tract is complete
C. Patient should return in 4–6 weeks for removal of catheter
    1. Catheter is removed by inserting needle into sealed-stopper and drawing out fluid
    2. Catheter then withdrawn from incision and the wound is cleaned

VII. **Complications**
   A. Continuous pain for 24 hours after insertion of catheter
      1. Bulb may be too large for cyst cavity
         a. May be corrected by withdrawing some of fluid and thus reducing size of bulb
         b. Must be careful to avoid piercing the stem with the needle
   B. **Cellulitis**
      1. Abscessed Bartholin gland may have cellulitis around vulvar opening of duct
      2. Simple incision and drainage may not resolve cellulitis; antibiotics may need to be prescribed for 48–72 hours after insertion of catheter
   C. **Deflation of catheter**
      1. If needle used to introduce water into catheter punctures stem of catheter, catheter gradually deflates and falls out before epithelialization is complete
   D. **Extrusion of catheter**
      1. If stab wound is too large, catheter will fall out
      2. May be necessary to suture stab wound around catheter to keep it in if stab wound is too large

SUGGESTED READING

1. Cohen SD, Wright F, Hernandez E, Dunton CJ: Management of the Bartholin abscess. Am J Gynecol Health 4:42–44, 1990.
2. Goldberg JE: Simplified treatment for disease of Bartholin's gland. Obstet Gynecol 35:109–110, 1970.
3. Heah J: Methods of treatment for cysts and abscesses of Bartholin's gland. Br J Obstet Gynecol 95:321–322, 1988.
4. Hill DA, Lense JJ: Office management of Bartholin gland cysts and abscesses. Am Family Physician 57:1611–1616, 1998.
5. Lashgari M, Curry S. Preferred methods of treating Bartholin's duct cyst. Contemp Obstet Gynecol 40:38–42, 1995.
6. Oliphant MM, Anderson GV: Management of Bartholin duct cysts and abscesses. Obstet Gynecol 16:476–478, 1960.
7. Word B: New instrument for office treatment of cyst and abscess of Bartholin's gland. JAMA 190: 777–778, 1964.

119. Diaphragm Fitting

Barbara S. Apgar, M.D., M.S.

The diaphragm is a barrier contraceptive device that mechanically blocks the entrance of the sperm through the cervical os. The diaphragm acts with spermicidal jelly to produce a theoretical contraceptive effectiveness rate of 98%. However, rates of 88–93% for new users and 97% for long-term users are more accurate representations of effectiveness. The diaphragm should be used by women who are familiar and comfortable with insertion and removal of this device.

   I. **Indications**
      A. Barrier contraception
  II. **Contraindications**
      A. Vaginal stenosis or pelvic abnormalities that preclude insertion and removal of diaphragm
      B. Allergy to spermicidal jelly
      C. Allergy to rubber
      D. Recurrent urinary tract infections associated with diaphragm use
      E. Aversion to touching genital area
      F. Fitting sooner than 6 weeks postpartum or before uterus has completely involuted
      G. History of toxic shock syndrome
      H. Current vaginal, cervical, or pelvic infections

III. **Patient Evaluation and Preparation**
   A. Explain procedure to patient
      1. How diaphragm is inserted, fitted, and removed by clinician
      2. How patient practices inserting and removing diaphragm
   B. Patient should not be menstruating or have vaginal, cervical, or pelvic infection at time of diaphragm fitting
IV. **Equipment**
   A. Three types of diaphragms (sizes 65–90)
      1. **Arching spring**
         a. Molded one-piece spring and dome with firm rim that forms arc when rim is compressed
         b. Needs no introducer
         c. Recommended for women with decreased pelvic support, cystocele or rectocele, or retroverted uterus; also for women who find firmer rim easier to insert
      2. **Coil spring**
         a. Molded one-piece spring and dome with soft flexible rim
         b. May be used with introducer
         c. Recommended for women with good vaginal support, no cystocele or rectocele or pelvic floor relaxation
         d. Cervix in midplane or anterior position
      3. **Flat spring**
         a. Molded one-piece spring and dome with soft rim for flexible compression
         b. May be used with introducer
         c. Recommended for smaller women with narrow or shallow pelvic shelf
         d. Excellent for nulliparous women
   B. Spermicidal jelly
   C. Diaphragm introducer (optional)
   D. Set of fitting rings or diaphragms (obtained from company usually at no cost to practitioners); full diaphragm preferable for fitting
V. **Technique**
   A. Place patient in lithotomy position
   B. Measure for correct size of diaphragm
      1. Hold index and middle fingers together and insert into vagina up to posterior fornix
      2. Raise hand to bring surface of the index finger in contact with pubic arch
      3. Use thumb to mark point directly under pubic bone and withdraw fingers from vagina holding thumb in position
      4. To determine the diaphragm size
         a. Place one end of diaphragm rim on tip of middle finger with opposite side of rim lying just in front of thumb tip
         b. This is approximate diameter of diaphragm needed
   C. Use lubricant on fitting rings or diaphragms to aid insertion and make procedure more comfortable for patient
   D. Prepare to insert fitting diaphragm or ring of approximate size into vagina by folding diaphragm in half by pressing middle of opposite sides together between thumb and fingers of one hand
   E. Hold vulva open with other hand and gently slide folded diaphragm into vagina and aim toward posterior fornix
      1. Proximal rim should fit behind pubic arch without undue pressure
      2. Cervix should be palpable through dome of diaphragm
   F. Diaphragm is removed from vagina when correct fit is determined by inserting index finger into vagina and hooking it under proximal rim of diaphragm
   G. Diaphragm is gently pulled down and out of vagina
   H. Patient practices inserting and removing diaphragm
   I. Patient is instructed on how to apply spermicidal jelly to rim and dome of diaphragm
      1. Spermicidal jelly supplies both contraceptive and STD protection
      2. Jelly applied to concave surface and rim of diaphragm so that uterus is sealed off mechanically as well as chemically

3. Approximately one teaspoon of jelly is placed in dome and thin layer is applied around rim

J. Patient is instructed to make sure diaphragm is firmly in place behind pubic bone with distal rim behind cervix; she should feel for cervix beneath dome of diaphragm

K. Patient is instructed to avoid douching or removing diaphragm for 6 hours after intercourse and to leave diaphragm in place and insert additional spermicidal jelly into vagina before additional coitus in this 6-hour period

L. Patient should walk around exam room with diaphragm in place to ensure comfortable fit

VI. **Postprocedure Care**

A. Fittings of diaphragms are cleaned by soaking in disinfectant solution such as Cidex; then autoclaved and disinfected

B. Patient should clean diaphragm in mild soap and water solution

C. Diaphragm should be rinsed in clear water and carefully dried

D. Diaphragm should be dusted with cornstarch and stored in original container; it should not be exposed to extreme heat, direct sunlight, or petroleum products

E. Diaphragm should be removed no sooner than 6 hours and no longer than 24 hours after intercourse; 8 hours is preferable

F. New diaphragm should be obtained every year or when rubber becomes brittle

VII. **Complications**

A. **Improper fit**

1. If diaphragm is too small, it may not completely cover cervix

2. If diaphragm is too large, it may be uncomfortable and not provide tight seal in vagina

B. **Toxic shock syndrome** (TSS)

1. Reported cases in women who have worn diaphragms continuously for > 24 hours

C. **Failure to use spermicidal jelly**

1. Pregnancy rate is increased if spermicide is not used with diaphragm

D. **Weight gain or loss**

1. Change in weight (± 15 pounds) may alter fit of diaphragm, as may pregnancy and pelvic surgery

E. **Pressure ulcerations** caused by excessive pressure of diaphragm against lateral vaginal walls due to improper fit

F. **Urinary tract infections** (UTI)

1. A diaphragm that is too large may cause excessive pressure on the urethra and increase the risk of UTIs

2. Increased risk from bacterial vaginosis and *E. coli*

SUGGESTED READING

1. Baehler EA, Dillon WP, Cumbo TJ, Lee RV: Prolonged use of a diaphragm and toxic shock syndrome. Fertil Steril 38:248–250, 1982.
2. Craig S, Hepburn S: The effectiveness of barrier methods of contraception with and without spermicide. Contraception 26:347, 1982.
3. Edelman DA, McIntyre SL, Harper J: A comparative trial of the Today contraceptive sponge and diaphragm. Am J Obstet Gynecol 150:869–873, 1984.
4. Fihn SD, Latham RH, Roberts P, et al: Association between diaphragm use and urinary tract infection. JAMA 254:240–245, 1985.
5. Foxman B: Recurring urinary tract infection: Incidence and risk factors. Am J Public Health 80:331–333, 1990.
6. Gillespie L: The diaphragm: An accomplice in recurrent urinary tract infections. Urology 24:25–30, 1984.
7. Jaffe R: Toxic shock syndrome associated with diaphragm use. N Engl J Med 305:1585, 1981.
8. Lanes SF, Poole C, Dreyer NA, Lanza LL: Toxic shock syndrome, contraceptive methods, and vaginitis. Am J Obstet Gynecol 154:989–991, 1986.
9. Leibovici L, Alpert G, Laor A, et al: Urinary tract infections and sexual activity in young women. Arch Intern Med 147:345–347, 1987.
10. Strom BL, Collins M, West SL, et al: Sexual activity, contraceptive use and other risk factors for symptomatic and asymptomatic bacteriuria. Ann Intern Med 107:816–823, 1987.

120. Placement of the Intrauterine Contraceptive Device

Barbara S. Apgar, M.D, MS.

The intrauterine contraceptive device (IUD) has not increased in popularity despite testimony to its effectiveness and safety. Although litigation against the currently marketed IUDs is minimal, the most common reason for clinician reluctance to insert IUDs is fear of litigation. All IUDs approved by the Food and Drug Administration have been removed from the market except the progesterone IUD (Progestasert) and Copper T (ParaGard T). The decision to discontinue marketing of most IUDs was based on economic rather than medical factors. The severity of IUD litigation results from the public perspective that the IUD is not safe. Sequelae of pelvic inflammatory disease (PID), alleged to have resulted in permanent infertility, account for 89% of the cases tried against Planned Parenthood. Legal counsel for Planned Parenthood have emphasized that successful defense of an IUD case depends on the clinician's full compliance with the manufacturer's recommended protocol and the use of complete informed consent.

Unlike other contraceptive methods, which have higher use-failure rates than method–failure rates, the method– and use–failure rates for IUDs are similar. First–year failure rates range from 2–3%. Correct fundal placement is key to successful contraception. The risk of adverse sequelae from the IUD decreases as the age of the wearer increases.

I. **Indications**
   A. Reversible contraception
II. **Contraindications**
   A. **Absolute**
      1. Pregnancy or suspected pregnancy
      2. History of ectopic pregnancy
      3. History of pelvic inflammatory disease, current sexually transmitted diseases such as gonorrhea or chlamydia, or postpartum endometritis
      4. Active vaginitis, cervicitis, or pelvic infection
      5. Undiagnosed vaginal bleeding
      6. Known or suspected cervical or endometrial carcinoma, including unresolved cervical dysplasia
      7. Abnormal uterine anatomy
      8. Multiple sexual partners
      9. Immunodeficiency state
      10. Allergy to copper
      11. Wilson's disease
      12. Uterus that sounds < 6.5 cm from external os
   B. **Relative**
      1. Severe dysmenorrhea
      2. Abnormal uterine bleeding associated with menstrual cycle
      3. Congenital or valvular heart disease
      4. Nulliparity
III. **Mode of Action**
   A. Is the IUD an abortifacient?
      1. Recent research demonstrated that IUD exerts effect outside uterus by interfering with reproductive process before fertilization occurs
         a. No fertilized eggs recovered from uterine cavities of IUD users
      2. Rate of recovery of tubal eggs is substantially lower in IUD (all types) users compared with controls and least frequent in users of Copper T device
      3. Possible explanations
         a. Failure of release of oocyte from ruptured follicle
         b. Failure of oocyte pick-up by fimbria
         c. Accelerated transport through tube

      d. Alterations in biochemical and/or cellular composition of tubal fluid leading to premature lysis of egg

    4. Because no fertilized eggs were found in fallopian tubes of IUD users, it is postulated that primary mode of action of IUDs is by method other than destruction of live embryos

  B. Reflux of fluid from uterus to fallopian tubes allows mixing of fluids

    1. Copper concentrations in fluid of uterus and tubes of copper IUD users are similar

    2. Mixing of fluid may explain how copper exerts effect on oocyte

  C. Rise in human chorionic gonadotropin does not occur after ovulation in users of copper IUDs compared with controls and indicates that IUD users do not retain natural fertility

  D. Other substances may be produced or released by uterus, such as lysozymes, that interfere with oocyte maturation in IUDs without copper

  E. Primary mode of action of IUD may be production of a local sterile inflammatory reaction in uterine cavity

    1. Breakdown products of inflammatory cells may be toxic to sperm

    2. Copper IUDs increase inflammatory response and are superior for long-term use over other metals, such as zinc, which become inert after short time in uterus

IV. **Preoperative Evaluation**

  A. Optimal candidates for IUDs

    1. Women who have had at least 1 child

    2. Women in mutually monogamous relationship

    3. Women at low risk for sexually transmitted disease

    4. Women who do not desire permanent sterilization

  B. Clinician should be thoroughly familiar with manufacturer's package insert information

  C. Both patient and clinician must sign informed consent

  D. IUD may be inserted anytime during menstrual cycle provided patient is not pregnant

  E. IUDs can be inserted immediately after delivery of placenta

    1. Postpartum expulsion of device varies from 6–37% at 6 months

    2. Rate may be decreased with intensive training and practice of proper fundal placement

  F. Use of prophylactic antibiotics administered at time of insertion is not recommended by many experts however consensus has not been obtained

    1. Antibiotics should not be used in order to insert IUD in woman with existing cervicitis or upper genital tract disease

    2. If STDs are prevalent in the community:

      a. Doxycycline, 200 mg orally 1 hour before insertion and 200 mg orally 12 hours later, *or*

      b. Erythromycin, 500 mg orally 1 hour before insertion and 500 mg orally 6 hours later

  G. Analgesics or antiprostaglandin agents can be given before insertion to lessen cramping

V. **Equipment**

  A. IUD in manufacturer's packaging

  B. Tenaculum

  C. Uterine sound

  D. Ring forceps

  E. Cotton balls or gauze pads

  F. Antiseptic solution (question about allergy to iodine)

  G. Speculum

  H. Scissors

VI. **Technique for Inserting ParaGard T 380A**

  A. Pelvic examination is performed to ascertain position, size, and shape of uterus

  B. Sterile vaginal speculum is placed

  C. Samples for chlamydia and gonorrhea should be obtained in high-risk patients prior to insertion

    1. If evidence of vaginal, cervical or uterine infections is present, IUD should not be placed

D. Cervix is cleansed with antiseptic solution
E. Tenaculum is placed and gentle traction is applied to correct uterine angle and to stabilize cervix during insertion
F. Uterine sound is inserted along axis of endocervical canal through internal os to determine depth and direction of uterine cavity
   1. If uterine cavity measures < 6.5 cm or > 10 cm, IUD should not be inserted
   2. Blue stop (flange) on outside of introducer tube is placed at correct measurement for length of uterine cavity
     a. Horizontal arms of IUD and long arms of flange should be in same plane
G. IUD is loaded into inserter tube under sterile technique
   1. With sterile gloves or inside package container
   2. Do not wait longer than 5 minutes to insert IUD after it is loaded because it will not return to its original shape after insertion
   3. Arms of IUD should be inserted only deeply enough into tube(until copper sleeve is reached) to ensure that they will not come out prematurely
H. Tip of inner plunger rod is placed at tail end of IUD (at blue tip of IUD)
I. IUD is inserted through cervical os until fundus is reached and flange is against external os
   1. When IUD is at fundus, introducer rod is pulled toward curled end of plunger rod (about 1 cm)
   2. Inserter rod must be held against tail of IUD to release arms of IUD from introducer tube
   3. Plunger rod is pushed up to meet introducer rod (about 1–2 cm)
     a. IUD is thereby placed high in fundus to ensure correct placement
     b. IUDs placed in the lower uterine segment tend to have higher rates of expulsion and failure
J. Inserting tube and rod are removed and string of IUD is cut 1.5–2 inches from cervical os
   1. Tenaculum is removed and speculum is removed

VII. **Postprocedure Care**
A. Patient recovers in the exam room
B. Patient is instructed to call if she experiences fever, excessive cramping, or expulsion of IUD
C. Patient should be instructed on proper procedure for checking string of IUD
D. Patient should return to office after first menstrual period so placement can be checked
   1. If menstrual period is missed, pregnancy should be ruled out

VIII. **Removal of IUD**
A. Indications for removal
   1. Abnormal uterine bleeding
   2. Increasingly severe dysmenorrhea
   3. Pelvic pain
   4. Pregnancy
   5. Suspected or documented pelvic infection
   6. Presence of *Actinomyces* species
   7. Desire for pregnancy
B. Progestasert replaced annually; Copper T replaced every 10 years
C. Technique of removal
   1. String of IUD is grasped with ring forceps as close to external os as possible
   2. Gentle traction is applied to string until IUD is removed
   3. Failure to visualize IUD string
     a. Pregnancy should be ruled out before probing
     b. After pregnancy ruled out, endocervical canal should be gently probed with cytobrush or uterine sound to find string
       i. If this is not successful, ultrasonography or hysteroscopy should be performed to ensure that IUD is still in uterine cavity and has not perforated through myometrium
       ii. If in abdominal cavity, IUD should be removed by laparoscopy

IX. **Complications**
  A. **Perforation**
    1. Rate varies from 1–3 per 1,000 insertions, depending on skill of clinician inserting IUD
      a. Highest rate if inserted postpartum
      b. No increased risk if inserted immediately after first-trimester abortion or immediately after delivery of placenta
    2. May be complete or partial
      a. Complete perforations through myometrium should be surgically assessed as soon as possible
      b. Laparoscopy or hysteroscopy can accomplish removal
      c. Failure to remove perforated IUDs may result in
        i. Adhesion formation
        ii. Peritonitis
        iii. Perforation of abdominal structures such as bowel
        iv. Infection and abscess formation
  B. **Pelvic inflammatory disease** (PID)
    1. Risk of PID is highest in first month after insertion
      a. Risk is directly related to introduction of pathogens from vagina and endocervix during insertion
    2. After 5 months, risk of PID is the same as for general population
    3. If PID arises while IUD is in place, it should be removed and appropriate antibiotics started
    4. Risk of PID is highest when patient has multiple sexual partners
  C. **Infection with *Actinomyces* sp.**
    1. Anaerobic gram-positive bacteria
    2. Detected on a Pap smear in IUD users
    3. Increases with duration of IUD use, regardless of type of IUD
    4. Options for treatment
      a. Remove IUD and repeat Pap smear in 3 months
        i. If still present, treat with penicillin or ampicillin
      b. Leave IUD in place and treat with antibiotics (least recommended)
        i. Repeat Pap smear in 3 months
        ii. If infection still present, remove IUD
  D. **Pregnancy with IUD present**
    1. Increased risk of spontaneous abortion, premature onset labor, and infection if not removed
    2. Incidence of spontaneous abortion in patient who conceives with IUD in place is about 55%, about 3 times greater than in controls
    3. IUD should be removed if possible
      a. Removal may result in spontaneous abortion
      b. If IUD is removed, incidence of spontaneous abortion decreases to 29%
      c. If string is not visible
        i. Leave in for duration of pregnancy
        ii. Advise patient of increased risk
        iii. Treat aggressively if infection occurs
    4. No associated risk of fetal anomalies due to copper
    5. IUDs do not offer protection against ectopic pregnancies
  E. **Expulsion**
    1. Higher rate if IUD is placed between 1–8 weeks postpartum
    2. Approximately 5–12% spontaneously expel IUD
  F. **Increased menstrual blood loss**
    1. Highest loss associated with loop devices (not currently on market), intermediate with copper devices, and lowest with progesterone devices
    2. Mefenamic acid administration during menstruation has been shown to decrease blood loss significantly
  G. **IUDs have no apparent effect on subsequent fertility status of users**

1. Return to fertility is not dependent on
   a. Age
   b. Duration of IUD use
   c. Timing of insertion
   d. Type of device used
2. 90–94% of women conceived within 1 year of removal of IUD

SUGGESTED READING

1. Alvarez F, Brache V, Fernandez E, et al: New insights on the mode of action of intrauterine contraceptive devices in women. Fertil Steril 49:768–773, 1988.
2. American College of Obstetricians and Gynecologists: The intrauterine device. ACOG Tech Bull 104:1–5, 1987.
3. Diagnostic and Therapeutic Technology Assessment Panel: Intrauterine devices. JAMA 261:2127–2130, 1989.
4. Eschenbach DA: The IUD and infertility. Fertil Steril 57:1177–1179, 1992.
5. Farley TMM: The IUD and PID. Lancet 339:785–788, 1992.
6. Grimes DA: Intrauterine devices and pelvic inflammatory disease: Recent developments. Contraception 36:97–102, 1987.
7. Gupta BK, Gupta AN, Lyall S: Return of fertility in various types of IUD users. Int J Fertil 34:123–125, 1989.
8. Sinei SKA, Schulz KF, Lamptey PR, et al: Preventing IUCD-related pelvic infection: The efficacy of prophylactic doxycycline at insertion. Br J Obstet Gynaecol 97:412–429, 1990.
9. Zhang J, Chi I, Feldblum PJ, Farr MG: Risk factors for copper T IUD expulsion: An epidemiologic analysis. Contraception 46:427–433, 1992.

121. Subdermal Contraceptive Implants

Gary R. Newkirk, M.D.

I. **Introduction**
   A. The Norplant contraception system consists of six levonorgestrel-containing silicon capsules
   B. Released by the Food and Drug Administration for use in the U.S. in early 1991
   C. Extremely low failure rates—in first year less than vasectomy, injectable progestogens, oral contraceptives. The average annual gross pregnancy rate over 5 years is less than 1%
   D. Slightly higher failure rate in the second and third year in women weighing over 70 kg, but still much less than competitive methods overall
   E. Continuation rates vary. In the U.S. the continuation rate for the first year is 82%; for the second year, 65%; for the third year, 50%; and for the fourth year, 44%
   F. Cumulative 5-year expense comparable to oral contraceptives
   G. Multiple mechanisms of action
      1. Suppression of ovulation in most cycles
      2. Thickening of cervical mucus
   H. Prevents conception within 24 hours after insertion if inserted within the first 7 days of menstrual cycle
   I. Totally reversible: 76% conception rate by 12 months, 90% by 24 months
   J. Should be removed if pregnancy desired, intolerable side-effects experienced, or after 5 years

II. **Indications**
   A. Reversible, longer-term contraception
   B. Candidates for subdermal implants
      1. Estrogen contraindicated
      2. Breastfeeding after 6 weeks
      3. Reproductively older women with risk for estrogen use (i.e., smoking, hypertension, diabetes)

III. **Contraindications**
   A. Current pregnancy
   B. Active thrombophlebitis or thromboembolic disorders
   C. Undiagnosed abnormal genital bleeding
   D. Acute liver disease
   E. Benign or malignant liver tumors
   F. Known or suspected carcinoma of the breast
IV. **Morbidities**
   A. Irregular bleeding patterns
      1. Most notable during first 6 months of use, almost universal in occurrence
   B. Headache, depression (some feel it should not be used with major depressive disorder)
   C. Nervousness, nausea, dizziness, dermatitis, acne, appetite change, weight change, mastalgia, hirsutism, hair loss
   D. Ectopic pregnancy rate is not increased, but if method fails, likelihood of ectopic pregnancy is higher
   E. Decrease in total cholesterol and triglyceride levels
   F. Both increases and decreases in HDL levels have been reported
   G. No significant change in diabetic or hypertension control
V. **Preinsertion Issues**
   A. Counseling, consent
      1. Patient selection and counseling are critical for successful outcomes
   B. Insert within first 7 days after menses or at any time if back-up contraceptive method is used
   C. Patient must not be pregnant
   D. Complete history, systems review, physical examination (including breast, pelvic, and Papanicolaou screening)
VI. **Insertion Method**
   A. Equipment
      1. Norplant kit
      2. Examining table for the patient to lie on
      3. Sterile gloves, antiseptic solution
      4. Local anesthetic (1% lidocaine)
   B. Patient lies supine with nondominant arm flexed at elbow and externally rotated so that her hand is lying by her head
   C. Prepare upper arm with antiseptic solution
      1. Inside of upper arm about 8–10 cm above elbow crease
   D. Cover with fenestrate sterile drape
   E. Open Norplant kit and count capsules; sterile gloves must be used
   F. Using stencil fan, mark the insertion point and six tracts with methylene blue pen
   G. Using 10-ml syringe filled with anesthetic agent, inject the six marked tracks just below the dermis
   H. Make a 2-mm stab incision at the insertion site
   I. Insert the trocar into the 14-gauge Norplant insertion needle. Note the proximal and distal marks on the needle, which denote the insertion and withdrawal depth for the needle
   J. Insert the tip of the needle with trocar in place, needle level up at a shallow angle. Advance the needle in the subdermal space until the insertion mark is flush with the insertion hole skin edge. Tent the skin up, ensuring a subdermal location
   K. Remove the trocar and load the first capsule into the needle lumen
   L. Gently advance the capsule with the trocar toward the tip of the needle until the tip of the capsule reaches the end of the needle. Never force the capsule into place
   M. Holding the trocar steady, withdraw the needle back, essentially laying the capsule into place under the skin
   N. Withdraw the needle until the capsule is seen to fall away from the needle tip. This occurs as the second needle mark becomes flush with the insertion site
   O. Replace the trocar. Leaving the needle tip under the skin, redirect and insert the needle along another marked track, repeating the insertion process (Fig. 1)

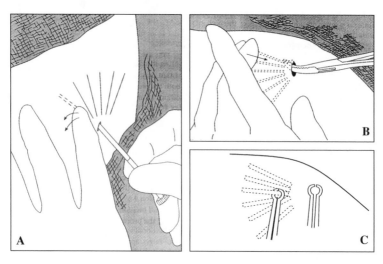

FIGURE 1. Techniques for insertion and removal of Norplant implants. *A*, Technique of pulling inserted implant away from the path of the trocar as the next implant is inserted. *B*, Use of hemostat to remove implant while clinician's finger pushes implant toward incision. *C*, U-technique for removing Norplant implants. (From Hatcher RA, Trusseu J, Stewart F, et al (eds): Contraceptive Technology, 17th ed. New York, Adrian Media, Inc., 1998, pp 491–495, with permission.)

      P. After the insertion of the sixth capsule, palpate the capsules to make sure that all six have been inserted in a simple linear, fan pattern
      Q. Apply steristrips to approximate the insertion wound edges
      R. Cover the insertion site with gauze, and apply a pressure wrap gauze
  VII. **Postinsertion Instructions**
      A. Leave the pressure dressing in place for 24 hours
      B. Leave the steristrips in place for several days
      C. Avoid direct shower contact for 48 hours
      D. Report signs of infection, bleeding
 VIII. **Removal Procedure**
      A. Preschedule when possible
      B. Allow for 30 minutes
      C. Locate the six capsules by palpation
      D. Mark capsule location with methylene blue pen
      E. Use antiseptic solution to clean removal site
      F. Inject local anesthetic under the distal one-quarter of the fan just deep to the capsule tips
      G. Make a 4-mm incision with scalpel close to the capsule ends
      H. Using a mosquito forceps (hemostat), vigorously spread tissue around the proximal capsule tips
      I. By massaging and palpation, extrude the proximal capsule tips through the skin incision. Use a scraping motion with the scalpel to scrape the adhesions at the end of each capsule tip. Grasp the capsule with the mosquito or fine-teeth forceps and withdraw the capsule
      J. Repeat this procedure for all six capsules, which can be removed in any order
      K. Avoid making additional removal incisions in the skin
      L. Close the skin, and apply a pressure dressing as for insertion
      M. Allow the patient to view the removed six capsules
      N. If all capsules cannot be removed, patient should use back-up contraception and another removal visit should be scheduled
  IX. **Removal Troubleshooting**
      A. Get formal training regarding insertion and removal techniques
      B. In general, removal session should not last over 30–60 minutes

1. Reschedule patient for another removal session. Allow swelling to resolve. If infection results from the first removal attempt, this must be completely resolved before further removal attempts
C. Before injection for removal, mark each capsule's proximal (toward axilla) and distal (elbow) tip with a methylene blue pen
D. Avoid overinjection of anesthetic agent for removal—limit of 1–2 ml at the distal one-third of each capsule. Too much anesthetic makes it more difficult to identify location of capsules
E. Vigorously break down adhesions distally with a small mosquito forceps prior to removing capsules
F. A U-flexed capsule requires identification before injection. This is accomplished by careful palpation
   1. Once identified, attempt to vigorously break down adhesions, allowing for grasping the capsule at the bottom of the "U" and removing by gentle traction
      a. Take care not to fracture this capsule; fractured capsules will require removal of each piece
      b. Only as a last resort should a separate incision be made to remove a capsule. This may be necessary for a widely displaced capsule or a capsule fragment
G. If all six capsules cannot be identified before injection, do not explore the subdermis to find the missing capsule
   1. Ultrasound can be used to locate lost capsules, which are often near the insertion site but too deep
   2. Soft-tissue radiographs can also identify lost capsules. At least two views are necessary to locate the capsule and indicate capsule depth
   3. A back-up method of contraception must be used until all capsules are removed

SUGGESTED READING

1. Berenson AB, Wiemann CM, McCombs SL, Somma-Garcia A: The rise and fall of levonorgestrel implants: 1992–1996. Obstet Gynecol 92:790–794, 1998.
2. Flattum-Riemers J: Norplant: A new contraceptive. Am Fam Physician 44:103–110, 1991.
3. Sivin I, Mishell DR Jr, Darney P, et al: Levonorgestrel capsule implants in the United States: A 5-year study. Obstet Gynecol 92:337–344, 1998.
4. Wyeth-Ayerst Laboratories: Norplant System: Prescribing Information. Philadelphia, Wyeth-Ayerst Laboratories, 1990.
5. Zibners A, Cromer BA, Hayes J: Comparison of continuation rates for hormonal comtraception among adolescents. J Pediatr Adolesc Gynecol 12:90–94, 1999.

122. Breast Examination

Cynda Ann Johnson, M.D., M.B.A.

Although controversy continues concerning the relative importance of mammography, breast self-examination, and breast examination by the health care provider, the fact is that all these screening modalities are extremely important. A combination of techniques used on a regular basis detects the greatest number of breast cancers at the earliest, most frequently curable stages.

I. **History**
   A. Previous breast disease, biopsies
   B. Breast symptoms, including pain, masses, discharge, relationship to menses
   C. Family history of breast cancer, other breast disease, biopsies
   D. Regular breast self-examination (BSE)
      1. Women who perform BSE
         a. Should be done monthly after, not before, menstrual period
         b. Ask patient to demonstrate her technique

    2. Women who do not perform BSE—common reasons
       a. Patient does not know how to perform BSE—demonstrate and provide hand-out
       b. Frightened—offer reassurance and suggest another trusted person perform exam
       c. Patient does not believe she will know when she finds abnormality
          i. Practice on breast model with palpable lumps
          ii. Patient with irregular breast tissue—important for woman to become familiar with her own breasts, lumps and all, in order to recognize when change has occurred
          iii. Encourage patient to seek consultation if she is unsure about physical finding

II. **Screening Breast Examination**
  A. Should take only 3 minutes
  B. Examiner should have warm hands
  C. Begin exam with patient sitting
    1. Inspection
      a. Symmetry and size
         i. Variance between breasts is typical
         ii. Patient usually knows if variance is her normal anatomy
      b. Nipple retraction
      c. Skin changes
      d. Vascular patterns
    2. Have patient flex pectoral muscles by pushing hands in on hips
      a. Accentuates abnormal thickening or tightening of tissue within breast
      b. Reinspect breasts
    3. Palpate for axillary, infraclavicular, and supraclavicular nodes
  D. Continue exam with patient in supine position
    1. Patient should put forearm of side to be examined under head which moves breast into flatter, more dispersed position on chest
    2. Area to be examined
      a. Vertically from clavicles to inframammary crease
      b. Horizontally from midaxillary line to midaxillary line
      c. Examine each breast from lateral side
      d. Majority of breast tissue falls into upper, outer quadrant
    3. Linear patterns of examination result in more complete breast exam than either concentric or radial patterns
      a. Palpate each strip from superior to inferior, beginning medially
      b. Use finger pads for palpation
      c. Expect softness behind areola in non-breastfeeding woman
      d. Squeeze nipple to determine if discharge is present
  E. **Abnormal findings**
    1. **Nipple discharge** (see Chapter 65)
      a. Describe discharge by color, consistency, odor
      b. Hemoccult test for blood
      c. Palpate surrounding ducts carefully to determine if discharge is emanating from single ductile region
    2. **Lump or fullness**—characteristics
      a. Size
      b. Is mass fixed to surrounding tissues? Discrete?
      c. Tenderness
      d. Shape
      e. Is area significantly different from other regions of breast?
    3. **Follow-up of abnormal findings**
      a. May have patient return after menses if exam is equivocal and patient is premenstrual
      b. Mammography
      c. Ultrasound defines whether mass is cystic or solid
      d. Breast cyst aspiration
      e. Fine-needle aspiration

4. Women who have irregular breast tissue on exam should not be told they have "fibro-cystic disease"
   a. "Fibrocystic" is nonspecific term, not clinical finding
   b. Patients who have irregular breast tissue without dominant mass do not have "disease"
5. Mass that can be palpated but not clearly identified on noninvasive or other studies should be biopsied

SUGGESTED READING

1. Baines CJ, Miller AB: Mammography versus clinical examination of the breasts. J Natl Cancer Inst Monogr 22:125–129, 1997.
2. Chalabian J, Dunnington G: Do our current assessments assure competency in clinical breast evaluation skills? Am J Surg 175:497–502, 1998.
3. Glass RH (ed): Office Gynecology, 4th ed. Baltimore, Williams & Wilkins, 1993.
4. Maurer F: A peer education model for teaching breast self-examination to undergraduate college women. Cancer Nurs 20:49–61, 1997.

123. Fine-needle Aspiration Biopsy of the Breast

Barbara S. Apgar, M.D., M.S.

Fine-needle aspiration biopsy of the breast is a procedure whereby cells are obtained from a palpable lesion with a thin needle using negative pressure through an attached syringe. Aspiration biopsy of the breast is safe, cost-effective, and accurate. Although the technique is deceptively simple, practice is required; both clinicians and pathologists should recognize that significant effort is required to gain proficiency. Aspiration biopsy complements rather than replaces histologic biopsy. The false-negative rate can be minimized by careful attention to collection and preparation of the sample.

The management of the results of the fine-needle biopsy is controversial. A conservative approach is to use the results only for preoperative assessment. Positive results allow the clinician and patient the opportunity to discuss treatment options before a definitive procedure such as mastectomy. With a negative result, it may be more appropriate to perform an open biopsy before definitive surgery. However, the practice of observing selected breast masses after a negative fine-needle biopsy, normal clinical exam, and mammography is common in some institutions. The decision about how best to use the result of fine-needle biopsy should be made by each clinician in concert with the surgeon and cytopathologist at his or her institution. An acellular specimen should always be interpreted as an unsatisfactory result.

I. **Indications**
   A. Palpable and clearly defined breast mass
II. **Contraindications**
   A. Nondistinct mass
   B. Mass < 1 cm in width
   C. Patients receiving anticoagulation therapy should be viewed with caution
III. **Equipment**
   A. Metal syringe holder
   B. Plastic syringe, 10 or 20 ml, with Luer-Lok tip
   C. 21- or 22-gauge needle
   D. Antiseptic
   E. Glass slides with frosted ends
   F. Sterile gauze pads
   G. Pressure dressing
   H. Lidocaine 1%

IV. **Preoperative Care**
  A. Mammography should be performed before procedure in patients who are candidates
    1. Mammography should be performed at least 4 weeks before fine-needle biopsy
      a. Avoids distortion of lesion's architecture
      b. Avoids having benign lesion appear malignant on mammography film due to hematoma formation
  B. Obtain informed consent
  C. Patient lies supine on exam table with arm that is closest to breast mass placed over head
  D. Breast mass is identified and palpated
    1. Size and depth of mass should be determined
      a. Failure to determine depth may result in unsuccessful attempts at aspiration
      b. Needle should not penetrate through mass
      c. If needle passes through mass, high false-negative results occur
  E. Area is prepped with antiseptic
V. **Technique**
  A. Needle is placed on syringe, which is snapped into metal syringe holder and locked
    1. Apparatus is checked for smoothness of movement
  B. **Simple aspiration of breast cyst**
    1. Breast mass may be cystic rather than solid mass
      a. Aspiration should be attempted before fine-needle biopsy
    2. Breast mass is immobilized with operator's nondominant hand
    3. Metal syringe holder with attached syringe and needle is held perpendicular to breast mass
      a. Metal syringe holder allows clinician to hold disposable syringe and create vacuum with same hand while immobilizing mass with other hand
    4. Needle is advanced into center of mass
      a. Needle should not go through mass
    5. Negative pressure is created by pulling backward on handle of syringe holder
      a. If mass is cyst, fluid is drawn into syringe
      b. Once cyst is completely aspirated, needle is withdrawn
    6. Pressure is applied over aspiration site with gauze pads
    7. Management of cyst fluid
      a. If fluid is not bloody or serosanguinous (yellow, dark green, or black), it does not have to be sent for pathologic analysis
  C. **Fine-needle biopsy of breast mass**
    1. Breast mass is immobilized with second and third fingers of nondominant hand
    2. Anesthesia
      a. Wheal of 1% lidocaine is produced over mass
        i. May make mass more difficult to palpate
    3. Needle is introduced quickly into mass perpendicular to skin
      a. Negative pressure is applied by pulling back all the way on metal syringe handle
    4. While maintaining negative pressure, needle is moved back and forth within mass in fanning motion
      a. Continuous suction must be achieved by constantly keeping negative pressure in syringe
      b. Sample material is drawn into needle
        i. Sample must not appear above hub of syringe or it will be lost
        ii. Sample is kept in needle
      c. Sample must not be diluted with blood
        i. If blood is obtained, start procedure again by attaching new needle onto syringe
    5. Before needle is withdrawn from mass, allow pressure in syringe to equalize by releasing handle of metal syringe holder
    6. Needle is quickly withdrawn
    7. Finger pressure is immediately applied to biopsy site
    8. Preparation of sample
      a. Needle is detached from syringe
        i. Syringe is filled with air

      b. Needle is reattached

      c. Needle is touched to a slide

          i. Drop of specimen is squirted onto slide

            (a) Another slide is used to smear aspirate in same way as blood smear is prepared

            (b) Successive slides are made in same way

          ii. One biopsy sample usually yields 5–6 slides

      d. Smears are allowed to air-dry

   9. Interpretation of results

      a. Acellular

      b. Benign nonspecific or benign specific

      c. Benign atypia

      d. Suspicious for malignancy

      e. Malignant

      f. Miscellaneous cells (lymph, fat, inflammatory)

VI. Postprocedure Care

   A. Patient wears pressure dressing for 24 hours

   B. Patient should call about hematoma formation, infection, excessive pain

   C. Remaining mass should be examined in 2 weeks and consideration given to open biopsy or performance of mammography

VII. Recommendations for Fine-needle Aspiration of the Breast

   A. Obtain accurate history and perform physical exam that includes axilla

   B. Obtain good-quality smears that contain as large a representative sample as possible

   C. Understand limitations of procedure

   D. Obtain best cytopathologic interpretation

   E. Incorporate clinical impression and mammography with biopsy results

   F. Surgically excise lesions that are suspicious, despite negative fine-needle biopsy and mammography results

VIII. Complications

   A. Hematoma formation

      1. Pressure dressing should be applied after procedure and worn for 24 hours

      2. If hematoma forms, it may be necessary to incise and drain blood

      3. Hematoma may appear as suspect area on mammography

         a. Mammography should be obtained before procedure if at all possible

         b. If mammograms are needed after procedure, wait 1 month

         c. Inform radiologist of prior fine-needle procedure

   B. Dissemination of cancer cells

      1. No evidence suggests that performance of fine-needle biopsy of breast disseminates cancer cells if present at the time of procedure

   C. False-negative rate

      1. Decreased by careful attention to assessment of size of breast mass

         a. Masses < 1 cm usually yield unsatisfactory number of cells for evaluation

         b. Fine-needle aspiration of small breast mass encourages high false-negative rate because needle misses actual mass and samples surrounding tissue

         c. Unsatisfactory smear is worthless result

SUGGESTED READING

1. Abele J, Miller T, Goodson W, et al: Fine needle aspiration of palpable breast masses. Arch Surg 118:859–863, 1983.
2. Caruthers (Apgar) BS: Fine-needle aspiration biopsy of breast lesions. Postgrad Med 84:47–55, 1988.
3. Erickson R, Shank C, Gratton C: Fine-needle breast aspiration biopsy. J Fam Pract 28:306–309, 1989.
4. Sickles EA, Klein DL, Goodson WH, Hunt TK: Mammography after needle aspiration of palpable breast masses. Am J Surg 145:395–397, 1983.
5. Smith TJ, Safail H, Foster EA, et al: Accuracy and cost-effectiveness of fine needle aspiration biopsy. Am J Surg 149:540–545, 1985.

124. Management of the Victim of Sexual Assault

Jane L. Murray, M.D.

Victims of sexual assault may be female or male and of any age. The term "rape" is a legal, not medical, term and therefore is avoided in this chapter, which discusses only the management of adult female victims of sexual assault. Special procedures for evaluation of children and adolescents are available from other sources.

In general, emergency departments (EDs) are best prepared to provide initial medical care for victims of sexual assault. Each legal jurisdiction has slightly different requirements for evidence collection, special kits for handling specimens, and detailed protocols for evaluating victims. Some facilities have special teams of social workers and other support personnel to provide immediate psychological support 24 hours a day. ED personnel usually receive special training in handling patients in this difficult situation and are up to date on legal procedures.

Follow-up care, however, is often provided by the patient's primary care physician; thus it is reasonable for all primary care physicians to understand the basics of emergency management of sexual assault as well as issues to address and follow over the longer term. In addition, many victims of sexual violence do not present for medical care immediately and may wait days, weeks, or even years before reporting an incident.

I. **Prevalence and Incidence**
   A. Estimated that rape (i.e., police report of sexual assault) is reported every 6 minutes in the U.S.
   B. Rape also considered most underreported of all violent crimes against persons due to fear, uncertainty about legal and medical systems, or guilt feelings on the part of victim
   C. In surveys of women 18 years and older, as many as 41% report having been victim of sexual assault at some time in their life
   D. College students are in the age group with highest risk
      1. National survey of male college students revealed that 1 in 15 reported committing or attempting rape in preceding year
      2. One in six female students reported being victim of rape or attempted rape during same period

II. **Immediate Evaluation**
   A. Multidisciplinary team required: medical and nursing personnel, law enforcement, support personnel
   B. Ascertain extent of trauma and stabilize patient: methodical history; complete physical exam; special attention to oral, anal, and genital mucosa for trauma, seminal fluid, evidence of infection; attention to emotional state
   C. Essentials of treatment
      1. **Care for physical injuries**
      2. **Psychiatric intervention**
         a. Involvement of counselor skilled in dealing with sexual assault victim is invaluable
         b. Counselor should meet with victim in private place in ED upon arrival, help console and relax the victim, and prepare her before exam
         c. Ideally counselor should stay with victim throughout exam and subsequent police report
      3. **Documentation of forensic evidence**
         a. Careful, complete, compulsive exam for evidence collection and samples
            i. Cultures for chlamydia and gonorrhea from throat, urethra, cervix, and rectum
            ii. Semen samples from clothing, skin, posterior fornix of vagina for sperm and prostatic acid phosphatase analysis
            iii. Saliva and vaginal fluid for ABO antigen typing
            iv. Hair and fingernail scrapings
            v. Sperm motility (sperm remain motile in vagina for 3–6 hours)

       b. Clear procedures for maintaining integrity and chain of evidence must be followed
         i. Careful identification of specimens
         ii. Should not leave examiner's possession until turned over to police
   4. **Prevention of sexually transmitted diseases (STDs)**
       a. Indications include victim's request, perpetrator infected, multiple assailants, follow-up unlikely, high incidence of STD in community, or signs and symptoms of STD
       b. Cover chlamydia, gonorrhea, bacterial vaginosis, trichomoniasis
         i. Ceftriaxone, 125 mg intramuscularly, single dose, plus
         ii. Metronidazole, 2 gm orally, single dose, plus
         iii. Doxycycline, 100 mg orally twice daily for 7 days
       c. Consider tetanus prophylaxis
       d. Consider administration of hepatitis B immunoglobulin and vaccination for hepatitis B virus
       e. Consider prophylaxis for HIV
   5. Prevention of pregnancy
       a. Postcoital contraceptives indicated if risk of pregnancy
       b. Ethinyl estradiol/norgestrel (Ovral), 2 tablets orally, then 2 more tablets in 12 hours
   6. Other testing
       a. Serologic tests for syphilis, hepatitis B, human immunodeficiency virus (HIV)

III. **Follow-up**
   A. Patients should be scheduled for medical follow-up within 2 weeks
      1. Follow-up cultures for gonorrhea, chlamydia
      2. Wet mount exam for *Trichomonas* sp., yeast, *Gardnerella* sp.
      3. Ongoing counseling and support
        a. Many victims begin to experience disorganization of lifestyle at 2–3 weeks, including nightmares, phobias, fear of being alone, change of address or phone number
        b. Depression and anxiety common
   B. Follow-up at 12 weeks
      1. Venereal Disease Research Laboratory for syphilis, HIV testing
      2. Observe and intervene for rape trauma syndrome and/or posttraumatic stress disorder; counselors experienced in working with such patients are essential

IV. **Common Psychological Reactions**
   A. Initial shock and disbelief
   B. Sleep disturbances and nightmares
   C. Flashbacks
   D. Anxiety
   E. Anger
   F. Mood swings, depression common
   G. Difficulty in concentrating on routine activities
   H. Fears about personal safety common and long-term feelings of vulnerability
   I. Guilt and shame common
      1. Victims often blame themselves and doubt their own judgment
      2. Others' reactions and social misconceptions about sexual assault may reinforce such feelings
   J. Victims often feel they should avoid talking about assault, but they should not avoid talking, which over time helps them regain some control
   K. Professional counseling as soon as possible after assault is essential

SUGGESTED READING

1. Dunn SF, Gilchrist VJ: Sexual asault. Prim Care 20:359–373, 1993.
2. Hampton HL: Care of the woman who has been raped. N Engl J Med 332:234–237, 1995.
3. Moscarello R: Psychological management of victims of sexual assault. Can J Psychiatr 35:25–30, 1990.
4. Petter LM, Whitehill DL: Management of female sexual assault. Am Fam Phys 58:920–926, 1998.
5. Sexual Assault: An Overview. Washington, DC, U.S. Victims Resource Center, Department of Justice, 1987.

Index

Page numbers in **boldface** type indicate complete chapters.